Smart and Sustainable Nanomaterials in Digital Healthcare and Theranostic

Sudip Mondal • Prodyut Dhar • Junghwan Oh
Editors

Smart and Sustainable Nanomaterials in Digital Healthcare and Theranostic

Springer

Editors
Sudip Mondal
Digital Healthcare Research Center
Pukyong National University
Busan, Korea (Republic of)

Prodyut Dhar
School of Biochemical Engineering
Indian Institute of Technology Varanasi
Varanasi, Uttar Pradesh, India

Junghwan Oh
Department of Biomedical Engineering
Pukyong National University
Busan, Korea (Republic of)

ISBN 978-981-95-9385-9 ISBN 978-981-95-9386-6 (eBook)
https://doi.org/10.1007/978-981-95-9386-6

This Springer imprint is published by the registered company Springer Nature Singapore Pte Ltd.
The registered company address is: 152 Beach Road, #21-01/04 Gateway East, Singapore 189721, Singapore

Foreword

It is with great pleasure that I introduce this important and timely volume, *Digital Healthcare and Theranostic*, which brings together a rich collection of insights from experts around the globe. The Editors of this book *Smart and Sustainable Nanomaterials in Digital Healthcare and Theranostic*, by Springer, possess extensive research experience in the fields of nanomaterials, biotechnology, and digital health technologies. Their strong potential for publication in reputed international journals speaks to the high level of academic and scientific rigor evident throughout this work. Their contributions, along with those of a distinguished group of international specialists, have resulted in a book of significant depth, breadth, and value. This book comprises *18 well-structured chapters*, covering a comprehensive range of topics, including:

- Introduction to Smart and Sustainable Nanomaterials
- Synthesis and Fabrication Techniques
- Functionalization and Characterization of Smart and Sustainable Nanomaterials
- Harnessing Carbon Nano-architectonics for Advanced Prodrug Delivery
- Applications in Digital Healthcare and Drug Delivery
- Diagnostic Nanoprobes and Imaging Agents
- Nanomaterials for Regenerative Medicine
- Biosensor Technologies for Disease Diagnosis and Environmental Monitoring
- Nanocomposites for Implants and Wearable Monitoring
- Clinical Applications and Case Studies
- Ethical, Safety, and Regulatory Considerations
- Future Trends and Innovations

The book highlights the tremendous progress in smart and sustainable nanomaterials and their transformative applications in *digital healthcare and theranostics*. As healthcare systems worldwide face unprecedented challenges and opportunities, the integration of advanced nanotechnologies presents a new era of precision, sustainability, and personalization in medicine. Of particular importance is the book's focus on how these nanomaterials—engineered at the nanoscale—can be tailored to possess unique functional properties. The ability to customize materials at the molecular and atomic level represents a major advancement in how we approach patient care and medical technologies.

This publication offers a *valuable resource* for a broad readership, including professionals, graduate students, and researchers working in materials science, polymer science, composite technology, nanotechnology, and biotechnology. Whether one is engaged in fundamental research or practical applications, this book provides a solid foundation and forward-looking perspective on the integration of nanomaterials in the healthcare domain. I am confident that this volume will serve as a cornerstone reference and an inspiration for future work in this fast-evolving field.

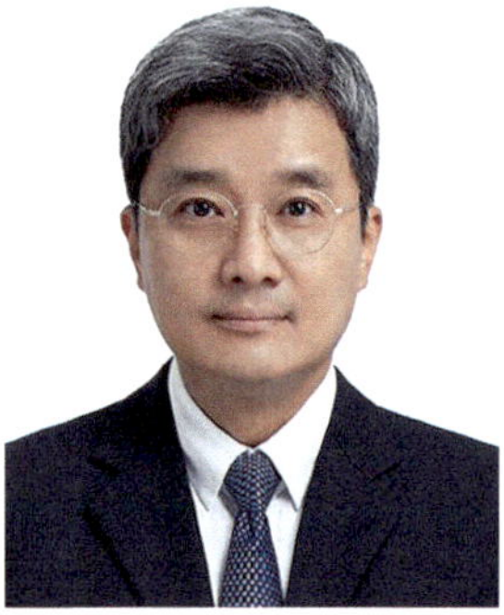

Professor, Pukyong National University Byeongil Lee
Busan, South Korea

Preface

It is our great pleasure to present this edited volume, *Smart and Sustainable Nanomaterials in Digital Healthcare and Theranostic*, which brings together a diverse collection of advanced research and innovative applications at the intersection of nanotechnology, materials science, and modern healthcare.

The rapid advancement of nanomaterials and their integration into biomedical systems have opened new possibilities for addressing some of the most critical challenges in healthcare—ranging from early disease detection and real-time monitoring to precision drug delivery and regenerative medicine. At the same time, the demand for sustainability and environmental responsibility has pushed researchers to explore smarter, greener, and more efficient solutions.

This book is structured into 18 chapters, carefully selected and contributed by leading experts across academia and industry. The contents span a wide range of topics, including the *synthesis, fabrication, and functionalization* of smart and sustainable nanomaterials; *drug delivery systems; biosensors for diagnostics and environmental safety; wearable monitoring technologies; clinical applications and case studies*; and critical discussions on *regulatory, ethical, and safety considerations.* The final chapters offer insights into *future trends* and *emerging innovations* in the field.

Our goal with this volume is to provide a comprehensive, practical, and accessible reference for researchers, graduate students, and healthcare professionals who are working at the forefront of biomedical materials. Each chapter presents both foundational knowledge and state-of-the-art developments, making this book suitable for both newcomers to the field and seasoned experts. We believe that *Smart and Sustainable Nanomaterials in Digital Healthcare and Theranostic* will contribute meaningfully to ongoing research and inspire future innovations that are not only technically sound but also socially and environmentally responsible. We would like to express our deepest gratitude to all contributing authors for their time, expertise, and dedication. Their work has made this book a rich and diverse collection of knowledge. We also extend our sincere thanks to Springer for their continued support and commitment to advancing scientific publishing.

We hope that this book serves as a valuable resource for the global scientific community and contributes to the development of next-generation healthcare technologies.

Busan, Republic of Korea — Sudip Mondal
Varanasi, Uttar Pradesh, India — Prodyut Dhar
Busan, Republic of Korea — Junghwan Oh

Acknowledgments

We would like to express our sincere gratitude to the President of Pukyong National University, Busan, South Korea, Professor Bae Sang-hoon, and the Director of the Indian Institute of Technology (IIT BHU), Varanasi, India, Professor Amit Patra, for their steadfast encouragement and institutional support, without which the realization of this book would not have been possible.

We extend our heartfelt thanks to all the contributing authors for their dedicated efforts and valuable insights across a wide range of disciplines, which have enriched the content and scope of this volume, *Smart and Sustainable Nanomaterials in Digital Healthcare and Theranostic*. Their collaborative spirit and academic rigor have been instrumental in shaping the quality and relevance of this work. Our sincere appreciation also goes to the students, research scholars, and staff members who contributed at various stages of this project, offering their time, technical expertise, and intellectual input. Their involvement was vital in coordinating the multifaceted aspects of this endeavor.

We warmly acknowledge the financial and institutional support that enabled this work to come to fruition. In particular, we are grateful for the generous support of the National Research Foundation of Korea (NRF) funded by the Korean government (MSIT), the Global Joint Research Program funded by Pukyong National University, and the Pukyong National University Research Fund in 2024. These contributions provided a solid foundation for the international collaboration and research dissemination facilitated by this book.

Most importantly, we would like to acknowledge the support from the Springer Book Publication team. Special thanks go to Lauren Kim, Springer Senior Editor, and Neeraja Padmanabhan, Springer Production Editor, for their continuous guidance, patience, and support throughout the preparation and publication process.

Finally, we are deeply thankful to all our colleagues and collaborators whose commitment to advancing knowledge in the field of nanomaterials and digital healthcare continues to inspire and propel this rapidly evolving scientific landscape.

Sudip Mondal
Prodyut Dhar
Junghwan Oh

Contents

About the Editors

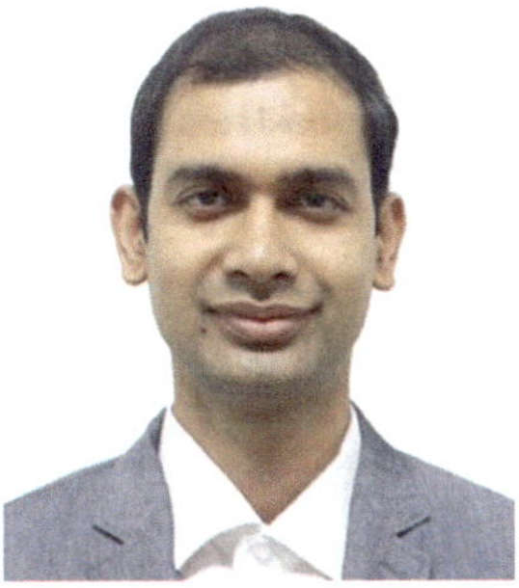

Sudip Mondal received his PhD in 2015 from the CSIR-Central Mechanical Engineering Research Institute and the National Institute of Technology Durgapur, India. He then joined the Autonomous University of Puebla, Mexico, as a Postdoctoral Fellow (2015–2017), and subsequently worked as a Research Professor at Pukyong National University, South Korea (2017–2023). He is currently serving as a full-time Assistant Professor at Pukyong National University, specializing in Photomedicine. His groundbreaking work in photothermal and photodynamic therapies has significantly advanced the field of disease treatment. His research interests include the synthesis of nanostructured materials, bioimaging, and various biomedical applications such as cancer therapy and tissue engineering.

ORCID ID:0000-0002-0638-9657

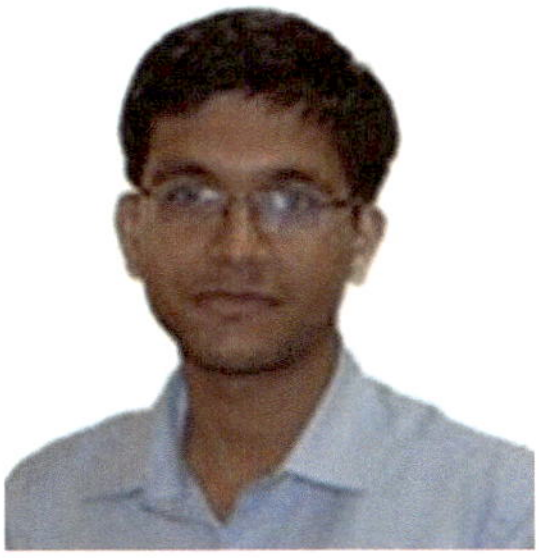

Prodyut Dhar is currently working as an Associate Professor in the School of Biochemical Engineering at the Indian Institute of Technology (IIT) BHU, Varanasi. His core areas of expertise include the design of smart and biodegradable polymers, protein-based biocomposites, bionanotechnology, and green materials, controlled-release systems, packaging, and sustainable agriculture. At IIT (BHU), he leads the Laboratory of Chem-Biosystems and Technologies, where his interdisciplinary team works on cutting-edge innovations such as 3D-printed food scaffolds, nanocellulose-based films, and biodegradable composites. He has published more than 50 peer-reviewed research papers in top international journals, also contributed several book chapters and filed patents on biodegradable straws, bagasse-based tableware, and textile coatings. He holds several national and international honors, awards, and fellowships. He currently holds two prestigious fellowships Har Govind Khorana-Innovative Young Biotechnologist Fellowship and Ramalingaswami Fellowship and was awarded prestigious Japan Society for the Promotion of Science (JSPS) Postdoctoral Fellowship (2018–2020), allowing him to pursue advanced research in forest and biomaterial sciences at Kyoto University, Japan. Through his translational research and innovation-driven pedagogy, he remains committed to addressing global sustainability challenges through science and engineering. He welcomes collaborative opportunities across disciplines and industries, aiming to develop smart, eco-friendly technologies for a better future.

ORCID ID: 0000-0001-9716-3866

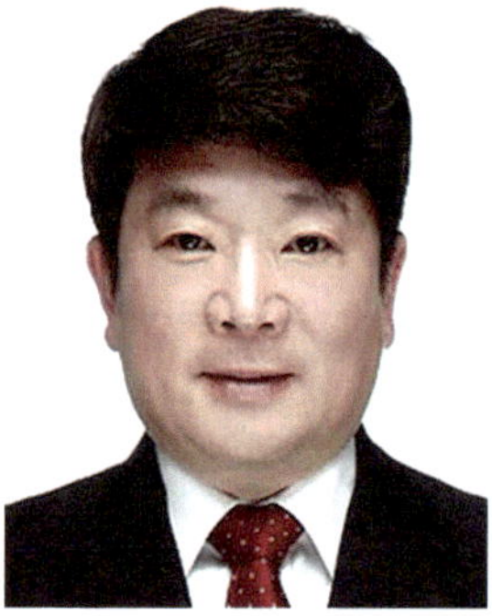

Junghwan Oh received the BS degree in Mechanical engineering from Pukyong National University in 1992, and the MS and PhD degrees in Biomedical engineering from The University of Texas at Austin, USA, in 2003 and 2007, respectively. In 2010, he joined the Department of Biomedical Engineering at Pukyong National University, where he is a Full Professor. He also serves as CEO of OhLabs Corporation. His current research interests include ultrasonic-based diagnostic imaging modalities for biomedical engineering applications, biomedical signal processing, and healthcare systems.

ORCID ID: 0000-0002-5837-0958

Chapter 1
Introduction to Smart and Sustainable Nanomaterials

Zareen Suhara Nazeer Ali, Mahalakshmi Manikandan, Sinduja Malarkodi Elangovan, Vaidhyanathan Baskaran, and Nazeer Abdul Azeez

Abstract The application of nanomaterials dates back to ninth century by the artisans in Mesopotamia, although the term nanotechnology was coined only in 1981 by the Japanese scientist Taniguchi. Since then, nanotechnology and nanomaterials have catalyzed the development of science and technology during the twenty-first century where the properties of these materials are well studied and optimized. Electron and X-ray dependent spectroscopy enabled the visualization of minute surfaces to elucidate their physical and chemical properties. The size of nanomaterials typically ranges from 1 to 100 nm rendering a high surface area to volume ratio spanning across 0–3 dimensions. This high surface area to volume ratio provides the quantum confinement of electrons for excellent catalytic, optical, and electronic applications. These enhanced properties enable their interactions with biological matter at the atomic level. The flexibility in tuning the size and properties of a nanomaterial has found promising applications in healthcare and diagnostics where they are widely being studied for targeted therapy, biosensing, and point-of-care devices. This chapter provides a timeline of nanomaterial application; probes into the physical, chemical, and optoelectronic properties of nanomaterials; and approaches to tuning each property for sensing, catalytic, biocompatibility, and toxicity masking for the biomedical and diagnostic applications primarily in the healthcare sector.

Keywords Nanomaterials · Biosensing · Catalysis · Healthcare · Theranostic

Z. S. N. Ali · M. Manikandan · S. M. Elangovan · V. Baskaran
Department of Biotechnology, Bannari Amman Institute of Technology, Sathyamangalam, Erode, India

N. A. Azeez (✉)
Department of Biotechnology, School of Bioengineering, SRM Institute of Science and Technology, Kattankulathur, Tamil Nadu, India

S. Mondal et al. (eds.), *Smart and Sustainable Nanomaterials in Digital Healthcare and Theranostic*, https://doi.org/10.1007/978-981-95-9386-6_1

1.1 Introduction

The terms "nanomaterials" and "nanotechnology" have gained prominence in the twenty-first century, yet the earliest traces of nanomaterials were found in meteorites formed at the time of the Big Bang. These nanodiamonds discovered on the surface of meteorites possibly date back beyond the formation of the solar system [22]. Since then, the progressive evolution of the definition of a nanomaterial paralleled with the advancements of human civilization. The first known use of nanomaterials was in Mesopotamia in the ninth century where artisans used copper and silver nanoparticles decoratively in pottery [76]. Pigments made from nanomaterials $CaCuSi_4O_{10}$ (Egyptian blue), $BaCuSi_4O_{10}$, SiO_2, and PdS_2 were used as colorants in ancient Egyptian, Roman, and Chinese civilizations [37, 79]. Similarly, Au-Ag nanoparticles embedded into the Lycurgus cup, a prominent Roman artefact, are responsible for the cup's color change from green to red under varying light conditions [30]. In 1857, Michael Faraday made the discovery that the color of a colloidal solution is manipulated by the gold nanoparticles present in it depending on the light directed onto it, which he coined as the Faraday-Tyndall effect [28]. Nanotechnology, the term to define the technology used to manufacture particles precisely on a nanoscale, was officiated by Norio Taniguchi [12]. It was during this period where nanotechnology started to gain ground in the scientific community.

The nanomaterials typically characterized by their size ranging from 1 to 100 nm, differing from bulk materials in terms of a high surface area to volume ratio and effects of quantum confinement [5]. The reduction of the bulk size to smaller than the size of an electronic orbit causes the confinement of electrons and holes, forming discrete energy levels and influencing band gap energies [27]. The extent of quantum confinement on a nanomaterial influences its physical, chemical, electronic, and optical properties. This affects the material's fluorescence, conductivity, melting point, dimension, and magnetic permeability [62]. Nanomaterials have surface charges that affect their stability and aggregate formation in colloidal solutions. Additionally, a high surface area to volume ratio influences magnetic behavior due to magnetic coupling with neighboring atoms resulting in superparamagnetic behavior [58]. Recent years have seen a surge in nanomaterials research owing to their catalytic properties. Surface charge and functional groups help adsorb substances onto the surface of nanomaterials where they exert their catalytic activity through redox reactions [21]. Tuning these properties resulted in diversified applications of nanomaterials.

The electronic properties of nanomaterials have been studied for their use in transistors, electrodes, nanowires, supercapacitors, fuel cells, touch screens, wearable electronics, and liquid crystal displays, to name a few [57, 69, 88]. Ongoing research in wastewater treatment utilizes catalytic and light harvesting properties of nanomaterials to effectively eradicate hazardous contaminants from aquatic bodies [36]. The presence of surface charge and functional groups in the surface of nanomaterials have made it a potential candidate in drug delivery applications. Administration of chemotherapeutic drugs in cancer patients causes unnecessary cytotoxic side effects in healthy cells, degrading the overall health of the patient [61]. Nanoparticle-mediated drug delivery systems target tumor-specific sites and release drugs that only eradicate neoplastic cells [83]. Similarly, nanomaterial-mediated thermal and photo ablation therapy scrutinizes the magnetic and optical properties of nanomaterials to eradicate tumor cells noninvasively [6]. Fluorescent and radiolabeled nanomaterials when functionalized attach to organs and tissues, providing scope in bioimaging applications [49]. Additionally, nanomaterials functionalized with enzymes and biomarkers aid in the detection of several biomolecules and pathogens [45, 56].

This chapter aims to shed light on nanomaterials' properties, which pave the way for their applications in the biomedical and theranostic fields. Through this chapter, we aim to provide insights into the intrinsic properties of nanomaterials that qualify them for smart and sustainable applications in the healthcare sector while also addressing current trends and future perspectives.

1.2 Properties

Nanoparticles offer improved catalytic activity and chemical stability due to their confined electronic movements and are thus used in various applications [29]. They are used as nanomedicines, which revolutionized medical treatments and therapies. They are being used in numerous fields such as imaging, tissue regeneration, and the formation of new compounds [17]. Nanoparticles can deliver drugs in optimal dosage, increasing therapeutic efficiency, and lowering side effects [68]. The core-shell nanocomposites and nanostructures vary in different shapes and sizes, like spherical, eEccentric, centric, star-like, and tubular. This difference causes changes in the properties of the particles, and the presence of different functional groups or coatings with other molecules will enhance the properties of the nanoparticles [4].

Nanoparticles usually vary in the 1–100 nm range; being small-sized particles, they serve as a better platform for medical devices and systems with novel properties. These particles are also used on a large scale, but the entire control of the system will remain at the nanoscale [26]. Possessing a large surface area, it is being used as an antibacterial agent (especially in wound healing) because it has more contact with microorganisms, thus increasing the surface area-volume ratios and increasing the efficiency [35]. The important parameter of a particle used for drug delivery is its biocompatibility. The shape and surface properties of the nanoparticles are optimized to improve the bioavailability. On applying the nanoparticles to brain tumor applications, it is necessary to check the surface charge property because it affects the behavior of the particle with biological moieties during penetration through the cell membrane and interaction with protein molecules [1].

Optical property is another important property of nanoparticles; thus, it is used in various parts of medical fields like optical sensing, imaging, and phototherapy. In conventional methods, dyes like rhodamine are used to fluoresce the cells because these can easily bind to the cells through ligand/receptor interaction. To bring the best alternative, quantum dots for these dyes were introduced. These are types of nanoparticles consisting of inorganic semiconductor materials that emit fluorescence under ultraviolet light. This is a unique property; thus, these semiconducting particles derive this from the "band gap" [59].

Drug delivery into the specific sites of the body is a complex part of the medical field, but nanoparticles were not suitable for this treatment because the polymers were not biodegradable. Soon after the development of nanodevices with biocompatible and biodegradable polymers like albumin, poly alkyl cyanoacrylate, polylactate-co-glycolate, and chitosan nanoparticles, it was used in the oncology field. Nanoparticles reduce the complexity of cancer treatment by delivering the drug specifically at the target site at a controlled rate, protecting it from degradation or metabolization and improving cellular uptake [19].

The surface chemistry of nanoparticles makes it interact with the biological systems in the body. Initially, nanoparticles were considered to be beginning carriers, but later after a lot of studies, it demonstrated the interaction of serum proteins and cell membrane receptors with nanoparticles in influencing cell uptake, gene expression, and toxicity. These nanoparticles act like a scaffold that dictates the interaction of multiple ligands from the surface of the particle with the receptors that increase the avidity and cell signaling [2].

Magnetic nanoparticles are used in the medical field due to the presence of unique magnetic properties and small dimensions (less than 20 nm). The overall magnetic field of the particle can be randomized to zero without any external source; thus, the fluctuation in the magnetic field makes the dispersion of the particle stable in a physiological solution and facilitates the coupling of nanoparticles with biological material to use it as a regenerative medicine [31]. Heat introduced non-remotely is more effective as the radio frequency waves pass with low-frequency heating nanoparticles rather than normal cells. This uniqueness with the help of nanoparticles plays a vital role in treating deep-seated tumors [82].

A deeper understanding of the molding mechanism, strengthening process, and modification methods to improve the microstructure of the nanoparticle will increase the uniqueness of the particle which will increase its usage in different medical sectors [84]. However nano-based products face limitations in manufacturing, as they require large investments from medical device corporations. At the same time, it focuses on optimistic methods for the policymakers to design nano-based products with sustainable systems [71]. The applications of sustainable nanomaterials based on their respective properties are summarized in Table 1.1.

1.3 Surface Properties

Nanomaterials are being used in many branches of research and engineering including energy, the environment, medicinal applications, and other fields. The current state of the ecosystem is exceedingly awful and devastating with no relief from environmental calamities or global climate change [34]. Furthermore, industrial

Table 1.1 Superior properties of nanomaterials and their respective applications

Property	Superiority of nanomaterials	Applications	Example	References
High surface:volume ratio	Nanomaterials have significantly larger surface areas compared to bulk materials, enhancing reactions and interactions per unit mass	Catalysts for chemical reactions	Platinum nanoparticles for low-temperature dehydrogenation of perhydro dibenzyltoluene	[53]
		Energy storage (batteries, supercapacitors)	Graphene oxide nanoparticles as symmetric supercapacitor	[7]
		Sensors (gas, bio, etc.)	Zinc oxide nanowires for high-performance ethylene glycol sensing	[80]
Optical properties	Unique light absorption, scattering, and emission due to quantum size effects, unlike bulk materials that follow classical optics	Quantum dots for displays and imaging	CdSe quantum dots for LED digital dynamic color display	[33]
		Solar cells	Preovskite nanocrystals with power conversion efficiencies (PCE) of around 22–25%	[65]
		Photodetectors	Graphene oxide with nickel oxide nanoparticles for fast response UV-detection	[78]
		Fluorescent markers for bioimaging	Iron-doped polymer dots for enhanced fluorescence and dual enzyme activity in bioassays	[85]

(continued)

Table 1.1 (continued)

Property	Superiority of nanomaterials	Applications	Example	References
Biocompatibility	Can be engineered for controlled interaction with biological systems, enabling reduced toxicity and improved cellular integration	Drug delivery systems	Silver oxide nanoparticles for enhanced delivery of hydrophilic drugs	[8]
		Implants and prosthetics	Hydroxyapatite nanoparticles for bone repair treatments	[72]
		Bioimaging agents	Gold nanoparticles in theranostic applications	[11]
		Antimicrobial coatings	Nano-ZIF-8 metal organic framework coatings on catheters for pathogen resistance	[10]
Reactive surface chemistry	Higher reactivity due to a large fraction of atoms on the surface and tunable surface functionalization compared to bulk materials	Water purification	TiO_2 nanoparticles to break down organic pollutants in water	[39]
		Environmental remediation	Zerovalent iron nanoparticles for removal of Chromium VI	[9]
		Self-cleaning surfaces	TiO_2 nanoparticles in acrylic paints for self-cleaning surfaces	[3]
Magnetic properties	Enhanced magnetic behavior (e.g., superparamagnetism) due to confined electron motion and smaller domain sizes	Magnetic data storage	Magnetic nanofiber mats (Fe_2O_3/NiO) for data storage and transfer	[25]
		MRI contrast agents	Iron oxide nanoparticles as T1 contrasting agent	[75]
		Programmed drug delivery (magnetic nanoparticles)	Poly (ethylenimine) dendrimers grafted magnetic nanoparticles for pH and magnetic responsive delivery of cytarabine	[55]

(continued)

Table 1.1 (continued)

Property	Superiority of nanomaterials	Applications	Example	References
Strength of the material	Nanostructures, like carbon nanotubes and graphene, exhibit significantly higher strength-to-weight ratios than bulk materials	Aerospace components	Carbon nanotube reinforced epoxy resin for effective electromagnetic interference shielding	[87]
		Lightweight armor	ZnO nanorods for soft-body high-velocity ballistic impact armor	[16]
		Construction materials	Graphene composite for effective concrete	[81]

wastewater treatment captivates and challenges the true vision of worldwide science and engineering [64]. The functionalization of the fields of nanotechnology holds the prospect of developing new substances and gadgets that take benefit of the distinctive characteristics provided by nanoscale substances, as well as convenient solutions to overcome the disadvantages that prevent its entirety utilization of nanotechnology in the area of environmental protection. So far, several well-known approaches have shown to be feasible. For example, coating the nanoparticle core surface with a capping agent was proposed to protect nanomaterials from erosion, surface reactivity, and reduce their toxicity. Furthermore, composites of nanomaterials with different ferrites and natural magnetite that may be easily recovered using an external magnetic field have been developed to provide recoverable and reusable nanomaterials [23].

A variety of approaches are used to functionalize the materials' surfaces, including oxidation and harmless changes to the surface. In oxidative processes, oxidized nanomaterials serve as a kick-start base for chemical substitutions such as condensation, polymer grafting, esterification, and so on, whereas non-defensive surface modifications are achieved through polymer wrapping and encapsulation processes [70]. Furthermore, the primary goals of NP surface functionalization are to reduce toxicity, remove immune responses, and bind more complex and specific ligands to improve efficacy and specificity for objectives such as antipathogenic actions via NPs [66]. Microorganisms have recently experienced rapid structural and behavioral changes. The rise of resistant microorganisms due to greater antibiotic adaptation is a serious public health issue; thus, significant efforts are required to improve the effectiveness and efficacy of antimicrobial drugs. Surface functionalization of antibacterial NPs can increase their efficacy, and several studies have demonstrated their potential for application against resistant microbes. It also reduces the tendency to cluster together carbon compounds and enhances graphene-polymer interaction via covalent or ionic interactions [18].

Numerous researchers have published numerous investigations on NPs and their biological uses in response to current needs. The biological use of nanoparticles remains the most appealing feature for scientists seeking better therapeutic outcomes. Targeted medication and gene delivery diagnostic algorithmic therapy techniques increase effectiveness while minimizing negative effects. However, the prospective function of nanotechnology in battling various diseases is more dependable and technological than traditional antibiotic therapy. Metal nanoparticles (NPs) have received a lot of attention in biological research due to their unique adaptive physical and chemical characteristics.

Metal NPs have a unique interaction with light, providing a reliable method for tracking nanocomplex therapeutic carriers throughout the body, enabling more efficient treatments with fewer side effects than existing conventional therapies [38]. For ligands and NP surfaces to create covalent connections, many linker molecules are usually utilized. According to Pagels et al., PEG can be synthesized at the terminals with specific functional groups and utilized as heterofunctional linkers to bring out a range of functionalization properties. One positive inference of non-covalent interactions is their simplicity; they do not alter the target biological material's interactions or the structure of the molecules used. Non-covalent changes, however, are easily impacted by an array of factors, including alkalinity and the strength of the ions [63].

Bioimaging, medication delivery, tissue engineering research, and biomedical diagnostics are the primary areas that are anticipated to entail several applications. Seeking proof will also come from studies on stem cell differentiation and transplantation, targeted medicine administration, and real-time monitoring capabilities. Shortly, numerous biological medicines with low permeability, poor water solubility, and low bioavailability will be able to be used with nanoparticulate drug loading methods. NPs can mitigate some of the particular issues associated with these medications by maintaining their stability and structure. In clinical and agricultural experiments, NPs also enable targeted loading and controlled release, offering a more sophisticated treatment.

1.4 Applications

Nanoparticles are tunable at their molecular and atomic levels based on the application. Thus, it is used in various fields including medical applications, nanofluid, corrosive resistive coatings, antifungal paints, water treatment, catalysis, sensors, energy storage, etc. Nanofluids are a new material engineering made up of solid-liquid composites consisting of nanosized particles suspended in the base fluids. These fluids' properties are comparatively better than conventional fluids because of the Brownian movement created by the particles. The applications of the nanoparticles are illustrated in Fig. 1.1. It possesses electrical conductivity and high thermal properties with heat-transfer properties. The longer time stability of this material is the key issue in practical applications, but it is still under research period [48].

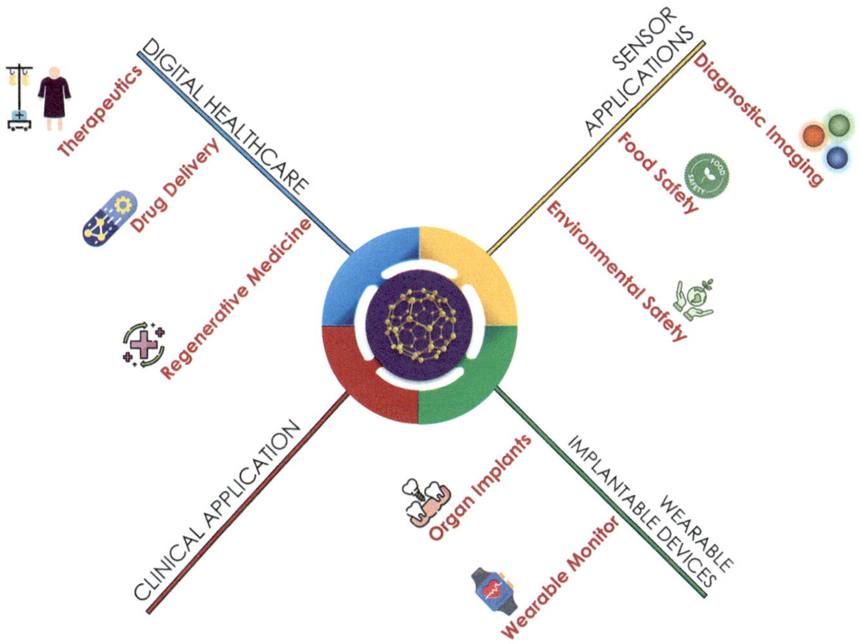

Fig. 1.1 Illustration of different applications of nanoparticles in healthcare

Unconventional water resources like waste, brackish water, and seawater cannot be consumed directly because they contain many pollutants that are harmful to living organisms. The high surface area and high porosity with an active site can adsorb molecules of varied sizes and, most significantly, have regenerative ability [44].

A heterogeneous reaction is something that occurs on the surface of the solid. The metal nanoparticles act as a catalyst in enhancing the reaction rate and are classified into transition metals (Fe, Co, Ni), IB metals (Cu, Ag, Au), and noble metals (Pd, Rh, Pt). These metallic nanoparticles can be synthesized using a liquid-phase fabrication method with tunable size, structure, and crystal phase. Sometimes new shapes are formed by the particles during their active participation in catalyst reactions due to the temperature changes and the reactive gases [48]. A typical class of slow-release (ultra-long-lived) trapped charge carriers towards recombination after cessation of external excitation energy is endowed in the nano-energy storage materials. For there are two different particles $CaAl_2O_4:Eu^{2+}$, Nd^{3+} and $SrAl_2O_4:Eu^{2+}$, Dy^{3+}, which are commercialized and used in various fields, especially in medical diagnostics. These provide longer luminescence and excite in both sunlight and room light. These properties show a way for the development of biosensors with improved stability and analytical behavior [52].

Nano-remediation is a new method developed to clean up the environment by playing a vital role in the detection, monitoring, radiation, and prevention of pollutants. This method can be remedied by both chemical reduction and catalysis to mitigate the pollutants of concern and is used constantly, as this remediation process is cost-effective. The main applications of nano-remediation are wastewater treatment, heavy metal detection, hydrocarbon remediation, and radioactive waste remediation [14]. There are a lot of water purification techniques, like chemical precipitation and coagulation, flocculation, electrochemical methods, photocatalytic degradation, membrane filtration, and ion exchange, but magnetic nanoparticles are the best because of the adsorption capacity and reuse efficiency. Magnetic nanoparticles present advantages due to their large surface area, size, and shape-dependent catalytic properties and can be separated from the aqueous solution with the use of a magnet field. This adsorption mechanism is the best for adsorbing the heavy metals present in the water, like Cd, Hg, As, and Cr, which are highly toxic and can cause DNA damage, lipid peroxidation, depletion of protein sulfhydryls, and other effects on living organisms [50].

Carbon nanotubes, graphene oxide, nanoscale zero-valent irons (NZVI), and many other metal oxide particles play a vital role in the decontamination of radioactive wastewater. Nanomaterials are functionalized with different functional groups for the targeted removal of radionuclides and solidification of radionuclides from large-volume aqueous solution [86]. Nanoparticles like silver, gold, and zinc oxide particles are used in the degradation of the dyes present in the effluent released from the textile industries. These dyes are highly toxic because of cerebral abnormality and intestinal cancer and cause mutation, which leads to tumor formation [60]. Other than this, metallic nanoparticles like titanium particles are used in the reinforcement of alloys for lightweight construction, having proper strength and hardness mainly in the aerospace and automotive sectors. Nanotechnology plays a vital role in various parts of civil engineering, especially in manufacturing construction materials with different properties, lighter weights, stronger composites, and self-disinfecting surfaces [77]. In the agricultural field, it is used as a nano-fertilizer. This increases the nutrient use efficiency (NUE) by three times as it contains n nutrients and growth promoters encapsulated in nanoscale polymers it builds carbon uptake, improves soil aggregation, and provides sustained, targeted release [42].

1.5 Future Prospects and Scope of Smart and Sustainable Nanomaterials

Smart and sustainable nanomaterials have the potential to expand the possibilities in diverse fields, with their enhanced functionalities, precision, and eco-friendliness. With their unique properties, such as high surface area, tunable reactivity, and scalability, nanomaterials are becoming integral in addressing global challenges in healthcare, environmental sustainability, energy storage, and electronics [41]. Their current applications range from advanced sensors for real-time monitoring to energy-efficient systems, biodegradable materials, and innovative solutions in wearables and implantable devices [20, 32, 67, 74]. These nanomaterials integrating with emerging technologies like AI, IoT, and robotics lead to transformative advancements across industries [15].

The future of nanomaterials in digital healthcare aims at remote monitoring and personalized medicine by enabling real-time health tracking through nanoscale biosensors and drug delivery systems [43, 51]. Specifically, quantum dots and graphene-based nanomaterials are studied to enhance bioimaging for early and precise detection of abnormalities in the human system [13, 24, 40]. These advancements promise to make healthcare systems more efficient, accessible, and patient-centric.

Nanomaterials with their unmatched sensitivity and specificity in sensor applications aim at efficient detection of biomarkers such as peptides in the brain, pathogens, and environmental toxins [46, 47, 73]. Innovations in nanosensors embedded with artificial intelligence and IoT capabilities can support predictive diagnostics, offering preventive measures in healthcare [15].

In clinical applications, the future scope is high on regenerative medicine and targeted therapies. Nanomaterial-based drug delivery systems for controlled release; magnetic nanoparticles for non-invasive cancer treatment through hyperthermia therapy; nanostructured scaffolds; and biocompatible materials in tissue engineering and organ regeneration [54].

Wearable and implantable devices are poised to benefit significantly from nanomaterials. Flexible, biocompatible nanomaterials like graphene and nanocellulose are being utilized in the development of wearable electronics that monitor vital signs, blood glucose levels, and cardiac health. Implantable devices, equipped with nanoscale sensors and actuators, provide real-time feedback, enhancing patient outcomes while reducing invasive interventions. Smart implants functionalized with self-healing and anti-biofouling nanocoatings further improve device longevity and safety.

Looking forward, the sustainability of nanomaterials will remain a priority, driving research into biodegradable, non-toxic, and energy-efficient alternatives. The fusion of nanotechnology with AI, 5G, and robotics holds immense promise for smarter, more sustainable solutions, ensuring equitable healthcare advancements globally. These innovations are not only shaping the future of medical science but also contributing to a healthier and more connected society.

1.6 Conclusion

Nanomaterials and nanotechnology have evolved from ancient practices to modern scientific innovations, playing a transformative role in almost every field. Their unique intrinsic properties, such as high surface-to-volume ratios, quantum confinement effects, and surface functionalization, have unlocked applications across medicine, energy, environment, and engineering. The sustained nanomaterials drive the progress in technology and improve the standard of human life. From enabling accelerated crop production to strong concrete roofs, from targeted drug delivery and bioimaging to revolutionizing water purification and agriculture, nanotechnology demonstrates immense potential for addressing critical challenges.

Despite these advancements, several hurdles remain, including the scalability, biocompatibility, and environmental impact of nanomaterials. Continued research, ethical considerations, and innovative solutions are essential to harness the full potential of nanotechnology sustainably. As we look ahead, nanotechnology promises to redefine industries and improve quality of life, bridging gaps between science, engineering, and societal needs. The following chapters will comprehensively deliberate on the application of the Smart and Sustainable nanoparticles in the digital healthcare and theranostic applications.

References

1. Adabi M, Naghibzadeh M, Adabi M, Zarrinfard MA, Esnaashari SS, Seifalian AM, Faridi-Majidi R, Tanimowo Aiyelabegan H, Ghanbari H. Biocompatibility and nanostructured materials: applications in nanomedicine. Artif Cells Nanomed Biotechnol. 2017;45(4):833–42. https://doi.org/10.1080/21691401.2016.1178134.
2. Albanese A, Tang PS, Chan WCW. The effect of nanoparticle size, shape, and surface chemistry on biological systems. Annu Rev Biomed Eng. 2012;14(1):1–16. https://doi.org/10.1146/annurev-bioeng-071811-150124.
3. Armaković SJ, Savanović MM, Šiljegović MV, Kisić M, Šćepanović M, Grujić-Brojčin M, et al. Self-cleaning and charge transport properties of foils coated with acrylic paint containing TiO2 nanoparticles. Inorganics. 2024;12(1):35.
4. Arvizo RR, Bhattacharyya S, Kudgus RA, Giri K, Bhattacharya R, Mukherjee P. Intrinsic therapeutic applications of noble metal nanoparticles: past, present and future. Chem Soc Rev. 2012;41(7):2943. https://doi.org/10.1039/c2cs15355f.
5. Asha AB, Narain R. Nanomaterials properties. In: Polymer science and nanotechnology: fundamentals and applications. Elsevier; 2020. p. 343–59.
6. Ashikbayeva Z, Tosi D, Balmassov D, Schena E, Saccomandi P, Inglezakis V. Application of nanoparticles and nanomaterials in thermal ablation therapy of cancer. Nanomaterials. 2019;9(9):1195.
7. Atta MM, Rabia M, Elbasiony AM, Taha EO, Abdel Hamid MM, Henaish AM, Zhang Q. Facile gamma-ray induced synthesis of reduced graphene oxide decorated with silver nanoparticles: A green approach for symmetric supercapacitor applications. Fullerenes Nanotubes Carbon Nanostruct. 2024;32(5):442–51.
8. Azeez NA, Saravanan M, Chandar NRK, Vishaal MK, Deepa VS. Enhancing the aspirin loading and release efficiency of silver oxide nanoparticles using oleic acid-based bio-surfactant from Enteromorpha intestinalis. Appl Organomet Chem. 2020;34(11):e5934.
9. Azeez NA, Dash SS, Gummadi SN, Deepa VS. Nano-remediation of toxic heavy metal contamination: hexavalent chromium [Cr (VI)]. Chemosphere. 2021;266:129204.
10. Azeez NA, Pahil S, Mahadevegowda SH, Vijaykumar SD. Metal-Organic Frameworks (MOFs) for the antimicrobial applications. In: Recent trends and the future of antimicrobial agents-part II. Bentham Science Publishers; 2023. p. 124–41.
11. Balasubramaniyan M, Nazeer AA, Vinayagam V, Vijaykumar SD. Smart Theranostic applications of metal nanoparticles against cancer. In: Handbook of research on Nano-strategies for combatting antimicrobial resistance and cancer. IGI Global; 2021. p. 319–36.
12. Barhoum A, García-Betancourt ML, Jeevanandam J, Hussien EA, Mekkawy SA, Mostafa M, Omran MM, Abdalla MS, Bechelany M. Review on natural, incidental, bioinspired, and engi-

neered nanomaterials: history, definitions, classifications, synthesis, properties, market, toxicities, risks, and regulations. Nanomaterials. 2022;12(2):177.
13. Baruah C, Deka B, Mahanta S, Sharma DK. Graphene-based nanomaterials as molecular disease theragnostic applications. In: Graphene-based nanomaterials. CRC Press; 2024. p. 219–32.
14. Bhandari G. Environmental nanotechnology: applications of nanoparticles for bioremediation; 2018. p. 301–15. https://doi.org/10.1007/978-3-030-02369-0_13.
15. Chaudhary V, Gaur P, Rustagi S. Sensors, society, and sustainability. Sustain Mater Technol. 2024;40:e00952.
16. Chu Y, Zhu B, Wang X, Min S, Chen H, Huang W, et al. Research on high-velocity ballistic impact of para-aramid sateen fabric with ZnO nanorods oriented to the development of soft body armor. Mater Des. 2024;248:113384.
17. Cormode DP, Gao L, Koo H. Emerging biomedical applications of enzyme-like catalytic nanomaterials. Trends Biotechnol. 2018;36(1):15–29. https://doi.org/10.1016/j.tibtech.2017.09.006.
18. Costa-Orlandi CB, Sardi JC, Pitangui NS, De Oliveira HC, Scorzoni L, Galeane MC, et al. Fungal biofilms and polymicrobial diseases. J Fungi. 2017;3(2):22.
19. Couvreur P. Nanoparticles in drug delivery: past, present and future. Adv Drug Deliv Rev. 2013;65(1):21–3. https://doi.org/10.1016/j.addr.2012.04.010.
20. Croitoru C, Bode F, Calotă R, Berville C, Georgescu M. Harnessing nanomaterials for enhanced energy efficiency in transpired solar collectors: a review of their integration in phase-change materials. Energies. 2024;17(5):1239.
21. Cuenya BR. Synthesis and catalytic properties of metal nanoparticles: size, shape, support, composition, and oxidation state effects. Thin Solid Films. 2010;518(12):3127–50.
22. Dai ZR, Bradley JP, Joswiak DJ, Brownlee DE, Hill HGM, Genge MJ. Possible in situ formation of meteoritic nanodiamonds in the early solar system. Nature. 2002;418(6894):157–9.
23. Darwish M, Mohammadi A. Functionalized nanomaterial for environmental techniques. In: Nanotechnology in environmental science; 2018. p. 315–50.
24. Díaz-García D, Díaz-Sánchez M, Álvarez-Conde J, Gómez-Ruiz S. Emergence of quantum dots as innovative tools for early diagnosis and advanced treatment of breast cancer. ChemMedChem. 2024;19(16):e202400172.
25. Döpke C, Grothe T, Steblinski P, Klöcker M, Sabantina L, Kosmalska D, et al. Magnetic nanofiber mats for data storage and transfer. Nano. 2019;9(1):92.
26. Dreher KL. Health and environmental impact of nanotechnology: toxicological assessment of manufactured nanoparticles. Toxicol Sci. 2003;77(1):3–5. https://doi.org/10.1093/toxsci/kfh041.
27. Edvinsson T. Optical quantum confinement and photocatalytic properties in two-, one- and zero-dimensional nanostructures. R Soc Open Sci. 2018;5(9):180387.
28. Edwards PP, Thomas JM. Gold in a metallic divided state—from faraday to present-day nanoscience. Angew Chem Int Ed. 2007;46(29):5480–6.
29. Elahi N, Kamali M, Baghersad MH. Recent biomedical applications of gold nanoparticles: a review. Talanta. 2018;184:537–56. https://doi.org/10.1016/j.talanta.2018.02.088.
30. Freestone I, Meeks N, Sax M, Higgitt C. The Lycurgus cup - a Roman nanotechnology. Gold Bull. 2008;40(4):270–7.
31. Gao Y, Lim J, Teoh S-H, Xu C. Emerging translational research on magnetic nanoparticles for regenerative medicine. Chem Soc Rev. 2015;44(17):6306–29. https://doi.org/10.1039/C4CS00322E.
32. Hu J, Dong M. Recent advances in two-dimensional nanomaterials for sustainable wearable electronic devices. J Nanobiotechnol. 2024;22(1):63.
33. Huang L, Huang S. Controllable preparation of CdSe@ ZnS quantum dots and their applications in high-performance LED digital dynamic color display. J Opt. 2024;53(4):3829–39.
34. Hussain CM, editor. Handbook of nanomaterials for industrial applications. Elsevier; 2018.

35. Ibrahim M. Current perspectives of nanoparticles in medical and dental biomaterials. J Biomed Res. 2012;26(3):143. https://doi.org/10.7555/JBR.26.20120027.
36. Jangid P, Inbaraj MP. Applications of nanomaterials in wastewater treatment. Mater Today Proc. 2021;43:2877–81.
37. Johnson-Mcdaniel D, Barrett CA, Sharafi A, Salguero TT. Nanoscience of an ancient pigment. J Am Chem Soc. 2013;135(5):1677–9.
38. Khan SS, Ullah I, Ullah S, An R, Xu H, Nie K, et al. Recent advances in the surface functionalization of nanomaterials for antimicrobial applications. Materials. 2021;14(22):6932.
39. Kholief MG, Hesham AEL, Hashem FS, Mohamed FM. Synthesis and utilization of titanium dioxide nano particle (TiO2NPs) for photocatalytic degradation of organics. Sci Rep. 2024;14(1):11327.
40. Kumar DL, Azeez AN. Graphene-based nanomaterials in myriad bio-imaging applications in vitro and in vivo studies. In: Graphene-based nanomaterials. CRC Press; 2024. p. 168–84.
41. Kumar K, Raju NN, Nazeer AA. Facile synthesis of mesoporous zinc oxide nanoparticle as a drug delivery system evaluated by IVIVE in PBPK modeling. Adv Nat Sci Nanosci Nanotechnol. 2024a;15(3):035009.
42. Kumar R, Dhiman M, Sharma L, Dadhich A, Kaushik P, Sharma MM. Nanofertilizers: the targeted nutrient supplier and enhance nutrients uptake by pearl millets (*Pennisetum glaucum*). Biocatal Agric Biotechnol. 2022;45:102524.
43. Kumar S, Yadav R, Kumar R, Raturi A, Rao ALN, Kumar A, Boob NS. The role of nanomaterials in advancing sustainable healthcare practices. In: E3S web of conferences, vol. 511. EDP Sciences; 2024b. p. 01025.
44. Kumari P, Alam M, Siddiqi WA. Usage of nanoparticles as adsorbents for waste water treatment: an emerging trend. Sustain Mater Technol. 2019;22:e00128. https://doi.org/10.1016/j.susmat.2019.e00128.
45. Lara S, Perez-Potti A. Applications of nanomaterials for immunosensing. Biosensors. 2018;8(4):104.
46. Lata S, Bhardwaj S, Garg R. Nanomaterials for sensing and biosensing: applications in agrifood diagnostics. Int J Environ Anal Chem. 2024;104(16):4868–85.
47. Lee YY, Sriram B, Wang SF, Kogularasu S, Chang-Chien GP. Advanced nanomaterial-based biosensors for N-terminal pro-brain natriuretic peptide biomarker detection: progress and future challenges in cardiovascular disease diagnostics. Nano. 2024;14(2):153.
48. Li Y, Zhou J, Tung S, Schneider E, Xi S. A review on development of nanofluid preparation and characterization. Powder Technol. 2009;196(2):89–101. https://doi.org/10.1016/j.powtec.2009.07.025.
49. Lin J, Huang Y, Huang P. Graphene-based nanomaterials in bioimaging. In: Biomedical applications of functionalized nanomaterials: concepts, development and clinical translation; 2018. p. 247–87.
50. Liosis C, Papadopoulou A, Karvelas E, Karakasidis TE, Sarris IE. Heavy metal adsorption using magnetic nanoparticles for water purification: a critical review. Materials. 2021;14(24):7500. https://doi.org/10.3390/ma14247500.
51. Lu C, Luo S, Wang X, Li J, Li Y, Shen Y, Wang J. Illuminating the nanomaterials triggered signal amplification in electrochemiluminescence biosensors for food safety: mechanism and future perspectives. Coord Chem Rev. 2024;501:215571.
52. Luo X, Morrin A, Killard AJ, Smyth MR. Application of nanoparticles in electrochemical sensors and biosensors. Electroanalysis. 2006;18(4):319–26. https://doi.org/10.1002/elan.200503415.
53. Mahayni Y, Maurer L, Auer F, Hutzler A, Wasserscheid P, Wolf M. Structure sensitivity of the low-temperature dehydrogenation of perhydro dibenzyltoluene on supported platinum nanoparticles. Cat Sci Technol. 2024;14(18):5464–73.
54. Mahendiran B, Azeez NA, Muthusamy S, Krishnakumar GS. Polymer-based bionanomaterials for targeted drug delivery. In: Fundamentals of bionanomaterials. Elsevier; 2022. p. 241–71.

55. Mashak SF, Moniri E, Azarakhshi F, Shahsavari S, Fard NT. Surface PEGylation of Poly (Ethylenimine) dendrimers grafted magnetic nanoparticles as a pH and magnetic targeting responsive system for Cytarabine drug delivery. Chem Phys Lett. 2024;857:141722.
56. Menon JU, Jadeja P, Tambe P, Vu K, Yuan B, Nguyen KT. Nanomaterials for photo-based diagnostic and therapeutic applications. Theranostics. 2013;3(3):152.
57. Miao J, Miyauchi M, Simmons TJ, Dordick JS, Linhardt RJ. Electrospinning of nanomaterials and applications in electronic components and devices. J Nanosci Nanotechnol. 2010;10(9):5507–19.
58. Mohan Bhagyaraj S, Oluwafemi OS, Oluwafemi OS. Nanotechnology: the science of the invisible. In: Synthesis of inorganic nanomaterials: advances and key technologies; 2018. p. 1–18.
59. Murthy SK. Nanoparticles in modern medicine: state of the art and future challenges. Int J Nanomedicine. 2007;2(2):129–41. https://doi.org/10.2147/IJN.S2.2.129.
60. Nandhini NT, Rajeshkumar S, Mythili S. The possible mechanism of eco-friendly synthesized nanoparticles on hazardous dyes degradation. Biocatal Agric Biotechnol. 2019;19:101138. https://doi.org/10.1016/j.bcab.2019.101138.
61. Narayana K, Al-Bader M, Mousa A, Khan KM. Molecular effects of chemotherapeutic drugs and their modulation by antioxidants in the testis. Eur J Pharmacol. 2012;674(2–3):207–16.
62. Neikov OD, Yefimov NA. Nanopowders. In: Handbook of non-ferrous metal powders: technologies and applications. 2nd ed; 2019. p. 271–311.
63. Nobs L, Buchegger F, Gurny R, Allémann E. Current methods for attaching targeting ligands to liposomes and nanoparticles. J Pharm Sci. 2004;93(8):1980–92.
64. Palit S, Hussain CM. Functionalization of nanomaterials for industrial applications: recent and future perspectives. In: Handbook of functionalized nanomaterials for industrial applications. Elsevier; 2020. p. 3–14.
65. Reus MA, Krifa A, Akkerman QA, Biewald A, Xu Z, Kosbahn DP, et al. Layer-by-layer printed metal hybrid (Cs: FA) PbI3 perovskite nanocrystal solar cells. Adv Opt Mater. 2024;12(8):2301008.
66. Sanità G, Carrese B, Lamberti A. Nanoparticle surface functionalization: how to improve biocompatibility and cellular internalization. Front Mol Biosci. 2020;7:587012.
67. Sathiyaseelan A, Zhang X, Lu Y, l Azeez NA, Zhang L, Krishnakumar GS, Wang MH. Exploring the synthesis, properties, and potential of chitosan-functionalized metal-organic frameworks in emerging applications. Prog Mater Sci. 2024;148:101387.
68. Seaberg J, Clegg JR, Bhattacharya R, Mukherjee P. Self-therapeutic nanomaterials: applications in biology and medicine. Mater Today. 2023;62:190–224. https://doi.org/10.1016/j.mattod.2022.11.007.
69. Sengupta J. Application of carbon nanomaterials in the electronic industry. In: Handbook of nanomaterials for manufacturing applications; 2020. p. 421–50.
70. Sham ML, Kim JK. Surface functionalities of multi-wall carbon nanotubes after UV/ozone and TETA treatments. Carbon. 2006;44(4):768–77.
71. Sharma D, Hussain CM. Smart nanomaterials in pharmaceutical analysis. Arab J Chem. 2020;13(1):3319–43. https://doi.org/10.1016/j.arabjc.2018.11.007.
72. Shokri M, Kharaziha M, Tafti HA, Dalili F, Aghdam RM, Ghiassi SR, Eslaminejad MB. Melatonin-loaded mesoporous zinc-and gallium-doped hydroxyapatite nanoparticles to control infection and bone repair. Biomater Sci. 2024;12(16):4194–210.
73. Stoia D, De Sio L, Petronella F, Focsan M. Recent advances towards point-of-care devices for fungal detection: emphasizing the role of plasmonic nanomaterials in current and future technologies. Biosens Bioelectron. 2024;255:116243.
74. Su T, Zhao F, Ying Y, Li W, Li J, Zheng J, et al. Self-monitoring theranostic nanomaterials: emerging visual agents for real-time monitoring of tumor treatment processes. Small Methods. 2024;8(5):2301470.
75. Suh M, Park JY, Ko GB, Kim JY, Hwang DW, Rees L, et al. Optimization of micelle-encapsulated extremely small sized iron oxide nanoparticles as a T1 contrast imaging agent: biodistribution and safety profile. J Nanobiotechnol. 2024;22(1):419.

76. Sudha PN, Sangeetha K, Vijayalakshmi K, Barhoum A. Nanomaterials history, classification, unique properties, production and market. In: Emerging applications of nanoparticles and architectural nanostructures: current prospects and future trends; 2018. p. 341–84.
77. Sharma VP, Sharma U, Chattopadhyay M, Shukla VN. Advance Applications of Nanomaterials: A Review. Materials Today: Proceedings. 2018;5(2):6376–80. https://doi.org/10.1016/j.matpr.2017.12.248.
78. Walleni C, Hamdaoui N, Fadil D, Nsib MF, Llobet E. Synthesis and characterization of nickel oxide nanoparticles decorated graphene oxide for fast-response UV photodetector: unveiling of negative photoconductance. J Mater Sci Mater Electron. 2024;35(18):1205.
79. Walter P, Welcomme E, Hallégot P, Zaluzec NJ, Deeb C, Castaing J, Veyssière P, Bréniaux R, Lévêque JL, Tsoucaris G. Early use of PbS nanotechnology for an ancient hair dyeing formula. Nano Lett. 2006;6(10):2215–9.
80. Wang X, Wang X, Sui X, Zhang W, Jiang H, Liu G, et al. ZnO nanowire/NiO foam 3D nanostructures for high-performance ethylene glycol sensing. Sensors Actuators B Chem. 2024;400:134918.
81. Wang X, Liu X, Zhao C, Zhu P, Liu H. The permeability, mechanical and snow melting performance of graphene composite conductive-pervious concrete. J Build Eng. 2023;79:107929.
82. Wen D. Nanoparticle-related heat transfer phenomenon and its application in biomedical fields. Heat Transfer Eng. 2013;34(14):1171–9. https://doi.org/10.1080/01457632.2013.776877.
83. Wilczewska AZ, Niemirowicz K, Markiewicz KH, Car H. Nanoparticles as drug delivery systems. Pharmacol Rep. 2012;64(5):1020–37.
84. Wu Q, Miao WS, Du Zhang Y, Gao HJ, Hui D. Mechanical properties of nanomaterials: a review. Nanotechnol Rev. 2020;9(1):259–73. https://doi.org/10.1515/ntrev-2020-0021.
85. Wu D, Zhao Q, Zhang B, Tang X, Li Y, Sun J, Yang X. Iron-doped polymer dots with enhanced fluorescence and dual enzyme activity for versatile bioassays. Anal Chem. 2024;96(7):2929–38.
86. Zhang X, Liu Y. Nanomaterials for radioactive wastewater decontamination. Environmental Science: Nano. 2020;7(4):1008–40. https://doi.org/10.1039/C9EN01341E.
87. Zhang C, Ling Y, Zhang X, Liang M, Zou H. Ultra-thin carbon fiber reinforced carbon nanotubes modified epoxy composites with superior mechanical and electrical properties for the aerospace field. Compos A: Appl Sci Manuf. 2022;163:107197.
88. Zhu J, Hersam MC, Zhu J, Hersam MC. Assembly and electronic applications of colloidal nanomaterials. Adv Mater. 2017;29(4):1603895.

Chapter 2
Synthesis and Fabrication Techniques

Shibani Kataria, Soumyakanta Prusty, and Sanjeeb Sutradhar

Abstract The development of nanoscience and nanotechnology is driving the wave of the technology revolution and impacting the broad range of areas of digital healthcare and theranostic applications. Nanoparticles are the fundamental building block of nanomaterials and nanostructures for the synthesis and fabrication of smart and sustainable nanomaterials. A large number of nanomaterials and nanostructures have been developed that depend on nonrenewable resources as well as energy-intensive manufacturing processes. A wide variety of physical, chemical, and mechanical syntheses of nanomaterials are used for tuning the size and shape. Moreover, biological synthesis is found to be cost-effective, eco-friendly, and free of any chemical contaminants in comparison to other syntheses for medical and biological applications. The current scenario appears to us that the various important concepts have been established in digital healthcare as well as theranostic fields. In this area, new advances are uninterruptedly growing to improve efficiency, bio-specific stimulation functionalities, and nanomaterial sustainability. This chapter focuses on cutting-edge synthesis approaches and advanced manufacturing approaches for smart and sustainable nanomaterials in digital healthcare and theragnostic applications.

Keywords Smart materials · Nanomaterials · Digital healthcare · Theranostic · Biomedical · Fabrication

S. Kataria · S. Sutradhar (✉)
Department of Chemistry, Dr. B R Ambedkar National Institute of Technology Jalandhar, Jalandhar, Punjab, India
e-mail: sutradhars@nitj.ac.in

S. Prusty
Department of Chemistry, SAS, VIT-AP University, Amaravati, Andhra Pradesh, India

S. Mondal et al. (eds.), *Smart and Sustainable Nanomaterials in Digital Healthcare and Theranostic*, https://doi.org/10.1007/978-981-95-9386-6_2

Abbreviations

3D	3-Dimensional
CTAB	Cetyl trimethyl ammonium bromide
GPTMS	3-Glycidoxypropyl-trimethoxysilane
MMT	3-[4,5-Dimethylthiazol-2 yl]-2,5-diphenyltetrazolium bromide
MRI	Magnetic resonance imaging
MTES	Methyl-triethoxysilane
MTMOS	Methyltrimethoxysilane
PANI	Polyaniline
PEG	Polyethylene glycol
Span 20	Sorbitan laurate
TEOS	Tetraethyl orthosilicate
Tween 80	Poly(oxyethylene) sorbitan monooleate

2.1 Introduction

Nanoparticles are the central building block of the nanomaterials and nanostructures for developing smart and sustainable nanomaterials. The widely accepted definition of nanoparticles is "the material that possesses at least one of the dimensions within the range of 1–100 nm". The material with dimensions 1–100 nm could act as a bridge between molecular or atomic structure and bulk structure due to possessing remarkable physicochemical properties. These properties are possessed due to their small sizes, large surface area, and outstanding chemical reactivity at different sites of the structure [1–3]. The nanoscale materials with a high surface area to volume ratio might be used to control the reaction rate that depends on the surface defect or surface area [4]. Those nanoparticles or nanostructures that can be modulated in their physicochemical properties under external stimuli are called "smart materials." The external stimuli can be physical and chemical stimuli such as pH, enzymatic activity, redox reaction, sugar concentration, temperature, light interaction, magnetic field, electric field, and mechanical stresses, which are listed in Fig. 2.1 [5]. Smart materials with remarkable functionalities and physicochemical properties have been synthesized and fabricated into different nanostructures such as nanorods, micelles, nanogels, and nanoparticles for digital healthcare and theranostic applications. Nanostructures and nanomaterials are dispersion solutions of solid particles or atomic aggregates with nanometric scale dimensions [6–8]. Many research groups have made substantial contributions toward the progress in the synthesis and fabrication of nanomaterials and nanostructure over the past 25 years. Nevertheless, there is a lack of a comprehensive and detailed review of nanomaterial synthesis for biomedical applications.

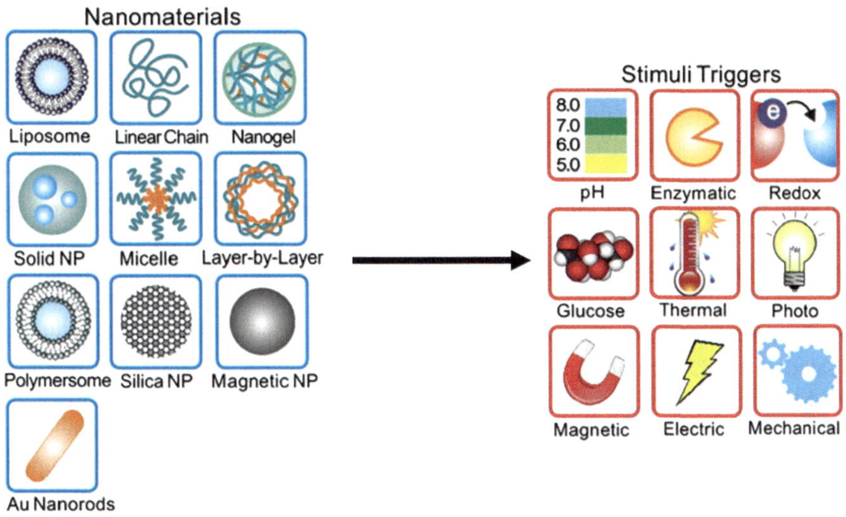

Fig. 2.1 Different nanomaterial structures with a wide variety of stimuli for smart nanomaterial synthesis and fabrication. (Reprinted with the permission from reference [5]. *Copyright © 2014 Elsevier B. V. All rights reserved*)

2.2 Cutting-Edge Nanomaterial Synthesis Methods

Currently, nanomaterial synthesis and fabrication use two methods i.e. top-down method and the bottom-up method for producing the desired size and shape of the nanomaterials [9]. In the top-down method, the fragmented bulk material is used for nanomaterial synthesis and fabrication. On the other hand, in the bottom-up method, the building blocks such as atoms, molecules, or clusters are used to produce nanomaterials using physical or chemical forces [10]. However, there are various specific techniques and various approaches included in these two methods. Those approaches as well as methods are chemical, physical, mechanical, mechanochemical, and biological [11]. The physicochemical properties, morphological, and structural features can be tunable with synthesis and fabrication strategies for applications in digital healthcare and theranostic [12–14]. Broadly, nanomaterials can be produced from three different methods such as chemical, physical, and biological synthesis methods.

2.2.1 Chemical Synthesis for Precise Control of Nanomaterials

Chemical synthesis approaches enable the development of stimuli-active nanomaterials by manipulating the chemical reaction conditions and offering control over the size, shape, morphology, and structure concerning the biomedical applications [15].

The common techniques included in the chemical synthesis are coprecipitation, sol-gel route, solvothermal and hydrothermal, pyrolysis, microwave-assisted, and microemulsion [16, 17].

Coprecipitation Technique The nanomaterial synthesis with coprecipitation technique is occasionally termed as chemical precipitation. It is a process by which two or more compounds precipitate out simultaneously in a suitable solvent [18, 19]. The precipitation occurs due to supersaturation that involves the continuous steps of nucleation, growth, and agglomeration of the particle formation as a precipitate in the solution [20, 21]. The salt of $FeCl_2.4H_2O$ and $FeCl_3.H_2O$ in the stoichiometric ratio of 1:2 in the presence of polymeric capping agent PEG and under the high basic condition produces iron oxide nanomaterials. This iron oxide nanoparticle coated with SiO_2 and oleic acid produced a less cytotoxicity nanomaterial measured by MTT assay [21]. Silver nanomaterial production is reported using trisodium citrate as a capping as well as a reducing agent. The aqueous solution changed the color upon heating at ~50 °C and was subsequently cooled down to room temperature for supersaturation. It was envisaged that this nanomaterial could be found in the treatment of brain tumors and breast cancer [22]. Gold nanomaterials were synthesized by adding gold solution to the boiling solution of sodium citrate as a reducing agent and PVP as a capping. The color of the solution was changed from pale yellow to deep red indicating the successful formation of gold nanomaterials. The PVP-capped gold nanomaterial was exhibited to show ultrasensitive detection of EHV-1 and EHV-4 in multiplex real-time PCR [23]. Further, the stability of the capped gold nanomaterial was enhanced with the alkylated and carboxyl terminated ligands by ligand surface reaction. The surface medication with mAb-anti *Listeria monocytogenes* was allowed to be used as a biosensor probe [24]. Under the UV light illumination (16 W, λ_{ex} = 253 nm), 12-phosphotungstic acid-modified PANI-coated TiO_2 nanomaterial activated the surface ligand for acting as a reducing agent. The activated surface layer 12-phosphotungstic acid was reduced to the $HAuCl_4$ for the fabrication of a ternary composite containing gold nanomaterials (cf. Fig. 2.2). The visual nanomaterial fabrication was indicated by the change in color from dark green to brown. The ternary composite was used for modification of GCE for photoelectrochemical detection of lactate [25]. Different magnetic iron-based smart materials were demonstrated as a contrast agent for MRI [26, 27]. The core/shell structure of iron/iron oxide nanomaterials was synthesized by the decomposition of iron precursor in the presence of capping agent polyamine and subsequently functionalized with meso-2,3-dimercaptosuccinic acid by ligand exchange reaction [28]. For chemical precipitation, the precursor solutions maintained alkalinity by adding ammonia solution, sodium hydroxide solution, and many more different types of bases. The size of nanomaterials could be controlled by controlling the ratio of the precursor, the temperature of the reaction, the pH of the solution, the reducing agent, and the type of base used.

Sol-gel Route Technique Sol-gel route technique is a wet chemical method for nanofabrication [29]. Sol-gel technique provides a unique approach for the prepara-

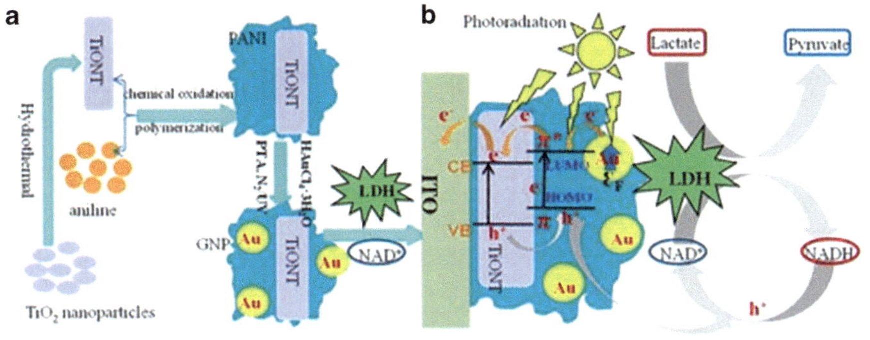

Fig. 2.2 A ternary composite-based TiO_2, PANI, and gold nanoparticle fabrication strategy for photoelectrochemical detection of biomolecules. (Reprinted with the permission from reference [25]. *Copyright © 2016, American Chemical Society*)

tion of smart materials due to the major advantages of simple procedure, high surface area, and stable surface [30]. Nanomaterial synthesis and fabrication by sol-gel route follow two two-step processes. In the first step, precursor solutions hydrolyze with either acid or base and in the second step, polycondensation occurs of the hydrolyzed products via an inorganic polymerization reaction. The second step allows phase change from liquid to gel phase and enhances the viscosity of the solution. Afterward, the gel phase changes to the powder phase due to condensation of water molecules [31]. It may require an additional higher temperature than room temperature to process the phase change. The major disadvantage of this method is the formation of the composite structure due to inorganic polymerization reaction and hence post-treatment is recommended for purification of the nanomaterials [32–34]. A hybrid organic-inorganic biomaterial with sol-gel coating methodology was developed by using MTMOS and GPTMS with different molar ratios. The acid was used as a catalyst for hydrolysis and exhibited to release silicon compounds under in vivo conditions [35]. The core-shell structure of the $CaO@TiO_2$-SiO_2 biomaterial was derived from sol-gel methodology, using tetrabutoxytitanium and tetraethoxysilane as a precursor solution in the phosphoric acid/butanol [36]. The presence of phosphoric acid allowed the formation of a calcium-phosphate layer on the biomaterial surface and accelerated its formation with the increase of the pH of the medium. This was allowed to release the calcium and silicon ions into the surrounding tissues [37]. The acid-catalyzed hydrolysis of MTMOS and TEOS precursors was used for the hybrid coating with different mole percentages of $MgCl_2$. Different substrates such as sandblasted and acid-etched grade-4 Ti discs are used for nanofabrication. The substrate-modified sample altered the protein adsorption pattern due to different mole percentage incorporation of Mg^{2+} in the sol-gel network [38]. Similarly, the concentration of $SrCl_2$ in the sol-gel coating of the polysiloxane network controlled the bone regeneration process [39]. A star block copolymer (DPE-*g*-OEGA-*b*-AA) was demonstrated for redox-responsive hydrogel with ferric ion (Fe^{2+}) instantaneously (cf. Fig. 2.3). The ionic-based crossed linking

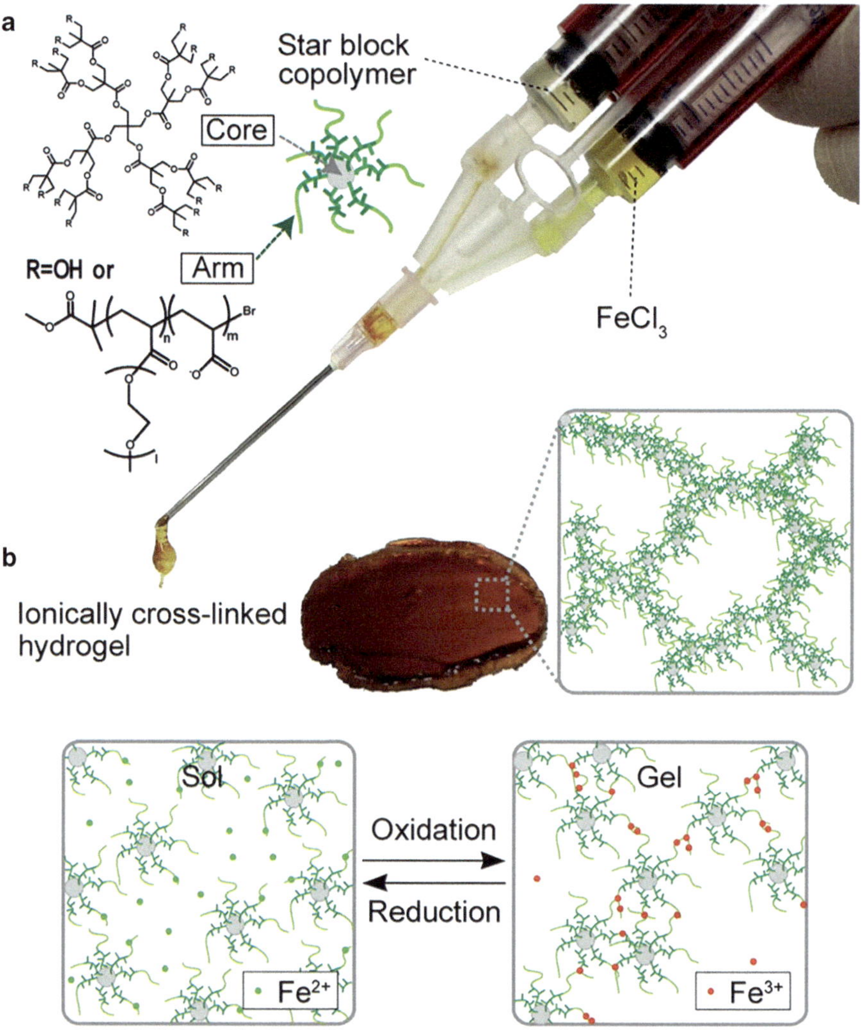

Fig. 2.3 (**a**) Schematic representation for the formation of star block copolymer hydrogel based on ionically cross-linked. (**b**) Schematic representation for redox-responsive stimuli transition from sol-gel to gel-sol. (Reprinted with the permission from reference [40]. *Copyright © 2017, American Chemical Society*)

with Fe^{3+} ion was able to control the hydrogel transition from sol-gel to gel-sol. The hydrogel showed excellent biocompatibility and injectability in vivo redox-responsive stimuli [40]. Two different sols were synthesized by using silicon alkoxides i.e. TEOS and MTES in the presence of acidulated water and alcohol (Sol A). Graphene nanoplatelets were used for functionalization of the sol (Sol B) by doping methodology. The magnesium AZ31 alloy substrate was modified with both sol A and sol B for anticorrosion and cytocompatibility assessment [41]. An aqueous polypeptide block copolymer with the moiety oligo(sulfamethazine) as pH-responsive, poly(γ-benzyl-L-glutamate) as temperature-responsive, and polyethylene glycol as hydrophilic characteristics was demonstrated to show sol-to-gel transition at physiological conditions with stimuli of pH and temperature. The cytotoxicity study of this hydrogel revealed the material are suitable for in vivo applications [42].

Hydrothermal and Solvothermal Techniques The hydrothermal technique can be defined as a chemical process or a transformation between precursors in an aqueous solvent (in a closed system) under high pressure and at a temperature higher than the boiling temperature of the solvent [43]. It is performed under high pressure and high-temperature reaction conditions in a Teflon-lined stainless-still autoclave to dissolve and recrystallize the materials that are relatively insoluble under ordinary experimental conditions [44–46]. However, the solvothermal technique uses the same process but the solvent is nonaqueous. The major advantage of using these techniques is the fabrication of good quality nanomaterial with the controlled composition of the nanostructure [47]. Fe^{2+} doped Fe(III)-polydopamine nanomaterials were fabricated using a hydrothermal strategy without the use of $FeCl_3$ for polymerization reaction (cf. Fig. 2.4). The nanomaterials were further functionalized with glucose oxidase for the generation of H_2O_2, which enabled the sequential Fenton reaction to produce hydroxyl radicals for cancer therapy [48]. Heteroatom-doped carbon nanomaterials were intensively fabricated using hydrothermal strategy for biomedical applications due to their low toxicity, high water solubility, and biocompatibility [49–51]. Boron-doped carbon nanomaterials were fabricated hydrothermally using phenylboronic acid and *L*-glutamic acid as the boron and carbon sources respectively in the presence of sulfuric acid [52]. Nitrogen-doped carbon nanomaterials were fabricated using immature seeds of elm trees and ethylenediamine as the source of carbon and co-reactant through a simple one-step hydrothermal technique for biological imaging and pH monitoring application [53]. Click chemistry was used for precursor preparation of Cd with ps-po DNA-N_3. The use of Te precursor and azide functionalized Cd precursor solutions were used hydrothermally for the fabrication of N_3-DNA functionalized CDTe: Zn^{2+} quantum dots for bioconjugation with dibenzocyclooctyne modified glucose oxidase The quantum dots complex could be used for glucose biosensor by the naked eye, spectroscopy, and paper-based analytical device [54]. This technique also allowed to fabricate carbon nanomaterials from a single precursor. Only the use of *p*-phenylenediamine in ethanol could be fabricated carbon quantum dots by hydrothermally for antibacterial properties [55].

Microwave-Assisted Technique Microwaves are electromagnetic radiation with a frequency range from 300 MHz to 300 GHz or wavelength range from 1 mm to 1 m [56]. The microwave-assisted technique for smart material synthesis is based on efficient heat absorbed by the reactants and solvent from the microwave dielectric heating i.e. ability to convert from microwave energy to thermal energy [57]. The mass conversion to the product is higher than the traditional heating method and

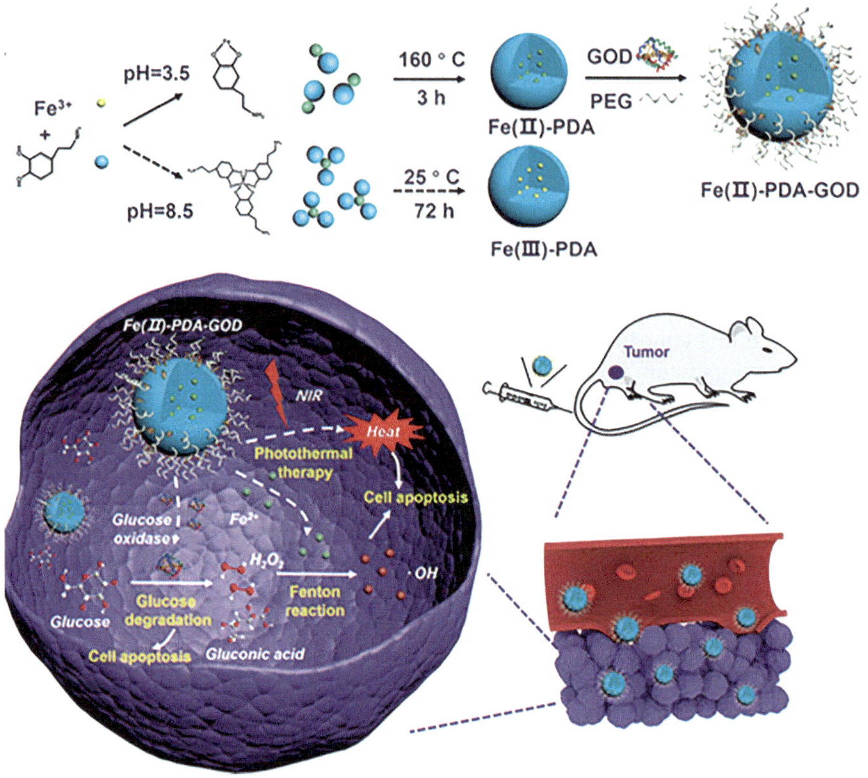

Fig. 2.4 Schematic representation of nanofabrication of Fe (III)-PDA under acidic (hydrothermal) and basic conditions. (Reprinted with the permission from reference [48]. *Copyright © 2019, American Chemical Society*)

produces fewer side products [58]. It can produce the next generation of advanced smart nanomaterials by controlling the microwave parameters such as temperature, pressure, and rate of increasing temperature [59]. Microwave-assisted techniques for synthesizing smart materials are increasingly more attractive due to enhancing reaction kinetics by controlling the microwave parameters [60, 61]. The neat reaction of $FeCl_2.4H_2O$, $FeCl_3.6H_2O$, ammonia solution, and PEG resulted in the formation of biocompatible iron oxide nanomaterials. The microwave-assisted nanomaterials synthesis could enhance the reaction kinetics within 5 min [62]. Treatment of gum kondagogu-derived solution with $AgNO_3$ solution upon microwave irradiation of power 750 W for 50–90 s led to the formation of silver nano materials. The as-synthesized nanomaterials could be found in the application for antibacterial and antioxidant activities [63]. Likewise, the treatment of aqueous solution of *Atalantia monophylla* leaves extract with anhydrous copper (II) sulfate under microwave irradiation power of 630 W for 10 min ensued copper nanoparticles. These nanoparticles demonstrated antioxidant, antibacterial, and anticancer applications [64]. Similarly, silver nanoparticles from pineapple waste were demon-

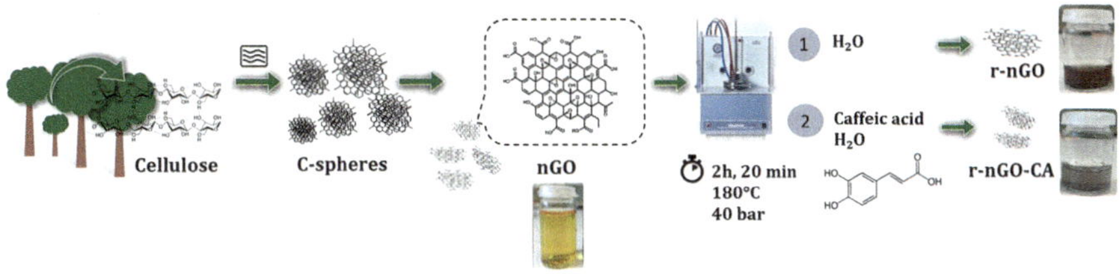

Fig. 2.5 Schematic representation for the two different syntheses of reduced nanographene oxide nanomaterials [68], an open-access article

strated using microwave irradiation power of 1100 W for 9 min [65]. Upconversion nanomaterials based on NaYF4: Yb were demonstrated by microwave-assisted solvothermal technique for bioimaging of HeLa cells as a marker of immunolabeling. The technique could produce a strongly fluorescent and highly crystalline material at a significantly lower temperature within 60 min [66]. Microwave-assisted polyol method was adopted for the synthesis of gadolinium doped carbon dots with microwave irradiation of 750 W for 50 s. The gadolinium-doped carbon dots could be used as a contrast agent for the magnetic resonance imaging application [67]. Reduced nanographene oxide and surface-functionalized reduced nanographene oxide with caffeic acid were synthesized with microwave irradiation of 950 ± 50 W for 120 min and at a pressure of 40 bar (cf. Fig. 2.5). The developed nanomaterial applied for toxicity behavior of the osteoblastic cells MG-63 and found the cell viability loss was dependent on pH of the medium [68].

Microemulsion Technique Microemulsion techniques are well-known for nanomaterial synthesis due to controllable nanostructure formulation without difficulty [69]. It is a colloidal system of self-aggregation in a controllable way with a remarkable application as a nanocarrier [70]. It is a highly thermodynamically stable, homogenous, and isotropic solution composed of at least three components, i.e., a polar phase, usually water; a non-polar phase, usually oil; and a surfactant (sometime uses fourth component as a co-surfactant). The formation of microemulsion is majorly of three types, i.e., water-in-oil microemulsion, where water is the dispersed phase; oil-in-water microemulsion, where oil is the dispersed phase; and water in sc-CO_2 (sc = supercritical) microemulsion. However, the surfactant solution in organic solvent has a tendency to form spheroidal aggregate, which is known as reverse micelle [71, 72]. Schematic representation of water-in-oil and oil-in-water structures are shown in Fig. 2.6. Water-in-oil microemulsion was prepared by using cetyl trimethyl ammonium bromide (CTAB) as the cationic surfactant, 1-butanol as a cosurfactant, and 1-hexanol as an oily phase. Iron salts and precipitating agent as 30% ammonia were added dropwise to form the superparamagnetic iron oxide nanomaterials. The as-synthesized nanomaterials were used for immuno-separation upon functionalization with liposomes [73]. A reverse microemulsion technique was adopted for the synthesis of Fe_3O_4–Ag_2S heteronanocrystals. Octyl polyethylene glycol phenyl ether as a surfactant, cyclohexane as an oily phase, and ammonia as a precipitating agent along with silver were used for reverse microemulsion formation (cf. Fig. 2.7). The modified Fe_3O_4–Ag_2S heteronanocrystals with sodium citrate solution were used for the magnetic resonance imaging in vivo [74]. Gold nanomaterials were synthesized by microemulsion technique with tetra-octyl ammonium bromide as a surfactant and aqueous solution of hydrogen tetrachloroaurate in the presence of reducing agent $NaBH_4$. A uniform nanomaterial size of 7–9 nm was obtained and demonstrated to show less cytotoxic toward HeLa cells upon functionalization with monohydroxy thioalkylated PEG ligand [75]. Silver nanomaterials were synthesized without using reducing agent in the microemulsion. The composition of the microemulsion contains ionic liquid, Tween 80, Span 20, and isopropyl myristate. However, $NaBH_4$ as a reducing agent was required for the synthesis of gold nanomaterials in this microemulsion [76]. Copper oxide (Cu_2O) nanomaterials using the reverse micelle technique were demonstrated to exhibit antimicrobial properties. It was used as a microbial surfactant, Bacillus cereus SPL-4 lipopeptide; n-butanol as a cosurfactant; n-heptane as an oil phase for the preparation of microemulsion; and $NaBH_4$ as a reducing agent [77]. The copper-based nanomaterials were reported by different surfactant molecules like CTAB and AOT and explored various biomedical applications [78, 79].

2.2.2 Biological Synthesis for Sustainable Nanomaterials

There are various chemical and physical techniques available to synthesize smart materials for digital healthcare and theranostic application [80–82]. These methodology designs involve reducing the metal ions, followed by stabilizing them with suitable organic ligand, surfactant, or complexing agent. The majority of these techniques are very expensive and use the toxic or hazardous chemicals that might pose

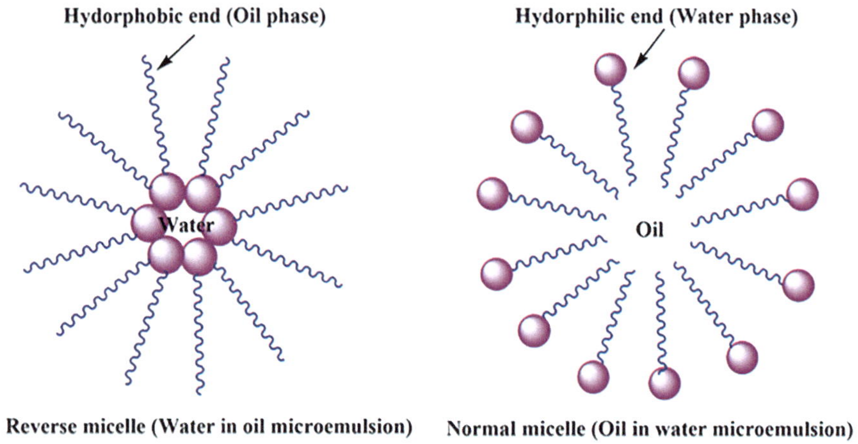

Fig. 2.6 Schematic representation for a microemulsion structure

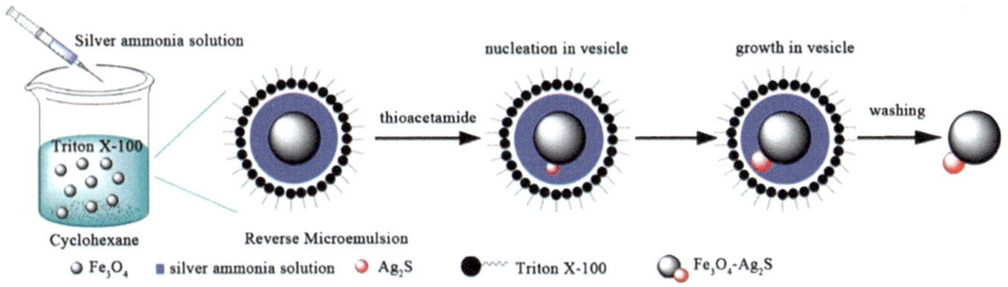

Fig. 2.7 Microemulsion technique for the synthesis of $Fe_3O_4-Ag_2S$ heteronanocrystals. (Reprinted with the permission from reference [74]. *Copyright © 2019, American Chemical Society*)

a potential threat to biological applications. Therefore, there is a demand for the use of ecofriendly and/or biocompatible substance for synthesis and fabrication of the smart materials. Nano-biotechnology is the branch of science that deals with the synthesis of smart nanostructures from the living or bio-organism [83–86].

Synthesis of Smart Materials from Plants Plant materials, viz., extracts from bark, roots, pericarp, leaves, flowers, and/or fruits, are widely known for synthesizing various nanomaterials due to the controllability of different sizes, shapes, and stability. Additionally, different plant materials act as reducing, capping, and stabilizing agents due to the presence of different rich natural compounds, viz., terpenoids, alkaloids, flavonoids, flavones, proteins, polyphenols, saponins, tannins, and steroids, as well as other nutritional compounds [80, 83]. It has potential advantages over other techniques that might eliminate the complex cell culture and maintain processes for digital healthcare and theranostic applications. A general schematic representation for the synthesis of metal nanomaterials from plant materials is shown in Fig. 2.8 [87]. Plant extracts from leaves of *Pistacia atlantica* and *Ficus hispida Linn. f.*, roots of *Salvadora persica*, as well as fruits of *Alpinia nigra* were used for the synthesis of silver nanoparticles. The as-synthesized nanomaterials by green reduction strategy have applications in antimicrobial, antibacterial activity, and antioxidant fields [88–91]. Gold nanoparticles were also synthesized using plant extracts from *Moringa oleifera* petals, *Artemisia vulgaris L.* leaves, and *Plumeria alba* flowers and demonstrated to apply in anticancer and antimicrobial, as well as larvicidal activity against dengue fever [92–94]. Similarly, platinum nanomaterials could be synthesized by using green reduction strategy with extract from pomegranate, black cumin seed, Saudi's dates, and *Xanthium strumarium* leaf for biomedical applications [95–98].

Synthesis of Smart Materials from Microbes Various microbial agents such as fungi, bacteria, viruses, microalgae, and actinobacteria could be used for nanomaterial synthesis due to their ability to reduce the inorganic metal to nanostructure either through intracellular or extracellular pathways [99]. The nanomaterials fabrication involves the absorption of precursors by the microbe at the extracellular or intracellular site, followed by enzyme-catalyzed bioreduction conversion to nano-

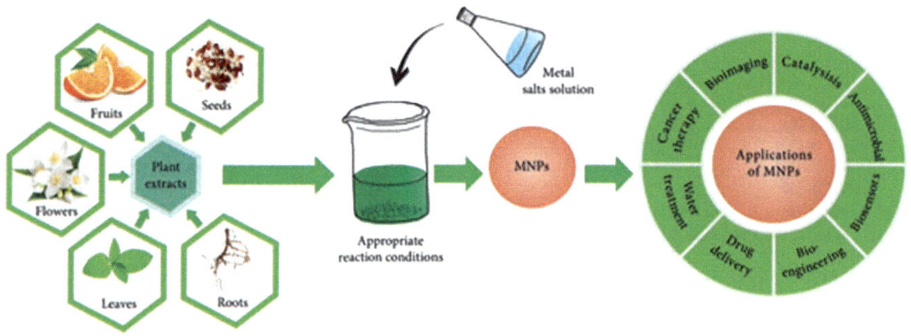

Fig. 2.8 General strategy for the synthesis of metal nanomaterials from different plant materials [87], an open-access article

structure. This approach of smart material synthesis is rapid, non-toxic, eco-friendly, and biocompatible. A large number of studies were carried out on the synthesis of biosynthetic metals such as gold, silver, copper, and zinc [100]. The various species of bacteria, such as, *Pyrococcus furiosus*, *Bacillus licheniformis*, *Pseudomonas deceptionensis*, *Pyrobaculum islandicum*, *Pseudomonas aeruginosa*, etc., were used for the synthesis of nanomaterials for digital healthcare and theranostic application [101]. Tobacco mosaic virus, cowpea chlorotic mottle viruses, and Benincasa hispida viruses were used for the gold, silver, and gold-silver hybrid nanomaterial fabrication [102–104]. Marine algae from seaweed extract was used for the fabrication of gold and silver nanomaterials and exhibited good antibacterial, anticancer, and antimicrobial activities [105–107]. Genetically modified Pichia pastoris contains the cytochrome b5 reductase enzyme and edible mushroom. *Pleurotus florida* contains riboflavin, which plays a major role in the bio-reduction of gold metal ions. These were produced well-dispersed in aqueous medium and in the 10–70 nm range size with uneven-shaped nanomaterials [108, 109].

2.3 Advanced Manufacturing Approaches

The advanced manufacturing approaches are those that support all current and emerging techniques in the manufacturing of smart nano- or micro-structure materials. Over the past few decades, 3D printing has gradually emerged as one of the potential advanced manufacturing approaches. It can fabricate smart materials in complex designs and/or shapes for digital healthcare and theranostic applications [110–112]. There are three steps to follow for fabricating a smart material using a 3D printing manufacturing approach. The first step is the groundwork after the creation of a 3D CAD file. In the second step, material as well as material properties are selected for actual printing in the device. In the third step, matching the specific instrumental skills with the properties of the smart nano- or micro-structure. The fabricated device or object can't be used until it has been finished such as by being cured, sanded, lacquered, and/or painted [113, 114]. Polydimethylsiloxane (PDMS) elastomer resin within a hydrophilic Carbopol gel demonstrated the 3D printing via freeform reversible embedding and is expected to expand to other biomaterials [115]. A complex 3D biological structure using soft protein and polysaccharide hydrogels as primary hydrogel embedded in secondary hydrogel as a thermoreversible, temporary, and biocompatible support was demonstrated for the 3D printing device for the coronary arterial tree [116]. A stretchable sensor based on 3D printing was demonstrated by tuning the rheological properties of the conducting carbon ink, filler fluid, and reservoir [117]. A piezoelectric sensor with polyvinylidene fluoride polymer was established by using integrated 3D printing and the corona poling process. It was exhibited to tune the piezoelectricity of the polyvinylidene fluoride polymer with the heating bed temperature [118].

Lithography is also one of the advanced manufacturing approaches. It relies on the interaction of light with polymer-based photo-resistive material to create a pattern on the substrate. There are various approaches to using lithography, viz., photolithography, electron beam lithography, proton beam lithography, ion beam lithography, soft lithography, etc. Photolithography is a geometric patterning approach on a device or substrate to print a complex architecture by using light (UV or X-ray) through a photomask. The light interaction allows the polymer-based photo-resist molecule to be removed or etched later on for unique geometric architecture. The electron beam is capable of changing the solubility of polymer-based photoresists and allows it to be removed selectively without using a mask. This type of lithography is termed electron beam lithography. Sometimes electrons might scatter due to the interaction of the electron beam with polymer-based resist molecules and create undesired architecture on the surface. In that instance, a proton can be used instead of an electron beam, termed proton beam lithography. Again, ions have better penetration power and less backscattering than electrons. Therefore, the ion can also be used in lithography, which is termed ion beam lithography. Moreover, soft or elastomeric molds can be used in the lithography to replicate the periodic architecture on the surface, termed soft lithography, which is again two types, i.e., nanoimprint and microcontact printing lithography [119–122]. Silver metal mesh/ $Ti_3C_2T_x$ MXene hybrid materials were demonstrated with angled-stencil lithography for the high-performance wearable thermotherapy. The fabricated material on lithography exhibited a fast response of 18–28 s with a homogeneous temperature distribution of 90 °C [123]. Introducing the liquid metal like EGaIn in the microfluidic channel simplified the soft lithographic fabrication process. The microfluidic channel was demonstrated to detect various variable motions such as beat, vibration, stretching, and friction used for glucose detection and therefore could be used as a biosensor for glucose detection [124]. There are numerous reports based on different lithography in the literature and recommended for interested readers [125–129].

A comparison table of different synthesis techniques for smart materials with benefits and limitations is shown in Table 2.1.

Table 2.1 Different smart material synthesis techniques with their benefits and limitations

Different synthesis techniques	Benefits	Limitation	References
Co-precipitation technique	It allows to tailor the precipitation of the smart materials by pH, temperature, and/or ionic strength	Less precursor impurity affects the precipitation	[20, 21]
Sol-gel route technique	It allows to prepare smart materials at low temperature with high yield (purity)	It can be difficult to control the size and shape with low temperature and requires more time to complete the reaction	[30, 31]
Hydrothermal and solvothermal techniques	It allows to prepare fine nanoparticle size, good crystal shape, and narrow size distribution	It requires very high temperature and pressure	[43–46]
Microwave-assisted technique	It allows preparing uniform distribution of nanoparticles, controlling the particle size and morphology, and low cost	Sometimes nanomaterial agglomerates	[58–61]
Microemulsion technique	It allows preparing materials very easily at room temperature and can be scaled up	It may be unstable for longer time, degrading the nanomaterial quality, and their formulation may sometimes be complex	[69, 70]
Biological synthesis for sustainable nanomaterials	It allows preparing materials with significantly reduced chemical reagents, cost-effective, less toxic, and eco-friendly	It may involve complex process to remove the excess or unessential biological entity that may interfere with the nanomaterial's properties	[80, 83, 99]
3D-printing technique	A complex design and shape-based can be synthesized on a various substrate	It is very expensive and well-trained manpower is required	[110–112]
Lithography technique	Different geometric patterns can be written on a substrate and can be synthesized on the substrate	It is also very expensive and well-trained manpower is required	[119–122]

2.4 Conclusions and Perspectives

In this chapter, cutting-edge and advanced approaches were discussed for the synthesis and fabrication of smart materials based on organic materials and inorganic nanomaterials. The biological approaches are more eco-friendly, sustainable, and inexpensive, and free of harsh chemicals as well as less toxic for digital healthcare and theranostic applications where the purity of synthesized product material is a major concern. Various significant advances have been established in the design, precursor, stabilizing agents, or capping agents for stimulus response for exerting a therapeutic action. Researchers are now paying attention to the development of smart materials with multifunctional, i.e., multiresponsive to enhance the efficiency of these materials in the challenging microenvironment. The ultimate aim of these materials is to make an effort to produce autoregulating therapeutic agents that make the most of physiological cues and external localized energy sources.

Acknowledgments SK and Dr. SS acknowledge the Department of Chemistry, Dr. B R Ambedkar National Institute of Technology Jalandhar for providing facilities and support (Project No.: NITJ/DRC/4710, Dated: 21/08/2024). Dr. SP acknowledges to Department of Chemistry, Vellore Institute of Technology, Andhra Pradesh, for funding through the RGEMS scheme (VIT-AP/SPORIC/RGEMS/2022-23/002) and facilities.

References

1. Hussain I, Singh NB, Singh A, Singh H, Singh SC. Green synthesis of nanoparticles and its potential application. Biotechnol Lett. 2016;38(4):545–60.
2. Mohanty A, Parida A, Raut RK, Behera RK. Ferritin: a promising nanoreactor and nanocarrier for bionanotechnology. ACS Bio Med Chem Au. 2022;2(3):258–81.
3. Baig N, Kammakakam I, Falath W. Nanomaterials: a review of synthesis methods, properties, recent progress, and challenges. Mater Adv. 2021;2(6):1821–71.
4. de Dios M, Barroso F, Tojo C, Blanco MC, López-Quintela MA. Effects of the reaction rate on the size control of nanoparticles synthesized in microemulsions. Colloids Surf A Physicochem Eng Asp. 2005;270–271:83–7.
5. Lu Y, Sun W, Gu Z. Stimuli-responsive nanomaterials for therapeutic protein delivery. J Control Release. 2014;194:1–19.
6. Blum AP, Kammeyer JK, Rush AM, Callmann CE, Hahn ME, Gianneschi NC. Stimuli-responsive nanomaterials for biomedical applications. J Am Chem Soc. 2015;137(6):2140–54.
7. Zhang C, He W, Liu C, Jiao D, Liu Z. Cutting-edge advancements of nanomaterials for medi-translatable noninvasive theranostic modalities. View. 2021;2(3):20200144.
8. Campora S, Ghersi G. Recent developments and applications of smart nanoparticles in biomedicine. Nanotechnol Rev. 2022;11(1):2595–631.
9. Mekuye B, Abera B. Nanomaterials: an overview of synthesis, classification, characterization, and applications. Nano Select. 2023;4(8):486–501.
10. Abid N, et al. Synthesis of nanomaterials using various top-down and bottom-up approaches, influencing factors, advantages, and disadvantages: a review. Adv Colloid Interf Sci. 2022;300:102597.
11. Kolahalam LA, Kasi Viswanath IV, Diwakar BS, Govindh B, Reddy V, Murthy YLN. Review on nanomaterials: synthesis and applications. Mater Today Proc. 2019;18:2182–90.
12. Malik S, Muhammad K, Waheed Y. Emerging applications of nanotechnology in healthcare and medicine. Molecules. 2023;28(18):6624.
13. Zhu W, Wei Z, Han C, Weng X. Nanomaterials as promising theranostic tools in nanomedicine and their applications in clinical disease diagnosis and treatment. Nanomaterials (Basel). 2021;11(12):3346.
14. Lim EK, Kim T, Paik S, Haam S, Huh YM, Lee K. Nanomaterials for theranostics: recent advances and future challenges. Chem Rev. 2015;115(1):327–94.
15. Kuchur OA, Tsymbal SA, Shestovskaya MV, Serov NS, Dukhinova MS, Shtil AA. Metal-derived nanoparticles in tumor theranostics: potential and limitations. J Inorg Biochem. 2020;209:111117.

16. Wang N, Fuh JYH, Dheen ST, Senthil Kumar A. Synthesis methods of functionalized nanoparticles: a review. Bio-Des Manuf. 2021;4(2):379–404.
17. Hachem K, et al. Methods of chemical synthesis in the synthesis of nanomaterial and nanoparticles by the chemical deposition method: a review. BioNanoScience. 2022;12(3):1032–57.
18. Li Z, et al. An overview of synthesis and structural regulation of magnetic nanomaterials prepared by chemical coprecipitation. Meta. 2023;13(1):152.
19. Bang LT, et al. Effects of silicate and carbonate substitution on the properties of hydroxyapatite prepared by aqueous co-precipitation method. Mater Des. 2015;87:788–96.
20. Huang B, He H, Liu H, Wu W, Ma Y, Zhao Z. Mechanically strong, heat-resistant, water-induced shape memory poly(vinyl alcohol)/regenerated cellulose biocomposites via a facile co-precipitation method. Biomacromolecules. 2019;20(10):3969–79.
21. Mohammadi H, Nekobahr E, Akhtari J, Saeedi M, Akbari J, Fathi F. Synthesis and characterization of magnetite nanoparticles by co-precipitation method coated with biocompatible compounds and evaluation of in-vitro cytotoxicity. Toxicol Rep. 2021;8:331–6.
22. Dasaradhudu Y, Arunachalam Srinivasan M. Synthesis and characterization of silver nano particles using co-precipitation method. Mater Today Proc. 2020;33:720–3.
23. Ghoniem SM, ElZorkany HE, Hagag NM, El-Deeb AH, Shahein MA, Hussein HA. Development of multiplex gold nanoparticles biosensors for ultrasensitive detection and genotyping of equine herpes viruses. Sci Rep. 2023;13(1):15140.
24. Ngernpimai S, Puangmali T, Kopwitthaya A, Tippayawat P, Chompoosor A, Teerasong S. Enhanced stability of gold nanoparticles with thioalkylated carboxyl-terminated ligands for applications in biosensing. ACS Appl Nano Mater. 2024;7(11):13124–33.
25. Zhu J, Huo X, Liu X, Ju H. Gold nanoparticles deposited polyaniline-TiO2 nanotube for surface plasmon resonance enhanced photoelectrochemical biosensing. ACS Appl Mater Interfaces. 2016;8(1):341–9.
26. Na BHB, Song IC, Hyeon T. Inorganic nanoparticles for MRI contrast agents. Adv Mater. 2009;21:2133–48.
27. Martins PM, Lima AC, Ribeiro S, Lanceros-Mendez S, Martins P. Magnetic nanoparticles for biomedical applications: from the soul of the earth to the deep history of ourselves. ACS Appl Bio Mater. 2021;4(8):5839–70.
28. Cheong S, et al. Simple synthesis and functionalization of iron nanoparticles for magnetic resonance imaging. Angew Chem Int Ed Engl. 2011;50(18):4206–9.
29. Bokov D, et al. Nanomaterial by sol-gel method: synthesis and application. Adv Mater Sci Eng. 2021;2021:1–21.
30. Ciriminna R, Fidalgo A, Pandarus V, Beland F, Ilharco LM, Pagliaro M. The sol-gel route to advanced silica-based materials and recent applications. Chem Rev. 2013;113(8):6592–620.
31. Kulkarni N, et al. Emerging role of injectable dipeptide hydrogels in biomedical applications. ACS Omega. 2023;8(4):3551–70.
32. Hao S, Lin T, Ning S, Qi Y, Deng Z, Wang Y. Research on cracking of SiO2 nanofilms prepared by the sol-gel method. Mater Sci Semicond Process. 2019;91:181–7.
33. Owens GJ, et al. Sol–gel based materials for biomedical applications. Prog Mater Sci. 2016;77:1–79.
34. Fernandez-Hernan JP, Torres B, Lopez AJ, Rams J. The role of the sol-gel synthesis process in the biomedical field and its use to enhance the performance of bioabsorbable magnesium implants. Gels. 2022;8(7):426.
35. Juan-Díaz MJ, et al. Development of hybrid sol–gel coatings for the improvement of metallic biomaterials performance. Prog Org Coat. 2016;96:42–51.
36. Castro Y, et al. Sol–gel hybrid membranes loaded with meso/macroporous SiO2, TiO2–P2O5 and SiO2–TiO2–P2O5 materials with high proton conductivity. Mater Chem Phys. 2015;149–150:686–94.
37. Kozik VV, Borilo LP, Lyutova ES, Brichkov AS, Chen YW, Izosimova EA. Preparation of CaO@TiO(2)-SiO(2) biomaterial with a sol-gel method for bone implantation. ACS Omega. 2020;5(42):27221–6.

38. Cerqueira A, et al. Characterization of magnesium doped sol-gel biomaterial for bone tissue regeneration: the effect of Mg ion in protein adsorption. Mater Sci Eng C Mater Biol Appl. 2021;125:112114.
39. García-Arnáez I, et al. Development and characterisation of strontium-doped sol-gel coatings to optimise the initial bone regeneration processes. Mater Today Commun. 2022;33:104674.
40. Nakagawa Y, Ohta S, Sugahara A, Okubo M, Yamada A, Ito T. In vivo redox-responsive sol–gel/gel–sol transition of star block copolymer solution based on ionic cross-linking. Macromolecules. 2017;50(14):5539–48.
41. Fernandez-Hernan JP, Lopez AJ, Torres B, Martinez-Campos E, Matykina E, Rams J. Anticorrosion and cytocompatibility assessment of graphene-doped hybrid silica and plasma electrolytic oxidation coatings for biomedical applications. ACS Biomater Sci Eng. 2021;7(12):5861–77.
42. Turabee MH, Thambi T, Duong HTT, Jeong JH, Lee DS. A pH- and temperature-responsive bioresorbable injectable hydrogel based on polypeptide block copolymers for the sustained delivery of proteins in vivo. Biomater Sci. 2018;6(3):661–71.
43. Chen A, Holt-Hindle P. Platinum-based nanostructured materials: synthesis, properties, and applications. Chem Rev. 2010;110:3767–804.
44. Zeimaran E, Pourshahrestani S, Shirazi SFS, Pingguan-Murphy B, Kadri NA, Towler MR. Hydrothermal synthesis and characterisation of bioactive glass-ceramic nanorods. J Non-Cryst Solids. 2016;443:118–24.
45. Somasundaram G, Rajan J, Sangaiya P, Dilip R. Hydrothermal synthesis of CdO nanoparticles for photocatalytic and antimicrobial activities. Results Mater. 2019;4:100044.
46. Tooklang P, et al. Functionalization of silver nanoparticles coating cotton fabrics through hydrothermal synthesis for improved antimicrobial properties. Nano Express. 2024;5(2):025009.
47. Yoshimura M, Byrappa K. Hydrothermal processing of materials: past, present and future. J Mater Sci. 2007;43(7):2085–103.
48. Zhu Y, et al. Novel tumor-microenvironment-based sequential catalytic therapy by Fe(II)-engineered polydopamine nanoparticles. ACS Appl Mater Interfaces. 2019;11(46):43018–30.
49. Aiyer S, Prasad R, Kumar M, Nirvikar K, Jain B, Kushwaha OS. Fluorescent carbon nanodots for targeted in vitro cancer cell imaging. Appl Mater Today. 2016;4:71–7.
50. Lu S, et al. Hydrothermal synthesis of nitrogen-doped carbon dots with real-time live-cell imaging and blood-brain barrier penetration capabilities. Int J Nanomedicine. 2016;11:6325–36.
51. Zheng M, et al. Self-targeting fluorescent carbon dots for diagnosis of brain cancer cells. ACS Nano. 2015;9(11):11455–61.
52. Ozkasapoglu S, Caglayan MG, Akkurt F, Ensarioglu HK, Vatansever HS, Celikkan H. Boron-doped carbon nanodots as a theranostic agent for colon cancer stem cells. ACS Omega. 2023;8(33):30285–93.
53. Guo L, Li L, Wang X, Zhang Y, Cui F. Synthesis of pH-sensitive nitrogen-doped carbon dots with biological imaging function and their application in Cu(2+) and Fe(2+) determination by ratiometric fluorescent probes. ACS Omega. 2023;8(40):37098–107.
54. Mao G, et al. Novel method of clickable quantum dot construction for bioorthogonal labeling. Anal Chem. 2021;93(2):777–83.
55. Ye Z, Li G, Lei J, Liu M, Jin Y, Li B. One-step and one-precursor hydrothermal synthesis of carbon dots with superior antibacterial activity. ACS Appl Bio Mater. 2020;3(10):7095–102.
56. Fernandez-Barahona I, Munoz-Hernando M, Herranz F. Microwave-driven synthesis of iron-oxide nanoparticles for molecular imaging. Molecules. 2019;24(7):1224.
57. Bilecka I, Niederberger M. Microwave chemistry for inorganic nanomaterials synthesis. Nanoscale. 2010;2(8):1358–74.
58. Chikan V, McLaurin EJ. Rapid nanoparticle synthesis by magnetic and microwave heating. Nano (Basel). 2016;6(5):85.

59. Gawande MB, Shelke SN, Zboril R, Varma RS. Microwave-assisted chemistry: synthetic applications for rapid assembly of nanomaterials and organics. Acc Chem Res. 2014;47(4):1338–48.
60. Nikam AV, Prasad BLV, Kulkarni AA. Wet chemical synthesis of metal oxide nanoparticles: a review. CrystEngComm. 2018;20(35):5091–107.
61. Kaur N, Singh A, Ahmad W. Microwave assisted green synthesis of silver nanoparticles and its application: a review. J Inorg Organomet Polym Mater. 2022;33(3):663–72.
62. Aivazoglou E, Metaxa E, Hristoforou E. Microwave-assisted synthesis of iron oxide nanoparticles in biocompatible organic environment. AIP Adv. 2018;8(4):048201.
63. Seku K, Gangapuram BR, Pejjai B, Kadimpati KK, Golla N. Microwave-assisted synthesis of silver nanoparticles and their application in catalytic, antibacterial and antioxidant activities. J Nanostructure Chem. 2018;8(2):179–88.
64. Verma R, et al. Microwave-assisted biosynthesis of CuO nanoparticles using atalantia monophylla (l.) leaf extract and its biomedical applications. Chem Eng Technol. 2021;44(8):1496–503.
65. Anis SNS, Liew WC, Mohd Marsin A, Muhamad II, Teh SH, Md Khudzari AZ. Microwave-assisted green synthesis of silver nanoparticles using pineapple leaves waste. Cleaner Eng Technol. 2023;15:100660.
66. Mi C, Tian Z, Cao C, Wang Z, Mao C, Xu S. Novel microwave-assisted solvothermal synthesis of NaYF4:Yb,Er upconversion nanoparticles and their application in cancer cell imaging. Langmuir. 2011;27(23):14632–7.
67. Gong N, et al. Microwave-assisted polyol synthesis of gadolinium-doped green luminescent carbon dots as a bimodal nanoprobe. Langmuir. 2014;30(36):10933–9.
68. Erdal NB, Adolfsson KH, Pettersson T, Hakkarainen M. Green strategy to reduced nanographene oxide through microwave assisted transformation of cellulose. ACS Sustain Chem Eng. 2017;6(1):1246–55.
69. Richard B, Lemyre J-L, Ritcey AM. Nanoparticle size control in microemulsion synthesis. Langmuir. 2017;33(19):4748–57.
70. Malik MA, Wani MY, Hashim MA. Microemulsion method: a novel route to synthesize organic and inorganic nanomaterials. Arab J Chem. 2012;5(4):397–417.
71. Solanki JN, Murthy ZVP. Controlled size silver nanoparticles synthesis with water-in-oil microemulsion method: a topical review. Ind Eng Chem Res. 2011;50(22):12311–23.
72. Ganguli AK, Ganguly A, Vaidya S. Microemulsion-based synthesis of nanocrystalline materials. Chem Soc Rev. 2010;39(2):474–85.
73. Salvador M, Gutierrez G, Noriega S, Moyano A, Blanco-Lopez MC, Matos M. Microemulsion synthesis of superparamagnetic nanoparticles for bioapplications. Int J Mol Sci. 2021;22(1):427.
74. Liu D, Lai J, Wang R, Ye L, Tian Y. Reverse microemulsion synthesis of Fe3O4-Ag2S heteronanocrystals for dual-modal imaging-guided photothermal tumor ablation. ACS Biomater Sci Eng. 2019;5(11):6196–206.
75. Salabat A, Mirhoseini F. A novel and simple microemulsion method for synthesis of biocompatible functionalized gold nanoparticles. J Mol Liq. 2018;268:849–53.
76. Ghosh M, Kundu S, Pyne A, Sarkar N. Unveiling the behavior of curcumin in biocompatible microemulsion and its differential interaction with gold and silver nanoparticles. J Phys Chem C. 2020;124(6):3905–14.
77. Bezza FA, Tichapondwa SM, Chirwa EMN. Fabrication of monodispersed copper oxide nanoparticles with potential application as antimicrobial agents. Sci Rep. 2020;10(1):16680.
78. Camacho-Flores BA, et al. Copper: synthesis techniques in nanoscale and powerful application as an antimicrobial agent. J Nanomater. 2015;2015:1–10.
79. Naz S, Gul A, Zia M, Javed R. Synthesis, biomedical applications, and toxicity of CuO nanoparticles. Appl Microbiol Biotechnol. 2023;107(4):1039–61.
80. Noah NM, Ndangili PM. Green synthesis of nanomaterials from sustainable materials for biosensors and drug delivery. Sens Int. 2022;3:100166.

81. Gupta D, Boora A, Thakur A, Gupta TK. Green and sustainable synthesis of nanomaterials: recent advancements and limitations. Environ Res. 2023;231(Pt 3):116316.
82. Goswami AD, Trivedi DH, Jadhav NL, Pinjari DV. Sustainable and green synthesis of carbon nanomaterials: a review. J Environ Chem Eng. 2021;9(5):106118.
83. Khan N, Ali S, Latif S, Mehmood A. Biological synthesis of nanoparticles and their applications in sustainable agriculture production. Nat Sci. 2022;14(06):226–34.
84. Jamalipour Soufi G, Iravani S. Eco-friendly and sustainable synthesis of biocompatible nanomaterials for diagnostic imaging: current challenges and future perspectives. Green Chem. 2020;22(9):2662–87.
85. Patwardhan SV, Manning JRH, Chiacchia M. Bioinspired synthesis as a potential green method for the preparation of nanomaterials: opportunities and challenges. Curr Opin Green Sustainable Chem. 2018;12:110–6.
86. Saratale RG, et al. A comprehensive review on green nanomaterials using biological systems: recent perception and their future applications. Colloids Surf B Biointerfaces. 2018;170:20–35.
87. Bao Y, et al. Plant-extract-mediated synthesis of metal nanoparticles. J Chem. 2021;2021:1–14.
88. Veisi H, Kavian M, Hekmati M, Hemmati S. Biosynthesis of the silver nanoparticles on the graphene oxide's surface using Pistacia atlantica leaves extract and its antibacterial activity against some human pathogens. Polyhedron. 2019;161:338–45.
89. Ramesh AV, Devi DR, Battu G, Basavaiah K. A Facile plant mediated synthesis of silver nanoparticles using an aqueous leaf extract of Ficus hispida Linn. f. for catalytic, antioxidant and antibacterial applications. S Afr J Chem Eng. 2018;26:25–34.
90. Baruah D, Yadav RNS, Yadav A, Das AM. Alpinia nigra fruits mediated synthesis of silver nanoparticles and their antimicrobial and photocatalytic activities. J Photochem Photobiol B. 2019;201:111649.
91. Arshad H, Sami MA, Sadaf S, Hassan U. Salvadora persica mediated synthesis of silver nanoparticles and their antimicrobial efficacy. Sci Rep. 2021;11(1):5996.
92. Anand K, Gengan RM, Phulukdaree A, Chuturgoon A. Agroforestry waste Moringa oleifera petals mediated green synthesis of gold nanoparticles and their anti-cancer and catalytic activity. J Ind Eng Chem. 2015;21:1105–11.
93. Sundararajan B, Ranjitha Kumari BD. Novel synthesis of gold nanoparticles using Artemisia vulgaris L. leaf extract and their efficacy of larvicidal activity against dengue fever vector Aedes aegypti L. J Trace Elem Med Biol. 2017;43:187–96.
94. Mata R, Bhaskaran A, Sadras SR. Green-synthesized gold nanoparticles from Plumeria alba flower extract to augment catalytic degradation of organic dyes and inhibit bacterial growth. Particuology. 2016;24:78–86.
95. Sahin B, et al. Cytotoxic effects of platinum nanoparticles obtained from pomegranate extract by the green synthesis method on the MCF-7 cell line. Colloids Surf B Biointerfaces. 2018;163:119–24.
96. Aygun A, et al. Biogenic platinum nanoparticles using black cumin seed and their potential usage as an antimicrobial and anticancer agent. J Pharm Biomed Anal. 2020;179:112961.
97. Al-Radadi NS. Green synthesis of platinum nanoparticles using Saudi's Dates extract and their usage on the cancer cell treatment. Arab J Chem. 2019;12(3):330–49.
98. Kumar PV, Jelastin Kala SM, Prakash KS. Green synthesis derived Pt-nanoparticles using Xanthium strumarium leaf extract and their biological studies. J Environ Chem Eng. 2019;7(3):103146.
99. Koul B, Poonia AK, Yadav D, Jin JO. Microbe-mediated biosynthesis of nanoparticles: applications and future prospects. Biomolecules. 2021;11(6):886.
100. Iravani S, Varma RS. Biofactories: engineered nanoparticles via genetically engineered organisms. Green Chem. 2019;21(17):4583–603.
101. Salem SS, Fouda A. Green synthesis of metallic nanoparticles and their prospective biotechnological applications: an overview. Biol Trace Elem Res. 2021;199(1):344–70.

102. Kobayashi M, et al. Chiral meta-molecules consisting of gold nanoparticles and genetically engineered tobacco mosaic virus. Opt Express. 2012;20(22):24856–63.
103. Slocik JM, Naik RR, Stone MO, Wright DW. Viral templates for gold nanoparticle synthesis. J Mater Chem. 2005;15(7):749.
104. Thangavelu RM, Ganapathy R, Ramasamy P, Krishnan K. Fabrication of virus metal hybrid nanomaterials: an ideal reference for bio semiconductor. Arab J Chem. 2020;13(1):2750–65.
105. Gonzalez-Ballesteros N, Prado-Lopez S, Rodriguez-Gonzalez JB, Lastra M, Rodriguez-Arguelles MC. Green synthesis of gold nanoparticles using brown algae Cystoseira baccata: its activity in colon cancer cells. Colloids Surf B Biointerfaces. 2017;153:190–8.
106. Dhas TS, Kumar VG, Karthick V, Angel KJ, Govindaraju K. Facile synthesis of silver chloride nanoparticles using marine alga and its antibacterial efficacy. Spectrochim Acta A Mol Biomol Spectrosc. 2014;120:416–20.
107. Kathiraven T, Sundaramanickam A, Shanmugam N, Balasubramanian T. Green synthesis of silver nanoparticles using marine algae Caulerpa racemosa and their antibacterial activity against some human pathogens. Appl Nanosci. 2014;5(4):499–504.
108. Elahian F, Reiisi S, Shahidi A, Mirzaei SA. High-throughput bioaccumulation, biotransformation, and production of silver and selenium nanoparticles using genetically engineered Pichia pastoris. Nanomedicine. 2017;13(3):853–61.
109. Bhat R, Sharanabasava VG, Deshpande R, Shetti U, Sanjeev G, Venkataraman A. Photo-bio-synthesis of irregular shaped functionalized gold nanoparticles using edible mushroom Pleurotus florida and its anticancer evaluation. J Photochem Photobiol B. 2013;125:63–9.
110. Nadgorny M, Ameli A. Functional polymers and nanocomposites for 3d printing of smart structures and devices. ACS Appl Mater Interfaces. 2018;10(21):17489–507.
111. Lombardo D, Kiselev MA, Caccamo MT. Smart nanoparticles for drug delivery application: development of versatile nanocarrier platforms in biotechnology and nanomedicine. J Nanomater. 2019;2019:1–26.
112. Khoo ZX, et al. 3D printing of smart materials: a review on recent progresses in 4D printing. Virtual Phys Prototyp. 2015;10(3):103–22.
113. Mondal K, Tripathy PK. Preparation of smart materials by additive manufacturing technologies: a review. Dent Mater (Basel). 2021;14(21):6442.
114. Ji Y, Luan C, Yao X, Fu J, He Y. Recent progress in 3D printing of smart structures: classification, challenges, and trends. Adv Intell Syst. 2021;3(12):2000271.
115. Hinton TJ, Hudson A, Pusch K, Lee A, Feinberg AW. 3D printing pdms elastomer in a hydrophilic support bath via freeform reversible embedding. ACS Biomater Sci Eng. 2016;2(10):1781–6.
116. Hinton TJ, et al. Three-dimensional printing of complex biological structures by freeform reversible embedding of suspended hydrogels. Sci Adv. 2015;1(9):1–10.
117. Muth JT, et al. Embedded 3D printing of strain sensors within highly stretchable elastomers. Adv Mater. 2014;26(36):6307–12.
118. Kim H, Torres F, Wu Y, Villagran D, Lin Y, Tseng T-L. Integrated 3D printing and corona poling process of PVDF piezoelectric films for pressure sensor application. Smart Mater Struct. 2017;26(8):085027.
119. Handrea-Dragan IM, Botiz I, Tatar AS, Boca S. Patterning at the micro/nano-scale: polymeric scaffolds for medical diagnostic and cell-surface interaction applications. Colloids Surf B Biointerfaces. 2022;218:112730.
120. Glangchai LC, Caldorera-Moore M, Shi L, Roy K. Nanoimprint lithography based fabrication of shape-specific, enzymatically-triggered smart nanoparticles. J Control Release. 2008;125(3):263–72.
121. Liddle JA, Gallatin GM. Lithography, metrology and nanomanufacturing. Nanoscale. 2011;3(7):2679–88.
122. Probst C, Meichner C, Kreger K, Kador L, Neuber C, Schmidt HW. Athermal azobenzene-based nanoimprint lithography. Adv Mater. 2016;28(13):2624–8.

123. Hossain M, Sibin KP, Rao KDM. Angled-stencil lithography based metal mesh/Ti3C2Tx MXene hybrid transparent electrodes for low-power and high-performance wearable thermotherapy. J Mater Chem C. 2021;9(19):6257–67.
124. Zhang Y, et al. Construction of liquid metal-based soft microfluidic sensors via soft lithography. J Nanobiotechnol. 2022;20(1):246.
125. Ye Z, Nain AS, Behkam B. Spun-wrapped aligned nanofiber (SWAN) lithography for fabrication of micro/nano-structures on 3D objects. Nanoscale. 2016;8(25):12780–6.
126. Agrawal H, Garnett EC. Nanocube imprint lithography. ACS Nano. 2020;14(9):11009–16.
127. Cai Y, Cao Y, Nordlander P, Cremer PS. Fabrication of split-rings via stretchable colloidal lithography. ACS Photonics. 2014;1(2):127–34.
128. Wisser FM, Schumm B, Mondin G, Grothe J, Kaskel S. Precursor strategies for metallic nano- and micropatterns using soft lithography. J Mater Chem C. 2015;3(12):2717–31.
129. Ho D, Zou J, Zdyrko B, Iyer KS, Luzinov I. Capillary force lithography: the versatility of this facile approach in developing nanoscale applications. Nanoscale. 2015;7(2):401–14.

Chapter 3
Functionalization and Characterization of Smart and Sustainable Nanomaterials

Abbas Aziz, Kissa E. Zehra, Amna Abbas, Huma Shaikh, and Bakhtawar Javed

Abstract Nanotechnology has attracted considerable attention due to its wide-ranging applications in various fields such as agriculture, sensors, and biomedicine. At the nanoscale, materials exhibit unique physical, chemical, and biological properties—including thermal, mechanical, electrical, and antimicrobial characteristics—that differ significantly from their bulk counterparts. Healthcare remains a fundamental responsibility of every nation. Effective disease management requires accurate and timely identification and diagnosis. However, conventional diagnostic and therapeutic methods are often time-consuming and costly, limiting their effectiveness in the current technological era. Smart nanomaterials, which are sustainable and highly tunable, have emerged as promising candidates for advancing digital healthcare solutions. The fabrication of smart nanomaterials for specific applications is challenging, as it demands precise control over morphology and surface functionalization. Optimization of these parameters, typically achieved through spectroscopic and microscopic techniques, is essential for enhancing performance. This chapter provides a detailed discussion of various functionalization strategies for developing smart nanomaterials, along with an overview of various spectroscopic, microscopic, thermal, and mechanical characterization methods used for the classification of smart nanomaterials. The aim is to strengthen understanding of smart and sustainable nanomaterials for digital healthcare applications, while addressing current challenges and outlining future research directions.

Keywords Smart nanomaterials · Functionalization · Novel strategies · Characterization · Digital healthcare devices

A. Aziz (✉) · K. E. Zehra · A. Abbas · H. Shaikh
National Centre of Excellence in Analytical Chemistry, University of Sindh, Jamshoro, Pakistan

B. Javed
USPCAS-W, Mehran University of Engineering and Technology, Jamshoro, Pakistan

S. Mondal et al. (eds.), *Smart and Sustainable Nanomaterials in Digital Healthcare and Theranostic*, https://doi.org/10.1007/978-981-95-9386-6_3

3.1 Introduction

Nanotechnology is an emerging technology with a wide range of applications. By definition, nanotechnology involves the manipulation of materials at the nanoscale (1–100 nm), where at least one dimension of the material is in this size range. At the nanoscale, the dramatically increased surface-to-volume ratio gives rise to unique physical, chemical, and biological properties that are often markedly different from those of the corresponding bulk materials. Nanomaterials can be synthesized via two primary approaches—bottom-up and top-down. Bottom-up techniques entail assembling atoms and molecules to form nanostructures. Top-down methods break down massive materials into nanoscale structures. Because of their remarkable properties, nanomaterials have attracted considerable attention for diverse applications. However, in biomedical contexts, several challenges remain, including limited biocompatibility, insufficient photostability, complex fabrication processes, and non-specific distribution within the body. To address these limitations, researchers have begun developing a new generation of advanced nanomaterials designed to overcome these drawbacks.

Smart nanomaterials are nanoscale materials that can be triggered by external stimuli, resulting in significant changes in their functional properties [54]. These novel properties are usually achieved through the combination of different materials or by a coating that affects the functionalization and modification of the surface, thereby creating complex structures capable of multi-responsive behavior. Unlike conventional nanomaterials, smart nanomaterials often exhibit relatively simple internal structures, allowing them to respond predictably to external stimuli such as light, temperature, pH, pressure, and magnetic fields. In addition to their unique multi-functional properties, smart nanomaterials are generally more sustainable than traditional nanomaterials. Various methodologies have been developed to assess their sustainability. For example, the Nanoscan tool evaluates environmental, social, and economic benefits against potential risks and compares them with conventional materials of similar function [27]. These remarkable capabilities enable smart nanomaterials to be applied in diverse fields, including biosensors, targeted drug delivery, and the treatment of various diseases [71]. The COVID-19 epidemic has particularly accelerated research and treatment tools. Specifically, current research is focused on the stimuli-responsive properties of smart nanomaterials to develop targeted methods for delivering drugs, enhancing the presentation of antigens, and modulating the immune system [12]. Intelligent nanomaterials may have applications in medicine. Researchers are also actively investigating smart biosensing materials as a key component of next generation, nano-enabled systems for non-invasive point-of-care diagnosis [53]. These smart nanomaterials are categorized based on their physical [24], chemical [83], and biological response [77].

Smart nanomaterials do not always exhibit the desired properties at the required level, especially for biomedical applications. To address these limitations, functionalization and surface modification are often performed to enhance performance and make them more effective candidates. Surface functionalization involves the introduction of chemical groups (such as polymers or biomolecules) or functional groups (e.g., -OH, -COOH, -COOC-) onto the surface of nanomaterials. This process creates active sites on a surface to enable further interactions. Several approaches are commonly used for the functionalization of smart nanomaterials, including chemical functionalization, coating or encapsulation, biomolecule conjugation, doping, and plasma treatment. These strategies can be implemented through two primary methods: post-functionalization and in situ functionalization. Surface-functionalized smart nanomaterials can be coupled with molecular functionalities to create hybrid systems with enhanced performance. Surface functionalization offers several significant advantages, including improved targeting and selectivity, enhanced stability and dispersibility, increased biocompatibility and functionality, higher detection sensitivity, and various notable environmental benefits.

Following surface functionalization of smart nanomaterials, it is essential to confirm the successful attachment of the desired functionality on the surface by characterization. Characterization represents a crucial and fundamental step, as it enables the evaluation of the material's properties based on optimized parameters. Each property can be assessed using appropriate analytical techniques [75]. A wide range of techniques—spectroscopic, microscopic, thermal, electrical, and mechanical—are commonly employed to characterize these materials. These techniques include Fourier transform infrared (FTIR) spectroscopy, thermogravimetric analysis (TGA), UV–visible spectroscopy, differential scanning calorimetry (DSC), energy-dispersive X-ray spectroscopy (EDS), DC four-probe resistivity measurements, scanning electron microscopy (SEM), nanoindentation, dynamic mechanical analysis (DMA), and transmission electron microscopy (TEM). Collectively, these techniques facilitate the monitoring of the functionalization process and provide detailed insights into its effects on the properties of the nanomaterials [7].

3.2 Surface Modifications and Functionalization Strategies

Smart nanomaterials can be made more functional by altering their structure or surface to enhance specific performance characteristics. Various functionalization and modification approaches have been used for smart nanomaterials, as shown in Fig. 3.1. The selection of a particular method depends largely on the desired properties and intended functionalities of the final material. This section explores typical techniques for functionalizing and modifying intelligent nanomaterials.

3.2.1 Coating or Encapsulation

Coating and encapsulation are two essential methods for modifying smart nanomaterials, each offering distinct advantages depending on the intended application. Coating involves applying a thin functional layer on the surface of the nanomaterial

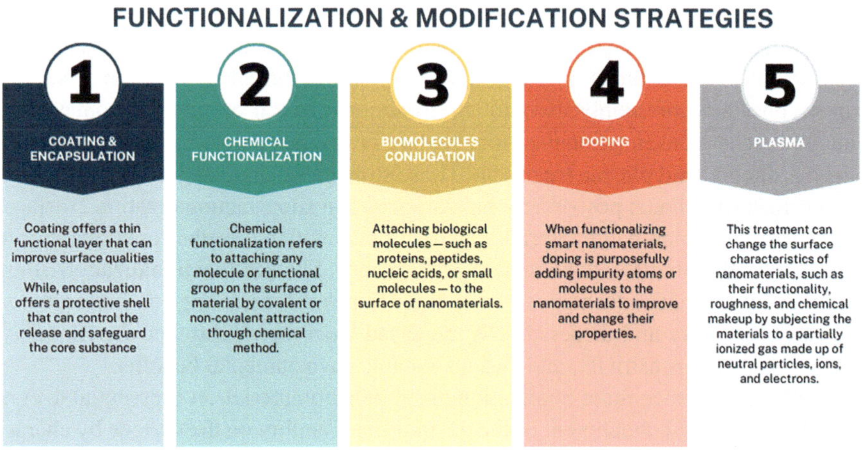

Fig. 3.1 The diagram shows the functionalization and modification strategies for smart nanomaterials

to enhance its surface properties, whereas encapsulation creates a protective shell around the core material, enabling controlled release and protection of the active substance. These approaches significantly expand the potential applications of nanomaterials in fields such as environmental science, diagnostics, medicine, and catalysis. For instance, Fatemeh Bazmi Zeynabad et al. developed a polymer–clay nanocomposite based on cationic silica for a multipurpose drug delivery. In this system, ciprofloxacin (CIP), an antibacterial drug, and two anticancer agents were loaded into a nanocomposite (NC). The release behavior of the three medications was pH dependent: at pH 4, the release was 100%, while at physiological pH 7.4, only 5–10% of the pharmaceuticals were released after 600 h. The difference was attributed to electrostatic interactions between the pharmaceuticals and the nanoparticles, which are stronger at lower pH and weaken as pH increases, thereby facilitating controlled release [88]. Conversely, smart coatings have also attracted considerable interest due to their multi-responsive behavior. These coatings can be applied to various surfaces and have diverse applications, including protective layers, sensors, biomedical devices, and self-healing materials. Coatings may consist of single, double, or triple layers. Zhou et al., for example, developed a pH-responsive layer-by-layer (LbL) hydrogel coating with dual functionality for both detecting and preventing bacterial infection. Coming from a commercial copolymer of methacrylic acid and methyl methacrylate, Eudragit S100 is a pH-responsive hydrogel with three layers: an outside layer of hydrogel, a middle layer of chitosan (CH), and an interior layer of hydrogel PAA (polyacrylic acid). By varying the pH levels of the solution, ciprofloxacin (CIP)-encapsulating polydiacetylene (PDA) vesicles were incorporated into the hydrogel layers of CH and PAA, which were deposited alternately through electrostatic interactions. Urease-producing organisms can hydrolyze urea, which raises the pH of the urine. One such species is *Proteus mirabilis*. At physiological temperature, the PDA vesicle system demonstrated a visible chromatic color change. In acidic fluid (pH <7), it became blue; in alkaline media, it showed purple at pH 7–8.8, and red at pH >8.8. This coating could limit the bacterial infection in addition to detecting its presence in the urine. In fact, the coated polymers did not release PDA vesicles, and no CIP was released at pH <7. However, as pH levels rose, the release rate increased because EudragitS100's trigger layer gradually diffused, releasing PDA vesicles into the surrounding media. After an overnight incubation period, this coating enabled a notable decrease in the original 7.105 CFU mL^{-1} viable *Proteus mirabilis* population. Since *Escherichia coli* lacks urease, it does not cause the medium to become alkaline for the EudragitS100 layer to subsequently degrade, in contrast to *Proteus mirabilis*. As a result, it served as a control species. It did not react to the covering as anticipated, and over time, there were more viable cells. Therefore, it has been demonstrated that this smart coating not only selectively detects the presence of pathogenic bacteria that produce urease in urine solution and generates a matching colorimetric signal when it does, but also inhibits the growth of these bacteria [91]. Both coating and encapsulation methods of modification of nanomaterials' surface are cost-effective and economically viable methods for surface modification of smart nanomaterials.

3.2.2 *Chemical Functionalization*

The chemical functionalization is based on two approaches: covalent (Chemisorption) and non-covalent (Physisorption).

3.2.2.1 Covalent Functionalization

Covalent bonds that are utilized to functionalize nanoparticles are comparable to those that occur naturally. Most surface functionalization techniques rely on covalent bond formation, which provides the benefit of strong bonding and surface group stability. A vast array of covalent and non-covalent techniques is used to functionalize graphene and its derivatives, utilizing an even greater variety of potential compounds. For example, DNA oligonucleotides and polymers such as polyethylene glycol (PEG) and polyetherimide can have their ends modified with amino or thiol groups, enabling the pendants of these molecules to covalently bind to graphene oxide (GO). In the same way, transition metal dichalcogenides (TMDs) are 2D nanosheets with an inert basal plane that allows the functional group to be attached covalently. Teng Liu et al. demonstrated the functionalization of MoS_2 nanosheets with LA-PEG (Lipoic acid modified PEG) for drug delivery applications. Since MoS_2 itself is not biocompatible, functionalization was required. PEG was selected for functionalization because it has a thiolated group. To achieve a stronger binding, lipoic acid was conjugated with PEG first and then functionalized covalently with MoS_2 (T. [43]). Furthermore, a popular functionalization technique for covalent modification of TMDs was introduced by

Damien Voiry et al., enhancing the passage of electrons between an organohalide reactant and metallic 1T TMDs. This enabled the attachment of covalently modified groups to the chalcogen atoms of TMDs [76].

3.2.2.2 Non-covalent Functionalization

Non-covalent functionalization is a technique wherein the ligand is adsorbed onto the nanomaterial's surface. Because of weak hydrogen bonds, hydrophobic interactions, van der Waals forces, and/or electrostatic interactions, the ligand-nanomaterial binding is often weak. Using polymers or surfactants as the capping layer, a technique known as *steric stabilization*, is a widely used approach to non-covalent surface functionalization. The steric repulsion of large ligand molecules in the surface coat prevents clustering by maintaining the integrity of the nanoparticle dispersion while also stabilizing individual nanoparticles in solution. An additional benefit of this method is the easier synthesis of monodisperse nanoparticles. The adsorbed polymer layer on the surface of the nanoparticles restricts the diffusion of growing species, resulting in diffusion-limited growth in the nuclei that follow. Livia E. Sima et al. reported the fabrication of functional graphene nano-colloids covalently functionalized with bovine serum albumin (BSA) for use as a drug carrier targeting melanoma cells by loading dabrafenib and trichostatin. The authors observed that melanoma cells showed a dose-dependent influence on target activity when exposed to GON-BSA coatings with an inhibitor compositional gradient. Such functional bio-platforms, which engineer the cell-biomaterial interface, hold significant promise for advancing personalized cancer therapy [69].

3.2.3 Biomolecules Conjugation

Biomolecule conjugation is a straightforward and effective strategy for modifying smart nanomaterials to enhance their specificity, functionality, and biocompatibility. With the ability to generate this library of biocompatible nanoplatforms, the branched polymers approach provides the basis for a wide range of uses in nanomedicine and nanotechnology, including targeted drug delivery, biosensing, imaging, diagnostics, theranostics, and biocatalysis. Conjugation of biomolecules, including tiny molecules, proteins, peptides, and nucleic acids to the surface of nanomaterials, is a process used in the functionalization of smart nanomaterials. The process must be performed to take advantage of the unique interactions and bioactivity of these biomolecules to enhance the functionality of the nanomaterials, which are especially useful in biomedical applications [40]. For example, a diphenylalanine (FF) peptide was thinned with a few drops of graphene dispersion solution and plated onto a sterilized material to be dried in an oven at 50 °C. Yang et al. tested the peptide nanowire (PNW) growth and self-assembly of the FF peptide on a graphene substrate. Hydrogen bonding and π–π interactions have been identified as the specific forces with which the FF peptide is able to self-assemble in water with graphene. The development of organized PNW arrays on the surface of graphene was promoted by intermolecular/molecule–graphene hydrogen interactions, while graphene supported π–π conjugations between peptides and graphene [41]. The biomolecules can be conjugated to nanomaterials through numerous strategies, and indeed, there exist several reasons that could affect biomolecular conjugation [79]. This strategy gives proper biocompatibility and stimulus-response that could be used in biomedical applications.

3.2.4 Doping

Doping is an essential tactic for functionalizing smart nanomaterials since it gives exact control over their characteristics and increases their range of applications. Nanomaterials can be tuned for use by doping them to change their electrical, optical, magnetic, and catalytic properties. This leads to improvements in industry and technology. When functionalizing smart nanomaterials, doping involves purposefully adding impurity atoms or molecules to the nanomaterials to improve and change their properties. The electrical, optical, magnetic, and catalytic properties of the nanomaterials can all be strongly altered by this method, which can improve their suitability for use. A fluorescent probe for the detection of pesticide traces was created by Chen et al. to create a novel proportional fluorescence detection technique. They created a composite probe using nitrogen-doped carbon quantum dots (N-CQDs), which produce blue light, with copper nanoclusters that emit red light. Even at extremely low concentrations, the probe system exhibits excellent detection performance due to its great sensitivity and selectivity [13]. In another project, Liu et al. conducted in vitro bioimaging studies using human cervical cancer HeLa cells. Dimethylformamide was used as both solvent and nitrogen source to synthesize nitrogen-doped graphene quantum dots (N-GQDs) via a solvothermal method. Without considerably accessing the nucleus, researchers found that N-GQDs successfully labeled the cytoplasm and cell membrane of HeLa cells. In conjunction with the cells' capacity to effectively absorb N-GQDs, N-GQDs can serve as a particular kind of 2-photon probe for an enhanced contrast in biological imaging (Q. [42]). Poly (N-isopropylacrylamide-co-acrylic acid) [p(NIPAm-co-AAc)] micro/nanogel was layered between two gold layers to create etalon structures. After that, etalons produced silver nanoparticles (AgNPs) by reducing them in situ with $NaBH_4$. Because of the micro/nanogel-based cavity's constructive and destructive interference, the etalons allowed light at specific wavelengths to be reflected; the wavelength of the reflected light depended on the size of the micro/nanogel particles. AgNPs were oxidized and converted to Ag^+ in the presence of H_2O_2, which caused the gel layer to enlarge. The reflectance intensity rose, and the reflectance peak moved to a higher wavelength as a result of the AgNPs' reduced absorption and the nano/microgels' larger diameter. The sensor demonstrated acceptable linearity in the 0.5–6 mM H_2O_2 concentration range [67].

3.2.5 *Plasma Treatment*

Smart nanoparticles can be functionalized by the effective process of plasma treatment, which offers a variety of surface alterations to improve the materials' functionality and adaptability. Through plasma treatment, surface properties can be changed without changing the bulk material, allowing for the development of customized functions for advanced nanomaterials used in environmental research, electronics, medicine, and other fields. When functionalizing smart nanomaterials, the process of plasma treatment involves exposing the materials to a partly ionized gas consisting of electrons, ions, and neutral particles. Without changing the bulk qualities, this treatment can modify the surface descriptions of nanomaterials, such as their functionality, roughness, and chemical makeup. A flexible and useful method for improving the functionality and suitability of nanomaterials in a range of industries is plasma treatment. Chandrima Karthik et al. reported a review that concluded that low-temperature plasma (LTP) treatment is a green method that allows for modifying the surface of biomaterials, which can be used in various applications. The process does not use any strong chemical agents, and there is no need for post-refinement [37]. The plasma treatment can also be used to fabricate high-performance fabric. H. Ahmed et al. reported the creation of a conductive natural high-performance fabric by plasma-assisted covering of cotton fabrics with several conductive polymers in the existence or non-existence of silver nanoparticles. After using the plasma activation approach, an in situ nanostructured thin layer of a derivative of polyaniline was created. Silver nanoparticles were produced by utilizing the conductive polymers' reduction capabilities to deposit silver nitrate solution. Changing the kind of conductive polymer and adding silver nanoparticles can result in high-performance textiles with enhanced or modified multifunctional qualities, including responsiveness, electrical conductivity, thermochromism, antibacterial properties, and acid sensitivity to metal ions. These properties offer diverse potential applications in areas such as geotextiles, biomedicine, and antistatic technology [2].

3.3 Characterization of Nanoscale Materials

Characterization is a crucial step that enables a comprehensive understanding of the properties of functionalized nanomaterials and facilitates their optimization according to specific requirements. A variety of analytical techniques are available to characterize the surface, composition, mechanical, optical, and electrical properties of the materials, as shown in Fig. 3.2.

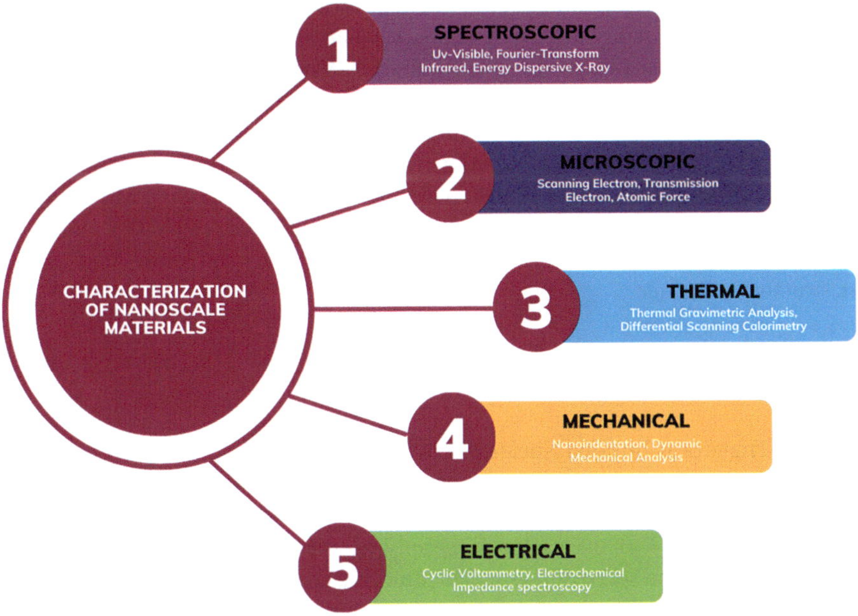

Fig. 3.2 The diagram shows the different analytical techniques that are used to characterize the nanoscale materials

3.3.1 Spectroscopic Characterization

Spectroscopic analysis is a critical tool for the categorization of materials, particularly functionalized nanomaterials. These techniques provide useful information about the composition, structure, and surface activity of nanomaterials. A variety of spectroscopic tools are currently employed to characterize specific properties of functionalized nanomaterials, including UV-visible spectrophotometers, energy-dispersive X-ray spectroscopy (EDS), X-ray photoelectron spectroscopy (XPS), Raman spectroscopy, and Fourier transform infrared (FTIR) spectroscopy.

3.3.1.1 UV-Visible Spectroscopy

UV-Visible spectroscopy is an analytical technique for evaluating the optical, surface, and functional properties of functionalized smart nanomaterials. The basic principle of this technique is to analyze, absorb, or transmit the specific wavelength from 200–800 nm provided by ultraviolet and visible sources, and show the characteristic peaks due to electronic transitions [58]. Smart nanomaterials need to be functionalized to perform better, especially for biomedical applications. Functionalization of ligands or surface functional groups of smart nanomaterials can be quantitatively optimized with the help of a UV-Visible spectrophotometer because the functionality absorbs specific wavelengths from 200–800 nm, and the Beer-Lambert law can be used to measure it. UV-Visible spectroscopy is also valuable for monitoring the size and shape of smart nanomaterials, since they exhibit plasmonic resonance, and their shift changes with a change in size and shape. The most fundamental parameter of functionalized smart nanomaterials is stability. The stability of functionalized smart nanomaterials can be measured by observing the change in absorption spectra. Compared to other characterization methods, UV-Visible spectroscopy is relatively inexpensive, most effective, and a nondestructive technique.

3.3.1.2 FTIR Spectroscopy

Fourier Transform Infrared Spectroscopy (FTIR) is a nondestructive method for analyzing different functional groups, surface chemistry, and interaction modes of smart nanomaterials, using infrared light between 400 and 4000 cm^{-1}. The principle behind it is that the molecule simply absorbs and transmits that specific wavelength, and the spectrophotometer prints out the transmittance or absorbance peak owing to the vibrational change in the absorption of the molecule [45]. It allows us to confirm the surface modification of a specific ligand or functional group qualitatively by comparing the peak intensity before and after the functionalization [16]. FTIR spectroscopy allows qualitative confirmation of the chemical bond existing between the smart nanomaterial and surface functionality, as well as intramolecular—functional group to functional group—bonds. It can also monitor the functionalization process through changes in peak intensity or the appearance of new absorption bands corresponding to the newly formed chemical entities. The right type of functionalization is essential, especially when using biosensors [50], electronics [15], and biomedical devices [1], where it can be used for quality control purposes to monitor accuracy. The technique is very useful, but it requires complex sample preparation processes.

3.3.1.3 EDS Spectroscopy

Energy dispersive X-ray spectroscopy (EDS) is an analytical technique utilized for the characterization of materials. It is not a standalone method but is typically integrated with scanning electron microscopy (SEM) or transmission electron microscopy (TEM) with a detector [30]. EDS determines the elemental composition of the material, including elements introduced during the functionalization of smart nanomaterials. In mapping mode, EDS can also reveal the spatial distribution of functional materials. While EDS is primarily a qualitative technique, certain researchers utilize it quantitatively by analyzing atomic percentage ratios. With EDS, the whole material elemental composition is provided, and even microimpurities are detectable with this method [51]. However,

EDS is most effective for elements with atomic numbers higher than that of oxygen. Ongoing research continues to improve the sensitivity and capabilities of EDS detectors [63].

3.3.2 *Microscopic Characterization*

Microscopy encompasses a range of techniques that enable the visualization of materials that are not visible to the naked eye under ordinary conditions [68]. Optical microscopy, also referred to as light microscopy, is the most common and widely accessible type. Light microscopes are relatively inexpensive, robust, and are generally associated with negligible interaction with the specimen under investigation, such that the specimen is not affected by the imaging process [10]. However, electron microscopy is often required for higher resolution imaging. For example, due to the low concentration of virus particles and the fact that only a small fraction (less than 10%) exhibits the characteristic five- or six-pointed star-formed particles, conventional electron microscopy can be an insensitive detection method [36]. Chemical interactions that occur at the interface between delivery systems and the target areas are influenced by surface morphology [22]. Smart healthcare systems have been in development for years, and because of this, tremendous scientific focus is on minimizing side effects and improving diagnostic accuracy [11, 20]. Both qualitative and quantitative characterization of nanoparticles—including surface morphology, size, structure, and shape—can be achieved using electron microscopy techniques, including SEM, TEM, and AFM [4].

3.3.2.1 Scanning Electron Microscopy

As with any type of microscopy, scanning electron microscopy (SEM) is employed to magnify minute features or structures that are otherwise not visible with the human eye. The term scanning electron microscope stands for getting images using a high-energy electron beam on the sample surface [74]. The resolution of any image relies on the characteristics of the electron beam and the way it interacts with the object of interest. The high-resolution potential of SEM is especially suitable for the analysis of nanomaterials in which the material properties and applications depend on the structural features of the constituent material that are measured at the nanoscale [49]. For example, Ali et al. developed a citric acid cross-linked hydrogel from Aloe vera leaves for sustained drug delivery [3]. SEM analysis revealed a highly porous structure capable of retaining large amounts of fluid, which is advantageous for on-demand or targeted drug release. In another study, Avossa et al. fabricated PCL/PHB membranes, which are both naked and packed, also coated with melanin-TiO_2/PCL/PHB, for use as moist wound-healing dressings. SEM images clearly showed a porous web-like network structure supporting cell transfer, proliferation, and differentiation. Consequently, it was found that the PCL/PHB mats have potential for use as dressings in wound-healing applications [5]. Jacob and his colleagues created a smart piezoelectric nanohybrid of barium titanate ($BaTiO_3$) and poly-(3-hydroxybutyrate-co-3-hydroxyvalerate) (PHBV) using electrospinning. The resulting electrospun pure PB and PB-BT nanofiber nanohybrids exhibited a highly porous chondrogenic nanostructure, a high aspect ratio, a large surface area, and a morphology closely resembling native tissue. The pore diameters of the PB and PB15-BT20 nanohybrids were approximately 1.139 μm and 1.52 μm, respectively, facilitating chondrocyte cell motion and nutrition transfer [33]. Goganian et al. developed smart superporous hydrogels (SPHs) from acrylamide and dimethylaminoethyl methacrylate monomers, with and without magnetic nanoparticles (MNPs), for gastroretentive DDS. SEM examination showed that the SPHs had a large particle size and a pore size resembling a honeycombed structure. However, at lengthy exposure times, cross-linking largely minimizes this shape. Thus, the materials' morphology and structure are controlled by the MNP concentration. However, increasing the MNP concentration led to a denser structure of the produced hydrogels with reduced porosity [26].

3.3.2.2 Transmission Electron Microscopy

Transmission electron microscopy (TEM) and scanning electron microscopy (SEM) operate on similar fundamental principles, but differ in how the information is collected from the sample specimen and differ in regard to the positioning of the detector relative to the sample [62]. TEM is a complicated piece of equipment with a resolution of approximately 0.07 nm, with ongoing efforts to improve it to 0.05 nm [19]. TEM is particularly useful for investigating the interaction of different nanomaterial structures with gaseous, liquid, or solid substrates at the nanoscale [81]. For example, Davoodbasha et al. developed copper/hydroxypropyl methyl cellulose nanobiocomposites with antibacterial and antioxidant properties. TEM analysis revealed that the CuO nanoparticles were well-dispersed within the hydroxypropyl methyl cellulose (HMPC) nanocomposites, with an average diameter of 2.5 nm. The smaller size of the NPs leads to more surface area and higher concentrations of chemisorbed surface oxygen species being available, which is why the antibacterial effectiveness is boosted [14]. Duarah et al. fabricated hyperbranched polyurethane (HPU) nanocomposites modified with starch and reduced carbon dots (RCD) for use as smart sutures for the first time. TEM images showed that RCD is evenly distributed across the HPU matrix, even at the maximum loading of the nanomaterial. The TEM image revealed that the RCD's lattice fringes exhibited an interplanar spacing of 0.30 nm [18]. Reddy et al. reported the first-time self-sensing performance of CNT/UHMWPE (ultra-high molecular weight polyethylene) nanocomposites. The TEM showed that the surface morphology of CNTs was entangled with the CNT's typical length of a few hundred microns, and its average diameter is around 30 nm [60]. Azadpour et al. synthesized chitosan-coated silver (Ag) nanoparticles that were successfully decorated by folic acid (FA-CS-AG) to serve as a smart drug delivery system. Upon loading the FA-CS-Ag into the nanocomposite, the particle diameter increased by approximately 100 nm in diameter, resulting in a small range of particle sizes, with an average of 10–50 nm. This size augmentation also confirmed the efficient drug filling into the nanocomposite [6]. It has been established that nanocomposites smaller than 200 nm are particularly suitable for targeted medication delivery to the cancer location [52].

3.3.2.3 Atomic Force Microscopy

Scanned-proximity probe microscopes include atomic force microscopy (AFM) [29, 66, 82]. Depending on the imaging and surface circumstances, AFM is capable of presenting pictures of surface descriptions at the minuscule scale, with vertical resolution in the picometres, and in general, lateral resolution falls between angstroms to tens of nanometers [72]. AFM offers quantitative measurements of different material properties at that exact scale, while simultaneously showing the surface topography with sub-nanometer spatial precision [73]. Mauro et al. fabricated hybrid nanoparticles (PLGA-CDs) comprising carbon-based nano-heaters that generate red light when inserted in a poly(lactic-co-glycolic acid) matrix. The goal of PLGA-CD nanoparticles is to present medication delivery within a single biodegradable and biodegradable nanoplatform. AFM revealed 1.5 nm-diameter nanodots on average, confirming the restricted size distribution that permits their possible use in biomedical applications [48]. Pooresmaeil et al. created a copolymer for novel stimuli-responsive brushes coated on the magnetic graphene oxide surface (MG-PB) for drug delivery applications. AFM was used to qualitatively assess the formation of copolymer brushes on the magnetic graphene oxide with triethoxyvinylsilane (MG-TEVS) surface. The MG-PB hybrid nanostructure displayed a greater thickness as compared to MG-TEVS, which may indicate that copolymer brushes are successfully growing from the MG-TEVS surface [57]. Khan et al. developed a smart pH-sensitive reduced graphene oxide/arabinoxylan/chitosan (rGO/ARX/CS) novel hydrogel for in vitro drug delivery, antibacterial activity, and other biological applications. AFM examination of the composite surface morphology revealed that samples ATC-4 and ATC-1 exhibited the highest and lowest roughness values, respectively. The reason for the rise in surface roughness is the presence of rGO aggregates both on top of and underneath the surface. Regarding the impact of rougher surfaces obtained by utilizing the composite rGO/ARX/CS, the results are quite promising [38].

3.3.3 Thermal Characterization

The methods employed in thermal analysis seek to identify the properties a material exhibits when heated, cooled, or maintained at a constant temperature. In 1887, Henry Le Chatelier initially proposed methods that are regarded as the inception of contemporary thermal analysis [86]. Thermogravimetric analysis (TGA) and differential scanning calorimetry (DSC), two of the most used thermal analytical methods, are covered in this section [56].

3.3.3.1 Thermogravimetric Analysis

In a furnace with regulated conditions, thermogravimetric analysis keeps track of the mass of the sample in relation to temperature or time. The sample is heated at a regulated pace in different environments—air, N_2, CO_2, He, Ar, and others—for thermogravimetric analysis (TGA). The substance's weight variation is noted in relation to temperature and/or time. For a material with an identified beginning weight, the temperature gradually rises. At different periods of time, the variations in weight in relation to temperature are documented. The core idea behind TGA is this plot of weight change versus temperature, which is known as the thermogravimetric curve or thermo-gram.

When heated to predefined temperatures and at predefined heating rates, thermogravimetric analysis is a useful technique for comprehending thermal phenomena related to nanomaterials and polymer composites [44]. According to Felipe López-Saucedo et al., the grafted film thermogram showed a 10% weight loss, which is faster than that detected in the polypropylene (PP) film's TGA curve, which is bare and not exposed to radiation. Pure PP exhibited a higher decomposition temperature (Td) compared to the grafted copolymers, with a 25% reduction observed for PP-g-MMA and a 19.5% reduction for (PP-g-MMA)-g-NVI. The grafted films exhibited a two-step degradation process, whereas the (PP-g-MMA)-g-NVI (19.5/6%) sample showed a three-step degradation with a total weight loss of 19.5%. However, although grafted films performed well at load and release temperatures, the study's findings of pristine PP's superior thermal stability are purely descriptive [46]. Another study reported that, according to the TGA data, TPU and C-TPU thermally degrade at 280 °C and 306 °C, respectively. The TGA research shows that TPU loses weight by 91% and C-TPU loses weight by 75% at 500 °C [28].

3.3.3.2 Differential Scanning Calorimeter

A thermoanalytical method called differential scanning calorimetry (DSC) is used to describe the thermal characteristics of materials, including transition temperature (T°) and enthalpy change (ΔH). Among its types, power compensation DSC measures heat flow via electrical power as a function of time or temperature. This technique maintains the sample's temperature and reference by adjusting the furnace heating rate. The sample and reference have different heat capacities, which causes a variation in heat flow that manifests as endothermic or exothermic peaks in the DSC trace [25].

Wang and colleagues developed a dual-stimuli-responsive—temperature and pH—phase-change microcapsule for intelligent drug delivery. The microcapsule comprises n-eicosane as the phase-change material (PCM) core, encapsulated within a poly (NIPAM-co-AA) layer. The phase-change characteristics and energy storage capacity (Ces) of the samples were characterized using differential scanning calorimetry (DSC), TA DSC/TA instruments. The melting and crystallization enthalpies of samples and PCMs are represented by ΔHm and ΔHC [87]. Another study examined the temperature transitions of the polymer carrier using differential scanning calorimetry (DSC) in a nitrogen atmosphere using a Q100 DSC equipment (TA Instruments) equipped with a refrigerated cooling system (RCS90). Samples were placed in aluminum pans and heated at a rate of 20 °C/min from −90 °C to a temperature that, for a fully amorphous polymer, was higher than the glass transition temperature (Tg). Conversely, the temperature was raised above the melting point (Tm) for semicrystalline polymers. In between heating scans, quenching or controlled cooling at a rate of 10 °C/min was used. Crystallization temperature (Tm) and exothermic peak maximum (Tc) were measured, while glass transition temperature (Tg) was determined at half-height of the glass transition heat capacity step [17].

3.3.4 Mechanical Characterization

A few smart nanomaterials lack sufficient mechanical strength for applications that require high tensile strength, such as electronics and sensors. In such cases, surface modification with polymers or biopolymers is necessary to enhance their mechanical properties. These modifications and the resulting functionalization can be quantitatively evaluated using mechanical methods, including nanoindentation, dynamic mechanical analysis (DMA), tensile testing, and compressive testing. Among these methods, nanoindentation and DMA are generally considered more powerful and informative than the others.

3.3.4.1 Nanoindentation

Nanoindentation is a versatile and powerful technique for evaluating the mechanical properties of both hard and soft materials, including alloys and biomaterials, particularly for elastic modulus and hardness. There are several tests that are carried out to determine these properties, such as tensile and flexural tests, but nanoindentation is more reliable and suitable for nanomaterials. The nanoindentation technique quantifies only two key parameters: indentation depth and loading force. From the resulting load-displacement curves, the elastic modulus and the hardness of the functionalized smart nanomaterials can be determined [23]. Functionalization plays a critical role in enhancing these mechanical properties and offers many benefits. Notably, the protein-functionalized gold nanoparticles have been shown to significantly improve the mechanical performance of nanomaterials [78].

3.3.4.2 Dynamic Mechanical Analysis

Dynamic mechanical analysis (DMA) is a powerful technique for evaluating viscoelastic properties of functionalized smart nanomaterials as a function of temperature, time, stress, and frequency. In a typical DMA experiment, a periodic force is applied to the sample under controlled parameters of stress, temperature, time, and frequency, and the material's response is measured [8]. Normally, stress refers to the applied force and the change in shape of the sample, referred to as strain. This way, loss modulus and elastic storage modulus may be determined with the help of stress and strain. The DMA is ideal for characterizing the mechanical behavior of functionalized nanomaterials, making it highly relevant to the present study [65].

3.3.5 Electrical Characterization

Electrochemistry is a major branch of chemistry that studies the relationship between chemical reactions and electrical phenomena, including the generation of electrical energy through chemical changes and the effects of electric current on chemical systems [55]. Electrochemical characterization is particularly vital for the study of nanomaterials [85], as a thorough understanding of their electrical properties is essential to optimize, minimize, or amplify specific performance properties. Electrical characterization techniques not only help reduce development costs but also improve material performance. These methods are critical in electronics, telecommunications, semiconductor devices, solar cells, military applications, and sensors [89, 64, 35, 39]. Smart nanomaterials exhibit unique electrical properties that may be optimized for different biomedical uses, including creating nanoscale biosensors to identify biomolecules or monitoring physiological changes within living systems. Several sophisticated characterization methods are used to study the electrical properties of smart nanomaterials. Among the most commonly used techniques for assessing the electrical properties of smart nanomaterials are cyclic voltammetry (CV) and electrochemical impedance spectroscopy (EIS). These methods provide valuable information to determine charge transfer resistance and capacitive behavior [34].

3.3.5.1 Cyclic Voltammetry

Cyclic voltammetry (CV) is one of the most widely used electrochemical methods for monitoring redox processes. It is a dynamic, potential sweep approach that provides valuable information about the cyclic voltammogram, which provides information on the mechanisms at the electrode surface and the chemically or electrochemically active species' reactivity. In addition to coupled chemical processes, the CV experiment provides direct insights into the kinetics of electrode reactions, encompassing both homogeneous and heterogeneous electron-transfer steps. In a typical CV experiment, the potential of an electrochemical cell is scanned, and the resulting current is plotted as a function of potential. A standard three-electrode setup is employed, consisting of a working electrode, a reference electrode, and a counter electrode. This configuration is particularly suitable for material research [61, 84].

Zhang et al. constructed a core-shell structure Au@PB NPs for flexible biosensors that exhibit excellent performance for biomarkers such as H_2O_2 and glucose. The CV curves of the Au@PB NPs/carbon ink-PET in electrolyte solution displayed a strong reduction effect upon addition of H_2O_2. The linear range of the H_2O_2 sensor was 1 μM to 1 mM H_2O_2. With a linear correlation coefficient (R) of 0.997, the sensor demonstrated an outstanding linear connection. Its sensitivity was 301.5 $\mu A{\cdot}mM^{-1}{\cdot}cm^{-2}$, and its detection limit was 0.28 μM. However, the pH value of 7 was more compatible with these barriers when considering the impact on enzyme activity and the expectation that it will be utilized for health monitoring [90]. A graphite-based electrochemical immunosensor for the identification of carcinoembryonic antigens was developed by Idris et al. Because the CNDTs accelerate the kinetics of electron transfer on bare exfoliated graphite, a 48% current augmentation was found on the working electrode modified with CNDTs; this electrode was designated as EG-CNDTs. Cyclic voltammetry was employed to evaluate every phase of the immunosensor's creation [31]. Erk et al. utilized functionalized multiwalled carbon ($MWCNT\text{-}NH_2$) for the sensitive and selective detection of Talazoparib (TLZ), an advanced electrochemical biosensing strategy in the field of cancer research. The electrochemical activity of both modified and unmodified electrochemical sensors was assessed using CV. Excellent repeatability, reproducibility, and high selectivity against a variety of interferences were exhibited by the MWCNT-NH2/GCE [21].

3.3.5.2 Electrochemical Impedance Spectroscopy

Electrochemical impedance spectroscopy (EIS) is a powerful technique for investigating mass transfer, charge transfer, and diffusion processes. It is particularly useful for analyzing linear time-invariant systems and provides detailed information about the intrinsic material features that impact an electrochemical system's capacitance, resistance, or conductance. In DC circuits, the impedance does not directly obey Ohm's Law, but the resistance does. To measure the impedance response, a tiny signal excitation is applied. The real and imaginary portions are the two components that make up the impedance expression. A *Nyquist plot* is produced by plotting the real component (Zreal) on the X-axis and the imaginary part (Zimag) on the Y-axis. One special benefit that EIS provides is the ability to conduct measurements at various potentials [47, 80]. Electrochemical impedance spectroscopy (EIS), one of the most sophisticated electroanalytical techniques, has several benefits over the widely used amperometry/potentiometry [9].

An innovative rGO-based microfluidic chip immunosensor was created for the label-free identification of the H1N1 influenza virus. EIS investigated the interfacial alterations brought about by the biological recognition events [70]. By assessing the Rct (charge transfer resistance), the electrodes' charge transfer process was examined. Following antibody immobilization, the Rct (1.01 kΩ) of CA/Au/RGO increased to 2.0 kΩ, demonstrating the antibody's macromolecular makeup and insulating qualities, which prevent electron transport. The fact that the Rct value of 2.5 kΩ for the combination of Ab, BSA, CA, RGO, and Au electrodes increased further suggests that every non-specific area of the electrodes was covered with BSA and hindered the transmission of electrons. Ilkhani & Fahad [32] fabricated a new sensing device that uses enzyme-amplified detection to diagnose Ebola viral DNA. The Rct value is altered by the DNA immobilization on the surface of the electrode. Optimizing the immobilization period and capture probe concentration resulted in the biosensor's great performance. The 45-minute immobilization period was chosen as the ideal duration since it was both sufficiently brief and efficient. The free sites on the surface electrode were covered and deactivated using MCH (6-mercapto-1-hexanol). Given that it had the highest Rct value, the 60-minute incubation period was the ideal duration for MCH. Using AuNPs, CNPs, and CNFs, Ranjbar and Shahrokhian created an aptasensor for identifying Staphylococcus aureus in human blood. Using EIS measurements on the surface of three distinct modified electrodes, the impact of carbon nanoparticles and cellulose nanofibers on aptasensor performance was examined. AuNPs/CNPs provide a good substrate for the thiolated S. aureus aptamer to self-assemble in the produced nanocomposite-based electrode, while CNFs improve attachment to GCE. As a result, the aptamers become more immobilized and are prevented from being released from the electrode surface. In fact, CNFs have enhanced the apt sensor's stability and durability at a comparatively low cost [59].

3.4 Current Challenges and Future Directions

Although functionalized nanomaterials offer unique benefits in many fields, researchers, engineers, and scientists are still working to advance the technology. Several key challenges must be addressed.

3.4.1 Challenges in Functionalization and Characterization

One of the biggest challenges in the case of smart nanomaterials is the high degree of difficulty in regulating the functionalization process. Advanced plasma and chemical functionalization techniques are particularly preferable to other strategies. These two can be used for control functionalization, but they have their own drawbacks, including long-term monitoring and chemical costs. On the other hand, no method can be accepted for converting to the large-scale synthesis method from the OTS synthesis method. As such, the remarkable properties of nanomaterials in the biomedical applications market are still in search of these gross manufacturers. The stability of functionalized nanomaterials remains a significant challenge. For example, biomolecule conjugation is often sensitive to environmental factors, which can compromise the stability of the conjugate. Although functionalized nanomaterials typically perform specific functions, there is still considerable scope to develop multi-functional systems through integrating multiple functionalities. To date, no in situ technique has been established that can provide real-time information under operational conditions. Consequently, there is a pressing need for advanced methods capable of elucidating the underlying mechanisms, properties, and behavior of stimuli-responsive nanomaterials.

3.4.2 Future Directions

Despite significant progress, there is still a lack of effective biomimetic approaches capable of producing superior, more efficient, and highly biocompatible materials. Additionally, the development of advanced microscopes and spectroscopic techniques is needed to obtain dynamic, real-time data that can elucidate the mechanism and behavior of functionalized materials. In the era of advancing artificial intelligence, integrating AI and computational modeling with experimental functionalization and characterization offers great potential to accelerate discovery and reduce unnecessary experimentation. Finally, comprehensive safety guidelines and regulatory frameworks for functionalized materials should be developed.

3.5 Conclusion

To uplift technology, researchers, engineers, and scientists continue to develop new materials that can replace conventional ones that are expensive, time-consuming, and toxic. Stimuli-responsive nanomaterials have emerged as promising alternatives to conventional materials used in biomedical applications. These materials respond with significant changes in their properties when exposed to external stimuli such as magnetic fields, light, or temperature. Various strategies are available to functionalize and modify these nanomaterials, including coating and encapsulation, chemical and biological conjugation, plasma treatment, and doping. While each technique offers advantages as well as limitations, chemical and biological conjugation, along with coating and encapsulation, remain the most widely used approaches. However, achieving precise and controlled functionalization using these techniques is often difficult. To ascertain the properties of functionalized nanomaterials, there are various analytical techniques available, such as spectroscopic, microscopic, mechanical, electrical, and thermal. These tools provide valuable information on structural, compositional, electrical, and mechanical characteristics. Nevertheless, there is still a notable lack of techniques for dynamically monitoring the functionalization process and its underlying mechanisms in real time. To advance the field, there is an open opportunity to develop novel, cost-effective, and efficient biomimetic approaches to nanomaterials functionalization, supported by standard protocols suitable for biomedical applications. Additionally, significant opportunities exist for integrating advanced imaging techniques with computational and AI modeling to accelerate research, reduce experimental trial-and-error, and enhance understanding of these smart materials.

References

1. Aflori M. Smart nanomaterials for biomedical applications—a review. Nano. 2021;11(2):396. https://doi.org/10.3390/nano11020396.
2. Ahmed H, Khattab TA, Mashaly HM, El-Halwagy AA, Rehan M. Plasma activation toward multi-stimuli responsive cotton fabric via in situ development of polyaniline derivatives and silver nanoparticles. Cellulose. 2020;27(5):2913–26. https://doi.org/10.1007/s10570-020-02980-7.
3. Ali A, Hussain A, Haseeb T. Citric acid cross-linking of a hydrogel from Aloe responsive, superporous, and smart material for drug delivery. RSC Adv. 2024;14:8018–27. https://doi.org/10.1039/d4ra00095a.
4. Anuradha, Bhatia T. Novel nanomaterials in forensic investigations: a review. Mater Today Proc. 2021;50:1071–9. https://doi.org/10.1016/j.matpr.2021.07.466.
5. Avossa J, Pota G, Vitiello G, Macagnano A, Zanfardino A, Di Napoli M, Pezzella A, D'Errico G, Varcamonti M, Luciani G. Multifunctional mats by antimicrobial nanoparticles decoration for bioinspired smart wound dressing solutions. Mater Sci Eng C. 2021;123:111954. https://doi.org/10.1016/j.msec.2021.111954.
6. Azadpour A, Hajrasouliha S, Khaleghi S. Green synthesized-silver nanoparticles coated with targeted chitosan nanoparticles for smart drug delivery. J Drug Delivery Sci Technol. 2022;74:103554. https://doi.org/10.1016/j.jddst.2022.103554.
7. Ballauff M, Lu Y. "Smart" nanoparticles: preparation, characterization and applications. Polymer. 2007;48(7):1815–23. https://doi.org/10.1016/j.polymer.2007.02.004.
8. Bashir MA. Use of dynamic mechanical analysis (DMA) for characterizing interfacial interactions in filled polymers. Solids. 2021;2(1):108–20. https://doi.org/10.3390/solids2010006.
9. Bertok T, Lorencova L, Chocholova E, Jane E, Vikartovska A, Kasak P, Tkac J. Electrochemical impedance spectroscopy based biosensors: mechanistic principles, analytical examples and challenges towards commercialization for assays of protein cancer biomarkers. ChemElectroChem. 2019;6(4):989–1003. https://doi.org/10.1002/celc.201800848.
10. Brodusch N, Brahimi SV, Barbosa De Melo E, Song J, Yue S, Piché N, Gauvin R. Scanning electron microscopy versus transmission electron microscopy for material characterization: a comparative study on high-strength steels. Scanning. 2021;2021:5511618. https://doi.org/10.1155/2021/5511618.
11. Cassano D, Pocoví-Martínez S, Voliani V. Ultrasmall-in-nano approach: enabling the translation of metal nanomaterials to clinics. Bioconjug Chem. 2018;29(1):4–16. https://doi.org/10.1021/acs.bioconjchem.7b00664.
12. Chauhan G, Madou MJ, Kalra S, Chopra V, Ghosh D, Martinez-Chapa SO. Nanotechnology for COVID-19: therapeutics and vaccine research. ACS Nano. 2020;14(7):7760–82. https://doi.org/10.1021/acsnano.0c04006.
13. Chen L, Lu J, Luo M, Yu H, Chen X, Deng J, Hou X, Hao E, Wei J, Li P. A ratiometric fluorescent sensing system for the selective and ultrasensitive detection of pesticide resi-

dues via the synergetic effects of copper nanoclusters and carbon quantum dots. Food Chem. 2022;379:132139. https://doi.org/10.1016/j.foodchem.2022.132139.
14. Davoodbasha M, Raghunathan S, MohammedYasin A, Rasool Kamli M, S.M Sabir J, Lee S-Y, Kim J-W. Synthesis and characterization of hydroxy propyl methyl cellulose/copper nanobiocomposites for antibacterial and antioxidant smart materials. J Mol Liq. 2024;400:124542. https://doi.org/10.1016/j.molliq.2024.124542.
15. De S, Madhuri R. Functionalized nanomaterials for electronics and electrical and energy industries. In: Handbook of functionalized nanomaterials for industrial applications. Elsevier; 2020. p. 269–96. https://doi.org/10.1016/B978-0-12-816787-8.00011-9.
16. Dendisová M, Jeništová A, Parchaňská-Kokaislová A, Matějka P, Prokopec V, Švecová M. The use of infrared spectroscopic techniques to characterize nanomaterials and nanostructures: a review. Anal Chim Acta. 2018;1031:1–14. https://doi.org/10.1016/j.aca.2018.05.046.
17. Di D, In R, Biomedica I, Sistemi EEDEI. Alma Mater Studiorum – Università di Bologna Dottorato di Ricerca in Ingegneria Biomedica, Elettrica e dei Sistemi. 2021.
18. Duarah R, Singh YP, Gupta P, Mandal BB, Karak N. Smart self-tightening surgical suture from a tough bio-based hyperbranched polyurethane/reduced carbon dot nanocomposite. Biomed Mater. 2018;13(4):045004. https://doi.org/10.1088/1748-605X/aab93c.
19. Dudkiewicz A, Tiede K, Loeschner K, Jensen LHS, Jensen E, Wierzbicki R, Boxall ABA, Molhave K. Characterization of nanomaterials in food by electron microscopy. TrAC Trends Anal Chem. 2011;30(1):28–43. https://doi.org/10.1016/j.trac.2010.10.007.
20. Duncan R, Gaspar R. Nanomedicine(s) under the microscope. Mol Pharm. 2011;8(6):2101–41. https://doi.org/10.1021/mp200394t.
21. Erk N, Vural Ö, Bouali W, Ayse Genc A, Gnanasekaran L, Karimi-Maleh H. Smart and sensitive nanomaterial-based electrochemical sensor for the determination of a poly (ADP-ribose) polymerase (PARP) inhibitor anticancer agent. Environ Res. 2023;238:117082. https://doi.org/10.1016/j.envres.2023.117082.
22. Falsafi SR, Rostamabadi H, Assadpour E, Jafari SM. Morphology and microstructural analysis of bioactive-loaded micro/nanocarriers via microscopy techniques; CLSM/SEM/TEM/AFM. Adv Colloid Interf Sci. 2020;280:102166. https://doi.org/10.1016/j.cis.2020.102166.
23. Geetha M, Asokamani R, Amit Kumar J, Ramalingam M. Mechanical characterization of nanofiber composites. In: Nanofiber composites for biomedical applications. Elsevier; 2017. p. 117–55. https://doi.org/10.1016/B978-0-08-100173-8.00006-5.
24. Genchi GG, Marino A, Tapeinos C, Ciofani G. Smart materials meet multifunctional biomedical devices: current and prospective implications for nanomedicine. Front Bioeng Biotechnol. 2017;5:80. https://doi.org/10.3389/fbioe.2017.00080.
25. Ghanbari E, Picken SJ, van Esch JH. Analysis of differential scanning calorimetry (DSC): determining the transition temperatures, and enthalpy and heat capacity changes in multicomponent systems by analytical model fitting. J Therm Anal Calorim. 2023;148(22):12393–409. https://doi.org/10.1007/s10973-023-12356-1.
26. Goganian AM, Hamishehkar H, Arsalani N, Khiabani HK. Microwave-promoted synthesis of smart superporous hydrogel for the development of gastroretentive drug delivery system. Adv Polym Technol. 2015;34(2). https://doi.org/10.1002/adv.21490.
27. Gottardo S, Mech A, Drbohlavová J, Małyska A, Bøwadt S, Riego Sintes J, Rauscher H. Towards safe and sustainable innovation in nanotechnology: state-of-play for smart nanomaterials. NanoImpact. 2021;21:100297. https://doi.org/10.1016/j.impact.2021.100297.
28. Ha JH, Jeong Y, Ahn J, Hwang S, Jeon S, Kim D, Ko J, Kang B, Jung Y, Choi J, Han H, Gu J, Cho S, Kim H, Bok M, Park SA, Jeong JH, Park I. A wearable colorimetric sweat pH sensor-based smart textile for health state diagnosis. Mater Horiz. 2023;10(10):4163–71. https://doi.org/10.1039/d3mh00340j.
29. Habibullah H. 30 years of atomic force microscopy: creep, hysteresis, cross-coupling, and vibration problems of piezoelectric tube scanners. Measurement. 2020;159:107776. https://doi.org/10.1016/j.measurement.2020.107776.

30. Hodoroaba V-D. Energy-dispersive X-ray spectroscopy (EDS). In: Characterization of nanoparticles. Elsevier; 2020. p. 397–417. https://doi.org/10.1016/B978-0-12-814182-3.00021-3.
31. Idris AO, Mabuba N, Arotiba OA. An exfoliated graphite-based electrochemical immunosensor on a dendrimer/carbon nanodot platform for the detection of carcinoembryonic antigen cancer biomarker. Biosensors. 2019;9(1):39. https://doi.org/10.3390/bios9010039.
32. Ilkhani H, Farhad S. A novel electrochemical DNA biosensor for Ebola virus detection. Anal Biochem. 2018;557:151–5. https://doi.org/10.1016/j.ab.2018.06.010.
33. Jacob J, More N, Mounika C, Gondaliya P, Kalia K, Kapusetti G. Smart piezoelectric nanohybrid of poly(3-hydroxybutyrate- co −3-hydroxyvalerate) and barium titanate for stimulated cartilage regeneration. ACS Applied Bio Materials. 2019;2(11):4922–31. https://doi.org/10.1021/acsabm.9b00667.
34. Jagadeesh P, Rangappa SM, Siengchin S. Advanced characterization techniques for nanostructured materials in biomedical applications. Adv Indust Eng Polym Res. 2023; https://doi.org/10.1016/j.aiepr.2023.03.002.
35. Joshi P, Riley PR, Denning W, Shukla S, Khosla N, Narayan J, Narayan R. Laser-patterned carbon coatings on flexible and optically transparent plastic substrates for advanced biomedical sensing and implant applications. J Mater Chem C. 2022;10(8):2965–75. https://doi.org/10.1039/D1TC05176H.
36. Kang G. Viral diarrhea. In: International encyclopedia of public health. Elsevier; 2017. p. 360–7. https://doi.org/10.1016/B978-0-12-803678-5.00486-0.
37. Karthik C, Rajalakshmi S, Thomas S, Thomas V. Intelligent polymeric biomaterials surface driven by plasma processing. Curr Opin Biomed Eng. 2023;26:100440. https://doi.org/10.1016/j.cobme.2022.100440.
38. Khan MUA, Haider S, Raza MA, Shah SA, Razak SIA, Kadir MRA, Subhan F, Haider A. Smart and pH-sensitive rGO/Arabinoxylan/chitosan composite for wound dressing: In-vitro drug delivery, antibacterial activity, and biological activities. Int J Biol Macromol. 2021;192:820–31. https://doi.org/10.1016/j.ijbiomac.2021.10.033.
39. Kösemen A, Alpaslan Kösemen Z, Canimkubey B, Erkovan M, Başarir F, San SE, Örnek O, Tunç AV. Fe doped TiO2 thin film as electron selective layer for inverted solar cells. Sol Energy. 2016;132:511–7. https://doi.org/10.1016/j.solener.2016.03.049.
40. Li L, Xing H, Zhang J, Lu Y. Functional DNA molecules enable selective and stimuli-responsive nanoparticles for biomedical applications. Acc Chem Res. 2019;52(9):2415–26. https://doi.org/10.1021/acs.accounts.9b00167.
41. Li P, Chen X, Yang W. Graphene-induced self-assembly of peptides into macroscopic-scale organized nanowire arrays for electrochemical NADH sensing. Langmuir. 2013;29(27):8629–35. https://doi.org/10.1021/la401881a.
42. Liu Q, Guo B, Rao Z, Zhang B, Gong JR. Strong two-photon-induced fluorescence from photostable, biocompatible nitrogen-doped graphene quantum dots for cellular and deep-tissue imaging. Nano Lett. 2013;13(6):2436–41. https://doi.org/10.1021/nl400368v.
43. Liu T, Wang C, Gu X, Gong H, Cheng L, Shi X, Feng L, Sun B, Liu Z. Drug delivery with PEGylated MoS 2 nano-sheets for combined photothermal and chemotherapy of cancer. Adv Mater. 2014;26(21):3433–40. https://doi.org/10.1002/adma.201305256.
44. Loganathan S, Valapa RB, Mishra R, Pugazhenthi G. Copyright. In: Thermal and rheological measurement techniques for nanomaterials characterization (Issue May); 2017. https://doi.org/10.1016/b978-0-323-46139-9.12001-8.
45. López-Lorente ÁI, Mizaikoff B. Recent advances on the characterization of nanoparticles using infrared spectroscopy. TrAC Trends Anal Chem. 2016;84:97–106. https://doi.org/10.1016/j.trac.2016.01.012.
46. López-saucedo F, López-barriguete JE, Flores-rojas GG, Gómez-dorantes S, Bucio E. Polypropylene graft poly(methyl methacrylate) graft poly(n-vinylimidazole) as a smart material for ph-controlled drug delivery. Int J Mol Sci. 2022;23(1). https://doi.org/10.3390/ijms23010304.

47. Magar HS, Hassan RYA, Mulchandani A. Electrochemical impedance spectroscopy (EIS): principles, construction, and biosensing applications. Sensors. 2021;21(19):6578. https://doi.org/10.3390/s21196578.
48. Mauro N, Utzeri MA, Drago SE, Buscarino G, Cavallaro G, Giammona G. Carbon Nanodots as functional excipient to develop highly stable and smart PLGA nanoparticles useful in cancer theranostics. Pharmaceutics. 2020;12(11):1012. https://doi.org/10.3390/pharmaceutics12111012.
49. Mayeen A, Shaji LK, Nair AK. Morphological characterization of nanomaterials. In: Characterization of nanomaterials. Elsevier Ltd; 2018. https://doi.org/10.1016/B978-0-08-101973-3.00012-2.
50. Miranda B, Rea I, Dardano P, De Stefano L, Forestiere C. Recent advances in the fabrication and functionalization of flexible optical biosensors: toward smart life-sciences applications. Biosensors. 2021;11(4):107. https://doi.org/10.3390/bios11040107.
51. Mishra RK, Zachariah AK, Thomas S. Energy-dispersive X-ray spectroscopy techniques for nanomaterial. In: Microscopy methods in nanomaterials characterization. Elsevier; 2017. p. 383–405. https://doi.org/10.1016/B978-0-323-46141-2.00012-2.
52. Moutabian H, Ghahramani-Asl R, Mortezazadeh T, Laripour R, Narmani A, Zamani H, Ataei G, Bagheri H, Farhood B, Sathyapalan T, Sahebkar A. The cardioprotective effects of nano-curcumin against doxorubicin-induced cardiotoxicity: a systematic review. Biofactors. 2022;48(3):597–610. https://doi.org/10.1002/biof.1823.
53. Mujawar MA, Gohel H, Bhardwaj SK, Srinivasan S, Hickman N, Kaushik A. Nano-enabled biosensing systems for intelligent healthcare: towards COVID-19 management. Mater Today Chem. 2020;17:100306. https://doi.org/10.1016/j.mtchem.2020.100306.
54. Munaweera I, Madhusha MLC. Smart nanomaterials. CRC Press; 2023. https://doi.org/10.1201/9781003366270.
55. Nnamchi PS, Obayi CS. Electrochemical characterization of nanomaterials. In: Characterization of nanomaterials. Elsevier Ltd; 2018. https://doi.org/10.1016/B978-0-08-101973-3.00004-3.
56. Ortiz Ortega E, Hosseinian H, Aguilar Meza IB, Rosales López MJ, Rodríguez Vera A, Hosseini S. Material characterization techniques and applications, vol. 19. Springer Singapore; 2022. https://doi.org/10.1007/978-981-16-9569-8.
57. Pooresmaeil M, Namazi H. Fabrication of a smart and biocompatible brush copolymer decorated on magnetic graphene oxide hybrid nanostructure for drug delivery application. Eur Polym J. 2021;142:110126. https://doi.org/10.1016/j.eurpolymj.2020.110126.
58. Quevedo AC, Guggenheim E, Briffa SM, Adams J, Lofts S, Kwak M, Lee TG, Johnston C, Wagner S, Holbrook TR, Hachenberger YU, Tentschert J, Davidson N, Valsami-Jones E. UV-vis spectroscopic characterization of nanomaterials in aqueous media. J Vis Exp. 2021;176:1–11. https://doi.org/10.3791/61764.
59. Ranjbar S, Shahrokhian S. Design and fabrication of an electrochemical aptasensor using Au nanoparticles/carbon nanoparticles/cellulose nanofibers nanocomposite for rapid and sensitive detection of Staphylococcus aureus. Bioelectrochemistry. 2018;123:70–6. https://doi.org/10.1016/j.bioelechem.2018.04.018.
60. Reddy SK, Kumar S, Varadarajan KM, Marpu PR, Gupta TK, Choosri M. Strain and damage-sensing performance of biocompatible smart CNT/UHMWPE nanocomposites. Mater Sci Eng C. 2018;92:957–68. https://doi.org/10.1016/j.msec.2018.07.029.
61. Rusling JF, Suib SL. Characterizing materials with cyclic voltammetry. Adv Mater. 1994;6(12):922–30. https://doi.org/10.1002/adma.19940061204.
62. Salame PH, Pawade VB, Bhanvase BA. Chapter 3 – Characterization tools and techniques for nanomaterials. Nanomaterials for green energy: Elsevier Inc.; 2018. https://doi.org/10.1016/B978-0-12-813731-4.00003-5.
63. Scimeca M, Bischetti S, Lamsira HK, Bonfiglio R, Bonanno E. Energy dispersive X-ray (EDX) microanalysis: a powerful tool in biomedical research and diagnosis. Eur J Histochem. 2018; https://doi.org/10.4081/ejh.2018.2841.

64. Şennik E, Ürdem Ş, Erkovan M, Kılınç N. Sputtered platinum thin films for resistive hydrogen sensor application. Mater Lett. 2016;177:104–7. https://doi.org/10.1016/j.matlet.2016.04.134.
65. Shen P, Jiang Z, Viktorova J, Pollard B, Kumar A, Stachurski Z, Connal LA. Conductive and self-healing carbon nanotube–polymer composites for mechanically strong smart materials. ACS Appl Nano Mater. 2023;6(2):986–94. https://doi.org/10.1021/acsanm.2c04370.
66. Shinato KW, Huang F, Jin Y. Principle and application of atomic force microscopy (AFM) for nanoscale investigation of metal corrosion. 2020;38(5):423–32.
67. Shu T, Shen Q, Wan Y, Zhang W, Su L, Zhang X, Serpe MJ. Silver nanoparticle-loaded microgel-based etalons for H_2O_2 sensing. RSC Adv. 2018;8(28):15567–74. https://doi.org/10.1039/C8RA02215A.
68. Shur J, Price R. Advanced microscopy techniques to assess solid-state properties of inhalation medicines. Adv Drug Deliv Rev. 2012;64(4):369–82. https://doi.org/10.1016/j.addr.2011.11.005.
69. Sima LE, Chiritoiu G, Negut I, Grumezescu V, Orobeti S, Munteanu CVA, Sima F, Axente E. Functionalized graphene oxide thin films for anti-tumor drug delivery to melanoma cells. Front Chem. 2020;8:184. https://doi.org/10.3389/fchem.2020.00184.
70. Singh R, Hong S, Jang J. Label-free detection of influenza viruses using a reduced graphene oxide-based electrochemical immunosensor integrated with a microfluidic platform. Sci Rep. 2017;7(1):42771. https://doi.org/10.1038/srep42771.
71. Singh R, Sharma A, Saji J, Umapathi A, Kumar S, Daima HK. Smart nanomaterials for cancer diagnosis and treatment. Nano Converg. 2022;9(1):21. https://doi.org/10.1186/s40580-022-00313-x.
72. Song J, Zhou Y, Huey BD. 3D structure–property correlations of electronic and energy materials by tomographic atomic force microscopy. Appl Phys Lett. 2021;118(8) https://doi.org/10.1063/5.0040984.
73. Stan G, King SW. Atomic force microscopy for nanoscale mechanical property characterization. J Vacuum Sci Technol B Nanotechnol Microelectron Mater Process Measur Phenomena. 2020;38(6) https://doi.org/10.1116/6.0000544.
74. Ul-Hamid A. A beginners' guide to scanning electron microscopy. Springer International Publishing; 2018. https://doi.org/10.1007/978-3-319-98482-7.
75. Vijayan JG. Design and characterization of smart supramolecular nanomaterials and their biohybrids. In: Bio-inspired nanotechnology. Bentham Science Publishers; 2023. p. 1–15. https://doi.org/10.2174/9789815080179123010003.
76. Voiry D, Goswami A, Kappera R, Silva C d CC e, Kaplan D, Fujita T, Chen M, Asefa T, Chhowalla M. Covalent functionalization of monolayered transition metal dichalcogenides by phase engineering. Nat Chem. 2015;7(1):45–9. https://doi.org/10.1038/nchem.2108.
77. Volpatti LR, Matranga MA, Cortinas AB, Delcassian D, Daniel KB, Langer R, Anderson DG. Glucose-responsive nanoparticles for rapid and extended self-regulated insulin delivery. ACS Nano. 2020;14(1):488–97. https://doi.org/10.1021/acsnano.9b06395.
78. Wampler HP, Ivanisevic A. Nanoindentation of gold nanoparticles functionalized with proteins. Micron. 2009;40(4):444–8. https://doi.org/10.1016/j.micron.2009.01.002.
79. Wang L, Gong C, Yuan X, Wei G. Controlling the self-assembly of biomolecules into functional nanomaterials through internal interactions and external stimulations: a review. Nano. 2019;9(2):285. https://doi.org/10.3390/nano9020285.
80. Wang S, Zhang J, Gharbi O, Vivier V, Gao M, Orazem ME. Electrochemical impedance spectroscopy. Nat Rev Methods Primers. 2021;1(1):41. https://doi.org/10.1038/s43586-021-00039-w.
81. Wang ZL. Structural analysis of self-assembling nanocrystal superlattices. Adv Mater. 1998;10(1):13–30. https://doi.org/10.1002/(SICI)1521-4095(199801)10:1<13::AID-ADMA13>3.0.CO;2-W.
82. Xia F, Youcef-Toumi K. Review: advanced atomic force microscopy modes for biomedical research. Biosensors. 2022;12(12):1116. https://doi.org/10.3390/bios12121116.

83. Xie X, Sun T, Xue J, Miao Z, Yan X, Fang W, Li Q, Tang R, Lu Y, Tang L, Zha Z, He T. Ag nanoparticles cluster with pH-triggered reassembly in targeting antimicrobial applications. Adv Funct Mater. 2020;30(17) https://doi.org/10.1002/adfm.202000511.
84. Yamada H, Yoshii K, Asahi M, Chiku M, Kitazumi Y. Cyclic voltammetry part 1: fundamentals. Electrochemistry. 2022;90(10):22-66082. https://doi.org/10.5796/electrochemistry.22-66082.
85. Yuan Chiu K, Xiang Su T, Hong Li J, Lin T-H, Liou G-S, Cheng S-H. Novel trends of electrochemical oxidation of amino-substituted triphenylamine derivatives. J Electroanal Chem. 2005;575(1):95–101. https://doi.org/10.1016/j.jelechem.2004.09.005.
86. Zainal NFA, Saiter JM, Halim SIA, Lucas R, Chan CH. Thermal analysis: basic concept of differential scanning calorimetry and thermogravimetry for beginners. Chem Teach Int. 2021;3(2):59–75. https://doi.org/10.1515/cti-2020-0010.
87. Zare M, Mikkonen KS. Phase change materials for life science applications. Adv Funct Mater. 2023;33(12) https://doi.org/10.1002/adfm.202213455.
88. Zeynabad FB, Salehi R, Mahkam M. Design of pH-responsive antimicrobial nanocomposite as dual drug delivery system for tumor therapy. Appl Clay Sci. 2017;141:23–35. https://doi.org/10.1016/j.clay.2017.02.015.
89. Zhang S, Zhao D. Aerospace materials handbook. CRC Press; 2016. https://doi.org/10.1201/b13044.
90. Zhang W, Ma J, Meng F, Jiang Y, Shen L, Sun T, Qin Y, Zhu N, Zhang M. Wearable biomolecule smart sensor based on Au@PB NPs with high electrochemical activity. J Alloys Compd. 2022;891:161983. https://doi.org/10.1016/j.jallcom.2021.161983.
91. Zhou J, Hou S, Li L, Yao D, Liu Y, Jenkins ATA, Fan Y. Theranostic infection-responsive coating to In situ detect and prevent urinary catheter blockage. Adv Mater Interf. 2018;5(24) https://doi.org/10.1002/admi.201801242.

Chapter 4
Harnessing Carbon Nano-Architectonics for Advanced Prodrug Delivery

Lalit Goswami, Anamika Kushwaha, Akhilesh Bind, Anshi, Karabi Roy, Seungdae Oh, Pankaj Verma, Kamin Alexander, and Rahele Khosravi

Abstract Carbon-based nanomaterials have arisen as potential candidates for medical applications due to their nanoscale dimensions, which allow for precise interactions with cellular structures. This compatibility is particularly beneficial for drug delivery, as these materials can target specific cells and tissues. Moreover, the unique optical properties of certain carbon nanostructures make them valuable tools for both diagnostic imaging and therapeutic interventions. Despite significant progress in nanotechnology, delivering anticancer drugs effectively to tumor cells still remains a major hurdle. One promising approach involves the development of nanostructures that encapsulate prodrugs—inactive compounds that are activated within

L. Goswami · S. Oh (✉)
Department of Civil Engineering, College of Engineering, Kyung Hee University, Yongin, Republic of Korea
e-mail: soh@khu.ac.kr

A. Kushwaha
Department of Chemical Engineering, Chungbuk National University, Cheongju, Republic of Korea

A. Bind
Department of Biochemistry and Biochemical Engineering, Sam Higginbottom University of Agriculture Technology and Sciences, Prayagraj, Uttar Pradesh, India

Anshi
University Institute of Biotechnology, Chandigarh University, Mohali, Punjab, India

K. Roy
Department of Chemistry, Salbari College, Baksa, Assam, India

P. Verma
Department of Biotechnology, IILM University, Greater Noida, Uttar Pradesh, India

K. Alexander
Department of Biological Sciences, Sam Higginbottom University of Agriculture Technology and Sciences, Prayagraj, Uttar Pradesh, India

R. Khosravi
Department of Chemical Engineering, Sahand University of Technology, Sahand New City, Tabriz, Iran

S. Mondal et al. (eds.), *Smart and Sustainable Nanomaterials in Digital Healthcare and Theranostic*, https://doi.org/10.1007/978-981-95-9386-6_4

the body. These prodrug-loaded nanoparticles offer several advantages, including increased absorption, high drug-carrying capacity, controlled release, and improved stability. This chapter summarizes the recent advancements in cancer therapies that utilize carbon nanomaterials in combination with prodrugs. The synthesis and characterization of these hybrid structures are included, further exploring current research efforts and addressing potential safety concerns associated with their use. Finally, we highlight the challenges and opportunities in this field and suggest future research directions.

Keywords Carbon nanomaterials · Cancer therapy · Nanotechnology · Anticancer drugs · Therapeutic interventions

4.1 Introduction

Regardless of the vast development attained in the past two decades, combating cancer continues to be an ongoing challenge for public health [105]. Despite the wide array of treatment approaches used in cancer therapy, current therapeutics have not yet met the desired level of effectiveness [52]. The ideal technique for cancer drug administration is the intravenous method owing to its complete and instant bioavailability [25]. In addition, most of these anticancer drugs are extremely noxious, and because of their widespread and imprecise distribution throughout the body, this results in reduced therapeutic efficacy and considerable undesired effects [67]. Presently, targeted cancer therapy is the prime area of research where targeting or inhibiting abnormal markers (in the case of some cancers) displays outstanding therapeutic outcomes along with low side effects on the normal tissues [95]. Inopportunely, in the case of most cancers, there is no specific marker [83]. In this respect, exploring a nano-platform that can enhance physicochemical properties, control drug release, and reduce drug toxicity is essential [17]. Therefore, the chief alternative to deal with this limitation is the utilization of prodrugs (PDs), which are recognized for a wide range of applications to either enhance or suppress the above-mentioned limitations [79].

The PDs are inactive precursor molecules of drug compounds that are designed to transform into their pharmacologically active counterparts when exposed to specific enzymatic processes or chemical conditions within the body [25]. The compound is created by the covalent bonding of the drug to a (macro) molecule. This combined structure is broken down through metabolic processes, releasing the drug in its active form in vivo [95]. PDs have a prodigious capability to address physiological obstacles, namely, the gastrointestinal tract, due to the structural characteristics of pharmaceutical compounds, such as their electrical charge distribution and ionizable functional groups, which have undergone alteration. Consequently, cancer treatments have evolved to be more precise. Traditional chemotherapy drugs like doxorubicin, camptothecin, and paclitaxel have been transformed into targeted PDs. This modification allows them to specifically attack cancer cells, enhancing their therapeutic efficacy while reducing collateral damage to healthy tissues [94]. This has led to an alternative to address challenges such as limited solubility, reduced stability, adverse effects, lack of specificity, ineffective tumor targeting, uncontrolled drug release, and incompetent cellular uptake of anticancer drugs [25].

Nanocarriers have significantly aided cancer treatment due to progress in nanotechnology and material science. Traditional PDs and nanoparticle drug delivery systems have inherent limitations in their clinical use. Traditional drug delivery systems face several challenges, including limited capacity for medication, stability issues during storage, unintended release post-injection, and possible harmful effects due to the increased use of biological materials. These materials are often used to make up for the low drug content. Additionally, smaller PD molecules may be eliminated from the body too rapidly or break down before reaching their target [13]. In this respect, the fusion of PD techniques and nanocarriers has led to the emergence of nano-based prodrug delivery systems (NPDS), currently attracting significant research interest [95].

This chapter deals with how carbon-based nanomaterials can be utilized in developing and delivering PD therapies. It explores the potential applications of these advanced materials in enhancing drug efficacy and targeting. Here, the discussion explores the relationship between PDs and carbon nanomaterials (CNMs) in the NPDS, the creation, analysis, and application of various CNMs, including graphene, carbon nanotubes (CNTs), nanodiamonds, fullerenes, and carbon dots. Further, the CNM's toxicity along with limitations and future perspectives are also discussed.

4.2 Prodrugs

PDs are pharmaceutically enhanced versions of small molecule drugs, biologically inert in their initial form but undergo transformation within the body to become therapeutically active drugs [112]. The design of PDs is based on the features that are much more abundant in cancer cells than in healthy cells, such as antigens, peptide transporters, or enzymes. This selectivity can be accomplished by connecting the drug to a tumor-specific binding molecule using a cleavable linker [25]. The parent drug is liberated when specific environmental factors, such as the occurrence of a specific enzyme or shifts in pH, induce the breakage of the linking component. Once released, the drug can then carry out its intended function (Fig. 4.1). Often, PD synthesis employs various linking structures that commonly encompass chemical bonds such as esters and amides.

Additionally, oximes and imines are utilized as linkers, while disulfide bonds serve as another option in this context. Furthermore, non-cleavable thioether bonds are sometimes incorporated as linking elements in PD design [25]. Here, the pro-moiety attached to the parent drug must possess a robust linker, ensuring its integrity is maintained until it arrives at the target cells. It is crucial that the bond connecting the pro-moiety to the parent drug remains stable, remaining unaltered

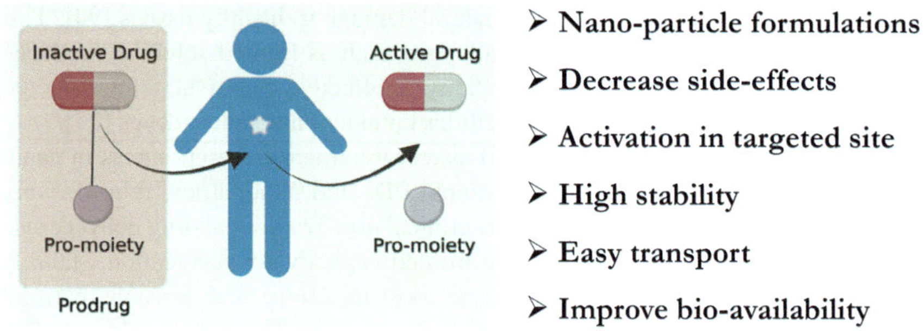

Fig. 4.1 Advantages and activation mechanisms of prodrug tactics

until reaching the intended cellular target. Therefore, further linkage optimization is required to maximize the stability and efficacy of the creation of PDs [41].

Usually, the PDs are utilized to disguise unsuitable functional groups on drugs that do not pass the medical studies owing to their very low bioavailability, side effects, inappropriate distribution, or ineffectiveness [71, 79]. The latest research indicates that modifying an active pharmaceutical ingredient to create a PD has demonstrated the ability to regulate crucial drug characteristics. This approach has subsequently led to improved clinical results as well. Thus, PD strategies have gained significant attention due to their growing market presence. Over the past 20 years, the proportion of PDs among marketed pharmaceuticals has increased, with roughly 10% of available drugs now being PDs [25].

4.3 Nanocarbon-Based Systems for Prodrug Delivery

Even though the NSPD research area is quite novel, elaborations on NSPD products are under development, further providing the signal while simultaneously favoring the advantages of the PD and nanoparticle techniques. Such complex phenomena are only considered if they have extravagant recompenses. Further enhancement in the PD's stability, bioavailability, accurate targeting, and release onto the site will boost the PD's efficacy and safety.

4.3.1 Carbon-Based Nanomaterials

Carbon nanomaterials (CNMs) have attracted significant interest since fullerene's (the first member of CNMs) groundbreaking discovery in 1985 [53]. Moreover, the discoveries of CNTs (1991) and graphene (2004) have sparked increased research focus on carbon-based nanoscale materials [42, 80]. Also, fullerenes, CNTs, and graphene are predominantly composed of sp^2 hybridized carbon atoms, which create conjugated systems. In contrast, carbon dots (CDs) incorporate both sp^2 and sp^3 hybridization, frequently featuring defects and heteroatoms. Additionally, nano-diamonds, which are chiefly made up of sp^3 C-atoms, have garnered considerable interest in the field [4, 73]. CNMs exhibit remarkable properties that are unimaginable in bulk carbon structures like graphite and diamond. These extraordinary characteristic features from quantum confinement effects in CNMs give rise to distinctive optical, magnetic, electrical, and chemical attributes. Consequently, CNM's novel properties make CNMs valuable for applications in electronics, photonics, renewable energy, and biomedicine [32, 33, 36].

Quantum confinement in carbon nanomaterials (CNMs) produces unique optical, magnetic, electrical, and chemical characteristics absent in bulk carbon forms like graphite or diamond [31, 54]f. Over the last 10 years, carbon nanomaterials (CNMs) have significantly progressed in biomedical uses. Their unique properties, including nanoscale dimensions, special optical features, and a high surface-to-volume ratio, have led to this advancement [11, 81]. CNMs possess dimensions that align with the specified criteria, providing an additional advantage as exceptional carrier nanomaterials for drug encapsulation and targeted in vivo delivery to specific sites. Furthermore, the unique optical characteristics exhibited by certain CNMs have garnered significant attention for their potential in therapeutic applications [38]. Here, initially, a concise overview of the methods used to create and analyze CNMs is provided. Following this is the explicit analysis of how various CNMs are utilized in PD-based therapeutic approaches, as illustrated in Fig. 4.2.

4.3.2 Synthesis Techniques

This section summarizes the recognized synthesis techniques for various carbon nanomaterials. Graphene is primarily produced through physical separation, chemical processes, and vapor deposition techniques (CVD) [12]. Graphene oxide (GO) production typically employs a top-down approach starting from graphite. However, this method

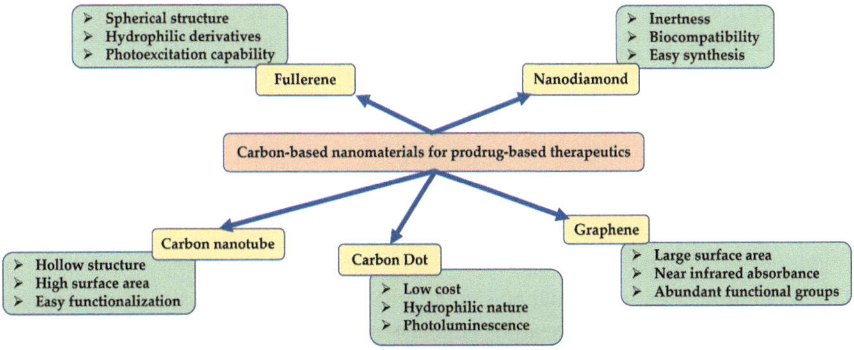

Fig. 4.2 Various carbon nanomaterial types and their significant attributes for prodrug therapies

faces challenges in terms of time efficiency and scalability. In general, the synthesis of GO typically employs the enhanced Hummers' technique. In brief, the process involves adding flaky or powdered graphite to a protonated solvent mixture, specifically H_2SO_4 and $NaNO_3$. The oxidation is then carried out using $KMnO_4$ as the oxidizing agent. Further, hydrogen peroxide is utilized for reacting the blend to eradicate any remaining metal ions. This leads to the color shift from dark brown to yellow. Thereafter, through centrifugation, washing, and lyophilization, GO is produced [97]. For fullerenes synthesis, various methods, including electric arc discharge, laser-based techniques, graphite electrode vaporization, and carbon material pyrolysis, are employed.

Among these, the arc discharge approach is most frequently employed [98]. The synthesis method utilizes an elevated-temperature oven in conjunction with a flowing buffer gas that passes through a silica conduit to heat-treat carbon aggregates. Usually, the tube is heated to 25 °C and is operated below 1000 °C. Carbon condenses and undergoes annealing to form fullerenes, which are collected in a water-cooled trap. Further, chromatography is then used to isolate fullerenes from the mixture [85]. For the synthesis of NDs, two techniques are more common: (i) transformation of graphite under extreme pressure and heat conditions and (ii) detonation of carbon-rich explosive materials [74]. CNTs can be produced through several manufacturing approaches. These include wet chemical methods like hydrothermal synthesis, gas-phase growth via chemical vapor deposition (CVD), and high-energy processes that utilize plasma, such as arc discharge and laser ablation techniques (also known as photoablation).

Among the conventional approaches for producing CNTs, CVD stands out as the most widely adopted method. Its popularity blooms from its versatility in yielding CNTs with diverse morphologies, ranging from powder to straight and coiled structures. The formation and expansion of CNTs can be readily accomplished by modifying the thermal conditions [7, 85]. Further, for the production of CDs, several bottom-up and top-down approaches are developed [110]. CDs can be synthesized primarily using two main approaches: (i) breaking down larger carbon-based materials, known as top-down methods, that include techniques such as chemical and electrochemical oxidation, as well as arc discharge and laser ablation processes, and (ii) bottom-up techniques, which focus on constructing carbon dots from smaller molecular components. This is typically achieved through various carbonization processes, including pyrolysis, hydrothermal treatment, solvothermal synthesis, and methods that utilize microwave assistance. These diverse approaches allow researchers to tailor CD production to specific needs and resources [104].

4.3.3 Characterization Techniques

The accurate evaluation of nanoparticle (NP) characterization stands as a crucial aspect of nanotechnology research. This task necessitates the use of advanced analytical techniques that can effectively identify and measure properties at nanoscale dimensions. Such sophisticated methods are essential for obtaining precise assessments of NPs, highlighting their significance in this scientific domain [33, 36]. The prime techniques employed to analyze crucial attributes of carbon nanomaterials, including their dimensions, surface electrical properties, morphology, light-interactive characteristics, and elemental makeup, are covered in this section. Dynamic light scattering (DLS) is an invasive technique that uses a laser for the quick and simple quantification of the size of NPs dispersed in the aqueous solution or suspension [7]. Further, the surface charge of CNPs in the colloidal solution can be quantified using the zeta potential technique. Here, the surface charge has a significant role in illustrating how stable the CNPs remain dispersed and the extent to which they aggregate [76]. To assess the surface characteristics of CNPs, researchers have employed various advanced microscopy techniques, including atomic force microscopy (AFM), transmission electron microscopy (TEM), and scanning electron microscopy (SEM) [27]. In comparison to the other prevailing techniques, SEM and AFM are more precise in representing the size, morphology, and other surface and morphological structures, while TEM is often used because of its high resolution and also projects 2D micrographs of 3D materials [46, 63]. The shape, size, aggregation state, and concentration of CNPs play a crucial role in determining their optical characteristics. These properties exhibit an exceptionally high degree of sensitivity to even minor changes. They are usually examined using UV-visible and fluorescence spectroscopies [6]).

All the aforementioned techniques used for the characterization of CNPs are performed without any significant alteration. For the physical observation of the microstructure and composition elemental analyses, numerous advanced analytical techniques—such as TEM and SEM often paired with energy dispersive X-ray spectroscopy (EDX),Fourier transform infrared (FTIR) spectroscopy, X-ray diffraction (XRD), X-ray fluorescence (XRF), and X-ray photoelectron spectroscopies (XPS)—can be utilized [9, 35, 55]. XRD analysis can be employed to elucidate the diffraction patterns of CNPs, while FTIR is useful for identifying the surface functional groups present in these particles [12]. In addition, Raman spectroscopy and vibrational spectroscopic techniques may analyze vibrational patterns in materials and offer comprehensive insights into the structural features, surface characteristics, and chemical makeup, whereas by using a vibrating-sample magnetometer (VSM), the magnetic behavior of the CNPs can be determined [34].

4.3.4 CNMs in Prodrug-Based Therapeutics

4.3.4.1 Graphene

In the last few years, graphene-based nanoparticles, mainly GO, have arisen as promising materials in drug delivery systems due to their unique structural and chemical properties [24, 99]. The extensive surface area of GO structures, combined with their carbon framework featuring sp^2 hybridization, contributes to their effectiveness. Additionally, these structures are rich in various functional groups, including hydroxyl, carboxyl, and epoxy moieties. These characteristics collectively result in an improved capacity for drug loading [47, 89]. Additionally, GO exhibits excellent thermal stability, optical properties, and strong near-infrared (NIR) absorbance, particularly after reduction, making it suitable for photothermal therapy (PTT). These attributes position GO as a versatile material for several biomedical applications, including drug delivery, PTT, biosensing, bioimaging, and 3D scaffolding [25, 64].

Huang et al. [41] developed PP-SS-DOX PDs by linking mPEG-PLGA (PP) and doxorubicin (DOX) via disulfide bonds. The incorporation of PEG-folic acid (FA) with GA (GO/PP-SS-DOX/PEG-FA) enhanced the system's active targeting capability. The GO's stability in physiological solutions was significantly improved by the addition of PP-SS-DOX, allowing the release of DOX in the reductive environment of cancer cells. PEG-FA also encouraged endocytosis via the folate receptor, aiming at cancerous tissues. The system displayed clear reductive sensitivity in vitro, with a cumulative release of 90% after 72 h, which was much higher than reported earlier, i.e., 40%. Targeting nanohybrids showed higher cytotoxicity compared to non-targeting types. In vivo studies in mice with B16 tumors confirmed the system's substantial antitumor effect with slight systemic side effects [41].

Researchers developed an advanced nanocomposite (PEG-NGO-Pt) by integrating three key components: a cisplatin PD, GO nanoparticles modified with polyethylene glycol, and a mechanism to detect programmed cell death. This sophisticated system combines multiple functionalities, allowing for precise drug targeting, heat-induced cancer treatment, chemotherapeutic action, and continuous monitoring of therapeutic efficacy within a unified platform. By merging these components, the nanocomposite offers a synergistic approach to cancer treatment, potentially improving therapeutic outcomes while providing continuous feedback on treatment effectiveness. The nanocomposite presented improved tumor targeting ability, enhanced cytotoxicity, and better therapeutic efficacy via apoptosis and cell death. This platform outpaced PTT and chemotherapy alone, efficiently removing tumors with nominal toxicity. A 3D supramolecular hydrogel combining PD-modified GO and α-cyclodextrin permitted the transport of anticancer drugs (both hydrophobic and hydrophilic), with a gel-to-sol transition activated by near-infrared irradiation [60].

Liu et al. [65] engineered a drug delivery system (DDS) utilizing GO as a foundation. This system was designed to incorporate a podophyllotoxin disulfide PD (DCM-S-PPT) through the implementation of a breakable disulfide bond. The biocompatibility of GO underwent enhancement through PEG functionalization, followed by the incorporation of DCM-S-PPT utilizing hydrophobic interactions and π-π stacking. Laboratory experiments demonstrated that GO-PEG/DCM-S-PPT exhibited superior inhibition of HeLa cancer cells compared to 293 T normal cells, attributed to variations in intracellular glutathione (GSH) concentrations. In tumor-bearing mice, GO-PEG/DCM-S-PPT displayed heightened anticancer effectiveness while producing fewer adverse effects when contrasted with DCM-S-PPT and podophyllotoxin (PPT) administered independently [65]. To overcome issues such as low drug stability and incomplete release of GO-based nanocarriers for cancer therapy, Ma et al. [68] established GO-prodrug nanohybrids (GO-PN). The PEG-PCL-SS-DOX prodrug, joined via a redox-sensitive disulfide bond, was used to decorate GO. The PD molecules enhanced dispersibility, stabilized GO, and ensured targeted release at tumor sites. In vitro results showed increased DOX accumulation in A549 and B16 cells, while in vivo studies confirmed significant tumor growth inhibition with reduced toxicity [68].

4.3.4.2 Fullerene

Fullerenes, composed of sp^2-hybridized carbon atoms, are typically soluble in organic hydrocarbons and halogenated solvents. Studies have focused on enhancing fullerene hydrophilicity for drug delivery applications. Covalently attaching DOX to a fullerene derivative improved the hydrophilicity and potential as a drug carrier [14, 66]. Fullerenes exhibit unique photosensitizing properties, enabling them to produce singlet oxygen ($^1O_2$) and other reactive oxygen species (ROS) when exposed to light. This characteristic enhances their cytotoxic effects. The scientists engineered a versatile anticancer PD platform with multiple functions using hydrophilic fullerene aggregates with doxorubicin (DOX) and folic acid (FA) for targeted dual-action treatment, combining pH-activated chemotherapy and light-triggered photodynamic therapy (PDT). This PD moves into cancer cells via the folate receptor (FR), activating intracellularly to destroy them. Light irradiation further boosts cytotoxicity. DOX fluorescence quenching occurs upon fullerene binding, with restoration signaling successful drug release and delivery [26].

GC-DMA-C60, a photosensitizer PD, was created by attaching glycol chitosan to 2,3-dimethyl maleic acid and linking this complex with fullerene. The resulting compound self-assembles into nanogels, combining hydrophilic GC/DMA segments with hydrophobic C60 components. The nanogels aggregated at pH 7.4 due to electrostatic interactions, but DMA blocks cleave, causing the aggregates to disintegrate at pH 5.0. Upon 670 nm light irradiation, the nanogels generate singlet oxygen ($^1O_2$), with higher production at pH 5.0 due to reduced photo-interference. This pH-responsive system makes GC-DMA-C60 a promising candidate for photodynamic therapy (PDT) and endosomal targeting in cancer cells [51]. The skin cancer therapy and brain tumor imaging agent 5-aminolevulinic acid (5-ALA), a PD, faced restricted use owing to its poor fat solubility. Researchers developed water-soluble fullerene nanomaterials, C60-ALA and C60-ALA-GA, to enhance 5-ALA delivery. HPLC, fluorescence, and qRT-PCR analyses verified biological activity, demonstrating the upregulation of ABCG2 and PEPT-1 genes. They also developed a combination photodynamic therapy (PDT) strategy using the ABCG2 inhibitor Ko143 alongside the fullerene conjugates [92].

4.3.4.3 NDs

Nanodiamonds (NDs) represent the sp^3-hybridized carbon nanomaterial form that can be concurrently modified with various molecules for purposes such as cellular markers and drug delivery. Studies indicate that NDs do not exhibit any significant toxicity or adverse impacts on biological systems [19, 119, 75]. Owing to their numerous intrinsic qualities, which garnered attention and increasing interest in their beneficial properties for their use in drug delivery systems (DDSs) utilizing NDs [87, 107, 120]. These properties include easy synthesis, nanoscale dimensions, chemical stability, a wealth of surface functional groups, compatibility with biological systems, and natural fluorescent properties; all these attributes make NDs versatile agents for a wide range of drug delivery applications [56].

In a recent study, researchers explored the development of an ND-based novel PD known as ND-ACA-HYD-DOX (NAHD), which incorporates aminocaproic acid. This PD exhibits pH-dependent fluorescence activation and demonstrates cytotoxic properties. More notably, remarkable stability was shown by synthesized PD at pH 7.4 and quenched DOX fluorescence, resulting in an "off" state. However, when exposed to the acidic environment typical of endosomes, NAHD undergoes a significant transformation. The acylhydrazone bond within the PD breaks down, leading to the release of a substantial amount of DOX. These observations are particularly noteworthy, as they suggest that the PD formulation does not compromise the drug's effectiveness and further exhibits a pronounced response to the tumor microenvironment. This targeted activation mechanism has the potential to significantly reduce the adverse side effects often associated with conventional chemotherapy, marking a promising step forward in cancer treatment strategies. Perhaps most importantly, the researchers established that the PD structure enables a localized activation within the tumor's specific environment, substantially minimizing undesirable systemic effects [15, 109].

A lysozyme-activated prodrug (NPGM) was created based on an ester linkage by linking glycidylated ND and methotrexate (MTX) via an ester bond. This prodrug (ND-PEG-GLY-MTX, NPGM) has been developed with the purpose of offering improved drug loading and controlled release. Newly synthesized NPGM nanoparticles exhibited stability under physiological conditions but released MTX in acidic, lysozyme-rich environments. It has a high drug loading capacity and releases MTX under an acidic environment or when lysozyme is present, triggered by ester bond cleavage in the nanoparticle-gel matrix. The cellular uptake of NPGM is time- and temperature-dependent but energy-independent, as elucidated using confocal microscopy and flow cytometry. Entry inside the cell occurs through caveolin-dependent endocytosis, localizing in the lysosomes, cancer cell lysozyme activates NPGM by cleaving the ester bond, triggering its toxic effects. NPGM exhibited enhanced anticancer efficacy versus free MTX, as evidenced by MTT and apoptosis assays, suggesting its greater therapeutic potential. By addressing common challenges in cancer chemotherapy, such as drug stability, targeted delivery, and controlled release, NPGM represents a promising advancement in cancer treatment strategies [122].

Gemcitabine (GEM) PDs enhanced pancreatic cancer treatment as proclaimed by the researchers. The choice of ND as a carrier is because of its incredible surface properties and biocompatibility. ND was coated with PEG, PEI, and PAA to improve the biocompatibility of carriers that employ electrostatic forces onto the surface of ND. GEM was linked to a glycine-phenylalanine-leucine-glycine (GFLG) peptide for enzyme-triggered release based on enzyme sensitivity. In vivo tests showed enhanced anticancer effects compared to free GEM therapy. Polymer-encapsulated nanodiamonds with enhanced surface capacity, combined with enzyme-triggered cellular gemcitabine release, boosted pancreatic cancer treatment effectiveness [114].

NDs functionalized with gemcitabine (GEM) prodrug-polymers were synthesized via grafting and strain-promoted alkyne-azide cycloaddition. It is an effective approach that enhances conjugation efficiency through covalent linkages between the polymers and surface moieties. The polymers were synthesized by combining gemcitabine PD with oligoethylene glycol methyl ether acrylate. These NDs showed accelerated drug release in acidic environments and variable cytotoxicity in AsPC-1 cells compared to physiological conditions. Researchers have demonstrated that NDs with higher OEGMEA content have IC50 values similar to the free gemcitabine, while those with less OEGMEA have higher IC50 values [56].

4.3.4.4 CNTs

Single-walled carbon nanotubes (SWCNTs) and multiwalled carbon nanotubes (MWCNTs) are forms of CNTs, both of which consist of graphene sheets rolled into nanoscale cylindrical structures [102]. CNTs are distinguished by their exceptional mechanical strength [50, 78], chemical stability [5], and electrical conductivity [30], which make them superior to other materials. In the medicinal field, the most important attributes are minuscule size, enormous surface area as well as hollow structure allowing them to carry and deliver substances effectively [116]. Functionalized CNTs show significant potential as tools for various biological applications due to their ability to effectively traverse biological barriers and accumulate within cells making them highly suitable for different applications [1]. Furthermore, their large surface area provides multiple sites for molecular attachments, making them ideal for precise targeting [49, 82].

CNTs have found applications as biological sensors, frameworks for regenerative medicine, and carriers for various bioactive substances, including medications involved in fighting cancer [25]. To ensure that therapeutic molecules remain active for a longer duration and facilitate controlled release, they can be attached to the outer surface of CNTs or enclosed within their structure [37, 72, 106]. Additionally, various techniques have been developed to enhance the biocompatibility of CNTs [10]. Oxidative enzymes have been shown to degrade modified CNTs, potentially enhancing their safety for biological use, according to new research [8].

A group of researchers developed a multifunctional, water-dispersal carbon nanotube-based anticancer PD system, featuring targeted delivery, pH-activated drug release, and photodynamic therapy capabilities. In this prodrug system, CNTs were functionalized with folic acid as a targeting moiety and doxorubicin via hydrazone linkage, creating a targeted prodrug delivery system. Ideally, this PD is designed to target cancer cells through folate receptor-mediated entry. Once inside, it responds to the tumor's acidic microenvironment by releasing the active drug intracellularly. Compared to conventional non-targeted systems, the targeted CNTs-based PD demonstrates a notable reduction in cell viability, specifically in folate receptor (FR^+) cancer cells. This enhanced targeting is due to the ability of the folate receptor to selectively bind folic acid, facilitating the uptake of the PD into cancer cells that overexpress these receptors. Additionally, the CNT carrier not only serves as a delivery vehicle but also possesses photodynamic therapy properties. When exposed to light irradiation, the CNTs generate reactive oxygen species (ROS), which can induce further cell death in FR^+ cancer cells [26].

In another study, researchers developed an innovative method for creating platinum-based compounds with integrated delivery and tumor-targeting capabilities. Their work demonstrated that a specific molecule (compound 1), featuring a folic acid variant as an axial ligand, preferentially binds to cancer cells overexpressing folate receptors. When combined with single-walled carbon nanotubes (SWCNTs), compound 1 exhibited significant enhancement in cytotoxicity, facilitating the process of endocytosis. SWCNT-bound compound 1 exhibits 8.6-fold higher cellular activity than free Pt when reduced. This results in predominantly forming 1,2-D(GpG) inter-strand cross-links in nuclear DNA. Internalization studies verified the SWCNT-1 conjugate's specific, high-affinity folate receptor binding [22]. A new approach was developed that employs tumor-targeting MWCNTs to encapsulate a non-reactive Pt (IV) PD, enabling exact proportions of Pt and DOX for endometrial cancer therapy. Once inside the cell, entry triggers Pt (IV) PD activation, concurrently freeing water-soluble platinum and equal quantities of DOX from their lipophilic surroundings. This results in a balanced delivery of these synergistic drug components, improving their combined therapeutic effects against cancer cells [18].

Scientists used multiwalled carbon nanotubes tagged with two fluorescent labels: mitochondria-targeting rhodamine-110 (MWCNT-Rho) and non-specific fluorescein (MWCNT-Fluo). Despite structural likeness between the dyes, only MWCNT-Rho accumulated in mitochondria, while MWCNT-Fluo did not show such ability. Despite the structural similarities between the two constructs, MWCNT-Rho demonstrates preferential mitochondrial localization, whereas MWCNT-Fluo does not exhibit comparable targeting capabilities. This divergence is likely attributed to the rhodamine moiety in MWCNT-Rho, which possesses physicochemical properties such as positive charge and lipophilicity that promote mitochondrial accumulation. In contrast, MWCNT-Fluo lacks these mitochondrial targeting attributes. MWCNT-Rho exhibits a higher capacity for encapsulating Pt (IV) compared to its counterpart. Notably, the unloaded MWCNT-Rho does not impact cellular viability nor disrupt mitochondrial membrane potential; furthermore, the cell excretes a portion of it. Owing to these advantageous properties, MWCNT-Rho was employed for the simultaneous encapsulation of Pt (IV) and 3-bromopyruvate. Studies across various cell lines demonstrated that this platform exhibited superior efficacy compared to the free Pt (IV) drug. Significantly, the mitochondrial membrane potential was reduced by half, suggesting that targeting the mitochondrial components resulted in greater mitochondrial damage [115].

In another study, researchers examined Pt (IV) encapsulation in two types of functionalized MWCNTs with varying diameters. They compared the resulting Pt (IV)-CNTs complexes to unbound drugs, assessing their performance in HeLa cells and RAW 264 murine macrophages. After 72 h of CNT exposure, cell mortality occurred in HeLa cultures following a 3D-CNT treatment for both specimen types. Notably, CNTs with larger diameters exhibited greater cytotoxicity toward HeLa cells, whereas smaller diameter CNTs enabled sustained drug release, thereby enhancing the long-term anticancer effect. Pt (IV)-CNT formulations exhibited minimal macrophage toxicity. TEM and flow cytometry confirmed efficient cellular uptake of both CNT samples. Compared to free drug complex treatment, Pt (IV)-CNT carriers enhanced intracellular Pt accumulation. The study demonstrates that by altering CNT diameter, CNTs' efficacy as nanocarriers amplifies anticancer drug accumulation and controlled release in tumor cells while minimizing inflammatory responses [77].

4.3.4.5 CDs

One of the emerging fluorescent carbon nanoparticles is CDs of size <10 nm inclusive of special properties such as quantum confinement effects, biocompatibility, and highly tunable photoluminescence with the sp^2 carbon core. These CDs are easy to prepare [44, 45] and have water dissolution ability and chemical reaction ability stemming from the presence of many polar functional groups like -OH, -COOH, and $-NH_2$ groups.

In recent years, carbon dots (CDs) have emerged as a standout among self-assembling nanomaterials. Their unique combination of properties, including exceptional stability, characteristic optical behavior, and compatibility with biological systems, has set them apart. CDs also boast excellent water solubility, resistance to photobleaching, cost-effectiveness, and straightforward synthesis methods making them eligible for a myriad spectrum of biomedical applications [29, 86, 93]. For instance, PTT agents can serve as carriers for chemotherapy medications, functioning as drug delivery systems. Their ability to dissolve in water and emit fluorescent light makes them promising for medical imaging applications, i.e., treatment and visualization [3, 27, 88, 113]. Fabrication of RCDs (near-infrared-active CDs) with Pt (IV) PD was achieved through covalent linkage for the creation of RCD-Pt complex, the surface of which was coated with the PEG-chitosan-2,3-dimethylmaleic anhydride polymer (PEG-CS-DA) to produce a multifunctional nanoprobe (RCD–Pt (IV)/PEG–CS–DA) for targeting tumors. RCD-Pt (IV) was rapidly released in tumor cells due to the hydrolysis of RCD-Pt(IV)/PEG-CS-DA under the acidic environment of cancer cells.

The elevated level of glutathione in cancer cells are due to the reduction of tetravalent platinum to its divalent state which leads to the gradual release of RCDs, eventually facilitating visualization of cancerous tissue and liberation of Pt (II) compounds. Simultaneously, when exposed to near-infrared light, the carbon-based nanostructures in tumor areas produce substantial thermal energy, swiftly eliminating malignant cells, and the accumulation of Pt (II) in tumor tissues enables targeted chemotherapy. As a result, this approach combines targeted drug delivery, diagnostic imaging, and a synergistic treatment utilizing both chemotherapy and photothermal therapy (PTT) concurrently [39].

Biotinylated CDs, covalently tethered with Fe^{2+} (FCD_b), have found their usage in cancer therapy as a precursor for PD, assist in diagnostic procedures, and serve as a carrier to precisely deliver the anticancer drug PTX. FCDs (CDs doped with Fe^{2+}) were formed by the hydrothermal process, which was covalently modified on the surface with biotin to produce FCD_b. Two compounds are employed as biological markers for B16F10 cancer cells: FCD and a substance that produces blue fluorescence under UV light. Of these, FCDb demonstrated superior efficacy due to the elevated biotin receptor expression in cancer cells. Furthermore, PTX-loaded FCDb selectively targeted and eliminated B16F10 malignant cells. OS generated from H_2O_2 with FCDb, combined with PTX's cancer-fighting abilities, synergistically increased B16F10 cell death 2.7–3.5-folds using FCD-PTX [20].

The advantage of using cyclodextrin-based (CD) compounds for diagnosis and treatment is their ability to be quickly cleared from the body via renal excretion owing to their small molecular size. Research demonstrates the application of cyclodextrin-derived nano-sponges to produce trackable PDs exhibiting fluorescence and a suitable size. PDs were synthesized to have a suitable size, with an average hydrodynamic diameter of approximately 120 nm, which was achieved through conjugation with about 19% of DOX to the nano-sponges using acid-sensitive bonds. The drug release mechanism was pH-dependent. This innovative approach to PD design, combining nano-sponge technology with stimuli-responsive drug release and built-in traceability, shows promise as a potential platform for future advancements in tumor therapy [59].

In another study, a novel cancer treatment approach was developed, utilizing luminescent CDs in a FRET-based ratiometric method to monitor anticancer PD activation, resulting in an effective and low-risk therapeutic system. Fluorescent CDs serve dual roles: they transport medications at the nanoscale while also functioning as energy donors in Förster resonance energy transfer processes. The Dabsyl group (a fluorescence quencher) was linked to the CD's surface via Pt (IV), which also acted as a model PD. Quenching of the blue fluorescence of CDs by the dabsyl unit occurred because of the FRET phenomenon. The reducing conditions within living cells promoted the transformation of Pt (IV) to Pt (II), which led to an enhancement of the carbon dots' blue fluorescence, while the green and red fluorescence intensities remained constant. Pt (IV) to Pt (II) transformation was tracked by observing the growing blue-to-green or blue-to-red fluorescence emission ratio. This ratiometric method, employing carbon dots' green/red fluorescence as a reference, helps counter complex biological matrix effects. Consequently, this method offers a novel strategy for monitoring Pt (IV) PD activation in cancer therapies [28].

Besides application as drug delivery systems, CDs have also been shown to be potent candidates for tumor imaging because of their distinct enhanced fluorescence characteristics. However, due to the limited utility of small particles, researchers created a pH/reduction-sensitive PEGylated CD-DOX conjugate PD named DOX-Hy-CD-SS-PEG, containing 28.5% DOX. This PD, combining PEG and hydrophobic acid-labile DOX-conjugated CD, formed distinct 127-nm micelles. These exhibited minimal drug leakage (9% over 150 h) and efficient pH/reduction-triggered release. Additionally, DOX release and de-PEGylation restored CD luminescence, indicating the potential for monitoring treatment response in real time [57, 58] (Table 4.1).

4.3.5 Toxicity of CNMs

Cytotoxicity is essential to evaluate potential toxicity thoroughly when introducing foreign materials or compounds into living cells. The toxic effects of CNMs are significantly influenced by their structural characteristics, including their shape, dimensions, and surface modifications [2]. Cytotoxicity of pure graphene can be attributed to two of the signaling pathways, namely, the TGF-β signaling cascade and the MAPK signaling network, both of which play crucial roles in how cells respond to this nanomaterial. Both signaling pathways activate apoptosis in response to oxidative stress and upregulate pro-apoptotic proteins [61]. However, modifying graphene through functionalization, particularly by creating GO or treating GO with various hydrophilic macromolecules, can significantly reduce its toxic effects on cells [38]. Fullerenes and their derivatives can pose significant toxicity risks to biological systems when exposed to oxygen and light. This toxicity stems from their ability to generate reactive oxygen species (ROS) such as singlet oxygen, superoxide anion, and hydroxyl radicals. These ROS can cause severe damage to crucial biomolecules, including DNA, proteins, and lipids. The same photochemical mechanisms that make fullerenes potentially useful for photodynamic therapy (PDT) and as antibiotics or antivirals also raise concerns about their potential harm to healthy cells and tissues [111]. Research has shown that unmodified fullerenes generally exhibit higher cytotoxicity compared to those with covalent modifications, such as hydroxylated C60 (fullerenols) or methano-fullerenes [90].

The hazardous properties of fullerenes that have been non-covalently functionalized with particular capping agents can be attributed to the creation of a charge-transfer complex between the core and the solubilizing covering molecules of fullerene [103]. A great number of cell types, for instance, neuroblastoma cells, macrophages, keratinocytes, and rat pheochromocytoma PC-12 cells have been found to remain unaffected by NDs, as NDs cause cellular oxidative stress compared to CNMs [70]. The MTT assay was used to evaluate how exposure to both unmodified and carboxyl-functionalized nano-diamonds (NDs) affected the mitochondrial function of the cells. The findings revealed minimal impact on

Table 4.1 Role of carbon nanomaterials in drug delivery systems

CNM	Function	Drug	Activation mechanism	In vitro toxicity	Reference
CNT	Carrier	Platinum (IV)	Redox	Ishikawa endometrial adenocarcinoma cells	[18]
	Carrier, PDT action	Doxorubicin	Acidic pH	HeLa cells	[26]
	Carrier	Platinum (IV)	Redox	HeLa cells and RAW 264.7 murine macrophages	[77]
	Carrier	Platinum (IV)	Redox	A2780 and MCF-7 cells	[115]
	Carrier	Droxidopa	Molecular study	Molecular study	[117]
Fullerene	Carrier, PDT action	Doxorubicin	Acidic pH	HeLa, L929, and A549 cells	[26]
	PDT action	Photosensitizer prodrug	Acidic pH	KB cells	[51]
	Carrier	Paclitaxel	Esterase hydrolysis	Panc1 and AsPC1 cells	[69]
	Carrier, PDT action	5-ALA	Carbon-nitrogen lyases	MCF-7, HCT 116, and A549 cells	[92]
	Carrier	Warfarin	Plasma enzymatic complex	Mouse plasma	[118]
GO	Carrier, PTT action Carrier	Doxorubicin	Redox	MCF-7, B16, and A549 cells	[41]
	Carrier	Doxorubicin	Acidic pH	Hep G2 and Hep 1–6 cells	[40]
	Carrier	Podophyllotoxin	Redox	HeLa cells	[65]
	Carrier	Doxorubicin, platinum (IV)	Acidic pH	CAL-27 and MCF-7 cells	[84]
	Carrier	Temozolomide	Biological pH	B16F10 Melanoma cells	[101]
	Carrier	Quercetin and lurbinectedin	–	A549 lung cancer cells	[62]
ND	Carrier	Doxorubicin	Acidic pH	HeLa cells	[15]
	Carrier	Gemcitabine	Acidic pH	AsPC-1 cells	[56]
	Carrier	Platinum (IV)	Acidic pH	U87MG and HeLa cells	[121]
	Carrier	Gemcitabine	Cathepsin B	BxPC-3 cells	[114]
	Carrier	Methotrexate	Lysozyme	HeLa cells	[121]
	Carrier	Mitoxantrone and Doxorubicin	–	HepG2 cells	[21]

(continued)

Table 4.1 (continued)

CNM	Function	Drug	Activation mechanism	In vitro toxicity	Reference
CD	Block of nanosponge, imaging	Doxorubicin	Redox, acidic pH	Hep G2 cells	[16]
	Carrier	Methotrexate	pH 5.5	HeLa and L929 cells	[96]
	Imaging	Doxorubicin	Acidic pH	Hep G2 cells	[23]
	Carrier, imaging	Doxorubicin	Redox, acidic pH	Hep G2 cells	[57]
	Carrier, imaging	Doxorubicin	Acidic pH	Only pH 7.4 and 5 evaluated	[58]
	Carrier, PTT action	Platinum (IV)	Redox, acidic pH	A549 cells	[39]
	Imaging-guided drug delivery	Docetaxel	pH 6.5	HER2-positive breast cancer cells	[108]

mitochondrial activity, suggesting that NDs exhibit excellent biocompatibility and do not induce significant cytotoxic effects [91]. The pristine CNTs, like SWCNT and MWCNT are not suitable for interaction with biomolecules because they have a pronounced tendency to agglomerate and form bundles, producing significant cytotoxicity to alveolar macrophages exposed to the substance for just 6 h [43]. However, modifying the surface properties can substantially decrease the toxic effects observed in vitro [48]. In comparison to the CNTs, CDs may not even require any extra surface modification by capping agents to be harmless [100]. The small size, oxidized form, and great water solubility of bare CDs are attributed to their less hazardous nature to the cells as compared to the unfunctionalized pure graphene. CDs are found to be potent candidates for fluorescence imaging applications in comparison to semiconductor quantum dots due to their low toxicity and biocompatibility [4].

4.4 Conclusions and Future Prospects

The combination of PDs and carbon nanomaterial (CNM) delivery systems represents an exciting frontier in drug development. This synergistic approach leverages the strengths of both technologies to create targeted delivery capabilities of CNMs with the enhanced pharmacokinetics of PDs, potentially leading to more effective and less toxic therapies. This chapter has explored the recent progress in this rapidly evolving field. CNMs are like tiny, versatile building blocks that can be shaped and changed to do all sorts of things, including carrying medicine to exactly where it needs to go. When paired with PDs, which are like clever disguises for medicines, they can make treatments more effective and less harmful due to their unique physical and chemical properties. But CNMs can do even more than just deliver medicine. Some of them can also use light to heat up or destroy cancer cells, making them even more powerful tools for fighting disease. Their carbon-based structure can be readily modified to enhance biocompatibility, meaning they are well tolerated by the body, and they can be easily modified to improve their properties and functionality. This versatility could lead to more comprehensive and efficient treatment strategies. Among the various CNMs studied, carbon dots have shown exceptional potential in PD applications. However, it is important to note that much of the current research remains at the preclinical stage.

More studies on animals are needed to make sure these treatments are safe and effective before they can be used in people. As research in this field progresses, it is crucial to consider the broader implications of nanomaterial-based therapies. Developing robust health, safety, and environmental protocols for the production and use of CNMs will be essential. With all the initial toxicity studies having been conducted, more comprehensive data are needed to inform regulatory guidelines and ensure the responsible development of these technologies. For example, CNM-based PD delivery systems could be used to treat cancer, infectious diseases, and rare genetic disorders. By delivering drugs directly to the affected cells, these systems could reduce side effects and improve treatment outcomes. In conclusion, while challenges remain, CNM-based PD delivery systems offer a promising path forward in therapeutic innovation. By addressing current limitations and expanding in vivo research, these technologies have the potential to lead to transformative advances in personalized medicine and targeted therapies.

References

1. Aslam J, Hussain CM, Aslam R. Functionalized carbon nanotubes for biomedical applications. John Wiley & Sons; 2023.
2. Ayardulabi R, Khamespanah E, Abbasinia S, Ehtesabi H. Point-of-care applications of smartphone-based microscopy. Sensors and Actuators A: Physical. 2021;331:113048.
3. Azad LM, Ehtesabi H, Rezaei A. Smartphone-based fluorometer for pH detection using green synthesized carbon dots. Nano-Struct Nano-Objects. 2021;26:100722.
4. Baker SN, Baker GA. Luminescent carbon nanodots: emergent nanolights. Angew Chem Int Ed. 2010;49(38):6726–44.
5. Balasubramanian K, Burghard M. Biosensors based on carbon nanotubes. Anal Bioanal Chem. 2006;385(3):452–68.
6. Barhoum A, García-Betancourt ML. Physicochemical characterization of nanomaterials: size, morphology, optical, magnetic, and electrical properties. In: Emerging applications of nanoparticles and architecture nanostructures. Elsevier; 2018. p. 279–304.
7. Barhoum A, Shalan AE, El-Hout SI, Ali GA, Abdelbasir SM, Abu Serea ES, Ibrahim AH, Kaushik P, Shalan AE, El-Hout SI. A broad family of carbon nanomaterials: classification, properties, synthesis, and emerging applications. Handbook of nanofibers. 2019:1–40.
8. Bianco A, Kostarelos K, Prato M. Making carbon nanotubes biocompatible and biodegradable. Chem Commun. 2011;47(37):10182–8.
9. Bind A, Goswami L, Prakash V. Comparative analysis of floating and submerged macrophytes for heavy metal (copper, chromium, arsenic and lead) removal: sorbent preparation, characterization, regeneration and cost estimation. Geol Ecol Landsc. 2018;2(2):61–72.

10. Boncel S, Zając P, Koziol KK. Liberation of drugs from multi-wall carbon nanotube carriers. J Control Release. 2013;169(1–2):126–40.
11. Brindhadevi K, Garalleh HA, Alalawi A, Al-Sarayreh E, Pugazhendhi A. Carbon nanomaterials: types, synthesis strategies and their application as drug delivery system for cancer therapy. Biochem Eng J. 2023;192:108828.
12. Bu Y, Kushwaha A, Goswami L, Kim BS. Green production of functionalized few-layer graphene-silver nanocomposites using gallnut extract for antibacterial application. Micromachines. 2022;13(8):1232.
13. Chakroborty S, Sahoo SK. Carbon-based nanomaterials in drug delivery systems. In: Environmental applications of carbon nanomaterials-based devices. 2021. pp. 375–394.
14. Chaudhuri P, Harfouche R, Soni S, Hentschel DM, Sengupta S. Shape effect of carbon nanovectors on angiogenesis. ACS Nano. 2010;4(1):574–82.
15. Chen L, Li L. Aminocaproylated nanodiamond prodrug for tumor intracellular enhanced delivery of doxorubicin. J Drug Delivery Sci Technol. 2020;60:102017.
16. Chen W, Xie P, Pei M, Li G, Wang Z, Liu P. Facile construction of fluorescent traceable prodrug nanosponges for tumor intracellular pH/hypoxia dual-triggered drug delivery. Colloid Interface Sci Commun. 2022;46:100576.
17. Chien HT, Prior H, Andrews L, Van Aerts L, Cauvin A, Clarke DO, van Meer P. Re-evaluating the need for chronic toxicity studies with therapeutic monoclonal antibodies, using a weight of evidence approach. Regul Toxicol Pharmacol. 2023;138:105329.
18. Chin CF, Yap SQ, Li J, Pastorin G, Ang WH. Ratiometric delivery of cisplatin and doxorubicin using tumour-targeting carbon-nanotubes entrapping platinum (IV) prodrugs. Chem Sci. 2014;5(6):2265–70.
19. Chow EK, Zhang XQ, Chen M, Lam R, Robinson E, Huang H, Schaffer D, Osawa E, Ho D. Nanodiamond therapeutic delivery agents mediate enhanced chemoresistant tumor treatment. Sci Transl Med. 2011;3(73):73ra21-73ra21.
20. Chowdhury M, Kumar Das P. Paclitaxel-loaded biotinylated Fe2+-doped carbon dot: combination therapy in cancer treatment. ACS Appl Biol Mater. 2021;4(6):5132–44.
21. Cui J, Zhao W, Wu J, Zhang D, Liu L, Qiao H, et al. Enhanced in vivo antitumor efficacy through the nanodiamond mediated co-delivery of drugs. J Drug Delivery Sci Technol. 2023;88:104984.
22. Dhar S, Liu Z, Thomale J, Dai H, Lippard SJ. Targeted single-wall carbon nanotube-mediated Pt (IV) prodrug delivery using folate as a homing device. J Am Chem Soc. 2008;130(34):11467–76.
23. Dong Y, Du P, Liu P. Absolutely "off–on" fluorescent CD-based nanotheranostics for tumor intracellular real-time imaging and pH-triggered DOX delivery. J Mater Chem B. 2020;8(35):8002–9.
24. Ehtesabi H, Kalji SO. Recent advancements in 3D graphene for electrochemical sensors. In: 3D graphene: fundamentals, synthesis, and emerging applications. Springer Nature Switzerland: Cham; 2023. p. 75–91.
25. Ehtesabi H, Kalji SO, Ahadian MM. Carbon nanomaterials in prodrug-based therapeutics. J Drug Delivery Sci Technol. 2023;88:104930.
26. Fan J, Zeng F, Xu J, Wu S. Targeted anti-cancer prodrug based on carbon nanotube with photodynamic therapeutic effect and pH-triggered drug release. J Nanopart Res. 2013;15(9):1–15.
27. Feng T, Ai X, An G, Yang P, Zhao Y. Charge-convertible carbon dots for imaging-guided drug delivery with enhanced in vivo cancer therapeutic efficiency. ACS Nano. 2016;10(4):4410–20.
28. Feng T, Chua HJ, Zhao Y. Reduction-responsive carbon dots for real-time ratiometric monitoring of anticancer prodrug activation in living cells. ACS Biomater Sci Eng. 2017;3(8):1535–41.
29. Ghosal K, Ghosh A. Carbon dots: the next generation platform for biomedical applications. Mater Sci Eng C. 2019;96:887–903.
30. Gooding JJ. Nanostructuring electrodes with carbon nanotubes: a review on electrochemistry and applications for sensing. Electrochim Acta. 2005;50(15):3049–60.

31. Goswami L, Kushwaha,A, Goswami S, Sharma YC, Kim T, Tripathi KM. Nanocarbon-based-ZnO nanocomposites for supercapacitor application. In: Nanostructured zinc oxide. Elsevier, 2021. pp. 553–73.
32. Goswami L, Kushwaha A, Shabbir M, Dikshit PK, Oh S, Bhan U. Covalent organic frameworks (COFs) and COFs-based hybrid architectonics: a promising material platform for organic micropollutants detection and removal from wastewater. Coord Chem Rev. 2025;527:216398.
33. Goswami L, Kushwaha A, Singh A, Saha P, Choi Y, Maharana M, Kim BS. Nano-biochar as a sustainable catalyst for anaerobic digestion: a synergetic closed-loop approach. Catalysts. 2022b;12(2):186.
34. Goswami L, Manikandan NA, Dolman B, Pakshirajan K, Pugazhenthi G. Biological treatment of wastewater containing a mixture of polycyclic aromatic hydrocarbons using the oleaginous bacterium Rhodococcus opacus. J Clean Prod. 2018;196:1282–91.
35. Goswami L, Manikandan NA, Taube JCR, Pakshirajan K, Pugazhenthi G. Novel waste-derived biochar from biomass gasification effluent: preparation, characterization, cost estimation, and application in polycyclic aromatic hydrocarbon biodegradation and lipid accumulation by Rhodococcus opacus. Environ Sci Pollut Res. 2019;26:25154–66.
36. Goswami S, Kushwaha A, Goswami L, Gupta NR, Kumar V, Bhan U, Tripathi KM. Nanobiochar-a green catalyst for wastewater remediation. In: Bio-based nanomaterials. Elsevier; 2022a. p. 109–32.
37. Heister E, Brunner EW, Dieckmann GR, Jurewicz I, Dalton AB. Are carbon nanotubes a natural solution? Applications in biology and medicine. ACS Appl Mater Interfaces. 2013;5(6):1870–91.
38. Hong G, Diao S, Antaris AL, Dai H. Carbon nanomaterials for biological imaging and nanomedicinal therapy. Chem Rev. 2015;115(19):10816–906.
39. Hu Y, Zhang L, Chen S, Hou L, Zhao S, Huang Y, Liang H. Multifunctional carbon dots with near-infrared absorption and emission for targeted delivery of anticancer drugs, tumor tissue imaging and chemo/photothermal synergistic therapy. Nanosc Adv. 2021;3(24):6869–75.
40. Huang C, Hu X, Hou Z, Ji J, Li Z, Luan Y. Tailored graphene oxide-doxorubicin nanovehicles via near-infrared dye-lactobionic acid conjugates for chemo-photothermal therapy. J Colloid Interface Sci. 2019;545:172–83.
41. Huang C, Wu J, Jiang W, Liu R, Li Z, Luan Y. Amphiphilic prodrug-decorated graphene oxide as a multi-functional drug delivery system for efficient cancer therapy. Mater Sci Envg C. 2018;89:15–24.
42. Iijima S. Helical microtubules of graphitic carbon. Nature. 1991;354(6348):56–8.
43. Jia G, Wang H, Yan L, Wang X, Pei R, Yan T, Guo X. Cytotoxicity of carbon nanomaterials: single-wall nanotube, multi-wall nanotube, and fullerene. Environ Sci Technol. 2005;39(5):1378–83.
44. Jia X, Pei M, Zhao X, Tian K, Zhou T, Liu P. PEGylated oxidized alginate-DOX prodrug conjugate nanoparticles cross-linked with fluorescent carbon dots for tumor theranostics. ACS Biomater Sci Eng. 2016;2(9):1641–8.
45. Jing HH, Bardakci F, Akgöl S, Kusat K, Adnan M, Alam MJ, Sasidharan S. Green carbon dots: synthesis, characterization, properties and biomedical applications. J Func Biomater. 2023;14(1):27.
46. Kaliva M, Vamvakaki M. Nanomaterials characterization. In: Polymer science and nanotechnology. Elsevier; 2020. p. 401–33.
47. Kalji O, Sefidbakht Y, Nesterenko AM, Uskoković V, Ranaei-Siadat SO. Colloidal graphene oxide enhances the activity of a lipase and protects it from oxidative damage: insights from physicochemical and molecular dynamics investigations. J Colloid Interface Sci. 2020;567:285–99.
48. Kam NWS, Jessop TC, Wender PA, Dai H. Nanotube molecular transporters: internalization of carbon nanotube-protein conjugates into mammalian cells. J Am Chem Soc. 2004;126(22):6850–1.

49. Kam NWS, Liu Z, Dai H. Carbon nanotubes as intracellular transporters for proteins and DNA: an investigation of the uptake mechanism and pathway. Angew Chem Int Ed. 2006;45(4):577–81.
50. Katz E, Willner I. Biomolecule-functionalized carbon nanotubes: applications in nanobioelectronics. ChemPhysChem. 2004;5(8):1084–104.
51. Kim S, Lee DJ, Kwag DS, Lee UY, Youn YS, Lee ES. Acid pH-activated glycol chitosan/fullerene nanogels for efficient tumor therapy. Carbohydr Polym. 2014;101:692–8.
52. Kouznetsov VV. Exploring acetaminophen prodrugs and hybrids: a review. RSC Adv. 2024;14(14):9691–715.
53. Kroto HW, Heath JR, O'Brien SC, Curl RF, Smalley RE. C60: Buckminsterfullerene. Nature. 1985;318(6042):162–3.
54. Kushwaha A, Goswami L, Kim BS. Nanomaterial-based therapy for wound healing. Nanomaterials. 2022;12(4):618.
55. Kushwaha A, Goswami L, Kim BS. An integrated chemical and biological approach for poly (ethylene terephthalate) depolymerization and biopolyol production. ACS Sustain Chem Eng. 2024;12(32):11866–78.
56. Lai H, Lu M, Lu H, Stenzel MH, Xiao P. pH-Triggered release of gemcitabine from polymer coated nanodiamonds fabricated by RAFT polymerization and copper free click chemistry. Polym Chem. 2016;7(40):6220–30.
57. Li G, Pei M, Liu P. DOX-conjugated CQD-based nanosponges for tumor intracellular pH-triggered DOX release and imaging. Colloids Surf A Physicochem Eng Asp. 2020a;603:125258.
58. Li G, Pei M, Liu P. pH/Reduction dual-responsive comet-shaped PEGylated CQD-DOX conjugate prodrug: synthesis and self-assembly as tumor nanotheranostics. Mater Sci Eng C. 2020b;110:110653.
59. Li G, Pei M, Liu P. Facile fabrication of fluorescent traceable hybrid prodrug nanosponges for tumor intracellular pH-triggered DOX release. Colloids Surf A Physicochem Eng Asp. 2021;611:125807.
60. Li J, Lyv Z, Li Y, Liu H, Wang J, Zhan W, Li X. A theranostic prodrug delivery system based on Pt (IV) conjugated nano-graphene oxide with synergistic effect to enhance the therapeutic efficacy of Pt drug. Biomaterials. 2015;51:12–21.
61. Li Y, Liu Y, Fu Y, Wei T, Le Guyader L, Gao G, Chen C. The triggering of apoptosis in macrophages by pristine graphene through the MAPK and TGF-beta signaling pathways. Biomaterials. 2012;33(2):402–11.
62. Liao R, Zhang Y, Mao W. Functionalized graphene oxide NPs as a nanocarrier for drug delivery system in quercetin/lurbinectedin as dual sensitive therapeutics for A549 lung cancer treatment. Heliyon. 2024;10(11).
63. Liao Z, Zi Y, Zhou C, Zeng W, Luo W, Zeng H, Luo Z. Recent advances in the synthesis, characterization, and application of carbon nanomaterials for the removal of endocrine-disrupting chemicals: a review. Int J Mol Sci. 2022;23(21):13148.
64. Lin J, Huang Y, Huang P. Graphene-based nanomaterials in bioimaging. In: Biomedical applications of functionalized nanomaterials; 2018. p. 247–87.
65. Liu Y, Lv X, Xia S, Hao B, Huang X, Shi P. PEGylated graphene oxide as a nanocarrier of the disulfide prodrug of podophyllotoxin for cancer therapy. J Nanopart Res. 2020;22:1–13.
66. Lu F, Haque SA, Yang ST, Luo PG, Gu L, Kitaygorodskiy A, Sun YP. Aqueous compatible fullerene– doxorubicin conjugates. J Phys Chem C. 2009;113(41):17768–73.
67. Luo C, Sun J, Sun B, He Z. Prodrug-based nanoparticulate drug delivery strategies for cancer therapy. Trends Pharmacol Sci. 2014;35(11):556–66.
68. Ma N, Song A, Li Z, Luan Y. Redox-sensitive prodrug molecules meet graphene oxide: an efficient graphene oxide-based nanovehicle toward cancer therapy. ACS Biomater Sci Eng. 2019;5(3):1384–91.

69. Mackeyev Y, Raoof M, Cisneros B, Koshkina NSBC, Berger CS, Wilson LJ, Curley SA. Toward paclitaxel-[60] Fullerene immunoconjugates as a targeted prodrug against cancer. Наносистемы. 2014;5(1):67–75.
70. Manus LM, Mastarone DJ, Waters EA, Zhang XQ, Schultz-Sikma EA, MacRenaris KW, Meade TJ. Gd (III)-nanodiamond conjugates for MRI contrast enhancement. Nano Lett. 2010;10(2):484–9.
71. Markovic M, Ben-Shabat S, Keinan S, Aponick A, Zimmermann EM, Dahan A. Lipidic prodrug approach for improved oral drug delivery and therapy. Med Res Rev. 2019;39(2):579–607.
72. Mendes RG, Bachmatiuk A, Büchner B, Cuniberti G, Rümmeli MH. Carbon nanostructures as multi-functional drug delivery platforms. J Mater Chem B. 2013;1(4):401–28.
73. Mochalin V, Shenderova O, Ho D, Gogotsi Y. The properties and applications of nanodiamonds. In: Nano-enabled medical applications; 2020. p. 313–50.
74. Mostofizadeh A, Li Y, Song B, Huang Y. Synthesis, properties, and applications of low-dimensional carbon-related nanomaterials. J Nanomater. 2011;2011(1):685081.
75. Moore L, Gatica M, Kim H, Osawa E, Ho D. Multi-protein delivery by nanodiamonds promotes bone formation. Journal of dental research. 2013;92(11):976–81.
76. Mourdikoudis S, Pallares RM, Thanh NT. Characterization techniques for nanoparticles: comparison and complementarity upon studying nanoparticle properties. Nanoscale. 2018;10(27):12871–934.
77. Muzi L, Ménard-Moyon C, Russier J, Li J, Chin CF, Ang WH, Pastorin G, Risuleo G, Bianco A. Diameter-dependent release of a cisplatin pro-drug from small and large functionalized carbon nanotubes. Nanoscale. 2015;7(12):5383–94.
78. Naief MF, Mohammed SN, Mohammed AM. Carbon nanotubes: a review on synthesis and drug delivery for cancer treatment. Inorg Chem Commun. 2024;159:111694.
79. Najjar A, Karaman R. The prodrug approach in the era of drug design. Expert Opin Drug Deliv. 2019;16(1):1–5.
80. Novoselov KS, Geim AK, Morozov SV, Jiang D-e, Zhang Y, Dubonos SV, Grigorieva IV, Firsov AA. Electric field effect in atomically thin carbon films. Science. 2004;306(5696):666–9.
81. Owida HA, Turab NM, Al-Nabulsi J. Carbon nanomaterials advancements for biomedical applications. Bull Electr Eng Inform. 2023;12(2):891–901.
82. Pantarotto D, Briand JP, Prato M, Bianco A. Translocation of bioactive peptides across cell membranes by carbon nanotubes. Chem Commun. 2004;1:16–7.
83. Passaro A, Al Bakir M, Hamilton EG, Diehn M, André F, Roy-Chowdhuri S, Peters S. Cancer biomarkers: emerging trends and clinical implications for personalized treatment. Cell. 2024;187(7):1617–35.
84. Pei X, Zhu Z, Gan Z, Chen J, Zhang X, Cheng X, Wang J. PEGylated nano-graphene oxide as a nanocarrier for delivering mixed anticancer drugs to improve anticancer activity. Sci Rep. 2020;10(1):2717.
85. Rao N, Singh R, Bashambu L. Carbon-based nanomaterials: synthesis and prospective applications. Mater Today Proc. 2021;44:608–14.
86. Rezaei A, Ehtesabi H. Fabrication of alginate/chitosan nanocomposite sponges using green synthesized carbon dots as potential wound dressing. Mater Today Chem. 2022;24:100910.
87. Rozhin P, Abdel Monem Gamal J, Giordani S, Marchesan S. Carbon nanomaterials (CNMs) and enzymes: from nanozymes to cnm-enzyme conjugates and biodegradation. Materials. 2022;15(3):1037.
88. Ryplida B, Lee G, In I, Park SY. Zwitterionic carbon dot-encapsulating pH-responsive mesoporous silica nanoparticles for NIR light-triggered photothermal therapy through pH-controllable release. Biomater Sci. 2019;7(6):2600–10.
89. Saharan R, Paliwal SK, Tiwari A, Babu MA, Tiwari V, Singh R, et al. Beyond traditional hydrogels: the emergence of graphene oxide-based hydrogels in drug delivery. J Drug Delivery Sci Technol. 2024;94:105506.
90. Sayes CM, Gobin AM, Ausman KD, Mendez J, West JL, Colvin VL. Nano-C60 cytotoxicity is due to lipid peroxidation. Biomaterials. 2005;26(36):7587–95.

91. Schrand AM, Huang H, Carlson C, Schlager JJ, Ōsawa E, Hussain SM, Dai L. Are diamond nanoparticles cytotoxic? J Phys Chem B. 2007;111(1):2–7.
92. Serda M, Gawecki R, Dulski M, Sajewicz M, Talik E, Szubka M, Musioł R. Synthesis and applications of [60] fullerene nanoconjugate with 5-aminolevulinic acid and its glycoconjugate as drug delivery vehicles. RSC Adv. 2022;12(11):6377–88.
93. Shakiba-Marani R, Ehtesabi H. A flexible and hemostatic chitosan, polyvinyl alcohol, carbon dot nanocomposite sponge for wound dressing application. Int J Biol Macromol. 2023;224:831–9.
94. Shan X, Zhao Z, Wang C, Sun J, He Z, Luo C, Zhang S. Emerging prodrug-engineered nanomedicines for synergistic chemo-phototherapy. Chem Eng J. 2022;442:136383.
95. Shi L, Lin S, Zhou F, Jiang H, Zhang J. Recent advances in engineering prodrug-based nanomedicines for cancer therapy. Mater Adv. 2024;5:4634–59.
96. Singh H, Dhar D, Das S, Halder M. Methotrexate-loaded manganese nitrogen dual-doped carbon quantum dots as targeted nano drug-delivery system for potential use in cancer theranostics. J Photochem Photobiol A Chem. 2024;455:115692.
97. Smith AT, LaChance AM, Zeng S, Liu B, Sun L. Synthesis, properties, and applications of graphene oxide/reduced graphene oxide and their nanocomposites. Nano Mater Sci. 2019;1(1):31–47.
98. Speranza G. Carbon nanomaterials: synthesis, functionalization and sensing applications. Nanomaterials. 2021;11(4):967.
99. Sundar LS, Ashraf MW. Synthesis and characterization methods of graphene oxide nanomaterial for biomedical and toxicity applications: a comprehensive review. Inorg Chem Commun. 2025;174:113936.
100. Tao H, Yang K, Ma Z, Wan J, Zhang Y, Kang Z, Liu Z. In vivo NIR fluorescence imaging, biodistribution, and toxicology of photoluminescent carbon dots produced from carbon nanotubes and graphite. Small. 2012;8(2):281–90.
101. Torabi M, Yaghoobi F, Shervedani RK, Kefayat A, Ghahremani F, Harsini PR. Mn (II) & Gd (III) deferrioxamine complex contrast agents & temozolomide cancer prodrug immobilized on folic acid targeted graphene/polyacrylic acid nanocarrier: MRI efficiency, drug stability & interactions with cancer cells. Colloids Surf A Physicochem Eng Asp. 2022;652:129797.
102. Trojanowicz M. Analytical applications of carbon nanotubes: a review. TrAC Trends Anal Chem. 2006;25(5):480–9.
103. Ungurenasu C, Airinei A. Highly stable C60/poly (vinylpyrrolidone) charge-transfer complexes afford new predictions for biological applications of underivatized fullerenes. J Med Chem. 2000;43(16):3186–8.
104. Wang R, Lu KQ, Tang ZR, Xu YJ. Recent progress in carbon quantum dots: synthesis, properties and applications in photocatalysis. J Mater Chem A. 2017;5(8):3717–34.
105. Wang Z, Zhang Y, Yang X, Zhang T, Li Z, Zhong Y, Lu M. Genetic and molecular characterization of metabolic pathway-based clusters in esophageal squamous cell carcinoma. Sci Rep. 2024;14(1):6200.
106. Wong BS, Yoong SL, Jagusiak A, Panczyk T, Ho HK, Ang WH, Pastorin G. Carbon nanotubes for delivery of small molecule drugs. Adv Drug Deliv Rev. 2013;65(15):1964–2015.
107. Wu Y, Ermakova A, Liu W, Pramanik G, Vu TM, Kurz A, Weil T. Programmable biopolymers for advancing biomedical applications of fluorescent nanodiamonds. Adv Funct Mater. 2015;25(42):6576–85.
108. Xu D, Guo D, Zhang J, Tan X, Deng Z, Hou X, Wang S. Innovative tumor interstitial fluid-triggered carbon dot-docetaxel nanoassemblies for targeted drug delivery and imaging of HER2-positive breast cancer. Int J Pharm. 2024;657:124145.
109. Xu J, Chow EKH. Biomedical applications of nanodiamonds: from drug-delivery to diagnostics. SLAS Technol. 2023;28(4):214–22.
110. Xu X, Ray R, Gu Y, Ploehn HJ, Gearheart L, Raker K, Scrivens WA. Electrophoretic analysis and purification of fluorescent single-walled carbon nanotube fragments. J Am Chem Soc. 2004;126(40):12736–7.

111. Yamakoshi Y, Umezawa N, Ryu A, Arakane K, Miyata N, Goda Y, Nagano T. Active oxygen species generated from photoexcited fullerene (C60) as potential medicines: O2-• versus 1O2. J Am Chem Soc. 2003;125(42):12803–9.
112. Yang B, Gao J, Pei Q, Xu H, Yu H. Engineering prodrug nanomedicine for cancer immunotherapy. Adv Sci. 2020;7(23):2002365.
113. Yang W, Wei B, Yang Z, Sheng L. Facile synthesis of novel carbon-dots/hemin nanoplatforms for synergistic photo-thermal and photo-dynamic therapies. J Inorg Biochem. 2019;193:166–72.
114. Ye W, Han H, Li H, Jin Q, Wu Y, Chakrabortty S, Ji J. Polymer coated nanodiamonds as gemcitabine prodrug with enzymatic sensitivity for pancreatic cancer treatment. Progr Nat Sci. 2020;30(5):711–7.
115. Yoong SL, Wong BS, Zhou QL, Chin CF, Li J, Venkatesan T, Ho HK, Yu V, Ang WH, Pastorin G. Enhanced cytotoxicity to cancer cells by mitochondria-targeting MWCNTs containing platinum (IV) prodrug of cisplatin. Biomaterials. 2014;35(2):748–59.
116. Yoosefian M, Etminan N. The role of solvent polarity in the electronic properties, stability and reactivity trend of a tryptophane/Pd doped SWCNT novel nanobiosensor from polar protic to non-polar solvents. RSC Adv. 2016;6(69):64818–25.
117. Yoosefian M, Jahani M. A molecular study on drug delivery system based on carbon nanotube for the novel norepinephrine prodrug, Droxidopa. J Mol Liq. 2019;284:258–64.
118. Zacchigna M, Klumpp C, Prato M, Bianco A. In vitro behavior of multifunctionalized fullerene-warfarin conjugates. J Nanosci Nanotechnol. 2009;9(10):6210–21.
119. Zhang Q, Mochalin VN, Neitzel I, Hazeli K, Niu J, Kontsos A, Zhang GJ, Pete IL, Gogotsi Y. Mechanical properties and biomineralization of multifunctional nanodiamond-PLLA composites for bone tissue engineering. Biomaterials. 2012;33(20):5067–75.
120. Zhao J, Lai H, Lu H, Barner-Kowollik C, Stenzel MH, Xiao P. Fructose-coated nanodiamonds: promising platforms for treatment of human breast cancer. Biomacromolecules. 2016;17(9):2946–55.
121. Zhao L, Xu YH, Qin H, Abe S, Akasaka T, Chano T, Chen X. Platinum on nanodiamond: a promising prodrug conjugated with stealth polyglycerol, targeting peptide and acid-responsive antitumor drug. Adv Funct Mater. 2014;24(34):5348–57.
122. Zhao W, Wei S, Zhao H, Li Y, Wu R, Wang J. Enhanced anticancer activity of an intracellularly activatable nanomedicine based on GLYlated nanodiamond. Diam Relat Mater. 2017;77:171–80.

Chapter 5
Smart and Sustainable Nanomaterials for Digital Healthcare: Application in Drug Delivery

Richa Pal, Rajesh Kumar, Trishant Kumar, Danveer Singh, and Kishant Kumar

Abstract Nanomaterials have revolutionized drug delivery, boosting therapeutic outcomes and reducing potential negative effects. Their distinctive characteristics, for instance, an extensive surface area, biocompatibility, and the capacity to tailor surface characteristics, enable precise and regulated drug delivery. Diverse nanomaterials like liposomes, dendrimers, nanotubes, and nanoparticles are engineered to enclose drugs, boosting their solubility and ensuring greater stability. Nanocarriers are tailored to activate in response to specific factors like pH variations, temperature, and electromagnetic signals, ensuring controlled drug release precisely at the target site. Furthermore, altering surface properties allows for active targeting of affected tissues, promoting cancer cell uptake while minimizing impact on healthy cells. Clinical research has highlighted the promise of nanomaterials for administering chemotherapeutic agents, biologics, and vaccines, offering a pathway to more efficient treatment strategies. This chapter summarizes the recent advancements and key developments, current obstacles, and potential future perspectives in utilizing nanomaterials for drug delivery applications, emphasizing their role in personalized medicine.

R. Pal · K. Kumar (✉)
Department of Chemical Engineering, Indian Institute of Technology Ropar, Ropar, India
e-mail: richa.23chz0016@iitrpr.ac.in; kishant@iitrpr.ac.in

R. Kumar
Department of Bio-Medical Engineering, Indian Institute of Technology, Ropar, India
e-mail: rajeshkumar@iitrpr.ac.in

T. Kumar
Department of Anaesthesiology & Critical Care Medicine, Patna Medical College & Hospital, Patna, India

Department of Anesthesia & Critical Care, Advanced Neuro Hospital, Patna, India

D. Singh
Department of Physics, Indian Institute of Technology Ropar, Ropar, India
e-mail: danveer.singh@iitrpr.ac.in

S. Mondal et al. (eds.), *Smart and Sustainable Nanomaterials in Digital Healthcare and Theranostic*, https://doi.org/10.1007/978-981-95-9386-6_5

Keywords Drug delivery · Nanomaterials · Nanoparticles · Stimuli-responsive · Cancer cells · Tumor

5.1 Introduction

Imagine a world where medicine knows exactly where to go in your body, only releases when and where it is needed, and adjusts the dose in real time based on your body's requirements. This is no longer a far-off dream but a reality made possible by smart and sustainable nanomaterials advances. As digital technology and healthcare come together, these innovative materials transform drug delivery, providing unmatched accuracy, efficiency, and personalized care. Targeted and regulated drug delivery is crucial as precision medicine becomes more important in modern healthcare. Drug delivery systems (DDSs) can significantly improve the pharmacological effects of generic and patented medications. DDSs can be efficiently implemented to cure several diseases that are almost impossible to cure using free drug intake due to its associated side effects. The targeted DDSs are proven to be effective because of their direct impact on the targeted tissues by controlled release of the drug molecules at the affected location. Traditional DDSs frequently result in unwanted side effects because they release drugs in an uncontrolled way and affect parts of the body not intended for treatment. In response to these challenges, innovative DDSs have been created to deliver medications directly to the intended site of action with high precision. In contrast to traditional systems, these advanced drug delivery methods minimize the frequency of administration and maintain a consistent drug level at the target site. This approach helps to minimize drug side effects that reduce fluctuations in drug levels and improve the overall effectiveness of the treatment [1]. Nanomaterials offer exciting advantages and new possibilities for smart DDSs. They are gaining attention due to their distinct nanoscale characteristics and specialized capabilities. For example, DDSs based on nanoparticles (NPs) can target and attach to disease sites more precisely and release drugs in a controlled way. Recent research has explored and highlighted several new ways to use these nanomaterials as smart drug carriers [2]. NPs are tiny solid particles made from larger molecules with sizes varying between 10 and 1000 nm. It is generally thought that NPs with diameters less than 100 nm in size are considered optimal for directing drugs to specific sites. They are stable in the bloodstream and can easily pass through small capillaries and are effective at crossing biological barriers [3]. They are utilized in medical applications because of their distinctive properties, which include a high surface area and customized pore structures that facilitate improved drug loading. NPs as drug delivery carriers should possess the following features: (i) size can easily be tuned to maintain the permeation barrier and retention rate, (ii) release kinetics, (iii) lipophilic drug molecules can be incorporated noncovalently, (iv) stable encapsulation of drug molecule to prevent it from premature release, (v) stimuli-responsive, and (vi) enhanced biocompatibility [4].

The term "smart material" (also known as "active," "adaptive," or "stimuli-responsive" material) describes a material that can swiftly and reversibly modify specific properties and activate certain functions in response to external stimuli [5]. Smart nanomaterials in DDS are designed so that drugs are not released until they reach the target-specific tissues or organs, releasing their contents only at the appropriate time and location. These advanced nanoplatforms are carefully designed to release the drugs precisely at the intended location in the body after they are administered.

Smart NPs are promising for targeted drug delivery, especially for compounds that do not dissolve well in water. They are also useful in combined cancer diagnosis and treatment systems known as theranostics [6]. They can evade the body's defense system (the reticuloendothelial system) [7] and cross the blood-brain barrier (BBB) [8], offering new possibilities for treating brain-related conditions. NPs have greatly improved drug delivery, especially with the development of liposomal-doxorubicin [9] and paclitaxel-albumin [10, 11] NPs. These early nanomedicines made it easier to deliver drugs like antibiotics and cancer treatments more effectively [12]. Initially, they were simple carriers such as liposomes that helped drugs spread more evenly. Over time, scientists have made these nanomedicines more advanced by adding special targeting features that help the drugs work better and reduce side effects [13]. In recent years, drug delivery NPs have greatly improved, making it easier to treat challenging diseases. These advanced NPs are specially designed to work in the challenging environment of tumors. For example, some NPs release drugs specifically when they encounter acidic conditions inside a tumor. Others shrink to penetrate deep into the tumor or are made larger to stay longer in the tumor. These improved NPs help deliver drugs more effectively and make treatments work better than before [14]. Stimuli-responsive smart nanomaterials (SNMs) alter their characteristics when exposed to environmental factors such as light, pH variations, temperature, ultrasound, magnetic field, electric field, and enzymatic activity. These changes can be reversible or irreversible, affecting their physical or chemical structure. Various types of SNMs have been developed including those made from magnetic, polymer, hydrogel, and metal-doped NPs, and they show great potential in the pharmaceutical field.

In this chapter, we explore the latest developments in nanomaterials for drug delivery, highlighting their innovative designs and applications. We cover a range of materials including liposomes, lipid NPs, metal-organic frameworks (MOFs), dendrimers, nanogels, chitosan, and carbon-based nanomaterials. Each offers distinct benefits for drug delivery: liposomes and lipid NPs improve drug solubility and targeting, MOFs provide high surface areas for drug loading, dendrimers offer precise drug attachment, nanogels adjust volume in response to environmental changes, and chitosan and carbon-based materials enhance biocompatibility. We then explore how these materials can be designed to react to different external triggers, including temperature, light, ultrasound, electric and magnetic fields, allowing for targeted drug release. Additionally, we examine the role of internal factors like pH and enzymatic activity in enhancing the precision of DDSs.

5.2 Nanoparticles for Drug Delivery Systems

In recent years, NPs have shown interest in DDS to overcome the existing limitations of direct drug intake. Several families of nanomaterials, such as liposomes, lipid NPs, MOFs, dendrimers, nanogels, chitosans, and carbon-based 2D and 3D materials, have been extensively explored in recent decades for their potential role as carriers in drug delivery systems. In this section, the mechanism of drug delivery through the use of potential NPs will be discussed in detail. In addition, the recent breakthroughs in these NPs for DDS will also be discussed in detail.

5.2.1 Liposome Nanoparticles

Liposomes are a class of phospholipid vesicles formed by concentric bilayers or multilamellar structures enclosing an aqueous environment. The size of such liposomes can range from 20 nm to a few micrometers depending on the thickness of the concentric phospholipid bilayer [15]. It has been investigated as a drug carrier particle for more than five decades due to its biocompatible nature. Liposomal-based DDS have been approved for clinical use because of their remarkable properties, such as high loading of hydrophobic and hydrophilic drugs in the bilayer and core of the liposome, respectively, as shown in Fig. 5.1. The phospholipid has a tail and head group that are assembled in such a manner that it helps to bind hydrophilic and hydrophobic drug molecules [16].

The basic component in the cell membrane is lipid, and therefore it eliminates the risk of toxicity in the body when used as a drug carrier. Despite its remarkable and fascinating properties toward the use as a drug carrier particle, it possesses some challenges when *administering* drug molecules at the targeted tissues. The main challenges were observed in the controlled and prolonged release of the drug molecule because of the limiting diffusion rate of the drug molecule across the phospholipid bilayer, which is a highly viscous region compared to the hydrophilic core of the liposome [18]. Therefore, several efforts are being made to improve the overall assembly of synthetic lipids by modifying the chemical environment of headgroups, hydrophobic and hydrophilic domains, and linkers to optimize the inter- and intramolecular forces, size, and diffusion of the drug across the phospholipid assembly. The design of a liposome for drug delivery application is mainly governed by the physical and chemical intuitions of lipid particles and their associated phase transition temperature (T_c). Physical and chemical intuitions include the size of the tail group and the chemical building blocks of head and tail groups, respectively, which can be tailored to achieve the target properties of liposomes. The value of T_c for any lipids governs the fluidity of the tail group and, hence, the overall liposome particle. Temperatures higher than T_c show a more diffusive nature of the liposome compared to that observed below T_c. Therefore, phase transition temperature is crucial for the movement and distribution of the liposome as a drug carrier in the body.

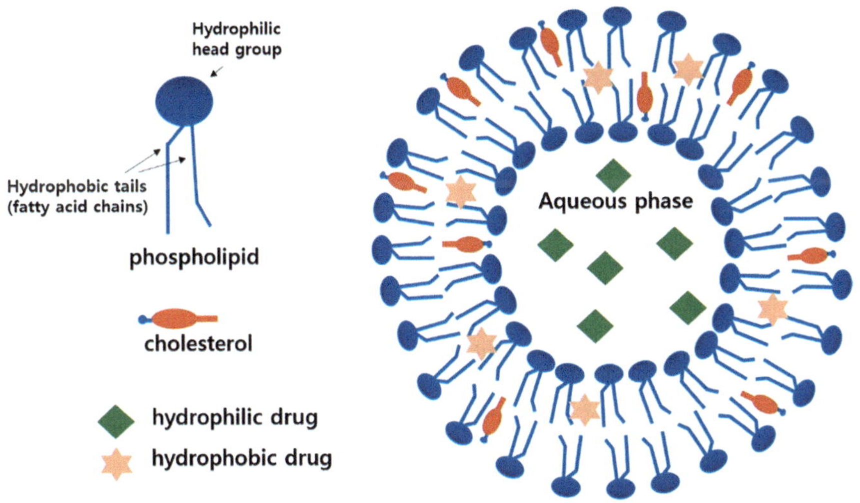

Fig. 5.1 Schematic of conventional liposome incorporating hydrophilic and hydrophobic drugs. (Reproduced with permission from ref. [17]. Copyright 2020, Multidisciplinary Digital Publishing Institute)

5.2.2 Lipid Nanoparticles (LNPs)

Lipid nanoparticles (LNPs) are versatile nanocarriers widely used in biomedical and pharmacological studies due to their capacity to encapsulate a variety of therapeutic substances, including small molecules, nucleic acids, and monoclonal antibodies. These nanocarriers enhance the solubility, targeted delivery, and distribution of drugs, effectively addressing common challenges such as drug inefficiency, enzymatic degradation, low bioavailability, and unintended effects. LNPs are designed to mimic cell membranes, allowing them to easily cross cellular barriers and deliver their therapeutic payloads directly into cells. LNPs are categorized according to the arrangement of core shells as shown in Fig. 5.2.

Cell membrane like LNPs biomimetic architecture can easily pass the cell membrane and transfer nanoparticle contents to internal regions. There are five primary types of LNPs, each with distinct structural features and applications. Liposomes, discovered in 1965, are nanosized lipid vesicles with concentric phospholipid bilayers. These structures are capable of enclosing hydrophilic drugs in their aqueous center and hydrophobic drugs within the lipid layers. Nanoemulsions consist of spherical droplets typically 50 to 500 nanometers in size and can be formulated as oil-in-water or water-in-oil droplets, making them suitable for delivering both hydrophobic and hydrophilic substances. These are often stabilized by surfactants or polymers and are particularly useful for topical drug delivery as shown in Fig. 5.2a, b. Solid lipid NPs (SLNs) are initially spherical particles featuring a solid lipid core that have evolved into various shapes, such as ellipsoids or discs, with the

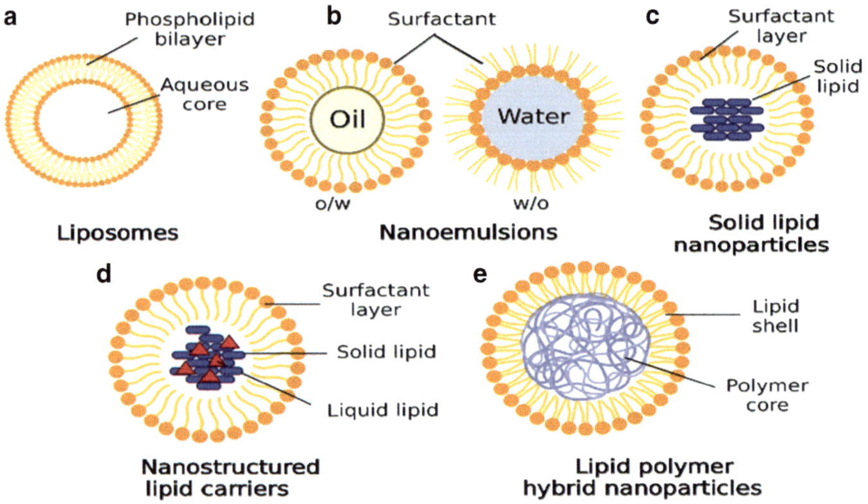

Fig. 5.2 A schematic representation displays various lipid nanoparticle (LNP) formations employed for transporting drugs. (**a**) Liposomes are microscopic spherical structures formed by phospholipid bilayers, capable of entrapping water-soluble materials in their inner core while sequestering fat-soluble molecules within the lipid bilayer. (**b**) Assembly of surfactant molecules in a nanoemulsion facilitates the oil phase in the aqueous medium, while the aqueous phase in the oil medium handles lipophilic and hydrophilic drug molecules, respectively. (**c**) Solid lipid NPs (SLNs) facilitate the encapsulation of hydrophobic drugs within their lipid core. (**d**) Nanostructured lipid carriers (NLCs) are cutting-edge systems that resemble solid lipid NPs (SLNs) but incorporate both rigid and fluid lipids, enhancing stability and increasing capacity for drug loading. (**e**) Lipid-based polymer composite NPs integrate lipid and polymer elements, combining the advantages of each. This combination improves drug encapsulation, enhances stability, and allows for controlled drug release. Every formulation variant delivers exceptional benefits and can be designed for accurate drug targeting, making it suitable for a diverse array of therapeutic substances. (Reproduced with permission from Ref. [19]. Copyright 2023, American Chemical Society)

ability to carry active ingredients in different parts of the nanoparticle. The use of cationic lipids in SLNs enhances their stability, targeting abilities, and effectiveness in delivering drugs across challenging barriers like the blood-brain barrier. Nanostructured lipid carriers (NLCs) represent an advanced form of SLNs, featuring a core composed of both solid and liquid lipids that creates a more disordered structure. This design increases drug-loading capacity and improves the control of drug release. NLCs can be further modified with ligands or polymers to achieve targeted drug delivery as shown in Fig. 5.2c, d. These NPs integrate the advantageous properties of lipids and polymers, offering a unique combination of benefits. These NPs have a drug-loaded polymer core encased in a lipid or lipid-PEG shell. This configuration enhances their biocompatibility and stability, making them well suited for sustained drug release and improved stability within the body [19] as shown in Fig. 5.2e.

The presence of the blood-brain barrier (BBB) makes the detection and cure of glioblastoma multiforme (GBM) difficult compared to extracranial tumors [21]. Temozolomide (TMZ) is considered a first-line drug against GBM. However, TMZ faces several challenges and limitations, such as fast degradation, limited solubility in serum, and limited solubility, resulting in poor efficacy against GBM. To overcome these shortcomings, pro-apoptotic peptides (PAPs) maybe used as a co-compound in DDS because they may facilitate the consumption of energy to destroy the mitochondria, leaving less energy available for the repair of the DNA. Unfortunately, PAP that cannot enter the brain tumor through the BBB makes DDS less feasible. Excipients such as 1, 2-distearoyl-sn-glycero-3-phosphoethanolamine polyethylene-glycol (DSPE-PEG2000-MA), cholesterol, and soy L-α-phosphatidylcholine (soy-PC) may be used to participate in the self-assembly of a liposome nanoparticle, making it easier for diffusion into the BBB. In this regard, the liposome, TMZ, PAP, and glucose surface were self-assembled to form Glucose-Liposome@TMZ&PAP (gLTP) as shown in Fig. 5.3a.

Zhang et al. [20] studied and demonstrated the synergistic effect of liposome NPs embedded with the TMZ, PAP, and glucose surface to target the GBM tumor. Administration of gLTP explores its effects in the GBM-bearing mice model. In the brain, glucose is essential for energy production facilitated primarily by the glucose transporter GLUT-1. This transporter allows glucose to enter the brain through endothelial cells and is found predominantly in glial cells, where it binds to glucose ligands on the surface. This interaction facilitates the delivery of liposomes across the blood-brain barrier (BBB). Once they enter the brain, the liposomes are directed toward acidic environments, such as those found in lysosomes. The acidic pH within the lysosomes causes the gLTP liposomes to release their contents: PAP and TMZ. PAP disrupts mitochondrial function, impairs DNA repair, and reduces ATP levels in GBM cells, making it harder for the tumor cells to survive. Meanwhile, TMZ targets the cell nucleus and interferes with DNA replication. PAP and TMZ work together to stop tumors from growing, effectively depicted in Fig. 5.3b.

5.2.2.1 In Vivo Analysis of gLTP Effects on GBM Mice

In the in vivo evaluation, both standard liposomes (LR) and glucose-functionalized liposomes (gLR) were injected into mice with subcutaneous glioblastoma (GBM) tumors using live imaging to track the liposomes. Both types of liposomes effectively targeted the tumors, with the highest concentration observed 24 hours after injection. After this peak, the amount of liposomes in the tumor gradually decreased. The mice were sacrificed after 48 hours, and their organs were retrieved for additional imaging analysis as shown in Fig. 5.4a, b.

Both LR and gLR mostly accumulated in the tumor with little distribution to other organs, which suggests that these liposomal formulations can effectively deliver their contents directly to the tumor, making them a promising option for brain tumor treatment. To test the antitumor effects, we created several glucose-modified liposomal formulations: gLT, gLP, gLTP, phosphate-buffered saline (PBS)

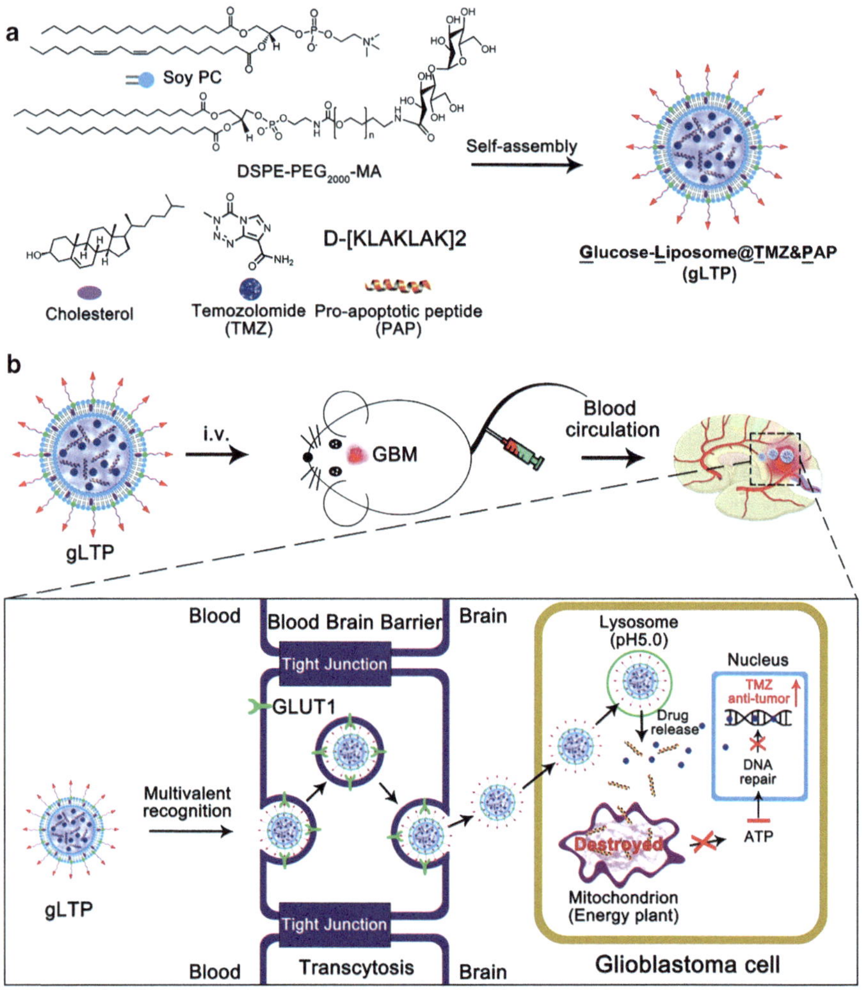

Fig. 5.3 A diagrammatic representation illustrating gLTP for GBM therapy. (**a**) Formation of glucose-liposome@TMZ&PAP through self-assembly. (**b**) Intravenous administration of gLTP into GBM-bearing mice leads to its transportation to the brain via the bloodstream. The glucose-based surface multivalent recognition of GLUT1 enables the liposome to cross the blood-brain barrier. In the low pH conditions of the microenvironment, TMZ and PAP are released in lysosomes. PAP disrupts mitochondrial function and depletes ATP production, impairing energy-dependent DNA repair mechanisms and enhancing TMZ's chemotherapeutic efficacy against GBM. (Adapted with permission from Ref. [20]. Copyright 2022, Royal Society of Chemistry)

solution, and a free drug mixture as control treatments, as shown in Fig. 5.4c, d. The mice received these formulations every 4 days with a total of 7 doses, and tumor growth was monitored periodically as shown in Fig. 5.4e. The results showed that tumors in mice treated with PBS grew quickly, indicating the aggressive nature of GBM. The free drug mixture had only a small impact on slowing down the tumor.

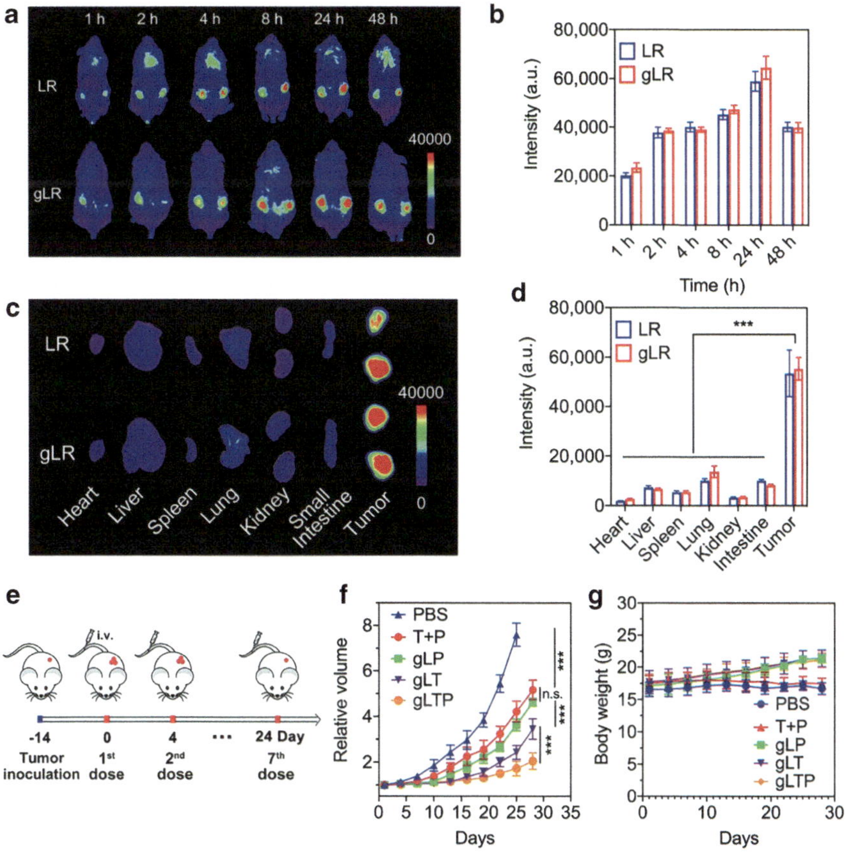

Fig. 5.4 In vivo evaluation of gLTP in mice bearing GBM. (**a**) Tumor accumulation of liposomes over time in mice with GBM. (**b**) Analysis of tumor growth corresponding to (**a**). (**c**) Ex vivo localization of liposomes within mice bearing GBM; (**d**) organ distribution assessed from the data in (**b**). (**e**) Animal treatment and a schematic illustration. Every 4 days, gLTP and control materials were delivered intravenously. (**f**) The gLTP and control groups showed antitumor effects on GBM-bearing mice. (**g**) Monitoring of body weight changes in treated versus control groups, with measurements of tumor volume and body mass, was recorded at 3-day intervals. Statistical analysis was performed, with n.s. indicating no significant difference; ***, $p < 0.001$. (Adapted with permission from Ref. [20]. Copyright 2022, Royal Society of Chemistry)

The gLP formulation was about the same as the free drug mixture but gLT worked better. The gLTP formulation, which combined TMZ and PAP, was the best at shrinking the tumors, as shown in Fig. 5.4f. Mice treated with the liposomal formulations did not lose weight, suggesting that the treatments were safe and had no harmful side effects. Overall, gLTP proved to be a promising option for treating brain tumors, as illustrated in Fig. 5.4g.

5.2.3 Metal-Organic Frameworks (MOFs)

Metal-organic frameworks (MOFs) represent a class of microporous polymer material that consists of metal clusters linked to organic ligands to develop a decorated one-, two-, or three-dimensional periodic structure. It possesses high surface area/volume ratios, excellent porosity, tunable pore size (diameter <2 nm), easy diffusion of small molecules within the pores through available windows, etc. MOFs have been designed and synthesized for application in gas storage and separation, sensing, water harvesting, biomedical industries, etc., [22] due to their high specific surface area (1000–8000 m^2/gm) [23] because of their tunable pore size, pore window, organic ligands, and inorganic cluster, they were observed to be emerging and promising candidates as drug carriers. Interestingly, the synthesis of uniform-size NPs is challenging for biomedical applications, which opens a window to introduce MOFs. NPs of the MOFs can be easily synthesized in varying sizes and shapes in a controlled manner.

Metal-organic frameworks (MOFs) are classified into four primary structural levels [24]. At their core, MOFs consist of metal ions or clusters connected to organic linkers, which commonly include functional groups like carboxyl or amine. These components form a crystal-like lattice with a regular repeating pattern. The second level involves secondary building units (SBUs) where multiple ligands coordinate with a metal ion to create structures that serve as templates for forming the MOF framework. The third level defines the internal structure where ligands connect these SBUs to create pores and cavities within the framework. This arrangement depends on the specific metal ions and ligands used. Finally, the fourth level encompasses the overall growth of the MOF framework and the encapsulation of molecules within it. MOFs are highly advantageous for drug delivery applications owing to their coordinatively unsaturated metal centers that function as Lewis acids, enabling efficient loading and controlled release of therapeutic agents as illustrated in Fig. 5.5a.

Visual representations of various MOF structures that highlight the metal ions (such as Zr, Fe, Cr, Zn, Mg, and Cu) and organic linkers that make up the framework are necessary to synthesize and describe the MOFs. The color-coded graphics (Zr: green, Fe: yellow, etc.) make it easier to understand how these components are organized, which contributes to our understanding of the chemistry and structure of MOFs [25]. These are crucial for their use in areas like drug delivery and catalysis, as depicted in Fig. 5.5b. MOF@lipid NPs are well absorbed by cancer cells, making them ideal for drug delivery and diagnostics. These NPs made from mesoporous iron (III) and chromium (III) carboxylates (i.e., MIL-100 (Fe) and MIL-101 (Cr), respectively) are enclosed within a lipid membrane layer [26]. The coating process involves controlled solvent exchange, forming a lipid layer on the MOF surface. This lipid bilayer not only encapsulates compounds within the MOF scaffold, preventing premature release, but also enhances the stability and absorption of the NPs by cancer cells, making them suitable for delivering therapeutic agents as depicted in Fig. 5.5c.

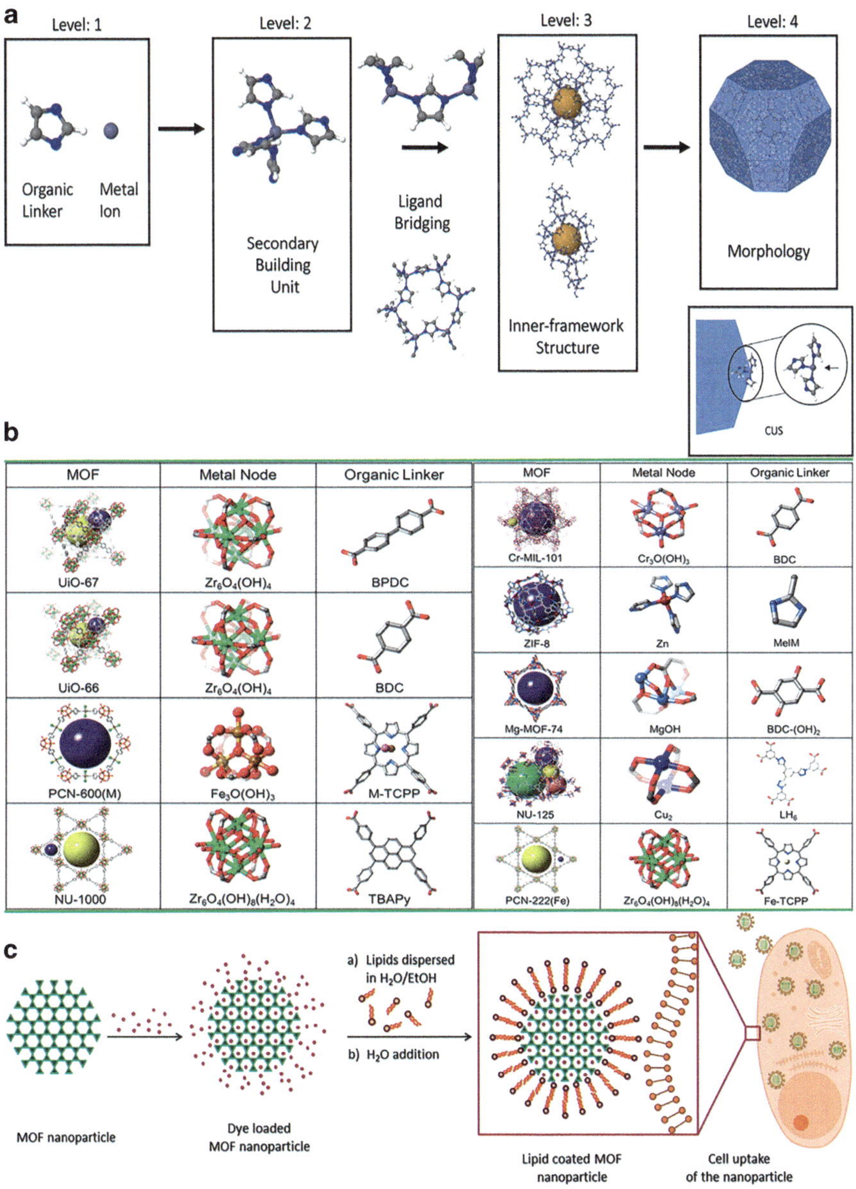

Fig. 5.5 (**a**) MOF structures can be analyzed at various structural and compositional levels: level 1 involves the linker and node, level 2 centers on the secondary building unit (SBU) and the coordination unsaturated site (CUS), level 3 relates to the underlying structural framework, and level 4 considers the overall morphology. (**b**) Illustrations of MOF structures, along with their associated node and linker components, are presented. The color representation includes Fe as yellow, Zr as green, Mg as blue, Cu as royal blue, C as grey, O as red, N as light blue, Cl as pink, and Zn as dark red. (**c**) A schematic diagram illustrates the creation of lipid bilayer-coated MOFs, NPs functionalized with dyes, and their absorption by cancer cells. (Adapted with permission from Ref. [24–26]. Copyright 2021, American Chemical Society(**a**); Copyright 2017, American Chemical Society(**b**); and Copyright 2015, Royal Society of Chemistry(c), respectively)

Fang et al. [27] prepared gold nanorods (Au-NRs) through a seed-mediated growth technique and modified them with specific functions with an aptamer to conjugate the DOX molecule. Thereafter, the functionalized nanorods loaded with drug molecules were impregnated in the synthesized ZIF-8. MOF was renamed as DOX-loaded Au-Aptamer@ZIF-8 NPs, and pathways can be seen in Fig. 5.6a. The detailed mechanism of photothermal-assisted drug delivery and cell apoptosis is illustrated in Fig. 5.6b. The drug release rate was determined under varying pH conditions to replicate the actual conditions of different organs of the body: cumulative release of DOX in artificially simulated blood (pH = 7.4), gastrointestinal fluid (pH = 6.5), tumor (pH = 4.5), and gastric fluid (pH = 1.2). The cumulative release rate of the drug after 24 hours and 48 hours of incubation varies depending on the pH level. After 48 hours, the release stabilizes with cumulative release rates of approximately 10.34, 15.86, 54.58, and 60.44% at different pH levels of 7.4, 6.5, 4.5, and 1.2, respectively. This indicates that drug release increases as the pH decreases, suggesting that DOX-loaded Au-Aptamer@ZIF-8 NPs are capable of releasing DOX effectively in the acidic environment of tumor cells

To evaluate the cellular uptake assay and to check if DOX-loaded Au-Aptamer@ ZIF-8 NPs target tumors effectively, fluorescence images were taken at different time intervals. Fluorescence images confirm that the NPs loaded with DOX molecules were efficiently internalized by MCF-7 cells after 2 hours of treatment. The

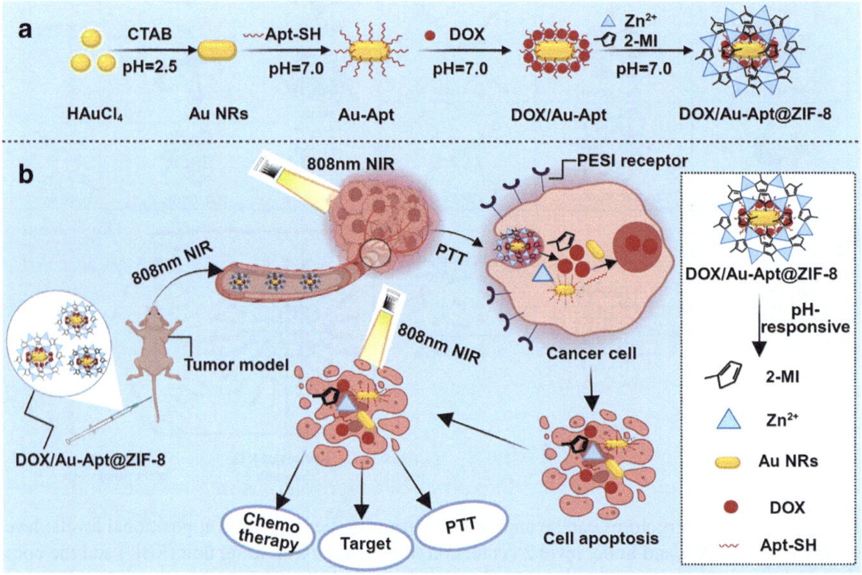

Fig. 5.6 Synthesis and working principle of DOX-loaded Au-Aptamer@ZIF-8 NPs (**a**) A diagrammatic depiction of the fabrication of DOX-loaded Au-Aptamer@ZIF-8 NPs (**b**) DOX-loaded Au-Aptamer@ZIF-8 NPs therapeutic mechanisms in the development of a tailored Nano-DDS and the multifaceted combination of chemotherapy and targeted PTT for antitumor applications. (Adapted with permission from Ref. [27]. Copyright 2024, American Chemical Society)

DOX-loaded Au-Aptamer@ZIF-8 NPs group showed stronger fluorescence compared to the DOX alone group with the red fluorescence mostly around the nucleus and nearby area (see Fig. 5.7a). After 6 hours of treatment of cancer cells, fluorescence images showed that DOX-loaded Au-Aptamer@ZIF-8 NPs delivered DOX into the cells more effectively and had a good ability to target tumor cells. Additionally, flow cytometry measured the mean fluorescence intensity in MCF-7 cells treated with DOX-loaded Au-Aptamer@ZIF-8 NPs over different times (0, 2, 6, and 12 hours).

As the treatment time increased, the mean fluorescence intensity of the cells also increased, as shown in Figs. 5.7b, c. This indicates that MCF7 cells absorbed DOX-loaded Au-Aptamer@ZIF-8 NPs more effectively over time with greater fluorescence intensity, suggesting more drugs were taken up by the cells.

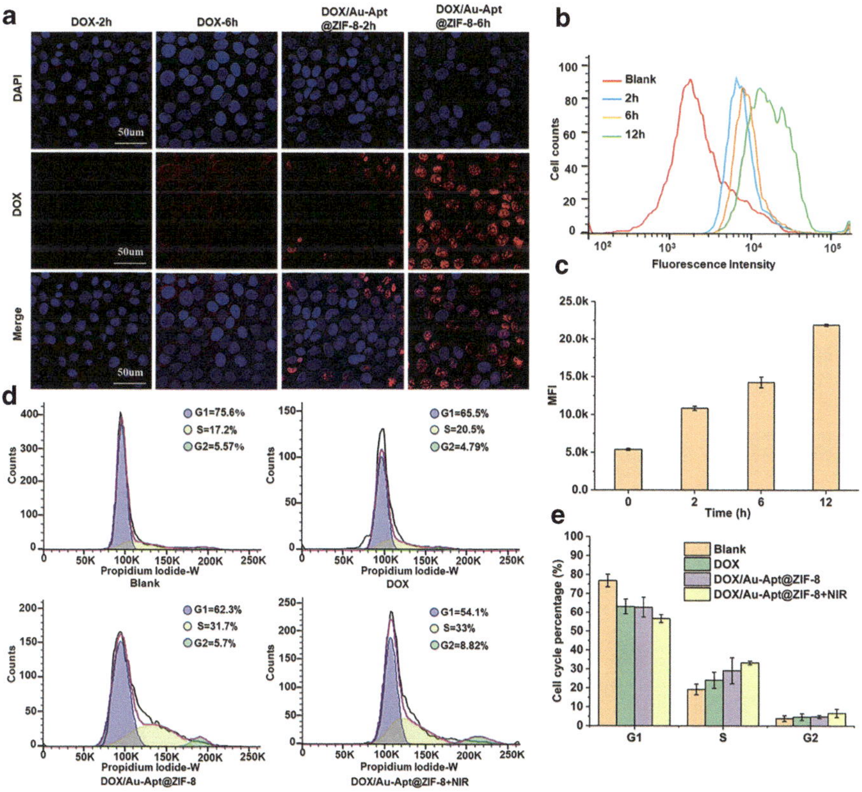

Fig. 5.7 (**a**) Images of DOX and DOX-loaded Au-Aptamer@ZIF-8 NPs were obtained using confocal laser microscopy. (**b, c**) Average fluorescence intensity of DOX-loaded Au-Aptamer@ZIF-8 NPs cell uptake at various treatment durations (0, 2, 6, and 12 hours). (**d, e**). MCF-7 cells exposed to DOX, DOX-loaded Au-Aptamer@ZIF-8 NPs, and DOX-loaded Au-Aptamer@ZIF-8 NPs + NIR underwent cell cycle analysis. (Adapted with permission from Ref. [27]. Copyright 2024, American Chemical Society)

DOX stops the cell cycle at the S and G2/M checkpoints by blocking topoisomerase, which is crucial for DNA replication. It also increases caspase activity, causing the cells to undergo death. The G1 stage of the cell cycle is reduced and the S phase is elevated in MCF-7 cells incubated with DOX or DOX-loaded Au-Aptamer@ZIF-8 NPs compared to the control group. The DOX-loaded Au-Aptamer@ZIF-8 NPs group shows a stronger effect, keeping more cells in the S phase. The addition of near-infrared (NIR) light to DOX-loaded Au-Aptamer@ZIF-8 NPs increases the S phase fraction by 4.17%, indicating that photothermal therapy (PTT) can boost the drug's effectiveness against breast cancer by making cells more sensitive to the treatment and disrupting the cell cycle depicted in Fig. 5.7d, e.

5.2.3.1 Effects of DOX-Loaded Au-Aptamer@ZIF-8 on In Vivo Cancer

In a model using nude mice with breast cancer tumors, the tumor size decreased in the DOX, DOX-loaded Au-Aptamer@ZIF-8 NPs, and DOX-loaded Au-Aptamer@ZIF-8 NPs + NIR groups in contrast to the control group as treatment continued. Figure 5.8a shows that DOX-loaded Au-Aptamer@ZIF-8 + NIR treatment was the most effective in reducing tumor growth. On day 14, tumors in the control group measured 1.35 centimeters, while those in the DOX-loaded Au-Aptamer@ZIF-8

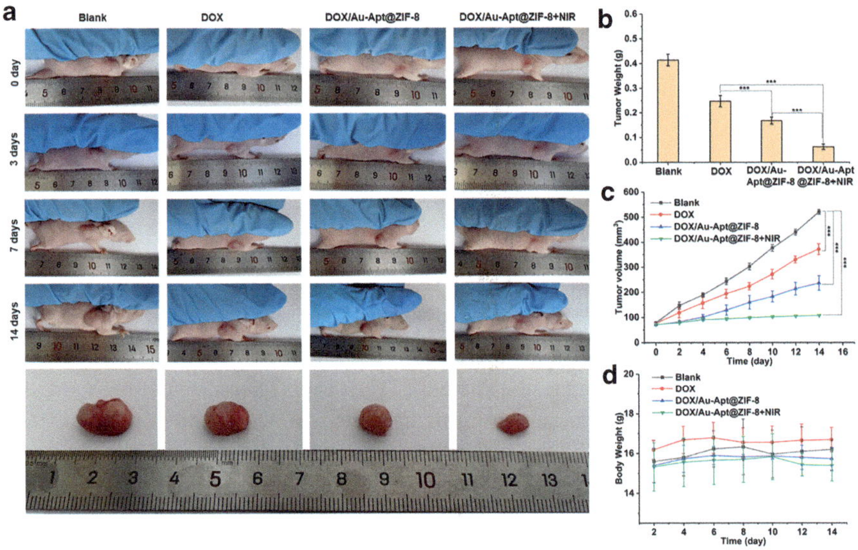

Fig. 5.8 Effects of DOX, DOX-loaded Au-Aptamer@ZIF-8 NPs, and DOX-loaded Au-Aptamer@ZIF-8 NPs + NIR on nude mice with breast cancer. (**a**) Changes in tumor diameter. (**b**) Relative tumor mass. (**c**) Changes in tumor volume. (**d**) Body weight variations in the mice are presented as mean ± standard deviation ($n = 3–5$). A significance level of $***P < 0.001$ denotes a marked difference from the control group. (Adapted with permission from Ref. [27]. Copyright 2024, American Chemical Society)

NPs + NIR group were only 0.7 centimeters. A decrease in tumor weight to 0.062 grams and a reduction in tumor volume to 109 mm^3 are shown in Fig. 5.8b, c. The DOX-loaded Au-Aptamer@ZIF-8 NPs + NIR treatment led to a slower tumor growth rate compared to the DOX group. Figure 5.8d shows that the mice's weight remained stable, indicating that DOX-loaded Au-Aptamer@ZIF-8 NPs were well tolerated with no significant side effects. The combination of photothermal therapy (PTT) and chemotherapy resulted in the slowest tumor growth and the most effective cancer treatment. Photothermal imaging showed that the tumor temperature increased to a maximum of 42.3 °C after about 5 minutes of exposure to 808 nm NIR light. In contrast, the temperature remained constant in the blank and DOX groups. This temperature rise was due to the efficient targeting of the drug carriers, particularly the Au-NRs, which concentrated at the tumor site.

5.2.4 Dendrimers

Dendrimers are categorized as polymer NPs that consist of globular shapes made from branched layers as seen in Fig. 5.9a. The outer layer of dendrimers can be modified with various functional groups like –COOH, $-COONa^+$,$-NH_2$, and –OH groups for a variety of applications. The controlled size of dendrimers can be easily synthesized with several functional groups on the outer surface, making it a promising candidate for DDS. The viability of drug loading, release, and biocompatibility can be attributed to several factors such as molar mass distribution, generation of branched chains, type of dendrons, and controllable nanoscale size. These dendrimers are produced using two distinct methods: the divergent and convergent approaches. In the divergent approach, first described by Tomalia et al. [28], the core of the dendrimers is developed sequentially, followed by radial growth by the addition of monomers. In the convergent approach, the dendrons first synthesize and emerge toward the core of the structure through several reactions. Dendrimers have a unique architecture consisting of three main components: consisting a central core to which dendrons are bound, branches attached to it, and an outer layer called generations. They can be divided into low- and high-generation categories. Low-generation dendrimers are typically more flexible and exhibit an open structure, while high-generation dendrimers are denser and tend to form a globular shape.

Several types of dendrimers were synthesized for different applications, which include lysine-dendrimers, poly (propylene imine) (PPI), poly (amido amine) (PAMAM), ether-amine, ester-amine, phosphorus, triazine, polyphenylene, and silicon-based dendrimers (see Fig. 5.9b).

Various families of dendrimers provide potential uses in the biomedical and pharmacological fields. Figure 5.9b 1 describes the first dendrimers created, which were lysine dendrimers (1). However, the first commercially available dendrimers were poly (propylene imine) (PPI) 5.9b 2 and poly (amidoamine) (PAMAM) dendrimers 5.9b (3–4). Ether amine-based dendrimers 5.9b 5 and ester amine dendrimers 5.9b 6 are cationic dendrimers with flexible cores, specifically engineered

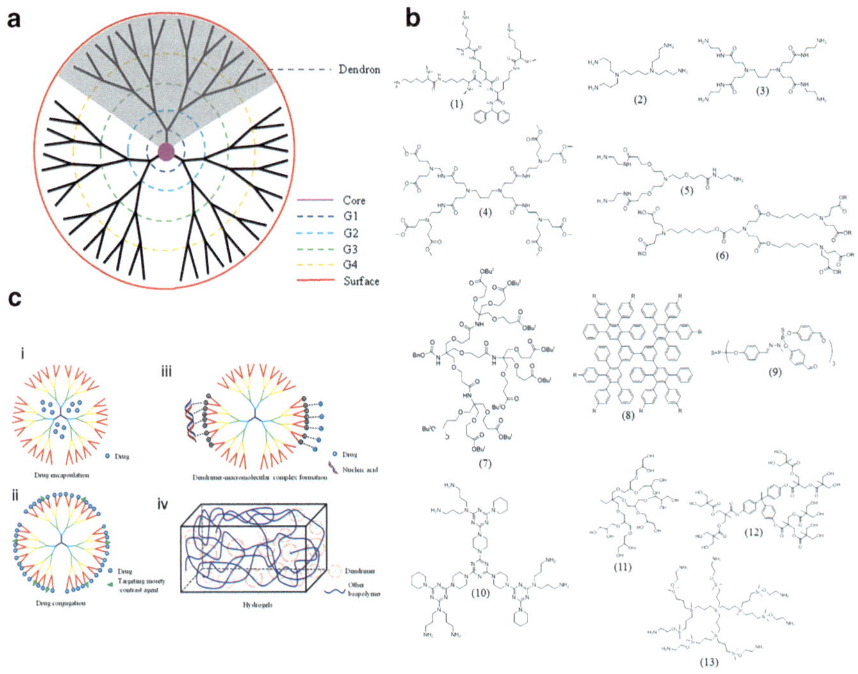

Fig. 5.9 (**a**) A schematic representation of dendrimer structure, with dashed lines indicating various dendrimer generations (G). (**b**) Selected dendrimer structures: (1) lysine-dendrimer with a benzhydryl amine core partially structured, (2) PPI G0 dendrimer, (3) PAMAM G0 dendritic structure, (4) PAMAM G0.5 dendritic structure, (5) ether-amine type dendrimer, (6) ester amine type dendrimer, (7) N Tris[(2[(tris[2(tertbutoxycarbonyl)ethoxy]methylmethyl)amino]carbonylethoxy) methyl]methylaminedendron, (8) polyphenylene-baseddendritic structure, (9) phosphorus-based dendrimer, (10) s-triazine-based dendritic molecule, (11) polyglycerol-based dendrimer, (12) polyester-derived dendritic molecule, and (13) silane-siloxane dendrimer. (**c**) Dendrimers have significant biomedical uses, such as: (i) functioning as carriers for encapsulating and delivering drugs and (ii) acting as versatile platforms for attaching ligands, targeting drug molecules, and linking reporter molecules like fluorescent markers or contrast agents. (iii) Dendrimers as platforms for the transport and compaction of nucleic acids; (iv) cross-linking dendrimers with biopolymers to facilitate tissue engineering. (Adapted with permission from Ref. [29]. Copyright 2015, American Chemical Society)

for the delivery of nucleic acids into mammalian cells. Other intriguing species with biomedical applications include structures produced from N-Tris [(2-[(tris[2-(tert-butoxycarbonyl) ethoxy]methyl-methyl) amino] carbonyl ethoxy)methyl] such as Methylamine dendron 5.9b7, phosphorus 5.9b9, s-triazine 5.9b10, polyglycerol 5.9b11, polyester 5.9b12, and silicon-based dendrimers 5.9b13. Polyphenylene-based dendrimers 5.9b8 are nonpolar branching macromolecules that have found applicability in numerous biological situations.

Dendrimers are versatile in medicine, as shown in several ways. First, they can encapsulate drug molecules within their internal cavities to deliver drugs safely at the targeted locations in the body. Second, dendrimers can be multifunctional, which helps to link different drugs, targeting molecules that guide the drug to specific cells, and reporter molecules used in diagnostics. This makes them useful for both treatment and diagnosis. Third, dendrimers can compact and deliver genetic material like DNA or RNA to cells, which is particularly important in gene therapy. In the end, they can cross-link with biopolymers to create structures that support tissue growth, aiding in tissue repair and regeneration as shown in Fig. 5.9c [29].

Targeted drug delivery is an advanced strategy that directs medications specifically to their intended sites. This can be achieved through two primary methods: endogenous targeting, where drugs bind to natural messengers that reach the target site, and exogenous targeting, which uses a carrier to transport the drug and release it precisely where needed. Extracellular vesicles (EVs) present a potential strategy for targeted drug delivery. These lipid-coated particles, which include microvesicles, exosomes, and apoptotic bodies, naturally carry substances like lipids, nucleic acids, and proteins. In cancer treatment, EVs from tumor cells are particularly effective due to their adaptability to the tumor environment and their ability to penetrate deep into tissues potentially improving treatment outcomes while minimizing side effects [30].

Dendrimers with their radial tree-like structure are ideal for precise drug delivery. Jiang et al. [31] developed a system named as amphiphilic dendrimers forming nanomicelles (ADNMs) using amphiphilic poly (amidoamine) (PAMAM) that work with tumor-produced extracellular vesicles (EVs) for enhanced drug delivery. These ADNMs utilize the enhanced permeability and retention (EPR) effect to target tumors, facilitating the deep penetration of drugs into the tumor tissue (see Fig. 5.10). Studies on pancreatic and colorectal cancer models show this method effectively halts tumor growth without side effects, highlighting its potential as an advanced cancer treatment.

Sun et al. [32] discuss a five-step process: circulation within the bloodstream (C), tumor accumulation through the enhanced permeability and retention (EPR) effect (A), deep tissue penetration (P), internalization by cancer cells (I), and subsequent drug release inside the cells (R) (CAPIR).

DOXIL is a special type of medicine that contains doxorubicin, a powerful drug used to treat cancer. It is packaged inside tiny bubble-like structures called liposomes, facilitating enhanced absorption of the drug within the body. It localizes effectively within the tumor's surrounding tissues but fails to penetrate the tumor itself, leading to limited therapeutic effectiveness. To achieve optimal therapeutic effectiveness, a range of bomb-like nanocarriers was engineered, combining the actions of their components to efficiently complete the CAPIR cascade. To improve its effectiveness, researchers developed a new type of nanocarrier designed to work like a "bomb" that can deliver drugs more efficiently. This new nanocarrier uses a combination of dendrimers and lipids. Dendrimers are tiny, organized molecules that carry drugs, while lipids help stabilize them in the bloodstream for effective tumor targeting. The fusogenic phospholipid DOPE coats the dendrimers, releasing the drug at the tumor site. To ensure stability and stealth, the nanocarrier is covered with DSPE-PEG, cholesterol, and lipids, enabling it to safely deliver its drug payload directly to the tumor. The self-assembling process of dendrimers containing

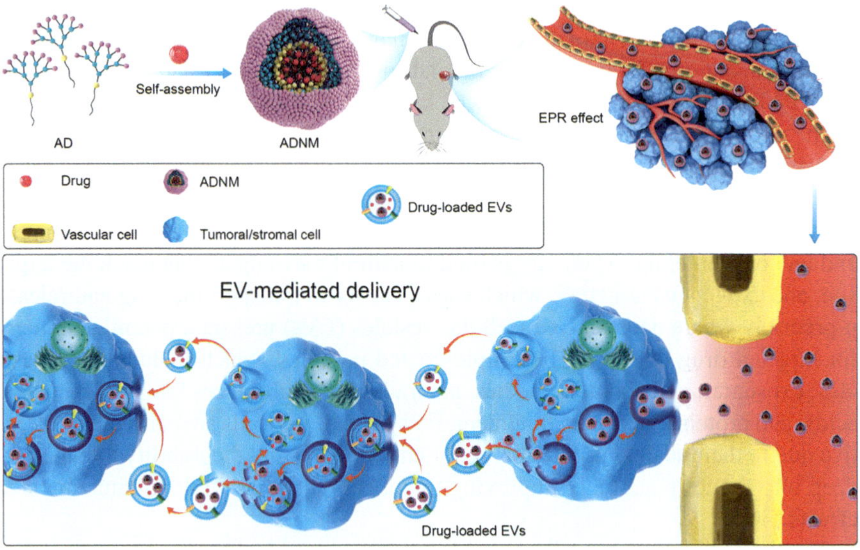

Fig. 5.10 Amphiphilic dendrimer-forming nanomicelles (ADNMs) are designed to enclose anticancer agents and facilitate targeted delivery to tumors through EV-mediated intercellular transport. These nanomicelles are formed by amphiphilic dendrimers (AD) loaded with anticancer agents and concentrate at tumor locations through the enhanced permeability and retention (EPR) effect. They leverage EV-mediated intercellular transport to facilitate in situ targeted drug transport for enhanced tumor infiltration. The EV-mediated delivery mechanism includes the following: (1) the absorption of ADNMs by tumor cells; (2) the incorporation of ADNM payload into extracellular vesicles (EVs); (3) the intercellular transport of these EVs; and (4) the absorption of EVs by recipient cells. (Adapted with permission from ref. [31]. Copyright 2023, Proceedings of the National Academy of Sciences)

DOPE lipid, cholesterol, and DSPE-PEG (commonly as D, L, C, and PEG in the nanoassembly label: DLC-PEG). This assembly consisting of 27 dendrimers is covered with a lipid layer. When loaded with DOX, DLC-PEG's diameter slightly increases. The nanocarrier can be lyophilized with trehalose and redispersed without size changes. DOX is released more slowly from DLC-PEG compared to other assemblies, indicating better encapsulation and reduced premature release. Sun et al. [32] evaluated the nanoassembly effectiveness in drug delivery for cancer treatment using the CAPIR method. The DLC-PEG nanoassembly with its lipid layer fuses with cell membranes to release dendrimers into tumor tissues. It proved stealthy and stable in the bloodstream, similar to PCL-PEG micelles, but with the added advantage of delivering DOX more evenly throughout the tumor, showing about ten times higher drug intensity compared to PCL-PEG micelles. The in vivo therapeutic efficacy of DLC-PEG conjugated with DOX was assessed in comparison to micellar PCL-PEG/DOX in mice bearing subcutaneous tumors of MCF-7 breast cancer cells exhibiting both drug sensitivity and resistance. DLC-PEG conjugated with DOX and free DOX significantly suppressed the growth of drug-sensitive MCF-7 tumors, outperforming PCL (2 k)-PEG (2 k)/DOX ($P < 0.005$). On day

19, DLC-PEG conjugated with DOX reduced tumor weight by 85%, compared to 40% with PCL (2 k)-PEG (2 k)/DOX. In MCF-7/ADR tumor models exhibiting drug resistance, neither free DOX nor PCL (2 k)-PEG (2 k)/DOX significantly decreased tumor growth, with reductions of only 32% and 21%, respectively.

5.2.5 Nanogels

A three-dimensional network formed by polymers containing hydrophilic groups covalently cross-linked in addition to hydrogen bonds and van der Waals interactions. Nanogels are found to be promising in drug delivery applications because of their remarkable properties, such as the ability to hold drug molecules covalently/physically, the ability to absorb water, the easy encapsulation of drug molecules, and the capability to respond to external stimuli. The specific behavior of such nanogels provides pathways to use them as DDS. Key characteristics include the following:

- Nanometric dimensions: This feature will enhance the surface area relative to the volume, enabling them to cross biological barriers followed by penetration into tissues and cells.
- Swelling behavior: This behavior in nanogel can be altered using temperature and pH response.
- Viscoelasticity: Nanogels are highly solvated by hydrophilic solvents, enabling the flow through nanochannels.

Ryu et al. [33] have developed a stable nanogel using a random copolymer with oligo ethylene glycol (OEG) units and pyridyldisulfide (PDS) groups. The OEG units make the nanogel, a biocompatible component for use as DDS. The PDS groups react with the thiol groups to form cross-links, creating the nanogel structure. These disulfide bonds can be cleaved through thiol-disulfide exchange interactions, allowing the release of any encapsulated molecules. This design ensures that the nanogels can hold and then release guest molecules, effectively making them suitable for drug delivery applications. The nanogel is created by using a random copolymer with pyridyldisulfide (PDS) and oligoethylene glycol (OEG) units. When the PDS groups in the copolymer are exposed to the reducing agent dithiothreitol (DTT), they break down, allowing the nanogel structure to form. The PDS groups are hydrophobic, so they tend to cluster together in water, creating larger aggregates. These aggregates can trap the lipophilic guest molecules. The copolymer's thiol groups react with PDS to form a disulfide bond that cross-links the polymers and stabilizes the nanogel. This design allows the nanogel to encapsulate and later release the guest molecules when the disulfide bonds are cleaved, as illustrated in Fig. 5.11a.

One of the nanogels is made using a random copolymer method consisting of 30% oligoethylene glycol methacrylate (OEG) and 70% PDS-derived methacrylate synthesized using RAFT polymerization. OEG units make the polymer water-soluble while PDS units facilitate cross-linking. The polymer was cross-linked with 20% dithiothreitol (DTT), and the nanogel encapsulates hydrophobic guest molecules like a dye molecule, i.e., Nile red, as shown in Fig. 5.11b. Glutathione (GSH) is used to break the disulfide bonds and release the dye. Low GSH concentrations lead to minimal dye release, while high GSH levels cause significant release. The nanogels showed excellent cell viability and potential for biological use due to their biocompatibility. When evaluated using MCF-7 human breast cancer cell lines, nanogels modified with a cell-penetrating peptide demonstrated improved internalization, highlighting their effectiveness for targeted drug delivery. In conclusion, a simple emulsion-free method was developed to create biocompatible nanogels using PDS-containing polymers. These nanogels

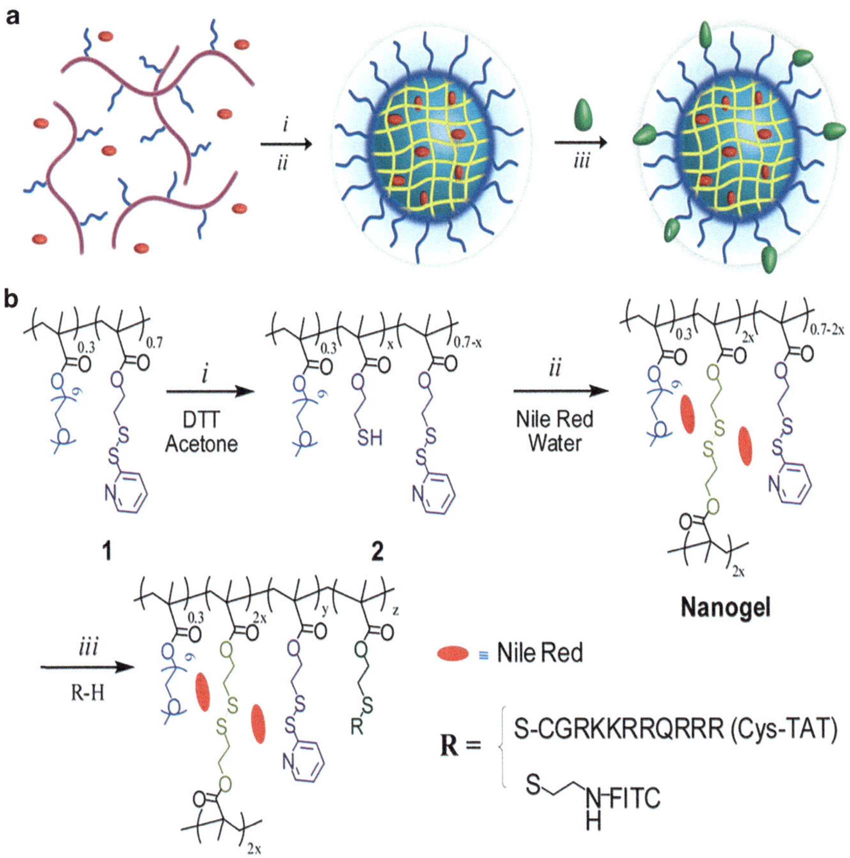

Fig. 5.11 Design, development, and synthesis of the NPs using polymers. (**a**) Development and synthesis of surface-modified biodegradable nanogels represented by a schematic diagram. (**b**) The polymer's chemical framework and the resulting nanogel are composed of: (i) Selective degradation of PDS groups with DTT. (ii) Formation of nanogels through cross-linking within or between polymer chains. (iii) Modification of nanogel surfaces using peptides conjugated with thiol groups or FITC. (Adapted with permission from Ref. [33]. Copyright 2010, American Chemical Society)

encapsulate hydrophobic guest molecules through disulfide bonds, which are biodegradable in alkaline environments, making them ideal for intracellular drug delivery. External factors can help release these guest molecules. The approach of using self-cross-linking polymers and enhancing the surface of nanogels improves their effectiveness for drug delivery and opens up new possibilities for their use in various biomedical applications.

Ryu et al. [34] have synthesized polymeric nanogels of high stability and demonstrated the precise delivery of drug molecules by altering the cross-linking density. The intracellular delivery of DOX was quantitatively assessed using three types of nanogels, labeled NG1, NG2, and NG3, with cross-link densities of 7%, 14%, and 35%, respectively. They found that the stability of DOX encapsulation increased with higher cross-link density, making NG3 the most stable.

From Fig. 5.12a, the nanogels were tested on 293 T human kidney cells at various concentrations for 24 hours. The results indicated that the nanogels were well tolerated, showing no significant induced toxicity at a concentration of 1 mg/mL, highlighting their potential for biological applications. In studies involving MCF-7 breast cancer cells, the DOX-loaded nanogels (NG1 and NG3) demonstrated drug loading of 24% and 20%, respectively, after a 72-hour incubation period. While the

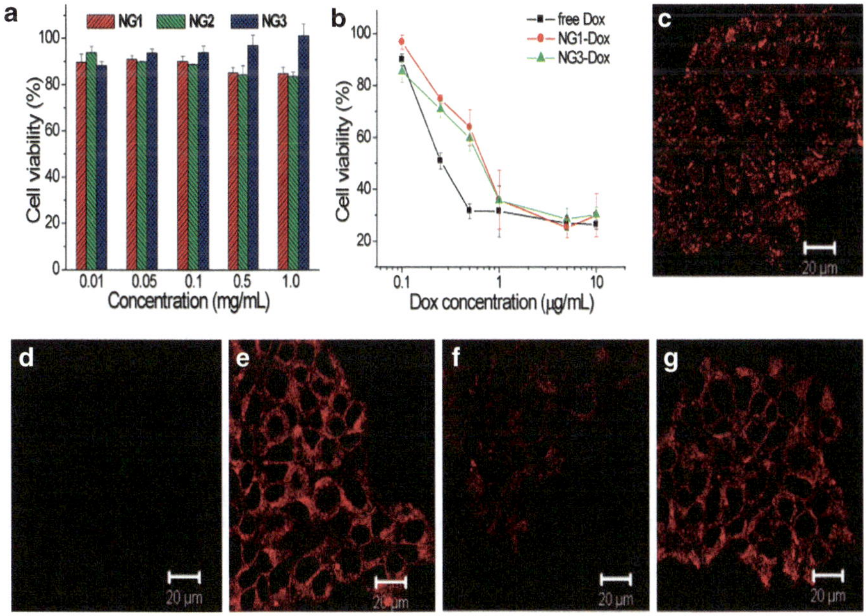

Fig. 5.12 (**a**) In vitro assessment of toxicity for 293 T cells on nanogels without payload during a 24-hour incubation period. (**b**) Confocal images showing MCF-7 cells treated with DOX-encapsulated nanogels for 72 hours showed the following. (**c**) DOX was found to be free after 3 hours. (**d**) NG1-DOX after 3 hours. (**e**) NG1-DOX after 4 hours. (**f**) NG3-DOX after 3 hours. (**g**) NG3-DOX after 4 hours. (Adapted with permission from Ref. [34]. Copyright 2010, American Chemical Society)

DOX-loaded nanogels did show some cell toxicity, it was lower compared to free DOX. The reduced toxicity is attributed to the slower release of DOX from the nanogels within the cells. The DOX-loaded nanogels showed lower levels of toxicity compared to free DOX. Figure 5.12b shows the reduced toxicity because free DOX quickly enters cells, whereas DOX released from nanogels inside the cells happens more slowly. This slower release is advantageous for targeting tumors more effectively in vivo, as the nanogels remain in the body longer, enhancing the drug's therapeutic effect. Free DOX quickly accumulated in the nucleus within 3 hours using confocal microscopy as shown in Fig. 5.12c. Nanogels NG1 and NG3 showed fluorescence in the cytoplasm after 3 to 4 hours. NG3-DOX reached the cytoplasm faster than NG1-DOX. The nanogels use disulfide bonds to encapsulate DOX, which can be triggered for release by glutathione (GSH) in the body, as shown in Fig. 5.12d–g. This controlled release and biocompatibility make the nanogels promising for targeted drug delivery, particularly in cancer therapy [34].

5.2.6 Chitosans

Chitosan (CS) is the linear, random copolymer formed by N-acetyl-D-glucosamine and β-(1–4)-linked D-glucosamine, which is linked through glycosidic bonds as a linear backbone [35]. The polysaccharide in CS contains protonated basic amine groups to develop a positively charged system, and hence it mostly behaves as hydrophilic. The varying number of acetylated monomers in the chains governs its solubility in aqueous medium. Such properties of CS in its solution show an ability to open epithelial tight junctions, pH-based stimuli response, and mucoadhesiveness. Such behavior has attracted attention to the application of CS in DDS [36].

The structure of chitosans consists of reactive functional groups as a key feature: amino groups at the C2 position and hydroxyl (OH) groups at the C3 and C6 positions (see Fig. 5.13a). Chitosan nanoparticles (ChNPs) are produced using various methods tailored to specific needs. Covalent cross-linking creates a 3D network by forming bonds between chitosan and cross-linkers such as glutaraldehyde. From Fig. 5.13b, self-organization involves assembling molecules into NPs through interactions like hydrogen bonding and hydrophobic forces, making it suitable for drug encapsulation. Ion cross-linking uses anionic cross-linkers under mild conditions, preserving sensitive bioactive molecules. Polyelectrolyte complex (PEC) formation relies on the electrostatic attraction between positively and negatively charged polyelectrolytes, resulting in stable structures without harsh chemicals. The emulsion technique, such as water-in-oil emulsification, produces NPs with high drug-loading efficiency and stability. Additionally, drying methods like spray and supercritical drying offer fast, simple, and adaptable solutions for various particle sizes and high stability. Each method has distinct advantages depending on the application requirements shown in Fig. 5.13b [37].

Chitosans loaded with drugs alone can be poorly controlled within the body to deliver at the targeted location. In this regard, superparamagnetic iron oxide NPs

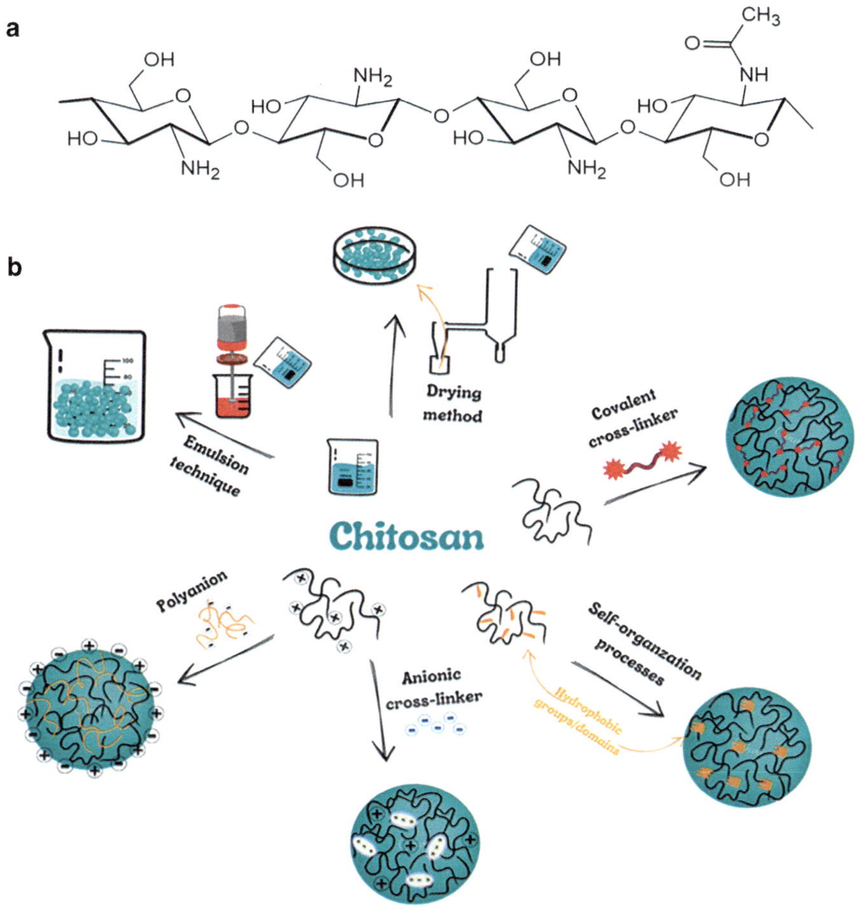

Fig. 5.13 (**a**) Chitosan's linear chemical structure is made up of polysaccharides. (**b**) The scheme depicts the most common techniques for producing chitosan NPs (ChNPs). (Adapted with permission from Ref. [37]. Copyright 2023, MDPI)

(SPIONs) are those that measure between 10 to 100 nm in diameter and can act as carrier NPs for targeted drug delivery. These SPIONs can be good carriers because of their easy control inside the body upon exposure to an external magnetic field. Superparamagnetic NPs are made of iron oxides such as magnetite (Fe_3O_4), maghemite (Fe_2O_3), and other ferrites. These NPs are of great concern because of their superparamagnetic behavior, biocompatibility, and surface modification properties. SPIONs are employed in a range of medical fields, including targeted drug delivery, cancer therapy, and as contrast agents in MRI [38].

Mistral et al. [39] developed to improve the biocompatibility of NPs. Chitosan (CS) coatings are applied to modify the properties of superparamagnetic iron oxide nanoparticles (SPIONs). Iron oxide NPs, especially (Fe_3O_4), are superparamagnetic, which means they become magnetized in the presence of a magnetic field but lose this magnetization once the field is removed. Chitosan, a biopolymer derived from chitin found in crustacean shells, is used to coat these NPs. This coating enhances the stability and functionality of the SPIONs, making them more biocompatible [40]. In the body, these SPIONs generate a magnetic moment only when subjected to an external magnetic field and can achieve much higher saturation magnetization compared to biological components. When exposed to a magnetic field, superparamagnetic (Fe_3O_4) NPs generate heat through the loss of hysteresis and relaxation processes. This property can be used to selectively increase the temperature of malignant tissues. Chitosan (CS) coatings can impact the effectiveness and application of SPIONs in magnetic resonance imaging (MRI) and magnetic hyperthermia. These coatings influence the physical, magnetic, and biological properties of SPIONs, affecting their performance in these applications.

(Fe_3O_4) SPIONs were synthesized using the chemical co-precipitation technique. This technique is simple and scalable for large-scale production. However, alternative methods such as flame spray pyrolysis and electrochemical processes are also available and can be scaled up. Iron (III) chloride hexahydrate ($FeCl_3.6H_2O$) and iron (II) chloride tetrahydrate ($FeCl_2.4H_2O$) were dissolved at a 2:1 stoichiometric ratio in deionized water at 60 °C under an inert atmosphere (Ar). HCl was added to the mixture to achieve a concentration of 0.1 M and stabilize the iron ions. To precipitate the iron ions and form magnetite, ammonium hydroxide (NH_4OH) was added dropwise until the pH reached approximately 10–11. The addition of (NH_4OH) caused the solution to change color from yellow to black, indicating the formation of magnetite. The SPIONs were then washed several times with deionized water and recovered using magnetic decantation until a neutral pH was achieved. Finally, the NPs were freeze-dried and stored at room temperature as shown in Fig. 5.14i.

A sensitive colorimetric test was used to assess cell viability for cell proliferation and cytotoxicity using Cell Counting Kit-8 (CCK-8) assay. The study examined the effects of magnetite-based superparamagnetic iron oxide nanoparticles (SPIONs) on canine fibroblasts at 24, 48, and 72 hours. Diluting the SPIONs improved cell viability by reaching over 80% at 125 μg/mL or lower concentrations. Bare magnetite SPIONs were toxic, with cell viability dropping to around 60% at a concentration of 1 mg/mL after 72 hours, as shown in Fig. 5.14ii. However, applying a chitosan (CS) coating reduced this toxicity.

This indicates that applying thin chitosan (CS) coatings helps to keep SPIONs biocompatible while maintaining their magnetic properties and reducing aggregation. Overall, chitosan coating improves the safety and effectiveness of magnetite-based SPIONs.

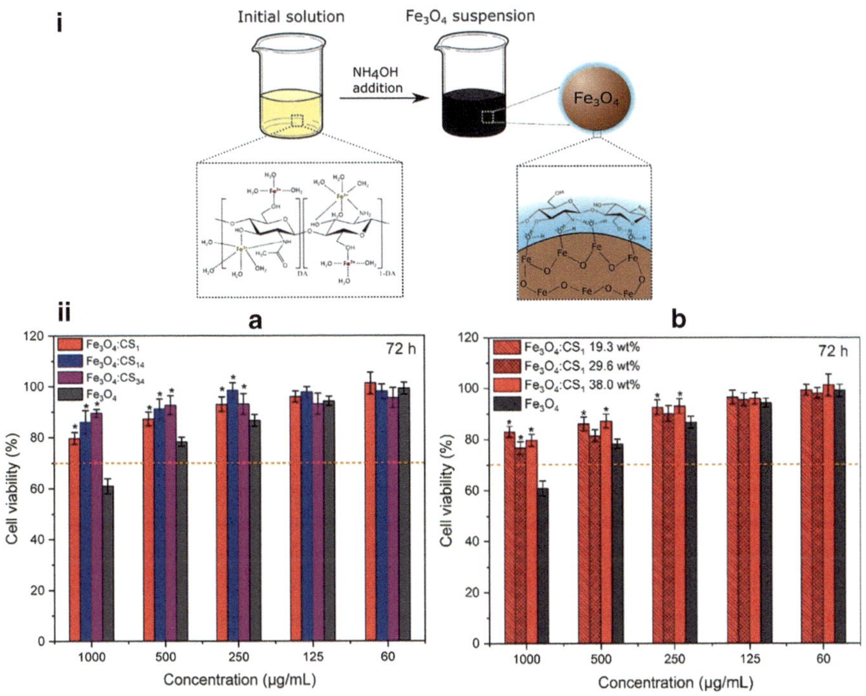

Fig. 5.14 (**i**) Chitosan-coated Fe_3O_4 NPs. (**ii**) Cell viability results of canine fibroblasts after 72 h of interaction time against (a) Fe_3O_4 and Fe_3O_4/CSDA SPIONs at different concentrations with the same amount of CSDA coating 38%, (b) Fe_3O_4 and Fe_3O_4/CS1 at different concentrations and different amounts of CS1 coating. * indicates statically different results of Fe_3O_4/CSDA from Fe_3O_4 SPIONs, using the Tukey test and p value <0.05. The orange dashed line marks the threshold for cell viability according to international standard procedures. ISO 10993-5. (Adapted with permission from Ref. [39]. Copyright 2024, American Chemical Society)

5.2.7 *Carbon-Based Nanoparticles (Carbon Nanotube, Graphene Oxide Sheet, and Nanodiamonds)*

5.2.7.1 Carbon Nanotube

Carbon nanotubes (CNTs) are assembled in the form of hollow cylinders of graphene sheets that possess remarkable mechanical, chemical, and physical properties, which make them suitable candidates for drug delivery to the target cells. The properties of CNTs mainly depend on the number of graphene layers incorporated to form the cylinder and the functionalized group attached to the edges and surface of the graphene. Single-walled nanotubes (SWNTs) possess a diameter of 1–2 nm, length of 50 nm to 1 cm, and surface area of 1300 m^2/g which permits the high loading of longer chains of drug molecules. The benzene ring-based drug molecules can bind with the nanotubes through π-π stacking. However, multi-walled NTs

(MWNTs) exhibit larger pore diameters compared to SWNTs allowing the loading of larger drug molecules [41].

Bhirde et al. [42] developed a successful in vivo killing of cancer cells using a DDS based on single-walled carbon nanotubes (SWNTs). This system showed higher effectiveness compared to nontargeted bioconjugates. The SWNTs were loaded with cisplatin and epidermal growth factor (EGF) to treat squamous carcinoma.

This demonstrated that using tailored drug delivery with SWNTs significantly reduces tumor size in mice. This DDS exploits EGF's strong binding to its receptor (EGFR), which is often overexpressed on squamous carcinoma cells to guide the therapeutic drug precisely to the cancer cells.

Carboxylated single-walled carbon nanotubes (SWNTs) are advanced drug delivery devices designed to target cancer cells, deliver chemotherapy medications, and provide imaging to monitor treatment progress. These nanotubes have carboxyl groups on their surfaces created by oxidizing the nanotubes. To attach therapeutic agents and imaging components to the SWNTs, a coupling agent called EDC (1-(3-(dimethylamino) propyl)-3-ethylcarbodiimide hydrochloride) is used. EDC forms amide bonds between carboxyl groups on the SWNTs and amine-containing compounds. This process allows the attachment of epidermal growth factor (EGF), cisplatin, and quantum dots (Qdots) to the carboxylated SWNTs.

EGF, a protein that targets cancer cells, is covalently bonded to the carboxylated SWNTs using EDC. Cisplatin, a chemotherapeutic drug, is also attached to the SWNTs through EDC-mediated coupling. Additionally, fluorescent quantum dots (Qdots) are chemically linked to the SWNTs.

Figure 5.15a, b shows a schematic of red carboxylated SWNTs that serve as the base for functionalization. The carboxyl groups interact chemically with EGF, cisplatin, and Qdots facilitated by EDC. These functionalized SWNTs are designed to deliver drugs specifically to cancer cells by binding to EGF receptors. EGF guides the nanotubes to the cancer cells, cisplatin provides the therapeutic effect, and Qdots enable imaging to track the treatment's effectiveness. The study used transmission electron microscopy (TEM) to examine the bioconjugation of nanotubes. Without EDC, the images showed striated nanotube bundles with diameters ranging from 1.0 to 1.4 nm, as shown in Fig. 5.15c. Adding EDC to the bioconjugation mixture resulted in visible tiny particles decorating the nanotubes. These particles are quantum dots (Qdots) that have an average diameter of 4 nm. The size of these spherical features matched the diameters observed in the nanotube bundles, as shown in Fig. 5.15d. Cisplatin was detected using scanning transmission electron microscopy. The final dispersion of SWNTs with cisplatin and EGF contained 1.3 M of cisplatin and 0.25 mg/mL of SWNTs, as shown in Fig. 5.15e.

Figure 5.16a–d depicts SWNT bioconjugates loaded with cisplatin that are used to specifically target in vitro cancer cells. To assess whether cell death caused by these bioconjugates depends on the EGF receptor (EGFR), siRNA-mediated EGFR silencing was carried out in HN13 cells, with the outcomes validated through Western blot analysis. The MTT assay was employed to assess cell proliferation. In Fig. 5.16e, the study compared the effects of SWNTs with cisplatin and EGF on

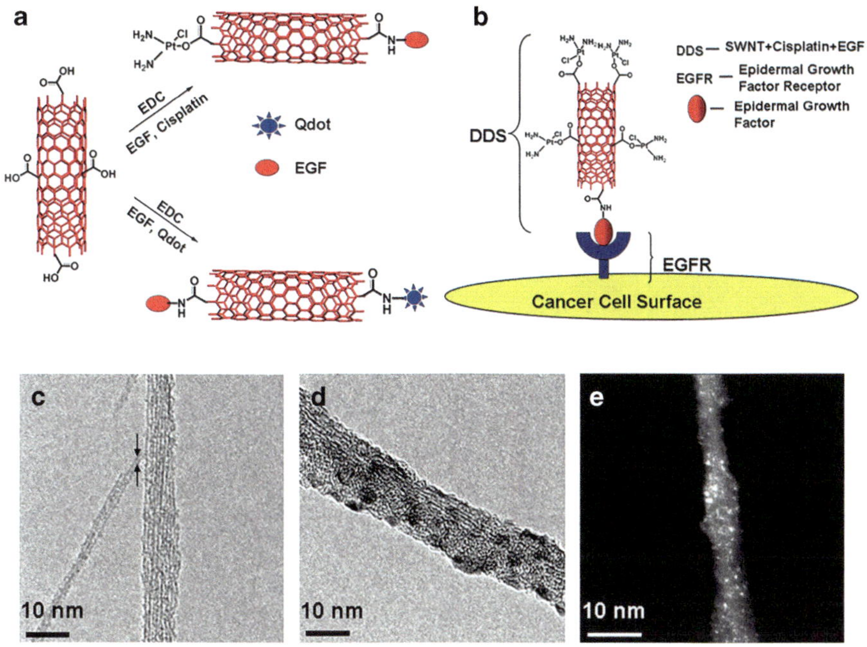

Fig. 5.15 Drug delivery system based on nanotubes. (**a**) Diagram showing the chemical reactions where EDC acts as a coupling agent to bind EGF, cisplatin, and Qdots to carboxylated SWNTs (depicted in red). (**b**) Illustration of SWNT bundles attached with EGF and cisplatin, aimed at the EGFR receptor on an individual HNSCC cell. Transmission electron microscopy images include (**c**) oxidized SWNT clusters, with arrows highlighting an individual SWNT, (**d**) SWNT-Qdot-EGF bioconjugate bundles, and (**e**) a STEM image showing a SWNT cluster, with cisplatin visible as luminous dots. (Adapted with permission from Ref. [42]. Copyright 2009, American Chemical Society)

HN13 cells, EGFR knockdown cells, and control cells treated with nontargeted siRNA. The concentration of cisplatin used in the experiments was similar to levels found in the serum of cancer patients. Cells treated with SWNTs and cisplatin or cisplatin alone without EGF showed minimal changes in growth. However, treatment with SWNT-cisplatin-EGF reduced cell growth by 25–50%. High doses of free cisplatin alone significantly inhibited cell proliferation, demonstrating the drug's effectiveness. Figure 5.16f shows the role of cisplatin incorported with SWNT-EGF (SCE) in majorly three different cell types viz. HN13, SAA, and NIH3T3 using cell viability test and observed to adversly effect the growth of HN13 and SAA cell compared to normal N1H3T3 cells. Additional studies were conducted on SAA cells including NIH3T3 cells with elevated EGFR expression and NIH3T3 cells with reduced levels of EGFR expression compared to HN13 cells. SWNT-transplatin-EGF effectively reduced cell proliferation in HN13 and SAA cells with high EGFR expression but did not affect NIH3T3 cells with reduced levels of EGFR expression. In contrast, nanotube-free cisplatin, SWNT-EGF, and SWNT-cisplatin showed no significant impact on cell proliferation. High doses of

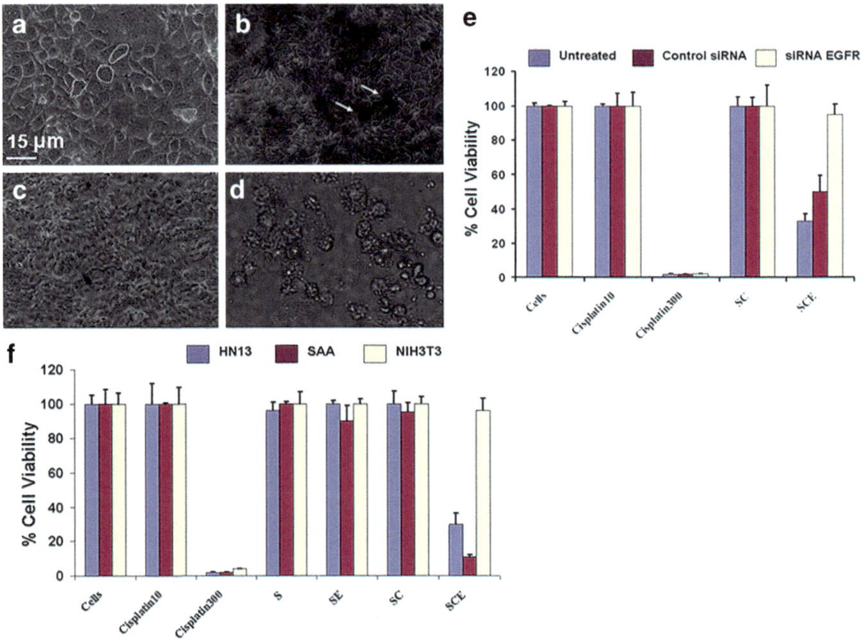

Fig. 5.16 Application of SWNT bioconjugates for targeted destruction of cancer cells. (**a**–**d**) Optical micrographs reveal the effect of SWNT-cisplatin-EGF (SCE) on HN13 cells: (**a**) Before treatment, cells are adhered to the plate and maintain their structural integrity. (**b**) Treatment with SCE for 10 minutes, showing dark regions where nanotubes are present. (**c**) After a 10-minute incubation with SCE, the cells were washed with PBS and resuspended in a DMEM medium for cell culture. (**d**) HN13 cells (after 10 minutes of SCE treatment and washing) were observed after 12 hours, appearing detached and floating. Parts **e** and **f** show cell viability assessments. (**e**) A cell proliferation assay was carried out to assess and compare the cell viability in HN13 normal cells, HN13 cells with suppressed EGFR expression, and untreated siRNA controls after 12 hours. The experimental conditions were as follows: "Cells" denotes the untreated control group; "Cisplatin10" denotes exposure to 10 µM of free-form cisplatin; "Cisplatin300" refers to exposure to 300 µM unbound cisplatin; "SC" indicates incubation with SWNT-cisplatin followed by a 10-minute PBS wash; and "SCE" represents incubation with SWNT-cisplatin-EGF concentration of (1.3 µM cisplatin) followed by a 10-minute PBS wash. (**f**) A similar assay was employed to examine the viability of HN13 normal cells, SAA cells, and NIH3T3 fibroblasts. The conditions tested included the following: "Cells" for untreated normal growth; "Cisplatin10" for treatment with an unbound cisplatin concentration of 10 µM; "Cisplatin300" for incubation with 300 µM unbound cisplatin; "S" for incubation with SWNTs for 10 minutes; "SE" for incubation with SWNT-EGF followed by PBS wash after 10 minutes; "SC" for incubation with SWNT-cisplatin followed by PBS washing after 10 minutes; and "SCE" for incubation with SWNT-cisplatin-EGF concentration of (1.3 µM cisplatin); subsequently, a PBS rinse was performed after a 10-minute interval. (Reprinted with permission from Ref. [42]. Copyright 2009, American Chemical Society)

free cisplatin were cytotoxic, significantly inhibiting cell proliferation. The SWNT-cisplatin-EGF dispersions outperformed free cisplatin in killing cancer cells, highlighting their enhanced effectiveness.

5.2.7.2 Graphene Oxide Sheet

Due to the 2D planar structure of graphene oxide (GO), it has a large surface area, mechanical stability, high conductivity, good biocompatibility, and tunable chemical and physical properties. It allows the drug molecule to effectively bind to the surface of the GO sheets through π-π stacking as well as functional moieties located at the edges and surface [43].

Zhang et al. [44] describe a synthetic method that has been used to create functional nanoscale graphene oxide (NGO), a new nanocarrier. Sulfonic acid groups functionalize the NGO and give it stability in physiological solutions. Then it binds covalently to folic acid molecules, enabling it to be directed specifically toward MCF-7 cells, which are FA-receptor-positive human breast cancer cells. It was studied how two anticancer medications, i.e., DOX and camptothecin (CPT), might be carefully loaded onto the FA-conjugated NGO (FA-NGO) through π-π interactions and hydrophobic forces. When compared to nonfunctionalized graphene oxide (NGO) loaded with DOX or camptothecin (CPT) alone, folic acid-functionalized graphene oxide (FA-NGO) loaded with these medications showed significantly higher cytotoxicity and selective destruction of MCF-7 cells. This suggests that anticancer drugs on graphene-based nanocarriers using targeted delivery could be highly beneficial in DDSs. To show how two or more medications can be loaded onto graphene at a regulated ratio of DOX to CPT, the study employed CPT and DOX as model pharmaceuticals. When combined, these medications exhibit a stronger anticancer impact and are frequently utilized in cancer treatment clinics.

5.2.7.3 Nanodiamonds

Nanodiamonds (NDs), a unique subset of inorganic carbon-based nanomaterials, are gaining attention for their potential in various applications. These materials exhibit a faceted, truncated octahedral morphology characterized by electrostatic fields across their surface facets. In the field of biomedicine, nanodiamonds are categorized into two main types: high-pressure, high-temperature nanodiamonds (HPHT) and detonation nanodiamonds (DNDs). The HPHT method is commonly employed to produce fluorescent nanodiamonds (FNDs), valued for their exceptional photostability, resistance to photobleaching, and enhanced fluorescence intensity. Despite these advantages, the HPHT technique can be less efficient, often requiring additional modifications to improve cost-effectiveness [45]. Alternatively, the detonation process offers a scalable approach to producing chemically robust DND particles with a uniform size of approximately 5 nm. In aqueous environments, these particles tend to form aggregates ranging from 50 to 200 nm and can organize into intricate, lace-like self-assembled networks. Their high surface area-to-volume ratio makes them particularly suited for drug loading and in vivo delivery applications. Nanodiamonds also exhibit unique surface electrostatic fields, which are advantageous for both drug delivery and imaging purposes. Their surfaces are populated with functional groups, such as hydroxyl, epoxide, phenolic, and pyrones, enabling strong covalent and hydrogen bonding with therapeutic agents. Additional functionalization can further enhance their drug-conjugation capabilities and delivery efficiency. Moreover, nanodiamonds demonstrate excellent water solubility attributed to their pronounced electrostatic fields and the formation of hydrogen bonds with water molecules, thereby solidifying their role in advanced biomedical applications [46].

A multi-component nanodiamond (ND)-based system is emerging as a powerful tool for drug delivery capable of targeting, imaging, and enhancing therapy. These nanodiamonds, which are 2–8 nanometers in diameter and have a truncated octahedral shape, show great promise in drug transport. They are biocompatible, meaning they are safe to use in the body, and they offer a range of functional properties thanks to their unique surface characteristics. In cancer therapy, nanodiamonds address several key challenges. Their ability to target specific cells provides imaging capabilities and improves the effectiveness of treatments, making them a valuable asset in advancing cancer care [47].

Tian et al. [48] propose multifunctional fluorescent nanodiamonds (FNDs) as innovative particles designed to both deliver drugs and detect free radicals. These particles are engineered with nitrogen vacancy centers and a diazoxide derivative, enhancing their ability to enter cells and deliver cancer medications effectively to HeLa cells. One key advantage of these FNDs is their ability to release drugs steadily over 72 hours, which is much longer compared to the free drug. They also offer a unique way to test how drugs affect free radical production. The optical properties of these nanodiamonds change in response to their magnetic environment allowing for precise measurement of spin noise from free radicals at the nanoscale. This approach provides subcellular resolution, which is compared to traditional fluorescence assays used for detecting reactive oxygen species. This method offers a new way to study the connection between drug release and cellular responses, specifically how drugs impact radical production or inhibition.

5.3 Exogenous Stimuli Responsive

5.3.1 Temperature Responsive

Temperature is an important stimulus for drug delivery, with clinical conditions causing regional or systemic rises in temperature and extrinsic energy sources enabling precise heating. Temperature is special among this range of stimuli in that it can be regarded as internal (certain tissues, such as tumors and infections, are normally at raised temperature) or external (heat is delivered from outside the body) [49]. Some polymeric materials contain a low critical solution temperature (LCST), which forms the foundation for most temperature-responsive nanocarriers and allows for precision-localized heating [50].

The lower critical solution temperature (LCST) and upper critical solution temperature (UCST) are critical temperatures for thermoresponsive polymeric materials that exhibit phase transitions in aqueous systems. To generate regulated DDS from a thermoresponsive nanocarrier for cancer treatment, the LCST has been increased to over 37 °C. To treat illnesses, invertebrates use temperature fluctuations ranging from 1 to 5 °C. Some thermoresponsive polymers, such as poly (N-isopropylacrylamide) (PNIPAAm), can improve their LCST by including hydrophilic regions [53]. A temperature-responsive polymer PNIPAAm exhibits consistent LCST behavior between 30 and 35 °C. Its hydrophilic media below and hydrophobic ones above have an impact on the LCST transition. Temperatures above the LCST cause the drug to release because they decrease the volumetric properties and solubility of the carrier medium. This reversible "swelling shrinkage" phenomenon results in concurrent drug release by making the carrier medium swell as a result of an increase in polymer solubility [54]. Among the many temperature-responsive polymers, poly (N-isopropylacrylamide) (PNIPAM) is one of the most popular. It is commonly used to create temperature-sensitive hydrogels because it responds very well to temperature changes [55]. PNIPAM can switch physical states based on temperature, known as LCST causing hydrogels to swell or shrink. This temperature-sensitive behavior is useful for controlled drug release [56]. However, chemically cross-linked PNIPAM hydrogels often release drugs slowly due to their gradual degradation. To improve this, decomposable cross-linkers like esters, peptides, or disulfide bonds (S–S) can be used. Disulfide bonds are particularly effective because they can be broken down by redox agents like dithiothreitol (DTT), glutathione (GSH), and reactive oxygen species (ROS), leading to faster and improved drug release [57].

Cheng et al. [51] developed a method incorporating disulfide bonds in hydrogels that allows for controlled drug release under different redox conditions, and some hydrogels respond to both temperature and redox changes. Diselenide bonds (Se–Se) are particularly promising because they break more easily than disulfide bonds under redox conditions. This makes them useful for creating hydrogels that can release drugs in response to oxidative environments. Diselenide-cross-linked hydrogels, due to their easier cleavage under milder conditions, offer a promising approach for precise drug delivery. A copolymer composed of 2-hydroxyethyl acrylate (HEA) and N-isopropyl acrylamide (NI-PAM) is being cross-linked with a diselenide-based agent to develop hydrogels that respond to both thermal and oxidative stimuli. These hydrogels can decompose into water-soluble polymers when exposed to oxidizing agents due to the diselenide linkages. Hydrogen peroxide (H_2O_2) was used to test how these hydrogels respond to temperature and oxidation. The results showed that the hydrogels can release drugs in a controlled manner in response to both temperature changes and oxidation. This makes it promising for use in DDSs where precise control over release is needed, as shown in Fig. 5.17a.

Mitochondria, often referred to as the cell's powerhouse due to their role in ATP production, play a crucial part in the advancement of multidrug-resistant cancers [58].

Targeting drug delivery to mitochondria has become increasingly popular because these organelles can be maintained at approximately 48 °C, and the variation in mitochondrial temperatures between normal and cancer cells can be exploited to bypass drug delivery barriers and specifically target cancer cells in mitochondria.

A mitochondrial temperature-responsive nanocarrier was used to address drug resistance in small cell lung cancer (SCLC) investigated by Ruan et al. [52]. Poly (N-isopropyl acrylamide) (PNIPAM) is used to create a thermoresponsive nanocarrier, while polyacrylamide (PAM) served as a nonthermal control. Integrins, which connect the cytoskeleton to the extracellular matrix, and Multidrug Resistance Protein 1 (MRP1), an efflux transporter, play significant roles in drug resistance. The nanocarriers were coated with (4-carboxymethyl) triphenylphosphonium

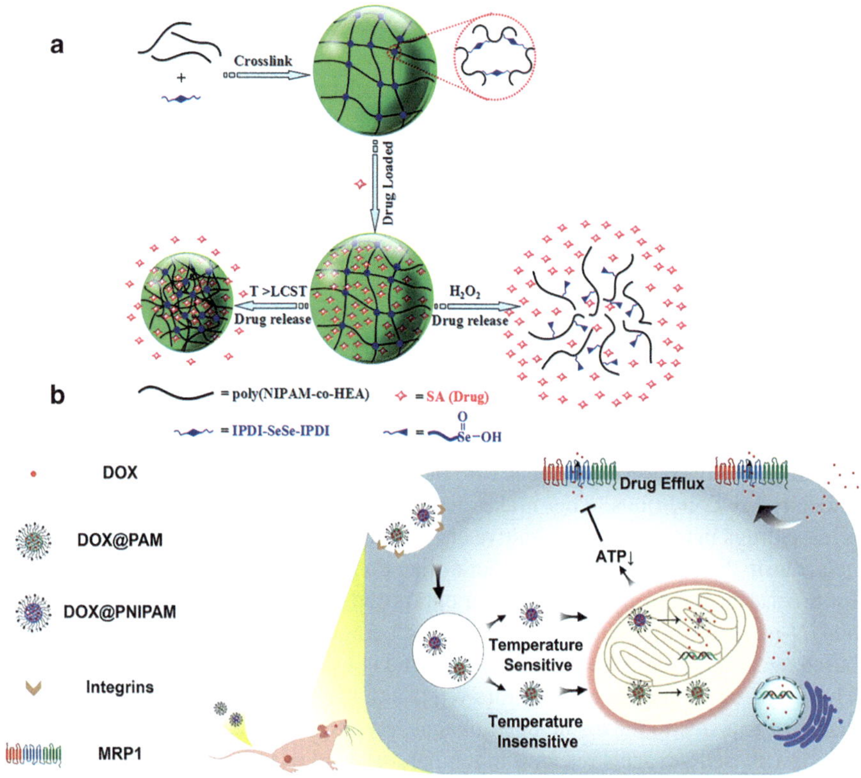

Fig. 5.17 (**a**) Diagram depicting the morphological transformations of poly (NIPAM-co-HEA) hydrogels cross-linked using diselenide linkages in response to thermal and oxidative stimuli. (**b**) Diagram depicting temperature-responsive drug delivery to mitochondria in a small cell lung cancer model resistant to DOX. Unlike the non-thermoresponsive PAM nanocarrier, the thermoresponsive PNIPAM nanocarrier releases DOX at elevated mitochondrial temperatures, causing mitochondrial damage and overcoming DOX resistance. (Adapted with permission from Ref. [51, 52]. Copyright 2015, Royal Society of Chemistry(**a**); Copyright 2022, Elsevier(**b**))

bromide (TPP), which facilitates entry into the mitochondrial membrane due to its negative membrane potential and helps the nanocarriers escape lysosomes. This approach uses a temperature-responsive system to deliver drugs specifically to mitochondria and overcome resistance, particularly to the chemotherapeutic agent DOX as shown in Fig. 5.17b. PNIPAM-based nanocarriers release their drug cargo in response to elevated temperatures within cancer cells. These PNIPAM nanocarriers specifically targeted the mitochondria, which often have slightly higher temperatures due to increased metabolic activity in cancer cells. When the internal temperature of cancer cells increased, PNIPAM released the encapsulated DOX leading to localized mitochondrial damage and subsequent cancer cell death.

5.3.2 Light Responsive

With the advancement in light, photothermal conversion efficiency (PCE) has become a key measure for evaluating how effectively NPs convert absorbed energy into heat. PCE is an important parameter to define the light-responsive nature of DDSs. The mathematical formulations used to measure PCE for a given frequency of light are calculated using Eqs. (5.1) and (5.2).

$$\tau_s = \frac{mC_{\mathrm{p}}}{hS} \tag{5.1}$$

$$\eta = \frac{hS\left(T_{\mathrm{max}} - T_{\mathrm{surr}}\right) - Q_s}{I\left(1 - 10^{-a_\lambda}\right)} \tag{5.2}$$

τ_s: System heat transfer time constant (s)
m: Mass of material (g)
C_p: Specific heat capacity of ultrapure water (J/(g·°C)
h: Heat transfer coefficient [mW/(m^2.°C)]
S: Surface area of heat transfer (m^2)
η: Heat transfer efficiency
T_{max}: Tmaximum temperature that the system can reach (°C)
T_{surr}: Initial temperature of the surrounding environment (°C)
Q_s: Heat dissipated by surrounding environment
I: Incident light radiation intensity mW/cm^2
a_λ: Photothermal material absorbance at a particular wavelength of λ

For instance, the PCE of different NPs under 808-nm laser irradiation has been measured with Au, Au-Pd, Fe, and Fe_3O_4 achieving values of 53.6, 41.9, 67, and 34.6%, respectively [59].

Medical devices can benefit from the unique qualities of electromagnetic waves, which are produced by coordinated oscillations of electric and magnetic fields. These waves span a broad range of wavelengths and include visible light, ultraviolet, X-rays, gamma, infrared, and radio waves. Photodynamic therapy (PDT) emerged as the minimally invasive technique for clinical treatments. It uses photosensitizers, light, and oxygen to induce tissue necrosis and cell damage through reactive oxygen species. It has a promising future in cancer therapy due to its high selectivity for cancer cells, microtrauma, high efficiency, and negligible resistance to drugs. Ji et al. [60] recently synthesized spiropyran nanoparticles (SP-NPs), the properties of which can be tuned by light responses in a reversible manner. SP-NPs are developed to meet the following requirements: (1) To regulate the generation of reactive oxygen species in solution or within cells in a reversible and light-controlled manner, without needing additional photosensitive substances. (2) Should not show any activity on exposure to natural light. (3) Cell imaging and cell killing must be possible upon exposure to light of particular intensity. The spiropyran unit possesses two isomers, i.e., SP and MC isoforms (merocyanine), isomers of which can be controlled by light irradiation. The exposure to LED UV-light irradiation of wavelength ($\lambda_1 = 365$ nm), power density of 2 $mWcm^{-2}$, and a time of 2 minutes led to a sudden change of isoform from SP to MC. However, MC to SP isomerization was observed during the exposure of LED visible light of wavelength ($\lambda_2 = 520$ nm) and a power density of 20 $mWcm^{-2}$. X-rays are frequently used in radiation treatment to treat cancer, specifically breast, prostate, brain, lung, and skin cancer. X-rays are utilized to image interior organs because of their high radiation energy (124 eV to 124 keV; 10 pm to 10 nm—atomic scale) and penetrating depth. The range of the IR (infrared radiation) spectrum is 700 nm (430 THz) to 1 mm (300 GHz). Skin tissue has a maximum light penetration of approximately 4–5 mm at 870 nm (NIR). DDSs that are infrared-sensitive have been created using this feature. Drug release from thermosensitive polymers has been triggered by surface plasmon resonance heat production in metal NPs (e.g., gold110, iron oxide111, and ruthenium112) [61].

Qiu et al. [62] developed an innovative approach to cancer treatment that incorporates the use of light to activate hydrogel nanostructures incorporating black phosphorus (BP). The BP photosensitizer converts light into heat, which softens the hydrogel, allowing precise control over drug release based on light intensity, exposure time, and hydrogel composition. BP's ability to penetrate tissues with near-infrared (NIR) light makes it effective for cancer therapy. This drug delivery system is both safe and biodegradable in vivo. When exposed to NIR light, the BP hydrogel nanocomposite comprising BPNS (BP nanosheets) and hydrogel can control the release of anticancer medications. BP offers distinct properties such as a tunable energy band gap, high photothermal conversion efficiency, ease of manufacture, and high chemical reactivity, making it a promising biological material for biomedical applications.

A smart NIR-light-regulated drug release BP@Hydrogel nanostructure is created by combining PEGylated BPNSs with low-melting-point agarose. After being injected into malignant tissue, the solid state of BP@Hydrogel changes into a gel

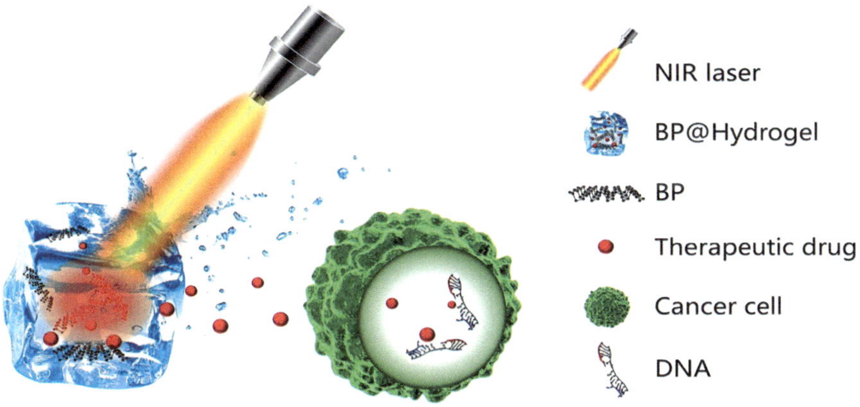

Fig. 5.18 Schematic illustration of the BP@Hydrogel mechanism. Upon NIR-light irradiation, BP@Hydrogel releases the encapsulated chemotherapeutic agents, leading to DNA strand breakage and triggering apoptosis. (Adapted with permission from Ref. [62]. Copyright 2018, Proceedings of the National Academy of Sciences)

state because of the decreased body temperature, as shown in Fig. 5.18. The rate at which drugs are released is advantageous for clinical use, as it can be regulated by both external and internal factors. Strong cancer-cell-killing and tumor ablation properties are demonstrated by BP@Hydrogel, which has minimal toxicity to a variety of cell types. The fact that the agarose hydrogel and BPNSs degrade after treatment gives them promise for use in clinical settings. The BP@Hydrogel drug delivery platform has potential applications for conditions including breast and melanoma malignancies.

5.3.3 Magnetic Responsive

Magnetic nanoparticle-based drug delivery uses magnetic particles such as iron oxide NPs to deliver medication to specific locations. Magnetic fields are a promising strategy in DDSs because of their potential use in micro- and nanomedicine. Magnetic fields span from low to high frequencies (<20 kHz). SPIONs are small particles that respond to magnetic fields. Upon exposure to an alternating magnetic field (AMF) at around 228 kHz, these particles generate heat due to a process called Néel's relaxation. This heat warms up the surrounding lipid membrane, causing the temperature around each SPION to rise significantly higher than the overall temperature. This local heating can make the lipid membrane more fluid in the area around the SPION while the rest of the membrane remains more solid. As a result, the membrane becomes more permeable, allowing drugs to be released. However, this effect is temporary; the drug release stops almost immediately after the magnetic field is switched off as the membrane quickly cools down, as shown in Fig. 5.19.

In a separate study examining the magnetic response, Chen et al. [64] presented a system utilizing a smart nanoparticle platform to control the release of drugs via the influence of an alternating magnetic field (AMF). The NPs have a core@shell structure: a core of superparamagnetic iron oxide surrounded by a mesoporous silica shell. This allows the NPs to generate heat efficiently under AMF, which helps in releasing the drug. A special gatekeeper made from a thermoresponsive aliphatic azo group is added to the silica shell to regulate the release of drug molecules. When exposed to AMF, the heat generated causes the gatekeeper to release its hold, allowing the drug to be discharged. The silica shell itself remains intact during this process. The duration of AMF exposure can be adjusted to control how much drug is released. Multiple exposures can further promote a higher release of the drug. The amount of drug released was shown to affect the death rate of pancreatic cancer cells, demonstrating that this method can be used to precisely control drug delivery.

Figure 5.20a depicts the mesoporous silica shell of the NPs that were functionalized with amine groups using 3-(aminopropyl)-triethoxysilane (APTS). This modification, known as Mag@MSNs-APTS, allows the NPs to load and deliver small drug molecules efficiently. The NPs were further modified by attaching a thermolabile gatekeeper, 4, 4′-azobis (4-cyano valeric acid) (ACVA), using chemical bonding agents. This created Mag@MSNs-ACVA with ACVA acting as a heat-sensitive switch to control drug release. Another modification involving 1-adamantylamine (AMA) was applied to the NPs, resulting in Mag@MSNs-AMA. This change kept the mesoporous structure intact, improving the encapsulation and transport of drugs. The gatekeepers on the NPs can bind to β-cyclodextrin (βCD) to block the pores and prevent drug leakage. Fluorescein, a model molecule, was used to test this system. β-CD was employed to cover the pores and trap the fluorescein inside. When heated in water baths, the fluorescein was released with magnetic heating, causing a more effective release. It shows that this system can precisely control drug delivery without overheating the entire solution. The thermal-responsive NPs offer a promising approach to developing targeted chemotherapy treatments [64].

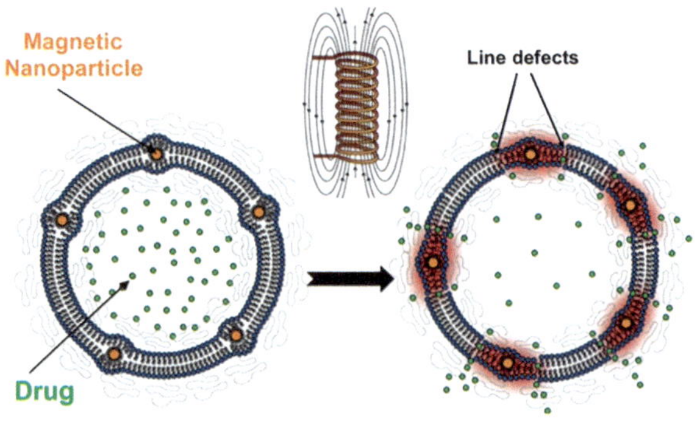

Fig. 5.19 A line defect in the membrane that divides the melting (liquid) from the solid domains is created by local heat generation from SPION through Néel's relaxation. (Adapted with permission from Ref. [63]. Copyright 2017, Nature Publishing Group UK London)

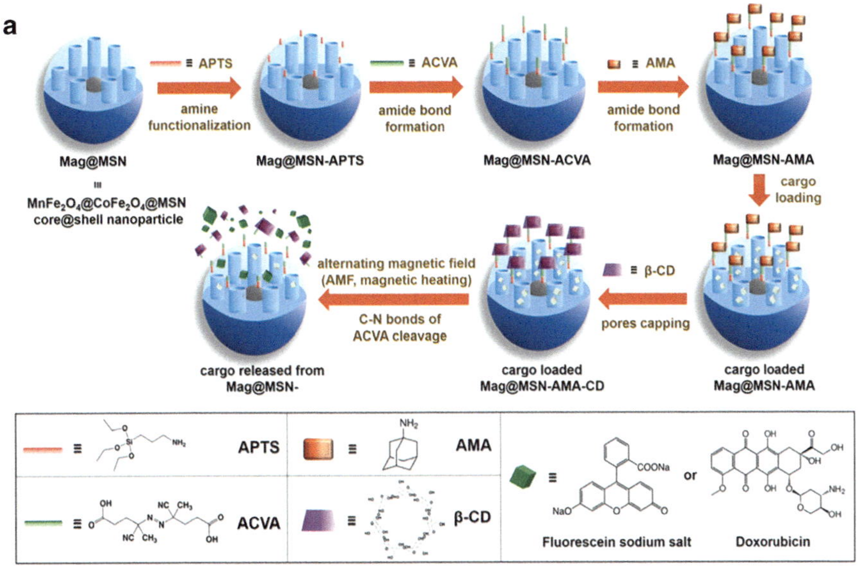

Fig. 5.20 Schematic representations of the platform's design and functioning: (**a**) The creation of mesoporous silica NPs with a core@shell structure with azo-based linkages with a snap-top configuration and its subsequent release induced by an alternating magnetic field exposure. Adapted with permission from Ref. [64]. Copyright 2019, American Chemical Society)

5.3.4 Ultrasound Responsive

High-frequency pressure waves resembling auditory sound at any localized region are known as focused ultrasound (FUS). Its frequency is above the human hearing threshold at 20 kHz or more. FUS can be used to trigger release at specific areas since it can focus on small volumes with dimensions as small as half the wavelength. FUS is a noninvasive technique that targets deep tissues with acoustic energy without the use of radiations and incisions. At present, thermal effects are being harnessed using high-pressure ultrasounds to ablate tissue. This is the most promising and futuristic technique in DDS, and clinical trials are in progress [65]. Another methodology is to use microbubbles with loaded drug molecules on their surface as drug carrier agents. These microbubbles oscillate or show a response under the influence of ultrasound, which leads to shrinkage and expansion followed by a collapse of the microbubble at the targeted location, as shown in the schematic diagram in Fig. 5.21.

Sun et al. [67] address the targeted ultrasound therapy facilitated by cavitation and microbubbles able to penetrate the blood-brain barrier (BBB) effectively and treat various neurological conditions. This approach uses a dual-transducer system operating at a frequency of 274.3 kHz to create a closed-loop cavitation-regulating system. Ultrasound waves generate localized heat and bubble cavitation, which helps nanostructures penetrate specific tissues and release medications. Unlike other external stimuli, ultrasound can deeply penetrate tissues and precisely target the area of interest. Polymer micelles and their assemblies are commonly used in ultrasound-activated drug delivery. Bubble cavitation can cause reversible destabilization of these micelles, allowing for controlled medication release. The amount of drug delivered can be adjusted by varying parameters such as power density, pulse length, and inter-pulse duration. This technique is often tested in animal models for tumor treatment using low-frequency ultrasound. Ultrasonography is used to monitor the delivery of micelles to target tissues. Once micelles accumulate in the targeted area, ultrasound helps release anticancer drugs, enhancing carrier accumulation through the enhanced permeability and retention (EPR) effect. This method improves drug delivery and anticancer efficacy by increasing the internalization of micelles, drugs, and genes into cells, facilitated by ultrasonic-induced cell membrane disruption (sonoporation).

In a distinct study examining ultrasound response, Hoang et al. [68] reported that reactive oxygen species (ROS) modulation in cancer therapy is gaining interest due to its capacity to cause oxidative stress in cancer cells, resulting in effective and cancer-specific cell death. In mildly acidic tumor environments, hydrogen peroxide (H_2O_2) is converted into hydroxyl radicals (•OH). However, the natural amount of (H_2O_2) is often too low for effective tumor treatment [69]. To address this, PEG-coated ZnO NRs are used to improve water solubility and extend circulation time in

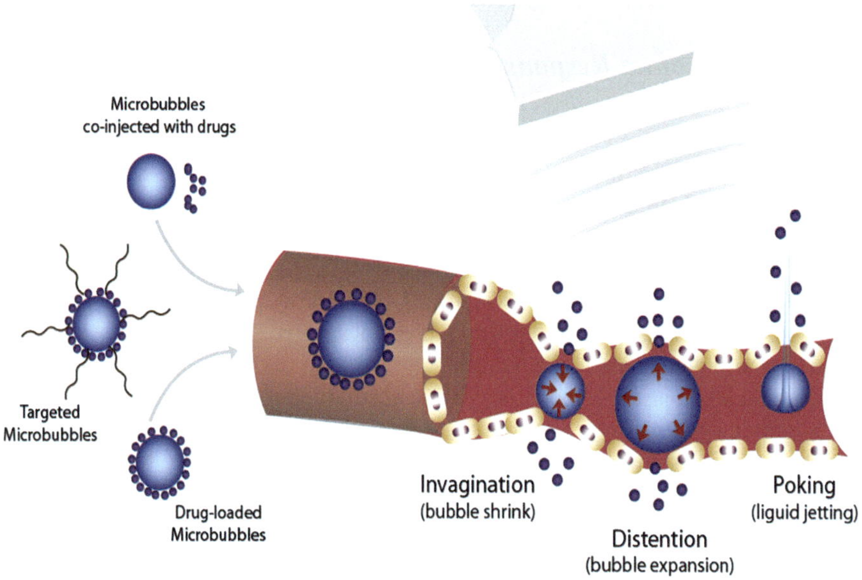

Fig. 5.21 Schematic illustration of ultrasound-assisted drug delivery. The ultrasound waves stimulate the oscillation of microbubbles, causing them to expand, contract, and eventually collapse. This process leads to blood vessel disruption and increased permeability, allowing for controlled and targeted drug release. Three distinct combinations of microbubbles and drugs are shown. (Adapted with permission from Ref. [66]. Copyright 2020, Elsevier)

the bloodstream. The PEG coating helps prevent protein attachment, which allows the nanorods to stay in the body longer. To further increase ROS production, Au NPs are added to the ZnO NRs, and (H_2O_2) is used as a substrate. The PL-loaded Au@P-ZnO NRs provide a combined chemopiezocatalytic therapy, producing high levels of ROS that specifically target and induce apoptosis in breast cancer cells.

Yet the concentration of H_2O_2 is insufficient for effective tumor elimination; thus, producing safe and efficient nanocatalysts with large ROS production is vital to efficient nanocatalytic cancer therapy. Piezoelectric ZnO NRs, which could generate ROS by charge carrier separation driven by FUS, were used as piezocatalytic nanocatalysts. ZnO NPs are not only capable of producing ROS, but they are also biodegradable to improve the water solubility of ZnO NRs.

ZnO nanorods (NRs) coated with PEG were synthesized using potassium hydroxide, with the PEG coating serving to reduce serum protein adsorption, thus prolonging the circulation time in the bloodstream. By adjusting the response time, the length of the PEGylated ZnO NRs was controlled. To enable a synergistic chemopiezocatalytic treatment, pro-oxidant PL was incorporated into the Au@P-ZnO NRs, as depicted in Fig. 5.22. This formulation is designed to enhance the generation of reactive oxygen species (ROS) and selectively induce apoptosis in breast cancer cells.

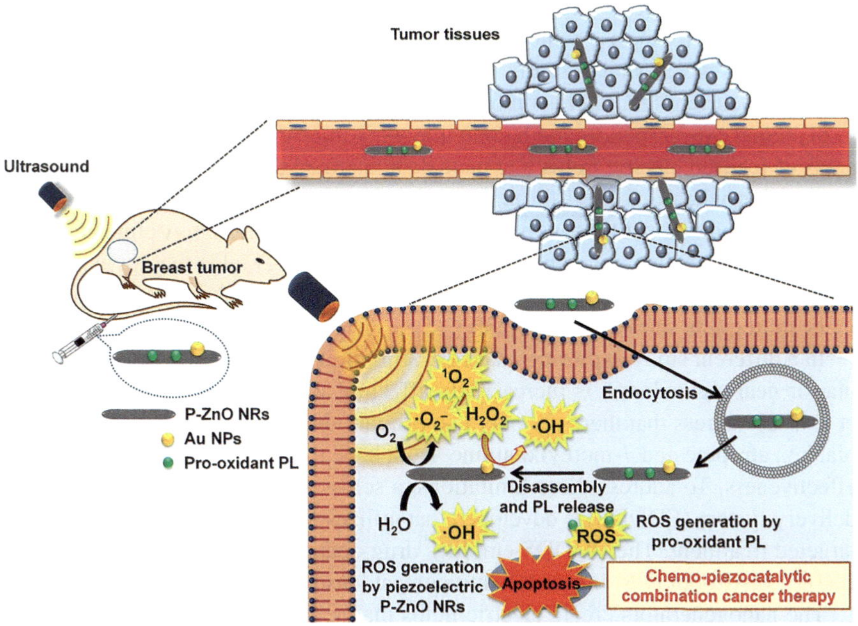

Fig. 5.22 A diagram illustrating the integrated synergistic chemopiezocatalytic actions of PL-coated Au@P-ZnO nanorods after intravenous injection into mice with breast tumors. Under pressure from ultrasonic cavitation, piezoelectric Au@P-ZnO NRs generate ROS and promote apoptosis. The pro-oxidant PL-induced ROS initiates apoptosis specifically in cancer cells, leading to effective chemopiezocatalytic combination therapy for cancer treatment. (Adapted with permission from Ref. [68]. Copyright 2022, Elsevier)

5.3.5 *Electric Responsive*

Electric fields can improve drug delivery through iontophoresis and electrophoresis in topical and transdermal techniques. In electroporation, a high-voltage pulse (>100 V) is applied to the skin surface for milliseconds to permeabilize, while in iontophoresis, a low-voltage galvanostatic electrode excitation (0.5 $mAcm^{-2}$) is used to move the medication through the skin or other tissues [70].

Typically, electric fields within cells range from 0 to 10 V/cm, though they can reach up to 10^5 V/cm in cell membranes. These fields can induce ion movement and polar molecules tend to align parallel to the uniform field's direction. In contrast, nonuniform electric fields create forces that drive polar molecules toward regions of higher field intensity, a phenomenon known as dielectrophoresis. Strong electric fields can stimulate nerves, muscles, and cardiac tissue. However, very strong electric fields can damage cells by generating heat, although they can also activate muscles, neurons, and heart muscle. In alternating current (AC) fields, which oscillate in direction, ionic movement and dipole rotation can vary. AC fields with frequencies of 100 kHz or higher generally have minimal biological effects other than heating, as their impact decreases with higher frequencies. AC fields between 100 kHz and 1 MHz can significantly impact dividing cells. These effects result from unidirectional forces generated by inhomogeneous fields at the interface between daughter cells during cytokinesis, which disrupt spindle tubulin orientation and induce dielectrophoresis as shown in Fig. 5.23a. Kirson et al. [71] explored the impact of alternating current (AC) fields on both resting and dividing cells in culture, as well as in animal cancer models and human tumors. Tumor-treating fields (TTFields) are areas of focused electric fields that have demonstrated their ability to inhibit tumor progression when delivered through insulated external electrodes, both in animal studies and among patients with recurrent glioblastoma (GBM). A clinical investigation on this challenging cancer type confirmed that TTFields therapy is safe and effective in reducing tumor growth, suggesting its potential as a novel cancer treatment strategy, as shown in Fig. 5.23b.

In a different study exploring electrical stimuli, it has been determined that myopia, or near-sightedness, is increasingly affecting young people worldwide. Jiang et al. [72] address that there are only two primary drugs available for treating myopia, i.e., atropine and 7-methylxanthine. Both have notable side effects or moderate effectiveness. To address these limitations, a self-generated electricity-driven drug delivery system (EDDDS) is developed that utilizes nanotechnology for precise and targeted treatment. The EDDDS employs drug-coated nanogenerators, specifically $BaTiO_3$ @Atropin NPs, integrated into contact lenses.

The nanogenerators create electric fields that activate the release of therapeutic agents like atropine directly into the eye when it is closed. This approach not only maximizes the drug's effectiveness but also reduces negative side effects. The mild electrical stimulation provided by the system also helps relax the ciliary muscle, further aiding in myopia control.

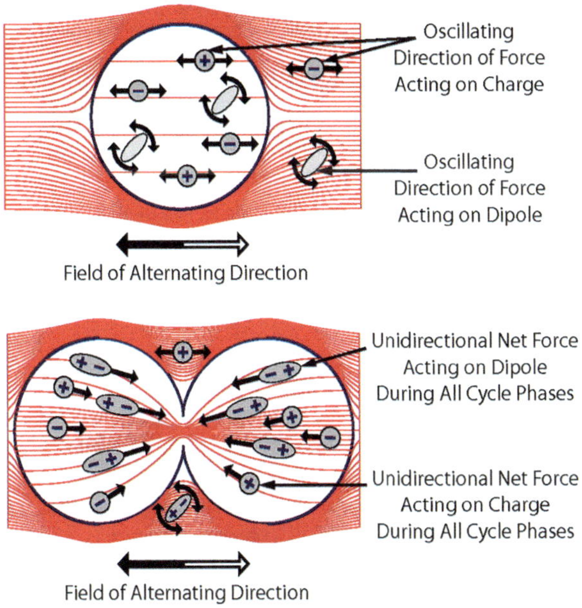

Fig. 5.23 The spread of the alternating current (AC) field, both within and surrounding stationary cells, has been investigated (**a**), and proliferating (**b**) cells vary significantly. In resting cells, the electric forces that oscillate exclusively are responsible for this effect, inducing the "vibration" of ions and dipoles, with the field within the cells being uniform (indicated by white and gray arrows showing forces during each half cycle). On the other hand, in proliferating cells, the nonuniform field generates forces that direct all dipoles toward the division furrow. It is important to note that, in the range of frequencies from 0.1 MHz to 1.0 MHz, the current penetration into the cells is limited due to the relatively high impedance of the cell membrane, as indicated by the density of the lines. (Adapted with permission from Ref. [71]. Copyright 2007, Proceedings of the National Academy of Sciences)

Figure 5.24 illustrates a synthesis of barium titanate NPs ($BaTiO_3$ NPs) through a hydrothermal synthesis process involving barium hydroxide and titanium isopropoxide. By adjusting the reaction time, the particle size can be controlled at nanoscale. The therapeutic ligand atropine was covalently attached to the surface of these NPs via a C-OC bond. $BaTiO_3$ is known for its piezoelectric properties, generating an electric charge under mechanical stress. This property is crucial for creating the necessary electric fields for drug release. The system is designed to work optimally when the eyes are closed, as the pressure from the eyelids induces mechanical stress, generating electricity. In order to enhance the bioefficacy of $BaTiO_3$@Atropine as a treatment for myopia, these NPs were coated onto specialized orthokeratology (Ortho-K) lenses. For the experiment, a lens-induced myopia (LIM) model was employed using guinea pigs. These guinea pigs were fitted with custom-designed soft contact lenses made from an acrylic-fluoro silicone material that provides high oxygen permeability (−10 diopters). The LIM-OK@$BaTiO_3$@

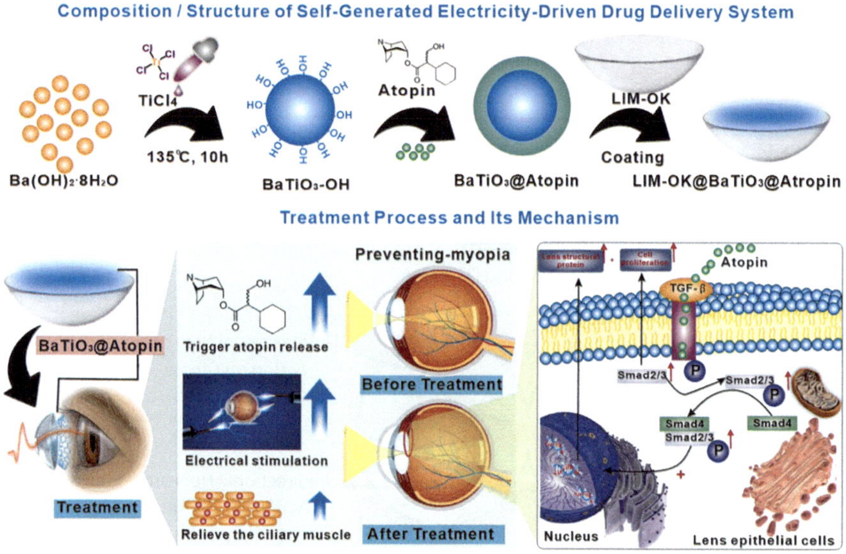

Fig. 5.24 The design and structure of the self-powered, electricity-driven drug delivery system, along with its functioning mechanism, are illustrated. This proposed system, known as LIM-OK@ $BaTiO_3$@Atropin, incorporates nanogenerators that produce electric fields. When the eyes are closed, these fields activate the release of medication, allowing for targeted treatment. Moreover, the application of a low voltage helps to reduce strain on the ciliary muscle, providing additional benefits for the treatment of myopia. (Adapted with permission from Ref. [72]. Copyright 2024, Elsevier)

Atropine system was designed to facilitate a controlled and progressive release of atropine. When the guinea pig's eyes were closed, the piezoelectric coating on the device generated a burst of voltage that disrupted chemical bonds, thereby releasing atropine. Both $BaTiO_3$ and $BaTiO_3$ @Atropin NPs effectively activate the TGF-β signaling pathway, which is important for regulating myopia. TGF-β signaling involves TGF-β binding to cell receptors activating SMAD proteins, which then enter the cell nucleus to influence gene expression related to growth and repair. The LIM-OK@$BaTiO_3$@Atropin system uses this pathway to enhance myopia treatment. This innovative system represents a significant advancement in myopia treatment, combining electrical stimulation with intelligent drug delivery to offer a more effective and tailored treatment approach.

5.4 Endogenous Stimuli Responsive

5.4.1 pH Responsive

The maintenance of cellular and tissue stability is closely tied to the regulation of pH levels. Lower pH levels are found in the inflammatory areas of primary tumors and metastatic cancers. After inflammation, the pH level within the affected inflammatory tissue drops from 7.4 to 6.5 because vigorous glycolysis in tumor cells in an oxygen-abundant environment shows an inverted pH gradient in the tumor microenvironment [73]. This phenomenon, referred to as the "Warburg" effect, lowers pH outside and inside intracellular acidic vesicles by enhancing glucose uptake, stimulating glycolysis, and producing lactic acid metabolites. These are the important features that govern pH imbalances in cancer cells [74]. The pH values of different fluids in the human body are depicted in Table 5.1 [75].

Liu et al. [76] developed a drug carrier to enhance the functionality incorporated in a pH-sensitive lipid called DSPE-PEOz into the platesome, enabling it to release its drug payload more quickly in acidic environments such as those found in tumors. The chemotherapy drug, i.e., DOX, was encapsulated within this hybrid vesicle through a process known as hydration. This process involved mixing two key components: PEOz-liposome-dox, a small and spherical vesicle loaded with doxorubicin and containing pH-sensitive lipids with platelet membrane vesicles (PMVs), tiny bubbles derived from platelet membranes. These components were fused during coextrusion to form the hybrid platesome. The resulting particles with sizes of 200 nm offer improved, effective, and stable tumor penetration.

After the PEOz-platesome-dox was prepared, it was injected into the bloodstream where its ability to target tumors is guided by the natural interactions between the platelet membrane and tumor cells.

A protein on the platelet membrane surface, i.e., CD62p, binds to CD44, a receptor commonly overexpressed on tumor cells. This specific binding directs the platesomes to the tumor site, increasing the concentration of the drug where it is needed most. The platesome pH-sensitive lipids are designed to respond to the acidic environment (pH = 5) typical of tumors. When the platesomes reach the tumor or enter acidic lysosomal compartments within tumor cells, the acidic conditions trigger the breakdown of the platesome, releasing DOX directly at the tumor site. Once

Table 5.1 pH values observed in physiological conditions

Site	pH value
Blood plasma	7.38–7.42
Salivary fluid	6.0–7.0
Gastric acid	1.0–3.5
Bile fluid	7.8
Pancreatic juice	8.0–8.3
Small intestinal fluid	7.5–8.0

released, DOX enters the tumor cells and inhibits their DNA replication, effectively killing the cells and slowing down the tumor growth and spread. This strategy improves treatment effectiveness by specifically targeting the area of interest, thereby reducing unintended side effects, marking a major progress in DDSs [76].

5.4.2 *Enzyme Responsive*

Enzymes in the body play an important role in creating and breaking polymer chains, which affect drug release rates and may cause disease states. Enzymes in healthy bodies can act directly on sensitive drug carriers, changing the rate at which the medication is released. Dysregulation of enzymes in the body, such as hypo- or hyperexpression, can cause disease and can be used to initiate medication release in affected tissues or sites.

Enzyme-responsive drugs need an enzyme-sensitive substance that can be either physically or chemically confined in the system. To be efficient, the DDS needs to reach the enzyme and expose the highly reactive group to it, particularly if the enzyme is connected with a particular tissue or is present in higher concentrations at a specific place [77].

Proteases, as reported by Medintz et al. [78], are enzymes that are broken down at specific peptide bonds within proteins and polypeptides. Proteases are essential in various biological functions and are linked to conditions like infections, cancer, and stroke. A new technique has emerged that utilizes luminescent quantum dot (QD) bioconjugates to monitor proteolytic activity via fluorescence resonance energy transfer (FRET). This approach involves attaching dye-labeled substrates specific to enzymes such as caspase-1, thrombin, collagenase, and chymotrypsin onto the QD surface, employing a modular peptide framework.

Proteolytic tests are performed with an excess of enzyme and substrate, allowing controlled FRET efficiency within the nanoassemblies. This approach not only enables the detection of proteases but may also be useful for monitoring other enzyme activities. The number of peptides attached to each QD nanoassembly can regulate FRET efficiency, and nanosensor models are developed based on this efficiency. These tests provide quantitative enzymatic data and insights into the mechanisms of enzyme inhibition, making them valuable tools in both research and diagnostic applications.

Poly(ethylene glycol)-b-poly(L-tyrosine) (PEG-b-PTyr) block copolymer structure has been developed as a promising drug delivery system for anthraquinone anticancer drugs like doxorubicin. DOX reported by this copolymer self-assembles into polytyrosine-based NPs (PTNs), which demonstrate exceptionally high drug-loading capacities and prompt enzyme-triggered drug release. The phenol groups present in the side chains of PTyr blocks, originating from the natural amino acid tyrosine, contribute to an increased drug loading capacity through π-π stacking, significantly improving the stability of PTNs as shown in Fig. 5.25. PEG2000-b-oligo(tyrosine) block copolymer forms nontoxic, biodegradable, and

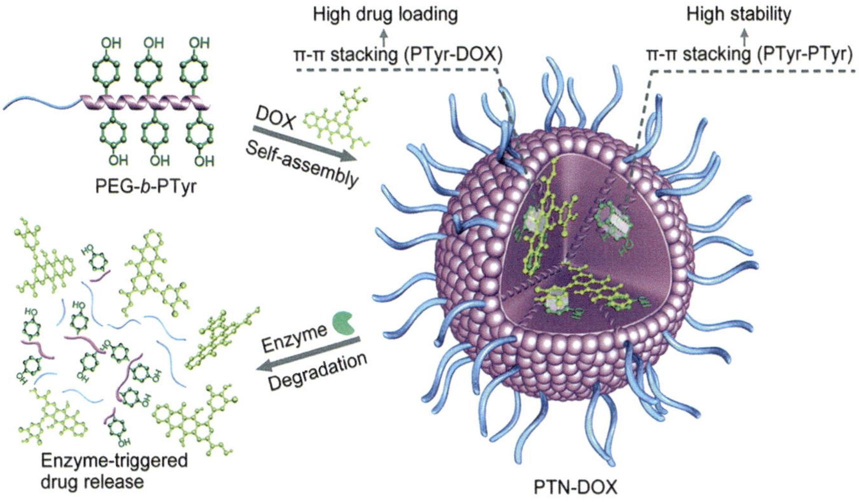

Fig. 5.25 A diagram depicting polytyrosine-based nanoparticles (PTNs) formed from a poly(ethylene glycol)-b-poly(L-tyrosine) block copolymer structure, which provides a significant drug loading capacity and allows for the rapid enzyme-triggered release of DOX. (Reproduced with permission from Ref. [79]. Copyright 2018, Royal Society of Chemistry)

thermoresponsive hydrogels. DOX-loaded PTNs demonstrate stability in physiological environments and effectively deliver and release DOX into HCT-116 human colorectal cancer cells. This results in a more effective antiproliferative response than the liposomal DOX (LP-DOX) formulation typically used in clinical practice. These enzyme-responsive polytyrosine nanoparticles present a promising platform for tailored cancer treatment [79].

5.5 Conclusion

Smart and sustainable nanomaterials are at the cutting edge of transforming digital healthcare, particularly in the realm of drug delivery for challenging diseases. This chapter has explored the innovative use of various nanomaterials and technologies to enhance therapeutic outcomes and address complex medical conditions. It is learned from the overview of the nanomaterials that some of the drugs containing carrier agents, such as liposomes, LNPs, nanogels, and dendrimers, are in clinical studies, while several of these have been authorized by the Food and Drug Administration. Nanomaterials such as MOFs, chitosans, and nanodiamonds are under research trials to bring them into clinical trials. Stimuli-responsive NPs were also discussed to investigate the emerging research in the field of targeted DDS in perspective to exogenous and endogenous stimuli-responsive NPs. Temperature, light, magnetic, ultrasound, and electricity come under the exogenous stimuli responsive to DDS. Among several routes of exogenous stimuli for drug delivery using NPs, light, magnetic, and ultrasound are proven to be smart choices in DDS with precision on controlled release of drug molecules. On the other hand, pH and enzyme-based stimuli-responsive routes are endogenous, for which selective design of NPs as carrier agents is very difficult to achieve for targeted DDS. Iron and gold NPs are being studied as promising delivery vehicles for precise and regulated drug targeting to cancer cells. Therefore, this chapter provides us a complete insight into recent advancements in the development of NPs for DDS.

References

1. Liu D, Yang F, Xiong F, Gu N. The smart drug delivery system and its clinical potential. Theranostics. 2016;6(9):1306.
2. Couvreur P. Nanoparticles in drug delivery: past, present and future. Adv Drug Deliv Rev. 2013;65(1):21–3.
3. Singh R, Lillard JW Jr. Nanoparticle-based targeted drug delivery. Exp Mol Pathol. 2009;86(3):215–23.
4. De Jong WH, Borm PJ. Drug delivery and nanoparticles: applications and hazards. Int J Nanomedicine. 2008;3(2):133–49.
5. Gottardo S, Mech A, Drbohlavová J, Małyska A, Bøwadt S, Sintes JR, Rauscher H. Towards safe and sustainable innovation in nanotechnology: Stateof-play for smart nanomaterials. NanoImpact. 2021;21:100297.
6. Wang Y, Chen L. Quantum dots, lighting up the research and development of nanomedicine. Nanomedicine. 2011;7(4):385–402.
7. Tang Y, Wang X, Li J, Nie Y, Liao G, Yu Y, Li C. Overcoming the reticuloendothelial system barrier to drug delivery with a "don't-eat-us" strategy. ACS Nano. 2019;13(11):13015–26.
8. Zhou Y, Peng Z, Seven ES, Leblanc RM. Crossing the blood-brain barrier with nanoparticles. J Control Release. 2018;270:290–303.
9. Tardi P, Boman N, Cullis P. Liposomal doxorubicin. J Drug Target. 1996;4(3):129–40.
10. Liu Y, Fang J, Kim Y-J, Wong MK, Wang P. Codelivery of doxorubicin and paclitaxel by cross-linked multilamellar liposome enables synergistic antitumor activity. Mol Pharm. 2014;11(5):1651–61.
11. Gradishar WJ. Albumin-bound paclitaxel: a next-generation taxane. Expert Opin Pharmacother. 2006;7(8):1041–53.
12. Green M, Manikhas G, Orlov S, Afanasyev B, Makhson A, Bhar P, Hawkins M. Abraxane®, a novel cremophor®-free, albumin-bound particle form of paclitaxel for the treatment of advanced non-small-cell lung cancer. Ann Oncol. 2006;17(8):1263–8.
13. Allen TM, Cullis PR. Liposomal drug delivery systems: from concept to clinical applications. Adv Drug Deliv Rev. 2013;65(1):36–48.
14. Zhou Y, Chen X, Cao J, Gao H. Overcoming the biological barriers in the tumor microenvironment for improving drug delivery and efficacy. J Mater Chem B. 2020;8(31):6765–81.
15. Mazur F, Bally M, Städler B, Chandrawati R. Liposomes and lipid bilayers in biosensors. Adv Colloid Interf Sci. 2017;249:88–99.
16. Pande S. Liposomes for drug delivery: a review of vesicular composition, factors affecting drug release and drug loading in liposomes. Artif Cells Nanomed Biotechnol. 2023;51(1):428–40.
17. Lee M-K. Liposomes for enhanced bioavailability of water-insoluble drugs: *in vivo* evidence and recent approaches. Pharmaceutics. 2020;12(3):264.
18. Lodish H, Berk A, Zipursky SL, Matsudaira P, Baltimore D, Darnell J. Diffusion of small molecules across phospholipid bilayers. Mol Cell Biol. 2000;1.

19. Mehta M, Bui TA, Yang X, Aksoy Y, Goldys EM, Deng W. Lipid-based nanoparticles for drug/gene delivery: an overview of the production techniques and difficulties encountered in their industrial development. ACS Mater Au. 2023;3(6):600–19.
20. Zhang Y, Qu H, Xue X. Blood-brain barrier penetrating liposomes with synergistic chemotherapy for glioblastoma treatment. Biomater Sci. 2022;10(2):423–34.
21. Abbott NJ, Patabendige AA, Dolman DE, Yusof SR, Begley DJ. Structure and function of the blood-brain barrier. Neurobiol Dis. 2010;37(1):13–25.
22. Altintas C, Altundal OF, Keskin S, Yildirim R. Machine learning meets with metal-organic frameworks for gas storage and separation. J Chem Inf Model. 2021;61(5):2131–46.
23. Al Sharabati M, Sabouni R, Husseini GA. Biomedical applications of metal-organic frameworks for disease diagnosis and drug delivery: a review. Nanomaterials. 2022;12(2):277.
24. Lawson HD, Walton SP, Chan C. Metal-organic frameworks for drug delivery: a design perspective. ACS Appl Mater Interfaces. 2021;13(6):7004–20.
25. Howarth AJ, Peters AW, Vermeulen NA, Wang TC, Hupp JT, Farha OK. Best practices for the synthesis, activation, and characterization of metal–organic frameworks. Chem Mater. 2017;29(1):26–39.
26. Wuttke S, Braig S, Preiß T, Zimpel A, Sicklinger J, Bellomo C, Rädler JO, Vollmar AM, Bein T. Mof nanoparticles coated by lipid bilayers and their uptake by cancer cells. Chem Commun. 2015;51(87):15752–5.
27. Fang T, Duan Z, Wan N, Zuo X, Pan Z, Zhang W, Ge F, Gui L. Goldaptamer-modified metal-organic framework drug delivery nanosystems for combined photothermal/chemotherapy of cancer. ACS Appl Nano Mater. 2024;7(10):12129–41.
28. Tomalia DA, Nixon LS, Hedstrand DM. The role of branch cell symmetry and other critical nanoscale design parameters in the determination of dendrimer encapsulation properties. Biomolecules. 2020;10(4):642.
29. Wu L-p, Ficker M, Christensen JB, Trohopoulos PN, Moghimi SM. Dendrimers in medicine: therapeutic concepts and pharmaceutical challenges. Bioconjug Chem. 2015;26(7):1198–211.
30. Herrmann IK, Wood MJA, Fuhrmann G. Extracellular vesicles as a next-generation drug delivery platform. Nat Nanotechnol. 2021;16(7):748–59.
31. Jiang Y, Lyu Z, Ralahy B, Liu J, Roussel T, Ding L, Tang J, Kosta A, Giorgio S, Tomasini R, et al. Dendrimer nanosystems for adaptive tumor-assisted drug delivery via extracellular vesicle hijacking. Proc Natl Acad Sci. 2023;120(7):e2215308120.
32. Sun Q, Sun X, Ma X, Zhou Z, Jin E, Zhang B, Shen Y, Van Kirk EA, Murdoch WJ, Lott JR, et al. Integration of nanoassembly functions for an effective delivery cascade for cancer drugs. Adv Mater. 2014;26(45):7615–21.
33. Ryu J-H, Jiwpanich S, Chacko R, Bickerton S, Thayumanavan S. Surfacefunctionalizable polymer nanogels with facile hydrophobic guest encapsulation capabilities. J Am Chem Soc. 2010;132(24):8246–7.
34. Ryu J-H, Chacko RT, Jiwpanich S, Bickerton S, Babu RP, Thayumanavan S. Self-cross-linked polymer nanogels: a versatile nanoscopic drug delivery platform. J Am Chem Soc. 2010;132(48):17227–35.
35. Croisier F, Jérôme C. Chitosan-based biomaterials for tissue engineering. Eur Polym J. 2013;49(4):780–92.
36. Herdiana Y, Wathoni N, Shamsuddin S, Muchtaridi M. Drug release study of the chitosan-based nanoparticles. Heliyon. 2022;8(1):e08674.
37. Jafernik K, Ładniak A, Blicharska E, Czarnek K, Ekiert H, Wiącek AE, Szopa A. Chitosan-based nanoparticles as effective drug delivery systems—a review. Molecules. 2023;28(4):1963.
38. Wahajuddin n, Arora S. Superparamagnetic iron oxide nanoparticles: magnetic nanoplatforms as drug carriers. Int J Nanomed. 2012:3445–71.
39. Mistral J, Ve Koon KT, Fernando Cotica L, Sanguino Dias G, Aparecido Santos I, Alcouffe P, Milhau N, Pin D, Chapet O, Serghei A, et al. Chitosan-coated superparamagnetic fe3o4 nanoparticles for magnetic resonance imaging, magnetic hyperthermia, and drug delivery. ACS Appl Nano Mater. 2024;7(7):7097–110.

40. Ul-Islam M, Alabbosh KF, Manan S, Khan S, Ahmad F, Ullah MW. Chitosan-based nanostructured biomaterials: synthesis, properties, and biomedical applications. Adv Indus Eng Polym Res. 2024;7(1):79–99.
41. Liu Z, Tabakman S, Welsher K, Dai H. Carbon nanotubes in biology and medicine: *in vitro* and *in vivo* detection, imaging, and drug delivery. Nano Res. 2009;2:85–120.
42. Bhirde AA, Patel V, Gavard J, Zhang G, Sousa AA, Masedunskas A, Leapman RD, Weigert R, Gutkind JS, Rusling JF. Targeted killing of cancer cells *in vivo* and *in vitro* with egf-directed carbon nanotube-based drug delivery. ACS Nano. 2009;3(2):307–16.
43. Shin SR, Li Y-C, Jang HL, Khoshakhlagh P, Akbari M, Nasajpour A, Zhang YS, Tamayol A, Khademhosseini A. Graphene-based materials for tissue engineering. Adv Drug Deliv Rev. 2016;105:255–74.
44. Zhang L, Xia J, Zhao Q, Liu L, Zhang Z. Functional graphene oxide as a nanocarrier for controlled loading and targeted delivery of mixed anticancer drugs. Small. 2010;6(4):537–44.
45. Chipaux M, van der Laan KJ, Hemelaar SR, Hasani M, Zheng T, Schirhagl R. Nanodiamonds and their applications in cells. Small. 2018;14(24):1704263.
46. Kuschnerus IC, Wen H, Ruan J, Zeng X, Su C-J, Jeng U-S, Opletal G, Barnard AS, Liu M, Nishikawa M, et al. Complex dispersion of detonation nanodiamond revealed by machine learning assisted cryo-tem and coarse-grained molecular dynamics simulations. ACS Nanosci Au. 2023;3(3):211–21.
47. Zhang X-Q, Lam R, Xu X, Chow EK, Kim H-J, Ho D. Multimodal nanodiamond drug delivery carriers for selective targeting, imaging, and enhanced chemotherapeutic efficacy. Adv Mater. 2011;23(41):4770–5.
48. Tian Y, Nusantara AC, Hamoh T, Mzyk A, Tian X, Perona Martinez F, Li R, Permentier HP, Schirhagl R. Functionalized fluorescent nanodiamonds for simultaneous drug delivery and quantum sensing in HeLa cells. ACS Appl Mater Interfaces. 2022;14(34):39265–73.
49. Shi Y, Cardoso RM, Van Nostrum CF, Hennink WE. Anthracene functionalized thermosensitive and uv-cross-linkable polymeric micelles. Polym Chem. 2015;6(11):2048–53.
50. Repasky EA, Evans SS, Dewhirst MW. Temperature matters! and why it should matter to tumor immunologists. Cancer Immunol Res. 2013;1(4):210–6.
51. Cheng X, Jin Y, Sun T, Qi R, Fan B, Li H. Oxidation-and thermo-responsive poly (n-isopropylacrylamide-co-2-hydroxyethyl acrylate) hydrogels cross-linked via diselenides for controlled drug delivery. RSC Adv. 2015;5(6):4162–70.
52. Ruan L, Chen J, Du C, Lu H, Zhang J, Cai X, Dou R, Lin W, Chai Z, Nie G, et al. Mitochondrial temperature-responsive drug delivery reverses drug resistance in lung cancer. Bioact Mater. 2022;13:191–9.
53. Constantin M, Cristea M, Ascenzi P, Fundueanu G. Lower critical solution temperature versus volume phase transition temperature in thermoresponsive drug delivery systems. Express Polym Lett. 2011;5(10):839–48.
54. Karimi M, Sahandi Zangabad P, Ghasemi A, Amiri M, Bahrami M, Malekzad H, Ghahramanzadeh Asl H, Mahdieh Z, Bozorgomid M, Ghasemi A, et al. Temperature-responsive smart nanocarriers for delivery of therapeutic agents: applications and recent advances. ACS Appl Mater Interfaces. 2016;8(33):21107–33.
55. Sun S, Hu J, Tang H, Wu P. Chain collapse and revival thermodynamics of poly (n-isopropylacrylamide) hydrogel. J Phys Chem B. 2010;114(30):9761–70.
56. Fujishige S, Kubota K, Ando I. Phase transition of aqueous solutions of poly (nisopropylacrylamide) and poly (n-isopropylmethacrylamide). J Phys Chem. 1989;93(8):3311–3.
57. Huo M, Yuan J, Tao L, Wei Y. Redox-responsive polymers for drug delivery: from molecular design to applications. Polym Chem. 2014;5(5):1519–28.
58. Cho H, Cho Y-Y, Shim MS, Lee JY, Lee HS, Kang HC. Mitochondriatargeted drug delivery in cancers. Biochim Biophys Acta. 2020;1866(8):165808.
59. Cui X, Ruan Q, Zhuo X, Xia X, Hu J, Fu R, Li Y, Wang J, Xu H. Photothermal nanomaterials: a powerful light-to-heat converter. Chem Rev. 2023;123(11):6891–952.

60. Ji J, Li X, Wu T, Feng F. Spiropyran in nano assemblies as a photosensitizer for photoswitchable ros generation in living cells. Chem Sci. 2018;9(26):5816–21.
61. Mirvakili SM, Langer R. Wireless on-demand drug delivery. Nat Electron. 2021;4(7):464–77.
62. Qiu M, Wang D, Liang W, Liu L, Zhang Y, Chen X, Sang DK, Xing C, Li Z, Dong B, et al. Novel concept of the smart nir-light–controlled drug release of black phosphorus nanostructure for cancer therapy. Proc Natl Acad Sci. 2018;115(3):501–6.
63. Shirmardi Shaghasemi B, Virk MM, Reimhult E. Optimization of magnetothermally controlled release kinetics by tuning of magnetoliposome composition and structure. Sci Rep. 2017;7(1):7474.
64. Chen W, Cheng C-A, Zink JI. Spatial, temporal, and dose control of drug delivery using noninvasive magnetic stimulation. ACS Nano. 2019;13(2):1292–308.
65. Carpentier A, Canney M, Vignot A, Reina V, Beccaria K, Horodyckid C, Karachi C, Leclercq D, Lafon C, Chapelon J-Y, et al. Clinical trial of blood-brain barrier disruption by pulsed ultrasound. Sci Transl Med. 2016;8(343):343re2.
66. Chowdhury SM, Abou-Elkacem L, Lee T, Dahl J, Lutz AM. Ultrasound and microbubble mediated therapeutic delivery: underlying mechanisms and future outlook. J Control Release. 2020;326:75–90.
67. Sun T, Zhang Y, Power C, Alexander PM, Sutton JT, Aryal M, Vykhodtseva N, Miller EL, McDannold NJ. Closed-loop control of targeted ultrasound drug delivery across the blood-brain/tumor barriers in a rat glioma model. Proc Natl Acad Sci. 2017;114(48):E10281–90.
68. Hoang QT, Ravichandran V, Cao TGN, Kang JH, Ko YT, Lee TI, Shim MS. Piezoelectric au-decorated zno nanorods: ultrasound-triggered generation of ros for piezocatalytic cancer therapy. Chem Eng J. 2022;435:135039.
69. Zhang C, Wang X, Du J, Gu Z, Zhao Y. Reactive oxygen species-regulating strategies based on nanomaterials for disease treatment. Adv Sci. 2021;8(3):2002797.
70. Banga AK, Bose S, Ghosh TK. Iontophoresis and electroporation: comparisons and contrasts. Int J Pharm. 1999;179(1):1–19.
71. Kirson ED, Dbal'y V, Tovaryš F, Vymazal J, Soustiel JF, Itzhaki A, Mordechovich D, Steinberg-Shapira S, Gurvich Z, Schneiderman R, et al. Alternating electric fields arrest cell proliferation in animal tumor models and human brain tumors. Proc Natl Acad Sci. 2007;104(24):10152–7.
72. Jiang L, Zhang L, Dai C, Zhao B, Yang Y, Wu Z, Qu C, Zou L, Lin Z-H, Miao Y-B, et al. A self-generated electricity-driven drug delivery system for precision management of myopia. Nano Energy. 2024;119:109040.
73. Zhang X, Lin Y, Gillies RJ. Tumor ph and its measurement. J Nucl Med. 2010;51(8):1167–70.
74. Webb BA, Chimenti M, Jacobson MP, Barber DL. Dysregulated ph: a perfect storm for cancer progression. Nat Rev Cancer. 2011;11(9):671–7.
75. Mu Y, Gong L, Peng T, Yao J, Lin Z. Advances in ph-responsive drug delivery systems. Open Nano. 2021;5:100031.
76. Liu G, Zhao X, Zhang Y, Xu J, Xu J, Li Y, Min H, Shi J, Zhao Y, Wei J, et al. Engineering biomimetic platesomes for ph-responsive drug delivery and enhanced antitumor activity. Adv Mater. 2019;31(32):1900795.
77. Shahriari M, Zahiri M, Abnous K, Taghdisi SM, Ramezani M, Alibolandi M. Enzyme responsive drug delivery systems in cancer treatment. J Control Release. 2019;308:172–89.
78. Medintz IL, Clapp AR, Brunel FM, Tiefenbrunn T, Tetsuo Uyeda H, Chang EL, Deschamps JR, Dawson PE, Mattoussi H. Proteolytic activity monitored by fluorescence resonance energy transfer through quantum-dot–peptide conjugates. Nat Mater. 2006;5(7):581–9.
79. Gu X, Qiu M, Sun H, Zhang J, Cheng L, Deng C, Zhong Z. Polytyrosine nanoparticles enable ultra-high loading of doxorubicin and rapid enzyme responsive drug release. Biomater Sci. 2018;6(6):1526–34.

Chapter 6
Diagnostic Nanoprobes and Imaging Agents

Tanvir Ahmed and Kazi Tasnuva Alam

Abstract The introduction of nanotechnology has enabled the development of highly sensitive and targeted diagnostic nanoprobes and imaging agents, transforming the field of medical diagnostics. The ability to precisely monitor and detect diseases early on has been difficult, and these nanoscale systems have brought about revolutionary changes in traditional diagnostic techniques. This chapter looks at the development, synthesis, and use of imaging agents and diagnostic nanoprobes, emphasizing theranostics and digital healthcare. We explored several kinds of nanoprobes, composed of gold, silver, magnetic, carbon, quantum dots, polymers, and lipids, highlighting their special optical, electrical, and magnetic characteristics that make them ideal for biomedical imaging. We also discussed the integration of these nanoprobes with cutting-edge imaging modalities such as fluorescence imaging, MRI, and PET, enabling the real-time and high-resolution visualization of disease biomarkers at the molecular level. The focus is on the development of smart and sustainable nanomaterials that improve the safety and efficacy of diagnostic processes while simultaneously tackling the issues of toxicity, biocompatibility, and environmental impact. This chapter intends to contribute to the continuing evolution of digital healthcare and theranostic approaches by offering a thorough overview of the recent developments and potential future developments in diagnostic nanoprobes and imaging agents. In the long run, this will improve patient outcomes and support sustainable healthcare practices.

Keywords Nanoprobes · Nanoparticles · Diagnostics · Imaging · Theranostics

---

T. Ahmed (✉) · K. T. Alam
Department of Pharmaceutical Sciences, School of Health and Life Sciences, North South University, Dhaka, Bangladesh
e-mail: tanvir.ahmed111@northsouth.edu

S. Mondal et al. (eds.), *Smart and Sustainable Nanomaterials in Digital Healthcare and Theranostic*, https://doi.org/10.1007/978-981-95-9386-6_6

6.1 Introduction

Since the dawn of time, scientists and researchers have been striving to enhance healthcare by exploring novel diagnostic and therapeutic methods to improve treatment for several diseases. In this journey, the development of nanotechnology has revolutionized the world of medicine and other industries, making it the greatest biomedical marvel of our time [1]. Nanotechnology is a versatile field of study that includes various disciplines and focuses on manipulating atoms and molecules at the nanoscale to develop, analyze, and create systems and devices. The term "Nanos" originates from Greek and means "dwarf." The nanoobjects used have a minimum dimension of around 100 nm or less, placing them in the realm of the infinitesimally small: one-millionth of a millimeter [2]. Nanotechnology is widely recognized as the most promising technology of the twenty-first century due to its extensive applicability in all aspects of the healthcare industry, ranging from disease diagnosis to disease monitoring. Nanoscience is based on the notion that materials can display distinct mechanical, electrical, optical, chemical, and physiological properties when their size is drastically reduced, as contrasted to their bulk counterparts. By using this concept, it is possible to fabricate structures and devices of various forms, dimensions, and desired characteristics. Presently, this radical technology finds its use in biosensors, implants, therapeutics, diagnostics and imaging, gene therapy tissue engineering, regenerative medicine, and personalized medicine.

Richard P. Feynman, a Nobel Prize-winning physicist, introduced the concept of nanotechnology in 1959, which involves using larger things and mechanical instruments on a smaller scale at the level of particles. He famously stated that "there is plenty of room at the bottom" [1]. Following the discovery of this emerging field, scientists from around the globe devised many methods to create nanostructures. These techniques can be categorized into two distinct groups: top-down and bottom-up. The top-down approach requires fragmenting large quantities of material into nanoparticles using techniques such as precision engineering and lithography. Conversely, the bottom-up strategy involves the step-by-step creation of nanostructures by systematically incorporating atoms or molecules through chemical and physical means within the nanoscale range of 1 to 100 nm [3]. In subsequent decades, several innovators in the field of nanotechnology emerged, disseminating their knowledge through the publication of several books on nanotechnology. They introduced groundbreaking concepts such as "self-assembly nanostructures," "nanobots," and other techniques for biomedical applications in their work. The famous term "nanomedicine" was used for the first time around that period [2]. The existence of nanotechnology dates back several centuries, and its proof can be found in objects of the ancient world, including the Lycurgus Cup, Damascene Swords, Italian Renaissance pottery, and medieval church windows. The intensive exploration and investigation of nanotechnology across various scientific disciplines have only occurred since the 1980s, with the invention of microscopes. In 1981, two physicists, Gerd Binnig and Heinrich Rohrer, developed the Scanning Tunneling Microscope (STM), a device that allows for the observation and manipulation of nanoscale particles with high precision, without the need for light or beams. The use of tunneling current in this technique enables the targeted disruption and development of chemical bonds to generate novel structures. This invention earned them the Nobel Prize in Physics in 1986. Following this remarkable development, the atomic force microscope (AFM) and scanning probe microscope (SPM) were introduced in later years for similar purposes, leading researchers to dive deep into the modern era of nanotechnology. In the meantime, Japanese scientist Iijima discovered the use of carbon in nanotechnology by observing carbon nanotubes using transmission electron microscopy (TEM). Due to their high robustness, flexibility, and thermal conductivity, such allotropes of carbon are widely used in different fields of biomedical science, including biosensors, drug delivery, drug analysis, gene therapy, and tissue engineering. In 2004, a more advanced carbon nanomaterial known as carbon dot (C-dot) was unintentionally discovered. It showed superior characteristics such as high biocompatibility and minimal toxicity, making it a highly suitable option for applications in the biomedical field [4]. Devices designed to view and functionalize nanostructures, combined with extensive interdisciplinary collaboration among different disciplines of science, have opened new doors for significant developments in nanomedicine that have had a large-scale transformative impact on the present-day healthcare system. Nanotechnology-based diagnostic tests and equipment are significant examples of this progress. By attaching nanoparticles to targeted biomarkers, researchers may augment the imaging capabilities of computed tomography (CT) scans, magnetic resonance imaging (MRI), and positron emission tomography (PET) scans. This will allow for more accurate and timely detection of cancer and other diseases. Biosensors are yet another impressive use of nanoscience that effectively turns a biological response into an electrical signal to detect biomolecules within our body. This technology has been widely employed in the early detection of diseases, treatment, monitoring, and managing patient health. In addition, as wearable ECG (electrocardiogram) and EEG (electroencephalogram) biosensors become more commonly used in the coming years, researchers predict that this revolutionary diagnostic tool will dominate the global biosensor industry. Another breakthrough in nano-diagnostics is the invention of microfluidic diagnostic chips. The precisely arranged microchannels in these chips, which resemble electrical circuits, specifically perform intricate functions like separation, dilution, detection, and extraction. Due to their exceptional sensitivity, minimal sample and reagent usage, excellent efficiency, and fast analytical speed, these systems show significant promise for replacing macrosystems in laboratory settings. An exemplary example of this technology is the Lab-on-Chip (LOC) system, which has proven effective in identifying serum biomarkers of infectious disorders such as HIV, hepatitis B, and hepatitis C. It offers the additional benefit of operating with tiny sample volumes such as 100 μL. Apart from these point-of-care (POC) diagnostic tools, nanoprobes, quantum dots, nanosomes, nanoshells, and nanopore sequencing are a few other applications of nanosystems in clinical diagnostics that detect disease proteins and DNA mutations and help visualize tumors inside our body. Therefore, by effectively integrating various tools and nanotechnologies, it is feasible to develop diagnostic processes with increased precision, minimized human errors, improved affordability, and greater user convenience [1, 5].

Nanotechnology has not only achieved great milestones in disease diagnosis but also has extensive applicability in drug delivery, thereby reshaping the field of pharmaceutical science and medicine. Nanotechnology-enabled drug delivery systems allow for targeted and controlled drug administration, minimizing off-target toxicity. As a result, there has been extensive investigation and advancement in the use of nano-carrier-based delivery systems for treating many diseases, including cancer. These nanocarriers selectively target tumor sites and infected areas without causing harm to nearby healthy cells, leading to successful drug delivery with minimal side effects. Using nanoparticles improves the solubility, stability, bioavailability, permeability, and life cycle of drugs while simultaneously reducing toxicity. These benefits suggest that the nanocarrier-based delivery system could potentially replace the current cancer treatment approach, where the main obstacle is chemotherapy-related drug toxicity. Several types of nanocarriers are currently used for drug delivery, such as liposomes, carbon nanotubes, dendrimers, micelles, lipids, inorganic nanoparticles, carbon dots, and biomimetic nanoparticles [6]. Nanotechnology has been integrated into gene therapy to deliver therapeutic genes to specific cells, aiming to address genetic abnormalities, malignancies, and infectious diseases. Nanoscale technology is crucial in gene therapy because it operates at the subcellular level, where disease prevention and genetic modifications occur. The nanocarriers shield the encapsulated DNA molecules from degradation and significantly boost therapeutic efficacy. Nanoscience has made notable advancements through its substantial contributions to regenerative medicine and tissue engineering as well. Researchers have created 3D-printed scaffolds that imitate organ structures of our body using nanoparticles. These scaffolds will aid in the development of implants for regenerating and growing tissue. Currently, such bioprinting technology has been used to address diverse orthopedic conditions by repairing damaged bones and promoting bone regeneration [7]. Another extraordinary breakthrough in nanotechnology is the introduction of nanorobots. These nanoscale robots can perform surgical procedures, administer anesthetics with high precision, monitor blood sugar levels, and deliver drugs to targeted locations. Scientists have a positive outlook on the use of nanobots in vaccination enhancement, killing cancer cells, repairing specific diseased cells, and developing personalized medicine for individuals in the near future. During the COVID-19 pandemic, nanomedicine played a pivotal role by using engineered nanoparticles for coronavirus detection, designing masks with nanoparticle coatings to entrap viruses, and introducing novel drug delivery methods like microneedle patches [8]. In addition to the above-mentioned accomplishments of nanotechnology in healthcare, there have been several other significant developments. One notable example is its application in dentistry for repairing teeth, restoring their natural state, and treating hypersensitivity using "dentifrobots." Implantable medical nanogenerators (IMGs) are introduced to provide power to medical devices such as pacemakers and neurostimulators. Nanobioelectric medicines are developed to stimulate the body's healing process for treating various conditions [1], and nanofiber dressings are specifically designed to promote wound healing. Last but not least, researchers today are trying to shift towards the field of green nanobiomedicine by combining eco-friendly nanoassemblies with drugs to minimize their adverse effects on both the environment and human well-being.

The application of nanotechnology in healthcare and medicine has the potential to significantly revolutionize the processes of disease diagnosis, treatment, and prevention. Nonetheless, this technology still has a long way to go, as many aspects of nanomedicine are under the research pipeline, and there are prevalent concerns regarding its safety and potential environmental impact. Globally, extensive nanotech research is underway to address these roadblocks. According to experts, it is likely that nanotechnology will soon become mandatory in the medical industry, transforming the current healthcare system's paradigm.

Diagnostic tests and procedures are instrumental in identifying a disease, obtaining prognostic data, and setting the course of treatment. Consequently, it assists healthcare professionals and patients in making well-informed decisions on the management of the condition. The element of time is critical in medical diagnosis, as there may be a minimal time interval between the initiation of a disease and its advancement. Therefore, it is crucial to identify problems at an early stage to halt their advancement, especially in the context of cancer progression. Medical diagnostics is advancing through the implementation of diverse nanotechnologies to create state-of-the-art diagnostic tools and tests, resulting in precise and prompt diagnosis. Among its several breakthroughs, the development of nanoprobes stands out as an exceptional innovation. Nanoprobes act as imaging agents and cell trackers, with nanoscale dimensions designed to help in the image formation of very small structures, such as the inside of cells and blood vessels. Nanoprobes enhance precision and efficacy when used in traditional diagnostic tools due to their exceptional physiochemical and optical properties, targeted cell recognition capabilities, biocompatibility, high volume/surface ratio, and multi-functionality. Therefore, over the years, these nanostructures have found application in the bioanalysis and diagnosis of a wide range of diseases, including cancer, brain diseases, heart problems, infectious diseases, diabetes, and many more. As explained in Table 6.1, major forms of nanoprobes used in the current healthcare systems are biosensors, quantum dots (QDs), inorganic nanoparticles, polymeric nanoparticles, nanotubes, nanowires, magnetic nanoparticles, and plasmonic nanoparticles. The distinctive characteristics of nanoprobes have gained increasing scientific attention, presenting opportunities for advancing nanodiagnostics through the development of cutting-edge diagnostic tools in the years to come [9].

Early and precise diagnosis of diseases is critical, as it enables the identification of the most appropriate treatment approach and prevents further progression of the disease. Medical imaging is a highly sophisticated technique used to obtain images inside the body at a subcellular level. It helps to identify and characterize tumors and other abnormalities present at different locations. Currently, computed tomography (CT), ultrasound imaging, MRI, optical imaging, positron emission tomography (PET), and single-photon emission CT (SPECT) scans are the most commonly used medical imaging tools. Diagnostic nanoprobes, which include nanoparticles, biosensors, nanocarriers, and microfluidic chips, function as contrasting agents or

Table 6.1 Types of diagnostic nanoprobes and their application in diagnostics

SL No.	Type of nanoprobe	Composition	Imaging modality	Application	Advantages	Challenges	Reference
1.	Metallic nanoparticles	Gold, silver	Optical imaging, CT scan, X-ray, PET scan, SPECT scan	Tumor imaging, stem cell tracking, imaging of cardiovascular diseases, biosensing, radiotherapy	Enhanced sensitivity and spatial resolution, Improved photostability, tunability of surface properties	Potential risk of cytotoxicity, limited penetration depth	[35]
2.	Carbon-based nanoparticles	Carbon nanotubes, quantum dots, graphene	MRI, photoacoustic imaging	Early diagnosis of cancer	Improved sensitivity, high mechanical strength, enhanced optical and electrical properties	Potential risk of cytotoxicity, photobleaching	[36]
3.	Magnetic nanoparticles	Iron oxide, cobalt, nickel	MRI	Tumor imaging in cancer, diagnosis of cardiovascular and neurological diseases	High spatial and temporal resolution, increased sensitivity of contrast	Potential risk of cytotoxicity, low biocompatibility	[37]
4.	Silica-based nanoparticles	Silicon dioxide, mesoporous silica nanoparticles (MSN)	Ultrasound imaging, PET scan	Diagnosis of infectious disease	Enhanced sensitivity, tunable surface properties, high biocompatibility, and biodegradability	Poor biodistribution	[38]

vehicles for these contrast media. These nanostructures improve current diagnostic tools by virtue of their advantageous size, exceptional mechanical, optical, and electrical properties; increased biocompatibility; high tissue penetrability; and adjustable surface characteristics. As a result, the contrast material is delivered in a targeted and immediate manner, resulting in improved contrasting ability and increased sensitivity in the diagnostic procedure. Therefore, it is reasonable to anticipate an early detection of the condition. The potential benefit of this advantage is highly valuable in the management of cancer, as timely identification of cancer assists in making informed decisions regarding the most suitable treatment strategy, enhancing the rate of survival, and improving the quality of life for patients. An instance of this is the integration of ultrasmall superparamagnetic iron oxide nanoparticles (SPIONs) and gadolinium-encapsulated silicon microparticles as contrast agents in magnetic resonance imaging (MRI). Results indicate that the high magnetic characteristics of SPIONs enable them to efficiently transport and distribute the payload, hence enhancing the contrast resolution and facilitating the early detection of malignancies. The progress in medical technologies is growing. Nanoparticles are generating significant interest as potential enhancers to traditional diagnostic methods. Nanoparticles possess inherent benefits over current modalities because they can be engineered to possess specific features. Practically, nearly all medical imaging techniques experience a deficiency in sensitivity and improved spatial resolution of images. Nanoprobes, when used in diagnostics, enhance the efficiency of diagnostic equipment by exhibiting exceptional selectivity towards the target, accommodating many payloads, and causing minimal toxicity. In addition, multiple biodegradable polymeric nanoparticles have been shown to display an enhanced permeability and retention (EPR) effect, allowing them to remain in circulation for an extended period. Moreover, many nanoparticles hinder the absorption by the reticuloendothelial system (RES), hence evading rapid clearance from the bloodstream. Nanomedicines have unique benefits, such as higher surface-to-volume ratios that let them selectively interact with, absorb, and transport small biomolecules to specific targets, enhancing the efficacy of both the probes and encapsulated drugs [10, 11].

6.2 Types of Diagnostic Nanoprobes

The field of nanomedicine has achieved several milestones, particularly in the use of nanoprobes in bioanalysis and diagnosis of many diseases. The following section discusses the important categories of diagnostic nanoprobes currently used in healthcare.

6.2.1 Metal-Based Nanoprobes

Considering their distinctive physiochemical characteristics, metal-based nanoprobes have emerged as strong candidates for use in the biomedical sector, particularly in imaging agents for diagnosing a variety of medical conditions. Metal nanoparticles can be manufactured by reducing the corresponding metal to its nuclear dimension using either the well-known bottom-up or top-down approaches. Generally, these conventional techniques have been proven to be hazardous and costly. Therefore, it is expected that there will be a move towards green chemistry for the production of metallic nanoparticles in the future. Current trends indicate the use of noble elements such as gold, silver, metal oxides of iron (Fe_2O_3), silicon (SiO_2), aluminum (Al_2O_3), titanium (TiO_2), and quantum dots in the development of state-of-the-art diagnostic tools, as well as in improving traditional diagnostic techniques for the treatment of various diseases. These metal nanostructures possess remarkable optical and plasmonic capabilities, making them ideal for sensor technologies employed in diagnostics. These nanoparticles are very stable, sensitive, and biocompatible, proving them ideal for use as contrast agents in various molecular imaging instruments and as drug carriers in drug delivery systems. To fully harness the potential of metal nanoparticles in biomedical applications, scientists still need to resolve the challenges of ensuring long-term stability and biodegradability as well as developing an eco-friendly and streamlined synthesis technique [12].

The following sections provide information on the key metal nanoprobes currently being used for diagnostic applications in the healthcare sector.

6.2.1.1 Gold Nanoparticles

The origin of gold nanoparticles (AuNPs) may be traced back to ancient times when red ruby glass first emerged. It was not until the late seventeenth century that they gained significant attention, eventually leading to their widespread application in numerous healthcare sectors today. Gold nanoparticles are made of clusters of colloidal gold atoms at the nanoscale level, suspended in water or other liquid mediums, and synthesized either by using physical methods of thermolysis, nanolithography, cutting, and milling to reduce the size to the desired nanoscale (5 to 400 nm) or by self-assembly of individual atoms through chemical processes. These particles show diverse shapes, including nanorods, nanostars, nanotriangles, and nanoshells. Typically, AuNPs show optical and electronic properties along with high redox potential, radioactivity, localized surface plasmonic resonance (LSPR), a high X-ray absorption coefficient, and good chemical stability. Remarkably, the aforementioned characteristics of AuNPs can be fine-tuned to obtain the desired shape, size, and function [12, 13].

These metallic nanostructures show a distinctive characteristic known as plasmonic resonance, wherein they absorb light in the blue-green range of the spectrum and reflect red light. This property enhances their ability to absorb and scatter light, making them excellent candidates in biosensor applications. In this particular use, the gold particles are stimulated by a light source while undergoing modifications in the surrounding reagents and size. This results in a plasmon amplification, which significantly enhances the sensitivity of the biosensors. Currently, biosensors use nanorod-shaped gold nanoparticles (AuNPs) to detect diseases. Additionally, AuNP-based optical biosensors monitor the interaction between the antigen (amyloid-derived diffusible ligands) and its corresponding antibodies to identify biomarkers for characterizing Alzheimer's disease. Calorimetric biosensors using gold nanoparticles show highly favorable thresholds for the detection of nucleic acids and proteins. The immobilization of glucose oxidase on gold nanoparticles serves as glucose biosensors to monitor blood glucose levels in individuals with diabetes. Besides its extensive application in biosensors, gold nanoparticles are also used in imaging techniques. For instance, it is known to us that optical imaging serves as a way to identify cancer cells, tumor angiogenesis, neuron functioning, and the presence of infectious molecules by capturing precise images of the corresponding tissues. However, the inherent emission of light compromises the sensitivity of this modality. Researchers use gold nanoparticles as contrast-enhancing dyes to address this limitation. Gold nanoparticles are very suitable for use as fluorescent dyes because of their exceptional optical properties. Therefore, optical imaging techniques such as endoscopy, Raman spectroscopy, and optical coherence tomography use gold nanoparticles infused with fluorescence dye to aid in bioimaging. Adding to this, AuNP-based contrast agents in MRIs are gaining increasing attention along with the use of gold nanocarriers for gadolinium chelate models in MRI techniques. Conventional radiation diagnostics and therapy have used mesoporous silica-coated gold nanorods for theranostic purposes. Gold nanoparticles are applied in biomarker analysis for the detection of several disorders. For example, researchers used the AuNP nanoextraction method to capture oxidized phospholipid, a biomarker for cardiovascular disease. Unfortunately, toxicity and stability-related issues limit the widespread applications of gold nanoparticles in biomedicine. These constraints present researchers with opportunities to further optimize gold-based nanoprobes, enabling their safe use in various diagnostic modalities in the future [13, 14].

6.2.1.2 Silver Nanoparticles

Silver was first used as an antimicrobial agent in ancient times and continues to find applications in various industries today, making it a highly valuable metal. Nevertheless, the process of bioengineering silver to produce silver nanoparticles represents a significant breakthrough in the domains of healthcare and medicine. The preparation of these nanostructures includes using various physical and chemical processes to reduce their size and facilitate the self-assembly of individual species. Nevertheless, such methods being deemed potentially toxic to the environment have led to the adoption of biological alternatives, which involve the use of different types of plants, bacteria, fungi, and algae as natural sources. Similar to other metal-based nanoparticles, silver nanoparticles (AgNPs) can be identified by their characteristic features such as size (ranging from 1 to 100 nm), shape, surface charge, surface/volume ratio, dissolving rate, coating, and agglomeration. These parameters heavily influence the cytotoxicity of AgNPs and are reasons why silver-based nanoparticles have widespread applications in several areas of biomedicine, including antibacterial, antifungal, antiviral, anticancer, diagnostic, drug delivery, water treatment, and even cosmetics [15].

Besides their impressive physiochemical attributes, AgNPs possess exceptional optical, electronic, and magnetic properties quite similar to those of gold nanoparticles (AuNPs). Scientists have been exploiting these unique microscopic features of silver for the last few decades, resulting in their enormous contributions as diagnostic nanoprobes in various technologies. For instance, the use of silver in imaging techniques enhances the acoustic reflectivity of images due to its nanoscale dimension, resulting in the generation of a more vivid and distinct image of tissues and organs. Nanosilver demonstrates a very distinguished optical property similar to gold, namely, its renowned ability to strongly absorb and scatter light in the regions of plasmon resonance wavelengths. This characteristic has been used in several imaging and biosensing applications for the optical analysis of molecular interactions between proteins, DNA, antibodies, and antigens for early detection of disease. Successful inquiry indicates that the use of AgNPs coupled with antibodies is applied for the identification of viral diseases such as HIV (human immunodeficiency virus), yellow fever, dengue, and Ebola. In addition to other diseases, silver-based nanoparticles are frequently used in the detection of cancer. One instance involves the use of silver-based biosensors to detect serum p53 indicators in head and neck squamous cell cancer. In addition, peptide-templated AgNP nanoprobes are used in electrochemical biosensors to identify PSMA (prostate-specific membrane antigen)-positive exosomes, which are diagnostic biomarkers of prostate cancer. Blood-dispersed silver nanoparticles are encapsulated within a protein-crown structure to identify new serum protein biomarkers for triple-negative breast cancer (TNBC). Silver nanoprobes have exceptional properties as contrast dyes in ultrasonography and photothermal imaging of tumors, owing to their remarkable absorbance and light scattering capabilities. The antibodies are attached to the AgNPs and then introduced into the tumor location, where they specifically bind to the antigens present. This interaction offers photoacoustic contrast specifically with healthy tissues, thus rendering it highly ideal for the in vivo assessment of cancers. A study conducted by Cheng et al. (2023) discovered that the combination of surface-enhanced Raman spectroscopy (SERS) using AgNP/porous silicon Bragg substrate and machine learning (ML) shows promise for the early detection of breast cancer biomarkers. Moreover, SERS-based silver-embedded magnetic nanoparticles are used in targeting breast cancer cells (SKBR3), indicating the applicability of silver nanoprobes in theranostic platforms. There have been findings suggesting that silver can be hazardous to living cells by inducing oxidative stress, and continuous exposure to silver might result in liver dysfunction. Thus, to use silver nanoparticles in medical diagnostics without causing harm to human health, scientists must carry out rigorous monitoring and develop strategies to evaluate their nanotoxicity [16, 17].

6.2.1.3 Quantum Dots

Discovered in the 1980s, quantum dots (QDs) are nanosized particles in a "quantum size regime," that is, with a diameter of less than 10 nm. They are composed of a heavy metal core (cadmium, selenium, or cadmium telluride) enveloped by an unreactive semiconductor shell and a customized outer coating of various biomolecules tailored for specific applications. They are identified as semiconductor crystals and are used in the medical field due to their unique optical features. Quantum dots, being far smaller than bulk semiconductors, show single-atom-like behavior, which directly affects their optical performance. Excited QDs with light sources can emit a rainbow of colors, where the relation between the size of the dot and the corresponding energy of the light is inversely proportional. Possessing such tuneable optical properties makes them ideal for biosensors and bioimaging modalities. By manipulating the core composition of quantum dots, it is possible to modify their particle size and emission spectra. Quantum dots (QDs), with their adjustable versatility and functionalization with ligands such as antibodies, serve as highly effective fluorescent probes for molecular labeling, cell-surface receptor imaging, immunoassays, detection of nucleic acids, detection of tumors, and in vivo and in vitro cell imaging. Fluorescence microscopes can easily identify the emission spectra produced, suggesting the capacity of quantum dots to improve the sensitivity of the imaging approach. In addition, researchers have created imaging probes using quantum dot (QD) technology, in which cancer-specific antibodies are linked to QDs that emit near-infrared light. These QDs are coated with a polymer to enhance their imaging capabilities, allowing for clear and detailed visualization of the specific tumor being targeted. Quantum dots are well-suited for use as biosensors because of their distinctive ability to chemically or physically bind a wide range of biomolecules to their surface. An example of this phenomenon is the use of the streptavidin-biotin complex coupled with quantum dots (QDs) to specifically target and analyze DNA molecules to diagnose different diseases at the genomic level. Additionally, due to their wide range of excitation spectra and limited range of emission spectra, these substances are highly effective as donors in biosensors that use fluorescence resonance energy transfer (FRET). Quantum dots show great potential for usage in many diagnostic applications due to their superior quantum yield and photostability in comparison to conventional fluorescent dyes. However, they encounter specific obstacles concerning their toxicity, limited stability, and degradability. By conducting thorough research on novel synthesis techniques and implementing intensive monitoring of quantum dots (QDs) in diverse applications, scientists are optimistic about fully unveiling the inherent capabilities of QDs as diagnostic probes [18, 19].

6.2.2 *Polymeric Nanoprobes*

Polymeric nanoparticle systems, made from natural or synthetic polymers, are another class of nanoprobes with substantial applications in the biomedical industry. Typically, protein, carbohydrate, nucleic acid, polyethylene glycol (PEG), poly (lactic-co-glycolic acid) (PLGA), and polyvinylpyrrolidone (PVP) are used in the composition of such nanoparticles. The synthesis of polymer nanoparticles generally involves processes like solvent evaporation, emulsification, and nanoprecipitation. Common characteristics of polymer-based nanostructures include size (100–300 nm), as well as their shape, crystallinity, zeta potential, surface area, pH, and surface chemistry. Over the past few years, there has been a mounting interest in adopting polymeric nanoparticles as bioimaging agents instead of small molecules to address the shortcomings of current therapeutics and imaging techniques. This is because polymeric nanoparticles can be easily modified on their surface and have a large surface area-to-volume ratio. These properties are advantageous for attaching fluorophores or targeting molecules, increasing their circulation time, and allowing them to build up at desired tumor sites due to the EPR effect. In addition, polymeric nanostructures are widely recognized for their exceptional ability to function as effective drug carriers for targeted drug delivery. Medical imaging techniques use this characteristic and create nanopolymeric imaging agents in which the contrast dyes or tracers are bound to the polymeric structure or enclosed within the polymer matrix. For example, researchers have created contrast agents made of polymers that incorporate gold, bismuth, and gadolinium. These agents are designed to enhance the sensitivity of CT imaging. Similarly, researchers are extensively investigating these polymer-based nanostructures as diagnostic and therapeutic agents in different imaging modalities, such as MRI, PET scans, optical imaging, and multimodal imaging [20].

The sections below focus on the present application of several biodegradable and non-biodegradable polymeric nanoparticles as drug carriers, imaging probes, and theranostic agents.

6.2.2.1 Biodegradable Polymers

Biodegradable polymers includes substances derived from both natural and synthetic origins. Like other inorganic particles, these polymeric substances are specifically designed through bioengineering to create nanostructures that have applications in different areas of healthcare. Biodegradable nanopolymers, especially the ones derived from synthetic sources, are widely available, biodegradable, compatible with living organisms, and replenishable, making them ideal for use as nanoprobes in imaging agents and drug delivery systems for the treatment and diagnosis of various conditions. Besides, biodegradable polymeric nanoprobes can be customized by altering their composition, structure, and internal volume and modified by conjugating them with bioactive ligands. This makes them excellent nanocarriers for targeted delivery of drugs, contrast agents, and radiotracers. Some examples of applications include the use of biodegradable nanoprobes as contrast dyes and theranostic agents for PET scans. In addition, a nanocapsule consisting of iodinated oil with methoxy-terminated poly (ethylene glycol)-block-poly (ε-caprolactone), or mPEG-b-PCL, has been designed to improve the contrast in CT scans. Additionally, researchers have created a nanoparticle system using gadolinium (Gd) and multiblock polymers made up of PLA (polylactic acid), PEG (polyethylene glycol), and PLL (polylysine) to improve MRI scans for hepatocellular cancer. These particles have proven to be promising theranostic agents. Apart from the imaging approaches stated earlier, researchers developed biodegradable plasmonic gold nanovesicles based on PEG-b-PCL for photoacoustic (PA) imaging and photothermal therapy, intending to reduce phototoxicity to neighboring organs. To surpass the limitations of various imaging techniques, scientists are eager to advance multimodal imaging. Biodegradable nanopolymers can be used in this novel imaging approach for their ability to transport several contrast agents to specific locations, enabling multimodal imaging and enhancing local contrast by distributing small molecules to the targeted site in vivo. In the context of medical imaging, synthetically derived biodegradable polymers are more commonly used. Among those derived from natural sources, chitosan is used as a tumor-targeting nanocarrier in the diagnosis of several cancer types. Although biodegradable polymeric nanoprobes show promise in biomedical imaging techniques and theranostics, researchers still need to work on improving several factors, including low drug loading efficacy, weak mechanical properties, rapid disintegration, and off-target toxicity [21, 22].

6.2.2.2 Non-biodegradable Polymers

Polymeric nanoprobes have favorable biological characteristics within the human body, making them highly suitable for drug delivery and imaging therapy. Non-biodegradable nanopolymers have limited usage in these areas due to their resistance to disintegration and ability to cause toxicity. Still, few cases can be found where non-degradable-based nanopolymers are used. For example, a few elastin-based nanopolymers are studied for their potential to be used as nanocarriers for antineoplastic drug delivery and gain higher specificity in PET imaging. In addition, a study was conducted on a non-degradable nanopolymer, namely polystyrene-polyacrylic acid (PA-b-PAA), to boost the effectiveness of drug delivery for antimicrobial drugs. These nanopolymers were investigated for their potential to overcome bacterial drug resistance and enhance the EPR effect within cells. Nevertheless, non-degradable polymers like poly(methyl methacrylate), poly(propylene), poly(ethylene), and polyurethane have other widespread biomedical uses, such as medical implants, orthopedic prostheses, hernia meshes, catheters, vascular grafts, and other medical devices, due to their robust mechanical properties and lack of reactivity [23]. The following section is about the lipid based nanoprobes and its types.

6.2.3 Lipid-Based Nanoprobes

Lipid-based nanoparticles, such as liposomes and solid lipid nanoparticles, have become vital tools in optimizing medical imaging modalities and biosensors for precise diagnosis and disease assessment. These nanoparticles serve as drug transporters and theranostic agents, playing a critical role in our healthcare sector. Structurally, lipid nanoparticles are spherical vesicles composed of ionizable lipids. They contain a core-shell, an inner shell, and an outer shell. The nanoparticle's core encloses the drug payload for transportation. The lipid core of the nanocarrier demonstrates the advantage of having a large storage capacity for trapping lipophilic drugs and contrast agents for both diagnosis and treatment. These structures produce negligible toxicity in living tissues, enable precise and sustained drug delivery, show low immunogenicity, and improve loaded drug molecules' solubility and biocompatibility [24].

As detailed in the sections below, liposomes and solid lipid nanoprobes are the most widely used nanocarriers at present for both diagnostic and theranostic platforms, due to their above-mentioned advantages.

6.2.3.1 Liposomes

The biomedical industry has extensively researched liposomes as delivery systems, documenting numerous recent breakthroughs in innovative liposomes over the last few decades. These lipid nanoparticles consist of phospholipids arranged in a bilayer configuration as a result of their amphipathic characteristics. Their dimensions range from 50 to 500 nm, and they can encapsulate drugs that are both hydrophilic and hydrophobic. Aside from phospholipids, additional substances like cholesterol can be incorporated into the framework to enhance the fluidity of the carrier and the permeability of the enclosed drugs. Liposomes typically serve as carriers through two mechanisms: active targeting and passive targeting. An impressive characteristic of these nanoparticles is their capacity to be modified with ligands such as PEG to enhance their effectiveness in delivering drugs and prevent deterioration within the body [25].

Liposomes are commonly used as carriers for encapsulating contrast agents in several imaging techniques, especially MRI. In particular, SPIONs and Gd-based contrast dyes are used in MRI for disease imaging. Gd is easily degraded in the cell, reducing the efficacy of the technique. Encasing these dyes within the liposomal core or conjugating them with liposomes has shown increased accumulation and longer retention time in blood, thus helping to gain a better visualization of the underlying pathophysiological processes [26]. Liposomes possess the distinct capability to transport several diagnostic compounds and can be enhanced by integrating multiple functionalities without compromising their stability within a living organism. Moreover, they offer a safeguarding shield for the compounds being transported and enable a non-intrusive imaging system. These characteristics make them ideal for PET and CT scans used in the diagnosis of many types of cancer. Liposomes are incredibly effective carriers of theranostic agents for cancer management, in addition to their extensive use in diagnostics. Theranostic liposomes grafted with ligands like antibodies can be selected as promising carriers of chemotherapeutic agents to promote both therapeutic and diagnostic effectiveness. These liposomes show improved tumor accumulation, greater permeability and retention effects, and prolonged circulation in the bloodstream [27]. Researchers are now developing liposomes as investigative tools for disease imaging and targeting with radiotherapeutic drugs for tumors and metastases. Furthermore, studies have shown that conjugating liposomes with radioactive and fluorescent markers enables the visualization and specific targeting of tumors in laboratory settings. To further the use of liposomes in diagnostics and disease management, researchers are looking into ways to develop novel liposomes with low production costs and increased half-life. Nevertheless, with their numerous benefits as drug carriers, it is anticipated that liposomes will find more applications in the biomedical industry in the coming decade [24].

6.2.3.2 Solid Lipid Nanoparticles

Solid lipid nanoparticles are a novel colloidal system consisting of physiological lipids that remain in a solid state at ambient or room temperature. Their particle size spans from 50 to 1000 nm. The solid lipid structure serves as a framework for enclosing drugs and can be stabilized by incorporating polymers or surfactants. Like liposomes, SLNs show properties such as controlled drug release, targeted drug delivery, biocompatibility, physical stability, and low systemic toxicity, making them a model candidate for use as nanocarriers in imaging and theranostics. The production and industrial scale-up of solid lipid nanoparticles (SLNs) are comparatively simpler than that of liposomes. The lipids used in this method are more cost-effective compared to liposomes. Besides the above-mentioned features, SLNs are capable of crossing the blood-brain barrier making them suitable tools to be used as a CNS MRI contrast agent. Apart from MRI, solid lipid nanoprobes are readily used in PET and CT scans as well for their precise delivery of contrast media to desired tissues without showing any signs of biotoxicity. SLNs show great potential for being used as highly efficient anticancer theranostics. Research indicates that using SLNs containing quantum dots (QDs) can be beneficial for detecting cancers and delivering a combination of paclitaxel and siRNA to treat such malignancies. SLNs can undergo functionalization with PEG and antibodies that possess an affinity for specific cell surface receptors. This enables the use of SLNs for in vivo imaging and the transportation of therapeutic drugs, particularly for conditions such as rheumatoid arthritis. Although there are some drawbacks concerning the crystallinity of lipids, drug loading efficiency, and dispersion of the nanocarrier formulations based on solid lipid nanoparticles (SLN) show significant potential for the advancement of therapy and diagnostics, due to their targeted delivery of therapeutic agents and simultaneous in vivo imaging [24, 28, 29].

6.2.4 Carbon-Based Nanoprobes

Carbon is an exceptional element in the periodic table because it has the remarkable ability to arrange its four valence electrons in various hybridization states and create amorphous forms. Different physical and chemical techniques are used to fabricate carbon nanostructures, retaining almost all the properties of the original element. In light of the extensive studies carried out over the last few years, numerous inherent characteristics of carbon-based nanoparticles have been uncovered. These include superior carrier mobility, high electrical conductivity, enhanced flexibility, optical transparency, exceptional mechanical resistance, structural diversity, and a high specific surface area. Exploitation of these features has led to the widespread use of carbon nanoprobes like fullerene, carbon nanotubes, graphene, and carbon dots in current medical diagnostics and therapeutics [30].

The subsequent sections explore two of the most commonly used carbon nanoprobes in the field of nanomedicine.

6.2.4.1 Carbon Nanotubes

Carbon nanotubes are a highly significant type of carbon nanoallotrope that show exceptional mechanical, chemical, electrical, and thermal characteristics. The discovery was made in 1991 by Sumio Iijima, a Japanese physicist. In this nanostructure, carbon atoms arranged in a graphene sheet essentially roll into a tubular shape at the nanoscale, showing exceptional features due to their highly symmetrical nanostructure. The number of walls in their tubular nanoformation categorizes CNTs into different types. These types include single-walled carbon nanotubes (SWCNT), double-walled carbon nanotubes (DWCNT), triple-walled carbon nanotubes (TWCNT), and multi-walled carbon nanotubes (MWCNT) [31].

Harnessing their unique properties, carbon nanotubes are becoming more prevalent in biosensor technology, medical imaging, and drug delivery systems. Carbon nanotubes (CNTs) possess exceptional electrical properties, rendering them ideal for use as a sensing component in electrochemical sensors for the identification and monitoring of many diseases, particularly diabetes and bacterial infections. Introducing carbon nanotubes (CNT) onto the electrode surface improves the biosensor's electron transport speed and sensitivity. Recent research has demonstrated that using carbon nanotubes (CNT) can improve the electrical conductivity of a non-enzymatic glucose detector, enabling faster screening of diabetics. Additionally, imaging techniques based on carbon nanotubes are becoming increasingly prominent. For instance, fluorescence-based single-walled carbon nanotubes (SWCNTs) are used in optical imaging to visualize blood vessels in depth and identify the presence of malignancies or other abnormalities. Similarly, carbon nanotubes (CNTs) are used in photoacoustic imaging, Raman imaging, and MRI to improve the contrast image resolution of the targeted region. Single-photon emission computed tomography imaging (SPECT) uses carbon nanotubes (CNTs) as carriers of the radioactive probes to detect and analyze problems inside the body. Through conjugation with other compounds, these carbon nanostructures can be modified to minimize the harmful buildup of radionuclides in healthy tissues and enhance the contrasts generated by different imaging techniques. Along with these applications, carbon nanotubes serve as carriers for drugs, particularly in the context of cancer therapeutics. Nanocarriers based on carbon nanotubes (CNTs) demonstrate exceptional transfection capability and exploit the enhanced permeability and retention (EPR) effect. Consequently, chemotherapeutic drugs can be enclosed within CNT carriers to specifically target tumors. For example, doxorubicin is incorporated into a carrier made of PEG-conjugated CNTs for anti-cancer treatment. Functionalizing with ligands such as PEG improves the hydrophilicity and duration of circulation of the nanocarrier throughout the body. Specific anticancer drugs that are coupled with carbon nanotubes (CNTs) demonstrate promise for both targeting tumors and imaging, suggesting the potential theranostic applications of CNTs. Nevertheless, carbon nanotubes in biomedicine still have some limitations to overcome. The primary concern is the high purity of CNTs, which can result in the release of toxic ions in a biological setting. To ensure the future development of carbon nanotubes that are both safe and biocompatible, it is imperative to address this matter concerning biosafety as early as possible [32, 33].

6.2.4.2 Graphene Oxide

Graphene oxide (GO) is a carbon nanomaterial that contains several functional groups on a carbon-based surface. GO is produced from graphite by a series of oxidation steps. The existence of several functional groups (hydroxyl, carbonyl, carboxyl, and epoxyl) on the surface of these materials contributes to their stability, solubility, and biocompatibility. Graphene oxide, similar to other carbon-based nanostructures, enables the modification of its surface using various compounds while allowing for tuning of its optical, mechanical, and electrical characteristics. These distinctive features of GOs have garnered the interest of researchers for their potential use in the biomedical domain [34].

Graphene oxides are commonly used as biosensors for in vivo monitoring of various biomolecules due to their strong fluorescence, high electrochemical reactivity, and ability to scatter Raman light. For instance, graphene oxide has been used in the design of DNA biosensors for the detection of both single- and double-stranded DNA molecules. Recently, a new method for detecting the hybridization of Mycobacterium tuberculosis DNA was proposed. This method involves using graphene placed on an SPR-sensing chip. Graphene oxides possess a large surface area, making them well-suited for transporting drugs in various anticancer treatments. Doxorubicin is frequently incorporated into PEG-conjugated GO nanocarriers to facilitate the specific transport of the enclosed anti-cancer medication. Subsequent CT and SPECT imaging demonstrated that the growth of tumors and the spread of cancer to the lungs were prevented by an increased abundance of cytotoxic CD8+ T cells within the system. In addition to this, a novel approach including Graphene

Quantum Dots (GQDs) is widely used as biosensors and drug carrier systems for several diagnostic and therapeutic purposes. Graphene oxides, despite their potential applications, can induce biotoxicity and immunogenicity in the body. Therefore, scientists must strive to improve the efficiency of GOs by tackling these critical limitations [33].

6.3 Imaging Techniques Enhanced by Nanoprobes

To detect and assess a disease within the body, it is crucial to be able to visualize the affected areas within our body. Molecular and diagnostic imaging facilitates the non-invasive visualization and analysis of biological processes within the human body by generating images of specific tissues and organs. This allows for the comprehension of complex biological processes, improves the knowledge of disease mechanisms at the molecular level, and promotes the identification of new biomarkers for disease diagnosis. Presently, multiple imaging techniques are widely used, such as magnetic resonance imaging (MRI), computed tomography (CT), ultrasound imaging, optical imaging, positron emission tomography (PET), and single-photon emission computed tomography (SPECT). In recent decades, nanotechnology has greatly benefited modern nanomedicine by playing a crucial role in both the diagnosis and treatment of diseases. In this regard, nano-based diagnostic probes are a highly notable breakthrough in the field of nanotechnology. When used in standard imaging methods, the unique physical properties of these nanostructures contribute to improving and optimizing the aforementioned imaging modalities, resulting in expedited and more accurate disease diagnosis. This, in turn, facilitates timely decision-making regarding the treatment strategy of the related disease.

6.3.1 Optical Imaging

Optical imaging is a valuable tool in the field of medical diagnostics that provides insights into the fundamental biological processes and facilitates disease identification. This diagnostic approach uses light of varying wavelengths to investigate and examine tissues, organs, and biomolecules. Optical imaging is widely preferred because of its biosafety, which minimizes patient exposure to hazardous radiation. Common optical techniques used in healthcare include fluorescence imaging, optical coherence tomography, photoacoustic imaging, and luminescence imaging. Despite its diverse potentialities, this modality has a few limitations, including a lack of penetration depth in the tissues due to autofluorescence, resulting in poor spatial resolution. Factors such as phase noise impede the sensitivity of the process. To address these challenges, nanoprobes with adjustable optical properties and high biocompatibility can be used in contrast dyes to enhance the contrast and image quality of the targeted areas in vivo. In addition, nanoparticles act as effective carriers that can transport contrast media to specific regions in optical bioimaging to achieve successful targeted delivery [14, 39].

6.3.1.1 Fluorescence Imaging

Fluorescence imaging is an optical technique that involves the stimulation of a fluorescent substance with light of a shorter wavelength, causing the emission of light with a longer wavelength. This principle is exploited to create molecular-level images of blood vessels, tissues, and organs inside our body. Typically, fluorophores use light in the near-infrared (NIR) of 650–900 nm for tissue imaging. However, this optical window fails to provide in-depth tissue penetration due to the phenomenon of natural emission of light (autofluorescence). In addition, it produces a low signal-to-background ratio, resulting in poor spatial resolution of the generated images. To tackle these issues, imaging nanoprobes that utilize light in the NIR-II window (1000 to 1700 nm) are employed. This allows for a high signal-to-background noise ratio and minimal autofluorescence, which aid in the visualization of deep tissue for accurate disease diagnosis. Probes for fluorescence imaging often rely on nanostructures that can modify their optical characteristics and are functionalized through structural modifications. These distinctive features, in return, make them useful for improving the sensitivity of fluorescence imaging systems. Gold nanoparticles and quantum dots frequently incorporate fluorescent dyes to enhance image visibility by improving contrast. Gold nanoprobes possess the remarkable quality of plasmonic resonance, which enables them to generate the specific optical characteristics necessary for fluorescence imaging. Quantum dots (QDs), in addition to gold, serve as ideal inorganic fluorophores for optical imaging given their precise size control, emitting diverse light spectra, and resisting photobleaching. The fluorescence emitted by excited single-walled carbon nanotubes (SWCNT) in the NIR-II region is used in optical imaging to visually detect biomolecules by penetrating deeper into the tissues. Alongside these, lipid- and polymer-based nanostructures are used as carriers for fluorescent dyes in optical imaging, do not elicit an immune response, are biodegradable, allow for site-specific delivery, and can evade rapid removal by the reticuloendothelial system (RES), leading to prolonged circulation within the body [32, 40].

6.3.1.2 Bioluminescence Imaging

Bioluminescence imaging is a versatile optical imaging technique that harnesses the fundamentals of bioluminescence, where live organisms emit light to create images. This form of imaging is mostly used to monitor cancer cells and study their biodistribution inside tissues. Bioluminescence imaging enables a higher signal-to-background ratio by the species emitting light rather than absorbing it. This modality is highly responsive and cost-effective. The majority of bioluminescence sensors emit light within the wavelength range of 400–600 nm, and their potential to penetrate deep tissues is limited, making them unsuited for deep tissue imaging. In recent decades, advanced nanoparticle-based technologies with high efficiency and sensitivity have been developed specifically for bioluminescence imaging, aiming to address this challenge. Bioluminescent resonance energy transfer-conjugated quantum dots (BRET-QDs) have recently become increasingly popular. BRET sensors use the bioluminescence produced by a luciferase enzyme present in the sea pansy to transfer energy to a fluorescence molecule, resulting in the emission of a detectable amount of fluorescence. This allows the continuous monitoring of changes in target molecules and live imaging within an organism with a high level of sensitivity. Furthermore, the use of D-luciferin conjugated magnetic nanoparticles in the field of bioimaging is currently under study to explore its potential in improving the functionality for bioimaging applications. Nevertheless, the potential toxicity risks concerning these nanoprobe-based techniques must be carefully considered during their development and subsequent optimization period [40, 41].

6.3.2 Magnetic Resonance Imaging (MRI)

Magnetic resonance imaging (MRI) is one of the most frequently used medical imaging tools in the healthcare industry. The process involves generating a strong magnetic field to align the hydrogen atom protons, which are then exposed to pulsed radio waves, causing the protons to spin. The movement of protons in the body produces a faint signal, which is then captured and analyzed by computers to form coherent images. Due to its superior sensitivity in comparison to other imaging techniques, it can generate images of almost every structure within the human body. In addition, MRI offers several other benefits, such as excellent temporal resolution, absence of radiotoxicity, and superior visibility of soft tissues. As a result, MRI is widely used for the detection of cancer, rheumatoid arthritis, injured ligaments, joint trauma, and diseases affecting organs such as the heart, brain, or stomach. Unfortunately, the full potential of MRI has yet to be used due to its limited specificity, resulting in an uncertain determination of the cancer stage. To improve the effectiveness of this system, various types of nanoparticle systems based on gold, iron, silver, metal oxides, carbon, lipid, and polymers, as well as superparamagnetic nanoparticles, are used as contrast agents and carriers. Their distinctive characteristics and capabilities not only enhance the sensitivity of MRI scans but also allow for accurate cancer staging [42, 43].

One of the applications of nanoprobe-based MRI procedures is illustrated in Fig. 6.1 below, stating the functionality of the UCNP (upconversion nanoparticle) @GA-FeIII probe used in MRI for tumor therapeutics and bioimaging in mouse models.

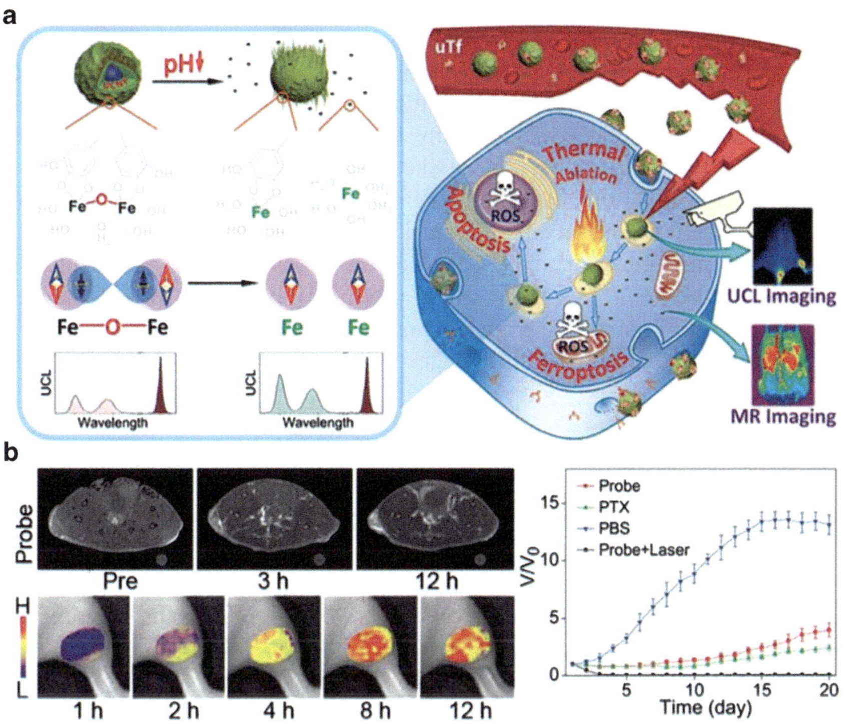

Fig. 6.1 (**a**) Diagram illustrating the UCNP@GA-FeIII probe's MRI-activatable function and its multi-pronged therapeutic action. (**b**)T1-weighted MR images of tumor-bearing animals were obtained at various intervals before and following the injection of the UCNP@GA-FeIII probe (upper), and Fe3+ release mapping determined by the upconversion luminescence's I475/I800 ratio (bottom). (**c**) the tumor growth curves following therapy in several mouse groups. (Reprinted from [44], Copyright © 2021 Yang, Yue, Qiao, Zhang, Jiang, Ning, Liu, and Hou. This is an open-access article distributed under the terms of the Creative Commons Attribution License (CC BY 4.0))

6.3.2.1 Superparamagnetic Nanoparticles

MRI is characterized by two proton relaxation parameters, specifically T1 and T2, which correspond to longitudinal and transverse relaxation, respectively. Substances that increase the T1 relaxivity cause a surge in signal intensity during imaging, while T2 agents decrease the intensity. Typically, chelated organic gadolinium III (Gd3+) is used as a contrast agent to extend the T1 relaxation time. However, employing superparamagnetic nanostructures such as superparamagnetic iron oxide nanoparticles (SPION) and ultra-small SPIONs (USPION) increases the T1 relaxation time by precise adjustment, hence enhancing the sensitivity of the process better than organic gadolinium. SPIONs contain a central core including many iron atoms, accompanied by a surface layer that serves to stabilize the magnetic nanoparticles. The core composition of SPIONs provides greater sensitivity compared to gadolinium complexes at the nanoscale range, making them strong contenders as contrast agents for MRI. Currently, SPIONs and USPIONs are widely used as T2 contrast agents due to the high sensitivity, biotolerance, and biodegradability of iron nanoparticles. Additionally, by regulating the size of the nanoparticles and the thickness of their outer shell, researchers can readily control the magnetic properties of superparamagnetic iron oxide nanoparticles (SPIONs), leading to greater MRI scan outcomes. Despite the benefits, there have been reports of SPIONs' potential toxicity and production of low-resolution images. Currently, scientists are endeavoring to enhance the functionality of these superparamagnetic nanostructures by incorporating compounds such as liposomes, poloxamers, PEG, and silicone to optimize their use in magnetic resonance imaging (MRI) [45, 46].

6.3.2.2 Contrast Agents

Contrast agents are highly essential and irreplaceable components of MRIs. These compounds improve the visibility of specific structures within the body, making it easier to differentiate between them. They not only facilitate biomedical imaging but also enhance the sensitivity of the process. As described in the previous section, the fundamental concept of contrast agents in MRI is influenced by two proton relaxation parameters, namely T1 and T2. As a result, two distinct types of contrast agents emerge: T1 and T2. A wide range of nanostructures are used as contrast agents for MRI for their adjustable structure and properties, as well as their ability to be functionalized by conjugation with other elements. Adding to this, nanostructures show enhanced EPR effects, biocompatibility, and reduced toxicity inside the body, which makes them highly suitable to be used in vivo.

Typically, Gd3+ chelates serve as a T1 contrast agent that generates a positive contrast effect in MRI scans. Nanoparticle-based T1 contrast agents are developed by conjugating Gd3+ chelates with inorganic nanoparticles, using nanotechnology. In addition, several nanostructures serve as carriers for these complexes' chelates, facilitating their selective accumulation at particular locations and improving the reliability of image diagnosis. Quantum dots have attracted significant interest as a semiconductor crystal for incorporating into the design of GD-chelated contrast dyes, thanks to their intense fluorescence and restricted emission spectrum. To enhance the performance of these nanosystems, they can be further improved by applying a PEG coating on their surface. This coating serves to prevent rapid removal by the liver. Additionally, the use of multi-walled carbon nanotubes (MWCNT) in conjunction with gadolinium has been shown to improve image quality in MRI when used as contrast agents, as opposed to employing gadolinium alone. Liposomes, gold, and biodegradable polymers are highly suitable for encapsulating the GD chelate agent. Such a nanoprobe-based carrier system serves the dual purpose of protecting the payload and facilitating precise delivery of the agent to the desired location. These nanostructures possess the ability to finely adjust their optical, mechanical, electrical, and structural characteristics. As a result, they are well-suited for usage as contrast agents and nanocarriers, aiding in the detection of diseases. Contrast dyes used in MRI may occasionally pose health and environmental risks, as well as an increased potential for toxicity due to their conjugation with nanostructures [13, 47, 48].

6.3.3 Computed Tomography (CT)

Computed Tomography (CT) is a non-invasive medical diagnostic technique that uses ionizing X-rays to generate cross-sectional and three-dimensional images of different parts of the body. This modality has a brief study time but yields high-resolution images, making it particularly suitable for visualizing bone structures. Even so, there is always a potential risk associated with being exposed to ionizing radiation during CT scans that may lead to adverse effects or long-term health issues in patients. Similar to MRI and optical imaging techniques, contrast dyes are used in CT scans to improve the visibility of specific parts of the body being scanned. Researchers and scientists today highly seek contrast agents that enhance the sensitivity of CT scans, thereby improving their ability to differentiate between various tissues, have a long retention time in the body, and permit unambiguous imaging of the specific tissue [49].

6.3.3.1 X-Ray Contrast Agents

CT scan uses X-rays and special X-ray digital detectors to obtain three-dimensional images of our body's internal structures. One of the important factors that influence the efficacy of this approach is X-ray attenuation. It refers to the extent to which the substance that the X-ray passes through weakens the incident beam. Greater image contrast is associated with a higher attenuation coefficient. To achieve greater X-ray attenuation than what is typically seen in tissues, elements with higher atomic numbers are added to the contrast agents. Iodine, with an atomic number of 53, has traditionally been the preferred element for CT imaging. Currently, there are multiple commercially available small-molecule iodinated contrast agents, such as iopromide, iothalamate, and iohexol. In addition, lanthanide-based contrast agents are available for CT scans, but their application is limited because of the extreme toxicity imparted by their free ions. Nevertheless, iodine exhibits minimal effectiveness in producing clear scans due to its short duration in the bloodstream and inadequate capacity to penetrate blood vessels. In addition, a substantial quantity of iodine is necessary to counterbalance the renal clearance process and get the desired concentration at the intended site, which may lead to systemic toxicity [49, 50].

6.3.3.2 Nanoparticle-Based Enhancements

To surmount the challenges associated with using X-ray contrast agents, scientists are turning to nanotechnology, which involves the incorporation of nanoparticles as contrast agents in CT scans, enabling improved image contrast and sensitivity of the scanning process. Nanoparticles encapsulating contrast agents can be engineered to specifically deliver the payload to desired locations and extend circulation. These nanostructures possess a greater capacity to transport a significant quantity of contrast material in comparison to small molecules, necessitating the use of relatively small amounts of contrast agents. This significantly reduces the risk of potential toxicity inside the body. The size of the nanoparticles allows them to evade renal clearance and uptake by macrophages. The design of nanoparticle-based iodine contrast agents leverages the aforementioned benefits to enhance the sensitivity of CT scanning. Presently, liposomes, micelles, polymeric nanoparticles, nanocapsules, nanoemulsions, and nanosuspensions are used to develop nanoparticle-based contrast agents. Among these, liposomes have demonstrated significant use as carriers of contrast agents. There is a potential risk of uptake by the reticuloendothelial systems (RES), leading to leakage of the contrast material and consequent renal damage. The distinct capacity of nanoparticles to be altered with multiple functionalities through size control and the addition of ligands or coatings like PEGylated sheaths to their framework can assist in overcoming this constraint. Researchers are currently studying a new method that uses self-assembling nanoparticles such as chitosan and folate labeled with contrast agents. The size of these specially designed structures helps to prevent renal clearance, extending the period they remain in circulation and facilitating the accumulation of the contrast media in tumors through passive targeting [51, 52].

6.3.4 Ultrasound Imaging

Ultrasound imaging has significantly transformed medical diagnostics in recent years, mostly because of its accessibility, affordability, lack of harmful radiation, and diagnostic effectiveness. This diagnostic tool uses high-frequency sound waves to penetrate the tissue via a probe. The probe reflects the pulses as echoes and converts them to electrical impulses. The monitor then converts these impulses into images, allowing us to visualize the internal structures of our body. Ultrasound possesses a remarkable capability to deeply penetrate soft tissues while providing a high level of spatial detail. This method offers live imaging, displaying the motion of the body's internal organs and the circulation of blood through the blood vessels, which acts as a guiding tool for treatments and biopsies. Ultrasound imaging facilitates the localized delivery of energy, which in turn aids in the release of drugs from carriers and expedites their impact in a specific area within a living tissue. This technology is extensively used in pregnancy to evaluate the development and health of the fetus. It is further used in the detection of tumors and abnormalities in organs such as the kidney, heart, liver, thyroid, uterus, and abdomen. Nonetheless, the image quality depends on operator skill and has limited depth for visualizing bone structure. Hence, ultrasound imaging uses contrast agents, such as microbubbles and nanoparticles, for efficient tissue penetration, precise tumor targeting, and the production of high-resolution images of the targeted tissues and organs [53].

6.3.4.1 Microbubbles

The well-known technique contrast-enhanced ultrasound imaging (CEUS) uses insoluble gases such as air, nitrogen, and perfluorocarbon microbubbles enclosed in protein, polymer, or lipid shells as contrast agents to visualize and analyze the internal structures of our bodies. Microbubbles act as agents that amplify the echo of ultrasonic waves, resulting in an increased level of ultrasound backscattering, a phenomenon present in all diagnostic ultrasonography techniques. Microbubbles are conjugated with ligands that bind to receptors in diseased tissues, enabling the microbubbles to collect specifically in those areas, resulting in the creation of high-resolution ultrasound images for early detection of diseases. These microsized gas-filled complexes boost the contrast of the images due to the echogenicity of their inner shell. They are particularly ideal for molecular imaging of blood vessels due to their size and tendency to remain confined in the bloodstream. Some commercially available contrast agents used today are Levovist, Sonazoid, Optison, Definity, and SonoVue. Unfortunately, these molecules have short circulation half-lives, which restrict their capacity to penetrate tumors and be targeted effectively. These contrast agents at a microscopic scale show instability when subjected to sonication. The limitations mentioned above necessitate developing and using nanoparticles as contrast agents, as they can effectively address most of the challenges imposed by microbubbles in ultrasound imaging [54].

6.3.4.2 Nanobubbles

Nanobubbles are sub-micron-sized particles that are enclosed by a shell made of lipid, protein, or biodegradable polymer. They are designed to address the challenges posed by microbubbles as contrast agents. Because of their nano size, ease of modification, enhanced stability, good permeability, and capacity to target tumors, nanoparticles are ideal to be used as contrast agents in ultrasound imaging. In addition, nanobubbles show stability under sonication, unlike microbubbles. Over time, researchers have developed a variety of nanosystems, such as liposomes, quantum dots, polymers, silica, and dendrimers, to serve as contrast agents and carriers in ultrasound imaging. Currently, there is significant research being conducted on lipid-shelled nanobubbles for their prospective use as diagnostic and therapeutic agents. They have demonstrated increased absorption and accumulation in specific tissues, as well as the ability to be optimized through surface modification. For instance, lipid-based nanobubbles have been developed consisting of lipid shells coupled with PEG and containing echo contrast gas perfluorocarbon. Surface functionalization of these liposomes with functional groups displays excellent compatibility with living organisms and remains in the bloodstream for a longer period. Similarly, biodegradable polymers like polylactic acid (PLA) are used to produce nanobubbles that transport SF_6 gas as contrast agents. The use of polymeric nanoparticles enhances the low echogenicity of the hydrophobic gas and demonstrates an improved permeability and retention impact within the body. Ultrasound imaging has achieved significant breakthroughs in the recent decade, such as developing a sophisticated dual imaging system that uses multimodal contrast agents and the use of copper oxide nanoparticles with enhanced acoustic properties. Scientists are hopeful that harnessing the unique benefits provided by nanosized particles will help create more optimized functionalized nanosystems, which will enhance the imaging sensitivity of ultrasound imaging by many folds in the future [54–56].

6.3.5 Positron Emission Tomography (PET) and Single-Photon Emission Computed

6.3.6 Tomography (SPECT)

Among other imaging techniques available, positron emission tomography (PET) and single-photon emission computed tomography (SPECT) have transformed medical diagnostics by allowing non-invasive imaging of the physiological activities of tissues and organs by the use of radioactive substances.

PET scan uses a radiotracer that detects any atypical metabolic activities in tissues or organs. A PET scan is mainly characterized by its capacity to evaluate physiological functioning in the human body by analyzing blood flow, metabolism, radiolabeled drugs, and neurotransmitters. One of the most prevalent applications of this method is in the detection of cancer, making it an essential diagnostic tool in the field of clinical oncology. The mechanism of action involves injecting a small amount of radiotracer into the peripheral vein via intravenous administration. Subsequently, the pet scanner traverses the specific region of the body under examination. When the radioactive substance collides with electrons in the tissues, it releases positrons that transform into photons. The scanning device converts the detected photons into electrical signals, consequently generating an image map on the computer. PET scans synthesize radionuclides by binding a radioactive atom to chemical compounds that the specific tissue metabolizes. For example, in PET scans of the brain, researchers administer a radioactive atom to glucose to produce a radionuclide known as fluorodeoxyglucose (FDG), given the brain's reliance on glucose for its metabolism. It is used to monitor chemical neurotransmitters to diagnose Parkinson's disease and detect cardiological disorders [57].

Single-photon emission computed tomography (SPECT) is a similar imaging technique to positron emission tomography (PET), with the only difference being the choice of radiotracer. Gamma-ray emitting radiotracers are used in SPECT scans. These gamma rays are detected by gamma camera detectors to capture 2D images from various angles. Subsequently, a computer is used to implement a tomographic reconstruction technique on the various projections, resulting in the generation of a three-dimensional (3D) image. This working principle of SPECT scans enables the evaluation of bodily functions, similar to PET scans, assisting in the diagnosis of brain disorders, cancers, heart disease, bone abnormalities, and various other conditions. While SPECT scanning may be more cost-effective, PET scans offer superior specificity and sensitivity, resulting in sharper images. Nevertheless, both techniques have the potential risk of subjecting patients to damaging radiation. In recent years, scientists have been endeavoring to revolutionize nuclear medicine and diagnostic imaging by integrating nanotechnology into PET and SPECT scans. Additional studies in this field can advance the utilization of improved PET and SPECT scans in molecular imaging and diagnosis [58].

6.3.6.1 Radiolabeled Nanoparticles

The integration of nanoscience into nuclear medicine is set to alter ways of disease evaluation and treatment, particularly in the context of cancer. The increasing number of annual publications about radiolabeled nanomaterials for biomedical applications substantiates the growing fascination with the subject. This technology labels nanoparticles with radioactive isotopes such as technetium-99 m, lutetium-177, gallium-68, iodine-125, carbon-14, copper-64, radium-223, gold-199, and many others. These targeting nanostructures act as carriers for the radiotracers, directing them toward the body parts under examination in PET and SPECT scans. The application of nanoparticle nuclear imaging modalities aims to enhance the efficiency of these processes. Using NPs as carriers enables precise targeting, improved EPR impact, extended circulation duration, increased biocompatibility, and the ability to load numerous agents onto a single carrier. In addition, the surface of nanoparticles can undergo surface modification by attaching biomolecules such as antibodies, aptamers, and peptides through covalent bonding. This allows for precise and active targeting of specific sites. This approach is frequently used to enhance the duration of circulation of nanoparticles in the body while reducing their uptake by the RES and promoting the uptake of radiotracers by the desired target. Technetium-99 m, copper-64, and lutetium-177 have been frequently used in radiolabeled nanoparticles for PET and SPECT scans. The applied nanostructures comprise gold particles, liposomes, micelles, polymers, silica, and iron. Although the use of radiolabeled nanoprobes is not widespread, there are numerous clinically approved agents available for nuclear imaging of several organs, such as lymph nodes, gastrointestinal tract, spleen, and liver, enabling the detection of carcinoma, the assessment of chemotherapy effects, the evaluation of biodistribution patterns, and assistance in molecular imaging of tissues. The indisputable potential of nano-radiotracers lies in their ability to change cancer therapies through early tumor diagnosis, disease staging, and treatment impact monitoring. Hence, it is imperative to achieve a harmonious balance in the forthcoming years between the evident benefits of nano-radiopharmaceuticals, such as their efficiency in loading radioisotopes, effectiveness in therapy and diagnosis, and possible drawbacks of unfavorable elimination from circulation, and challenges related to regulatory compliance [59].

6.3.6.2 Hybrid Imaging Modalities

In recent years, substantial research and development have focused on integrating various imaging techniques to generate a hybrid platform that enhances the effectiveness and sensitivity of diagnosis. One of the most prominent approaches is the integration of positron emission tomography-computed tomography (PET/CT) and single-photon emission computed tomography (SPECT/CT). They are used to image many organs and tissues such as tumors, heart, bones, thyroid, liver, lungs, brain, GI, and spleen to identify malignancies or any other abnormalities that necessitate medical intervention. This novel approach works by combining the images obtained from PET and CT scans. A single machine performs both scans simultaneously. As a result, the combined scans provide more intricate images of internal body regions than either individual scan alone. In addition, it allows for improving the detection of lesions, accurately locating malignant areas, characterizing abnormal lesions, and producing high-resolution images. Thus, the fusion of anatomic and molecular imaging allows for highly precise interpretations of PET/CT and SPECT/CT studies while offering reliable prognostic information. This, in turn, enables healthcare professionals to make a well-informed therapeutic decision. These strategies can be used during the initial diagnosis to evaluate the early response of the disease to treatment, post-treatment, and during the ongoing monitoring of patients. PET/MRI and SPECT/MRI are newly emerging techniques that integrate PET and SPECT scans with magnetic resonance imaging (MRI). In this process, PET and SPECT data are combined and merged with MRI data using specialist software to generate a unified image that includes both functional and structural information. This modality has high potential in the imaging of many diseases and conditions, especially neurological disorders. Multiple reports consistently show that PET/MRI scans show a superior ability to detect abnormal findings in comparison to PET/CT scans. Furthermore, PET/MRI substantially decreases patients' radiation exposure in comparison to PET/CT and SPECT/CT assessments. Nevertheless, the costly expense and complicated operational nature of PET/MRI restrict its regular application in clinical settings. Currently, the usage of MRI in cancer is considerably lower compared to that of CT. The hybrid technologies described above undoubtedly improve the sensitivity and effectiveness of imaging methods. It is crucial to further standardize and examine the risks associated with these technologies to expand their application in the biomedical field [60].

6.4 Design and Functionalization of Nanoprobes

Nanoprobes are crucial in disease detection, drug design, and drug delivery, shifting the paradigm of the healthcare sector for the better. Despite extensive research efforts in the development and production of nanomaterials for therapeutic uses, only a limited number have proven successful in clinical applications. The presence of a "protein corona" around nanoparticles, the risk of toxicity, inadequate delivery efficacy, manufacturing challenges, and various other issues hinder the widespread application of nanomaterials in the biomedical field. It is important to modify nanostructures through functionalization to harness their capabilities fully. The primary objective of this optimization is to improve and strengthen the molecular interactions between the nanoparticles and the surrounding environment in vivo. Consequently, this leads to controlled dispersion and organization, improved colloidal stability, strong compatibility with biological systems, greater tissue absorption, and precise delivery to specific targets. Presently, nanosystems for biomedical use are functionalized through the conjugation of several functional ligands, antibodies, aptamers, and other biomolecules with the surface of the nanoparticles [61].

6.4.1 Surface Modification Techniques

Nanoparticle surface modification entails using various physical and chemical techniques to alter the surface structure and functionality of the nanoparticles within the human body. This includes the alteration of characteristics such as functional groups, crystallinity, adsorption, electrical properties, surface energy, and other related attributes leading to enhanced stability, biocompatibility, surface reactivity, dispersion, targeting capability, and drug transportation of nanoprobes used in diagnostic imaging. Consequently, this improves the sensitivity and efficiency of all imaging modalities. Surface functionalization enables the attachment of biomolecules to the surface of nanoparticles through covalent and non-covalent bonding, coating, adsorption, or grafting. This, in turn, aims to modify and improve the capabilities of nanoparticles in the field of bioimaging [62].

The following section explores biomolecules used as ligands to modify the structural functionalities of nanoprobes used as imaging agents.

6.4.1.1 Functional Ligands

The surface functionalization of nanoparticles can be achieved by conjugating them with specific biomolecules referred to as functional ligands. These ligands have been shown to affect the surface charge, size, surface chemistry, hydrophobicity, and hydrophilicity of the nanoparticles, facilitating the optimization of diagnostic imaging tools. Peptides and polymers are widely accepted and used functional ligands that are conjugated onto the surface of the nanoprobes in medical diagnostics and theranostics. Polymers such as polyethylene glycol (PEG), dextran, starch, citrate, and polymeric micelles can be applied as a coating on the surface of nanoprobes to enhance their functionality. This conjugation leads to increased biodistribution within the tissues, improved cellular absorption, effective renal clearance, and extended circulation duration inside the bloodstream. It facilitates steric stability and imparts "stealth" properties to the surface, preventing protein adsorption [63].

Research conducted over time has indicated the extensive study and use of PEG in the surface functionalization of nanoparticles owing to its inherent physicochemical features. However, its use as a drug carrier conjugate has been restricted due to its low payload capacity. Polyethylene glycol, or PEG, is a hydrophilic polymeric chain made of its monomer, polyethylene glycol, which can be anchored onto the surface of the NPs through adsorption or covalent bonding. A significant issue in the application of nanoparticles is their absorption by pathogens through opsonization. Particular proteins attached to the nanoparticles' surface interact with phagocytes to initiate this process. PEG has been demonstrated to significantly decrease nonspecific contacts, thus inhibiting the release of opsonin and ultimately impeding phagocytosis, due to its chain length, hydrophilicity, and steric repulsion effects. Consequently, this leads to a longer residence time in the bloodstream and enhances the stability of the nanoparticle complex. Adding to this, PEG is nontoxic and demonstrates a high permeability into tissues due to its adjustable particle size and surface composition, allowing for efficient and targeted distribution. Exploiting the advantages of PEG coating as functional ligands, many types of nanoparticles, such as gold, silver, quantum dots, carbon, silica, and magnetic NPs, have been modified to serve as contrast agents in imaging techniques. For instance, PEGylated superparamagnetic iron oxide nanoparticles (SPIONs) are recognized for their ability to exhibit longer relaxation durations, hence improving the contrast of images in magnetic resonance imaging (MRI). Similar functionality is used in CT scans, where a PEGylated sheath enhances the performance of NP-based contrast agents. This coating prevents the contrast agents from being absorbed by the reticuloendothelial systems (RES), thus preventing contrast leakage and extending the time they circulate in the blood. This type of functionalized nanoparticle has an improved ability to penetrate the blood-brain barrier (BBB), making it more effective for targeting tumors during CT scanning. PEG is used to functionalize gold and lipid-based nanoprobes to improve the targeting effectiveness and contrast of the resulting CT scans. In addition to CT and MRI, other imaging modalities (ultrasound, PET, SPECT, optical imaging, etc.) use PEG, small molecules, chitosan, folate, and other polymeric particles to further enhance the efficacy of the NPs being used as contrast media. The added benefits imparted through functionalization help in achieving higher biocompatibility and improved resolution of contrast images, consequently boosting the sensitivity of the imaging process by many folds [62, 64].

6.4.1.2 Antibodies and Aptamers

The role of recognition elements for distinct targets is vital to achieving high-performance imaging in diagnostic imaging technologies. In this context, antibodies and aptamers serve as highly effective targeted ligands due to their active uptake through biomolecular recognition. Antibody-conjugated nanostructures have high efficacy in selectively binding to surface cell receptors, enabling the controlled release of encapsulated contrast media or drugs for disease detection or therapy. Monoclonal antibodies, in particular, have exceptional stability and strong binding affinity in cancer theranostic applications. On the other hand, aptamers have significant advantages over antibodies in targeting ligands in molecular imaging because of their inherent characteristics. Aptamers are nucleic acids, either DNA or RNA, that can fold into a wide range of secondary and tertiary structures. This allows them to attach with excellent sensitivity and specificity to different target biomolecules. Aptamers have a much smaller size compared to antibodies and other small molecules, allowing them to diffuse more rapidly in tissues. This characteristic enables the quick attainment of the highest signal-to-noise ratio, hence improving the contrasting ability of various imaging techniques. Aptamers can undergo conformational changes during interaction with the receptors on the targets. This allows the generation of signal output for biorecognition in various imaging modalities. Aptamers conjugated with nanoprobes have become highly regarded for their ability to effectively direct different imaging contrast agents toward specific tissues for various imaging techniques such as optical, magnetic resonance, computed tomography, ultrasound, and hybrid imaging. Nonetheless, clinical translation of aptamers is limited in molecular imaging due to their susceptibility to rapid degradation and clearance. To tackle these difficulties, researchers have devised an in vitro screening technique known as systematic evolution of ligands by exponential enrichment (SELEX), which engineers the aptamer in such a way that will increase their targeting efficacy and stability in vivo when used in molecular imaging [65].

6.4.2 Targeting Strategies

A principal rationale for using nanoparticles as carriers in diagnostic imaging is to achieve precise and efficient targeting of the contrast media. This is not always achievable because of several obstacles hindering the effectiveness of the nanostructures, such as the blood-brain barrier (BBB), absorption by the reticuloendothelial system (RES), and rapid clearance. Nanoprobes that have undergone surface functionalization with ligands are suitable carriers or vehicles in imaging tools due to their exceptional ability to specifically target specified tissues or organs. This is accomplished by actively and passively targeting specific tissues, thereby overcoming the aforementioned limitations. This further enables a greater accumulation of payloads and improves the potency of the nanostructure complex in medical imaging.

6.4.2.1 Passive Targeting

Passive targeting is a strategy that enables the payload to reach the desired tissue via its nanostructure carrier. This method involves the transportation of drugs or other substances into cells by using the interstitial space in capillary pores through passive diffusion or convection. A large number of authoritative research reveals that passive targeting is generally mediated by the enhanced permeability and retention effect (EPR), serving as the conceptual foundation for the passive targeting of nanodrugs to various types of tumors. The EPR effect is a distinct feature exclusive to solid tumors, corresponding to the unique pathophysiological phenomenon of the vasculature in these tumors. This feature is primarily defined by the increased permeability of the blood vessels that surround solid tumors as opposed to normal tissue, as well as the lack of functional lymphatic channels. The nanoparticles, ligand-conjugated nanostructures, or macromolecular drugs (with a size of approx. 250 nm) can accumulate in the tumor-vascularized area by passively diffusing via the pores of the tumor capillaries. This results in the targeted delivery and retention of nanoparticles containing anticancer agents in solid tumor tissue. Medical diagnostics, especially tumor imaging and assessment, extensively use functionalized nanoprobes with PEG or other ligands that deliver contrast media or drugs through a passive targeted delivery system. Examples of such nanostructures include polymeric NPs, liposomes, silicon dioxide NPs, and metal NPs. This targeting strategy takes advantage of the EPR effects, leading to enhanced bioavailability, selective accumulation of the payload, improved local effectiveness, and decreased toxic side effects [66].

6.4.2.2 Active Targeting

Active targeting refers to a targeting pathway that harnesses the ligand-receptor interaction to deliver drugs to the desired site in vivo. Ligands such as antibodies, aptamers, peptides, and small molecules alter the surface of nanoparticles to identify and bind to specific cell surface receptors at the targeted region, enhancing the precision of drug delivery. Diagnostic nanoprobes use an active targeting strategy to transport the enclosed contrast agent or drug to the specific area of the tissue being examined using various imaging techniques. The quest to find appropriate ligands for biomolecule recognition in diagnostics led to the selection of antibodies as the most preferred ligand for targeting receptors on cell surfaces. Antibodies can identify and bind to specific antigens on cells, enabling them to accurately release the payload enclosed within the nanovesicle. These molecules have a diminished toxicity profile and a longer plasma half-life, resulting in greater absorption of cancer cells compared to smaller particles. Examples of available agents for antibody labeling, especially for cancer imaging, include CT contrast agents, microbubbles, fluorophores, radioisotopes, and multimodality probes. Similarly, various imaging techniques such as MRI, CT, echography, Raman spectroscopy, and fluorescence imaging use aptamer-based targeted nanoparticles to transport diagnostic probes or therapeutic drugs, enabling the detection of infectious pathogens, tumors, biomarkers, and toxins. Aptamers can easily bind to the nanoprobes, rendering them a promising tool for diagnostic purposes. In addition, they possess advantageous qualities of improved tissue permeability, minimal immunogenic side effects, increased stability, and a greater ability to target less immunogenic antigens compared to antibodies. Peptides are used in bioimaging to modify nanoparticles. They possess the ability to specifically target proteins that are excessively produced on cancerous cells and effectively bind to them with accuracy. This enables contrast imaging and the administration of anti-cancer drugs to treat cancerous growths. PEGylation is a commonly employed peptide-based method to modify the surface of diagnostic nanoprobes. PEG-conjugated nanostructures have superior biodegradability, colloidal stability, and reduced cytotoxicity compared to other inorganic nanostructures. Small molecules conjugate with nanoparticles to selectively bind to receptors on cells in vivo using the active targeting strategy. Due to their small size and low molecular weight, they can more easily traverse biological barriers compared to other ligands. For instance, folic acid, small molecules based on benzothiazole motifs, and G-quadruplex (GQ)-stabilizing small molecules are used in NIR imaging, photoacoustic imaging, photothermal therapy, chemotherapy, PET scans, and MRI [66, 67].

Nanocarriers use both active and passive targeting mechanisms to efficiently transport the payload to the desired tissues in diagnostic imaging modalities. Nevertheless, both strategies have their advantages and disadvantages. Passive targeting possesses universality due to its reliance on the properties of tumor tissue to trap drugs, allowing the nanoparticles (NPs) to effectively target a diverse range of tumor types. It allows for greater bioavailability and imparts low toxicity in vivo. However, the extent of precision in targeting is restricted by the impact of tumor heterogeneity. Due to the constraints of passive targeting, researchers have intensively investigated the active targeting strategy. This approach facilitates the customization of nanoparticle surfaces with ligands. Consequently, it shows greater targeting effectiveness because the ligands have a higher affinity for cell surface receptors, resulting in more precise binding. Active targeting mechanisms enable drugs to penetrate tissues at the molecular level [66].

6.4.3 Biocompatibility and Toxicity Considerations

Nanoparticles have significantly transformed many different aspects of modern health care by facilitating diagnostic and treatment strategies. To enhance their versatility, nanoparticles undergo surface functionalization through several methods. This, in turn, allows them to sensitize and optimize the imaging and therapeutic modality. Hence, conducting a thorough assessment of the parameters that impact the biocompatibility and toxicity of nanoparticles is essential for ensuring the safe advancement of these novel compounds. Diagnostic nanoprobes demonstrate their functionality within living tissues through interaction with several types of biomolecules. This can occasionally lead to undesirable outcomes that pose a risk to human health. Therefore, it is essential to evaluate and track the compatibility of nanoparticles with their surrounding environment, as well as their nanotoxicological reactions, to fully exploit their potential in the field of biomedicine. Under the standard protocol, tests evaluating the hemocompatibility, histocompatibility, cytotoxicity, genotoxicity, pyrogenicity, immunotoxicity, and systemic toxicity of the nanoparticles are carried out to assess the biocompatibility and toxicity of engineered nanoprobes used in medical diagnostics and therapy [68].

6.4.3.1 In Vitro and in Vivo Assessment

Both in vitro and in vivo studies are conducted to assess the biocompatibility and toxicity of nanoprobes. Diagnostic nanoparticles come into direct contact with blood; hence, in vitro studies are conducted to evaluate the blood compatibility of the nanoparticles by examining blood cell aggregation and hemolysis. For the sample to be deemed safe for circulation in the bloodstream, its hemolytic ratio must be below 5%. The use of nanoparticles allows for precise transport within tissues, making it essential to assess their histocompatibility to prevent any kind of toxicity. Nanotoxicological research involves the use of various biological systems, such as primary human cells, to evaluate potential immunomodulatory effects. In a conducted investigation, primary peritoneal macrophages from rats and mice were subjected to 20 nm and 60 nm dextran-coated superparamagnetic iron oxide nanoparticles (SPIONs). As a result of this exposure, there was an increase in the secretion of anti-inflammatory cytokines. Generally, SPIONs do not exhibit any toxicity toward human macrophages and dendritic cells, and they do not have any detrimental effects on liver function. Likewise, studies have been carried out to assess the biocompatibility of gold nanoparticles within living organisms. The majority of engineered gold nanoparticles did not elicit any immunological responses but gold nanoparticles coupled with peptides triggered an immune response, as they were identified by murine macrophages [69].

The cellular interactions with the circulating NPs via active or passive mechanisms are not yet fully understood, and this complexity is further amplified when transitioning from in vitro to in vivo models. The nanotoxicological reactions depend on various criteria, including size, charge, surface chemistry, coating, agglomeration, and shape. Predicting the adverse effects of nanoparticles requires consideration of all these factors. Toxicological evaluations of nanoparticles are performed to assess their cytotoxic effects on different types of cells in our body, including those found in the lungs, liver, kidneys, and heart. Cytotoxic assays like the MTT, MTS, ELISA (enzyme-linked immunosorbent assay), and LDH (lactate dehydrogenase) tests are mainly done by considering a few parameters associated with damaged cells including impaired metabolism and cell-death markers. For instance, polymeric nanoparticles are extremely valuable as transporters of drugs because they have a high level of biodegradability. Additionally, it was found that the toxicity of PLGA NPs, which were stabilized by bovine serum albumin (BSA), significantly decreased in comparison to synthetic coating substances in laboratory-cultured lung cancer cells. Conversely, oxidative stress in living organisms causes numerous silica nanoparticles to clump together, leading to protein agglomeration. Researchers are extensively studying quantum dots (QDs) to evaluate their potential hepatotoxicity, revealing that the adverse effects caused by QDs are primarily due to the discharge of metal ions from the heavy metal core. Several established methods such as the Ames test, DNA laddering test, comet test, micronuclei test, and chromosome aberration test are used to assess the genotoxicity of NPs. Scientists have conducted research on various nanoparticles, including PEGylated NPs, carbon nanotubes, metal NPs, silica NPs, gold NPs, silver NPs, and others, to investigate their impact on nanomaterial immunomodulation, nanomaterial-induced fibrosis, and systemic toxicity. These tests are evaluated considering the factors related to protein corona formation, molecular interaction, and cellular interactions of the nanostructures with various organ systems in our body. To effectively harness the potential of nanoparticles in the biomedical field, researchers must improve our understanding of the toxicological and biocompatible assessments of nanostructures. This necessitates extensive research to investigate the relationship between the biological environment and nanoparticles, assisting in the development of a precise and practical toxicological profile for nanoparticles. The safe application of nanoparticles (NPs) in healthcare will ultimately benefit both patients and the environment [68, 70].

6.4.3.2 Regulatory Guidelines

The increased emphasis on nanoparticle safety in the healthcare sector has resulted in a growing focus of attention on the design, development, and implementation of toxicity evaluation models in the field of nanotechnology. The tests, experiments, and investigations conducted must comply with the regulatory criteria that are currently in place. These guidelines and standards aid in the safe development of toxicological models of NPs for use in healthcare and their implementation is strongly recommended by various regulatory bodies. The regulations on NP evaluation procedures differ across countries and agencies. For example, the International Organization for Standardization (ISO) provides multiple guidelines and standards to help researchers in evaluating and monitoring the hazards and ensuring the safety of nanoparticles. The U.S. Environmental Protection Agency (EPA) offers a framework for assessing the risks associated with nanoparticles, including examining the bioaccessibility, impact on the environment, physical and chemical properties, and systemic toxicity of nanoparticles. In addition, the European Chemicals Agency has implemented various approaches per EU (European Union) regulations to effectively assess the safety of toxicological research on NPs. The US FDA and ICH (International Council for Harmonization of Technical Requirements for Pharmaceuticals for Human Use) have recently established many standards to address the hazardous consequences concerning nanoparticle use. Upon failure to meet the safety and regulatory guidelines, each nanoparticle-based product will be subject to inspection by the relevant agencies [71].

6.5 Applications in Disease Diagnosis

6.5.1 Applications of Nanoimaging in Cancer Detection and Diagnosis

Global statistics indicate that cancer is the second most prevalent cause of death. Hence, it is imperative to diagnose and manage cancer promptly. Lung cancer is the most common type of cancer in the general population, followed by hepatic, colorectal, stomach, and breast cancer. Over the past decade, numerous cancer diagnostic and therapeutic techniques have emerged. Diagnosing cancer in laboratories is typically limited to advanced stages and specific forms. Hence, it is crucial to advocate for early diagnostic indicators. Conventional cancer treatment includes surgical procedures, radiation therapy, chemotherapy, and hormone therapy. Chemotherapies can be delivered through different administrative routes, including intravenous, oral, and topical routes. Cancer theranostics encompasses cutting-edge molecular diagnostics for identifying new biomarkers, innovative molecular imaging agents, and methodologies for early cancer diagnosis, and nanoplatforms that combine cancer imaging and therapy. Commonly used imaging modalities include PET, SPECT, and MRI. Imaging methods used in the realm of nuclear medicine Nanosystems labeled with radioisotopes have been administered using positron emission tomography (PET) and single-photon emission computed tomography (SPECT). These methods depend on the detectability of all particular substances or cells. Several genetic agents frequently used include photoproteins, PET, magnetic resonance detectable reporter genes, radiolabeled particles, fluorochromes, magnetic molecules like antibodies, small compounds, and biorthogonal agents. Conventional and biomimetic cancer nanotheranostics are currently available. Various nanocarriers, including liposomes, micelles, nanogels, and nanoparticles, show promise for cancer treatment. The imaging and diagnostic capabilities of these substances are limited because they need to be combined with fluorescent dyes or other active chemicals. To extend the lifespan of these systems, it is essential to incorporate poly(ethylene glycol) (PEG). Biomimetic nanosystems incorporating proteins, phospholipids, cholesterol, cell membranes, bacteria and viruses, apatite, and exosomes have gained considerable attention from researchers. Cancer nanotherapeutics harness the increased permeability and retention (EPR) effect to specifically accumulate nanoparticles (NPs) in tumor tissue rather than normal tissues. The occurrence of this phenomenon depends on the tumor's surrounding environment and is not universally seen in all types of cancers. Consequently, it restricts the precise delivery of drugs exclusively to the tumor. Studies have shown that most human cancers do not show the enhanced permeability and retention (EPR) effect. Thus, it is crucial to study cancer nanotheranostics in cancer models or tumors that are therapeutically relevant and demonstrate a significant EPR effect, like Kaposi sarcoma and head and neck tumors. Cancer nanotheranostics can be affected by various factors such as light, temperature, magnetism, and sound. Light or photo stimuli are used in photodynamic, photothermal, or phototriggered therapies.

Photodynamic therapy (PDT) involves the administration of a photosensitizing compound into the tumor, which may require biological synthesis. The agent is triggered by a specific wavelength of light. This therapy causes photochemical and photobiological reactions that lead to permanent damage to tumor tissues. PDT is not extensively applied in the field of cancer treatment. Photothermal therapy (PTT) is a technique that involves using electromagnetic radiation to raise the temperature of cancer cells, resulting in tissue damage. Phototriggered drug release uses a light-sensitive agent to modify the active molecule and enable the precise release of the drug at the desired time and dosage. A new tumor diagnostic system based on photonics has been recently developed. The use of liposomes, a gene probe, tirapazamine, and Chlorin e6 allows for the combination of photodynamic treatment with hypoxia-activated prodrug therapy. The field of optical imaging theranostics utilizes various imaging techniques, including phosphorescence, bioluminescence, fluorescence Raman, and photoacoustic imaging. After absorbing electromagnetic radiation, fluorescence imaging emits light of a specific wavelength. Fluorescence is a valuable tool for capturing molecular mechanisms and structures. This is achieved by using fluorescent dyes and proteins as markers. The researchers used PEG-b-poly(ε-caprolactone) nanoparticles to develop a nanoplatform for fluorescent image-guided surgery, incorporating silicon phthalocyanine. Animal studies have shown that activatable nanoparticles, when administered systemically, can accumulate at cancer sites and generate silicon phthalocyanine. The application of nanoparticles in combinatorial phototherapy effectively eliminated chemoresistant ovarian cancer tumors. Magnetite and iron oxide are examples of magnetic nanotheranostics. Nanotheranostics uses a magnetic field to effectively concentrate and retain nanocarriers at a specific malignant site. These substances are more commonly used in MRI to improve contrast, as well as in combination with hyperthermia chemotherapy. Additionally, they are used to provide magnetic force for cell labeling, tracking, and isolation. When exposed to a high-frequency magnetic field, magnetic nanotheranostics generate thermal energy that can eliminate cancer cells. Magnetic resonance imaging (MRI) is a commonly used diagnostic tool that produces highly detailed images of the body's structure and physiological functions without the need for invasive surgical procedures. Radiology frequently uses it. MRI scanners employ magnetic field gradients, radio waves, and strong magnetic fields to visualize organs. Compounds that contrast enhance can significantly improve sensitivity and enhance diagnostic accuracy in over 35% of clinical MRI scans. The objective of developing Prussian blue nanoprobes was to facilitate tumor imaging through photothermal therapy (PTT) and magnetic resonance imaging. The nanoprobes demonstrate exceptional biocompatibility and exhibit outstanding in vivo performance. Another instance involves the application of hollow manganese/cobalt oxide nanoparticles in cancer nanotheranostics. The nanoplatforms mentioned can respond to glutathione and can be used as contrast agents for both T1- and T2-weighted MRI imaging. Ultrasound nanotheranostics have demonstrated significant efficacy in cancer diagnosis. Ultrasound contrast agents are tiny gas-filled bubbles that generate strong echoes under ultrasound waves. Ultrasound has numerous advantages for tumor diagnosis. These include the ability to provide real-time imaging, its portability, the fact that it does not use ionizing radiation, and its ability to penetrate deep into tissue. In the field of cancer treatment, high-intensity-focused ultrasound and sonodynamic therapy are used. Contrast-enhanced ultrasonography improves the backscatter of ultrasonic waves, resulting in enhanced contrast of the sonogram. This is accomplished by using the notable difference in echogenicity. An ultrasound scan can provide valuable information regarding the blood flow, receptor density, and perfusion of a tumor. Ultrasound molecular imaging encompasses a range of techniques, including photoacoustic imaging, multi-modality imaging, phase-changeable imaging, tumor microenvironment-responsive imaging, and acoustic reporter gene imaging. Ultrasound-targeted therapy uses sonodynamic therapy and high-intensity US ablation. Ultrasonic theranostics uses various contrast agents, including perfluorocarbon NPs, noble metal materials such as Au, Ag, Pd, and Pt, carbon-based nanomaterials like carbon nanotubes, carbon dots, graphene, and graphene oxides, as well as silica-based nanoparticles. Indocyanine green (ICG), IR780, and IR825 are organic dyes known for their high efficacy in generating heat through light absorption. The dyes can absorb near-infrared (NIR) light and convert it into thermal energy. Many of the diagnostic procedures mentioned above can be used for the diagnosis and treatment of different diseases [72–77].

Figure 6.2 below depicts the process for developing a nanomaterial-based system for cancer diagnostics.

6.5.2 Nanoprobes Targeting Tumor Microenvironment

The tumor microenvironment exerts a substantial influence on tumor growth and the spread of cancer cells to far-off regions inside the body. The characteristics of the tumor microenvironment differ from those of normal tissues, with low oxygen levels (hypoxia) and elevated levels of proteases being notable examples. These characteristics serve a dual purpose in the identification and treatment of tumors. Optical imaging methods, such as magnetic resonance imaging (MRI) and positron emission tomography (PET), have been used to study the tumor microenvironment. A wide range of imaging probes have been extensively studied for their ability to selectively target pH, hypoxia, and proteases in the tumor microenvironment. Researchers are actively looking into ways to develop probes that can specifically target the tumor microenvironment through the use of non-invasive imaging techniques. Various nanoparticle-based strategies are now under development to create molecular imaging probes that can selectively target the tumor microenvironment. Nanoparticles, such as the pH-titratable superparamagnetic iron oxide particles (SPIOs), have demonstrated enhanced accumulation in acidic tumors. The application of an external magnet to control the movement of a liposome encapsulating magnetic nanoparticles can be used to specifically target the tumor microenvironment and improve the visibility of MRI scans, resulting in a substantial contrast. Nanoprobes are often created using receptor-ligand interactions to target the tumor

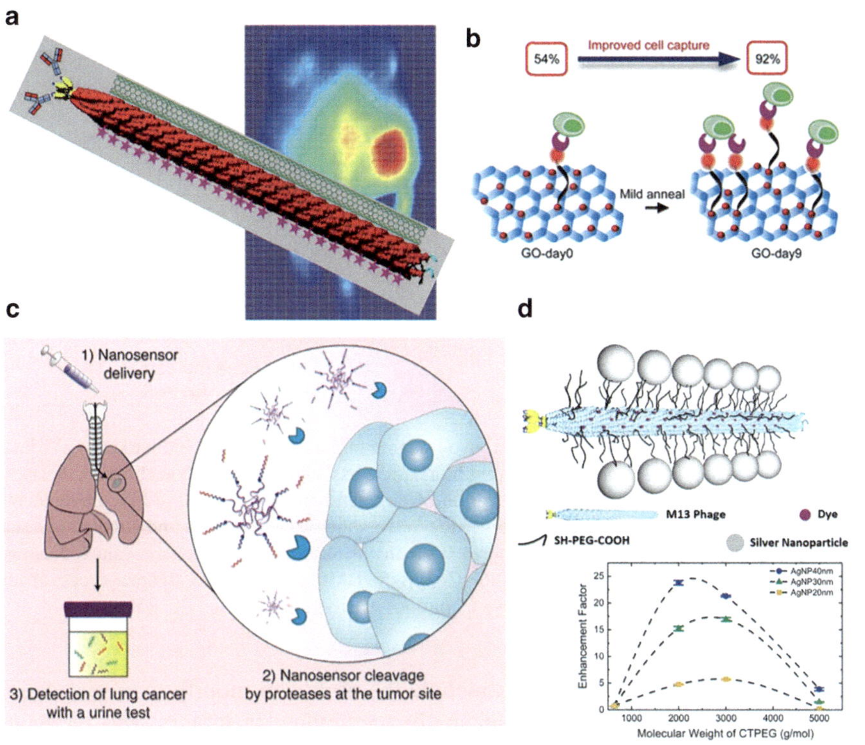

Fig. 6.2 The process for developing nanomaterials for cancer diagnostics involves the following steps: (**a**) Using an antibody to target an M13 bacteriophage nanoprobe (shown in red) to deliver a payload of interest, such as dye molecules (purple) or a carbon nanotube (green). Here is an example of how to image a bacterial infection in an intramuscular mouse model (the bright red area on the right flank). (**b**) A planar, microfluidic-free apparatus built on graphene oxide (GO) nanosheet substrates that have been treated to quickly and effectively extract cells from whole blood; the device's capture efficiency is increased from approximately 54% to 92% when a gentle thermal annealing procedure is used. (**c**) A "smart" activity-based nanosensor designed to detect lung cancer non-invasively using urine. The reporter molecules are transported to the lungs, where they are broken down by tumor-associated proteases and eliminated in the urine. (**d**) An illustration of how to use a nanotemplate to improve plasmonic fluorescence: by decorating M13 phage with dye molecules and Ag nanoparticles, fluorescence can be increased. (Reprinted from [78], Copyright, Springer Nature, 2022, This Open Access Article is licensed under a Creative Commons Attribution 4.0 International License)

microenvironment. Advanced fluorescent probes can be used to optically image the tumor microenvironment, along with standard MRI and PET imaging techniques [79, 80]. Additionally, multicolored nanoprobes play a crucial role in cancer diagnostics by enabling in vivo imaging targeted at specific biomarkers as illustrated in Fig. 6.3.

Fluorescent nanospheres and nanorods have proven to be highly essential tools for studying the impact of nanoparticle shape on tumor penetration in real-time. Fluorescence nanoprobes offer numerous advantages compared to small

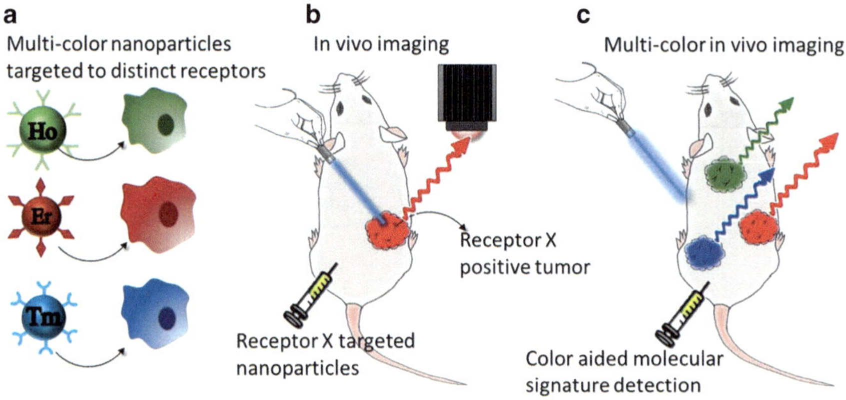

Fig. 6.3 Multicolored nanoprobes for in vivo imaging targeted at specific biomarkers. (**a**) Multi-colored nanoprobes were designed to target biomarkers associated with various breast cancer cell lines specifically. (**b**) The in vivo localization of targeted nanoprobes assessed in subcutaneous tumor models was examined using whole-body SWIR (short-wave infrared) imaging. (**c**) The sensitivity of multi-color nanoprobes to tumors expressing different biomarkers was evaluated using a bilateral tumor model. (Reprinted from [86], Copyright, BMC, 2020. This is an open-access article distributed under the terms of the Creative Commons Attribution License (CC BY 4.0))

molecular probes. These features include the ability to modify their circulation lifespan, the propensity to systematically accumulate in tumors, and increased sensitivity resulting from the attachment of multiple imaging molecules on a single nanoparticle. The pH-dependent fluorescence of the nanoprobes is caused by the Förster resonance energy transfer (FRET) phenomenon, which occurs as a result of the self-aggregation related energy transfer (SAET) effect. Quantum dots have been used as donors in pH nanoprobes, using Förster resonance energy transfer. The QD-dopamine-peptides possess the capability to establish a chemical connection with another substance, resulting in the formation of a pH probe that relies on charge transfer. The redox characteristics of the dopamine coating can be altered when oxidized at basic pH. This alteration can be used to track the pH reaction of the QD conjugates. Quantum dots (QDs) serve as donors in ratiometric pH probes that use Förster resonance energy transfer (FRET) pairs. Ratiometric pH probes based on quantum dots (QDs) have been created by coating the surface of QDs with organic dyes that are sensitive to changes in pH, such as fluorescein isothiocyanate (FITC), the pH dye SNARF (seminaphtharhodafluor), and fluorescent diblock copolymers. A recent discovery revealed that pH-sensitive fluorescent proteins coated on quantum dots (QDs) offer superior sensitivity and photostability compared to traditional fluorescent dyes for pH imaging. A separate research work used a pH-sensitive NIR nanoprobe based on dextran to conduct in vivo differential-absorption dual-wavelength photoacoustic imaging of cancers. The synthesis and examination of quantum dot nanoprobes were conducted to investigate their potential for delivering siRNA into cells and enabling real-time imaging [81].

In 2010, a group of researchers, Li et al., developed a nanoprobe called lnNP1, which is known for its exceptional sensitivity. The nanoprobe was used to study human glioblastoma U87MG cancer cells in a controlled laboratory environment, as well as subcutaneous U87MG xenografts in living organisms. The visualization was accomplished by using pH-activated NIR fluorescence. Zhou et al. introduced a group of micellar nanoprobes in their research, which are sensitive to changes in pH and may be modified accordingly. The nanoprobes are created by the self-assembly of micelles generated from ionizable block copolymers. The nanoprobes in question are categorized as SAET-type pH nanoprobes. A set of SAET probes was created by incorporating amine groups with different pKa values into the polymer backbone. The probes become activated at various pH levels due to the existence of protonated ammonium groups. The presence of these groups induces the micelles to separate into individual molecules, resulting in a significant enhancement in the emission of fluorescence. A fluorescent nanoplatform was developed using easily accessible dyes that remain unaffected by pH changes. The nanoplatform can change colors and adjust pH. The nanoplatform enables accurate manipulation of fluorescence wavelengths, spanning from green to the near-infrared (NIR) emission range of 500–820 nm. In addition, fluorescence can be activated or deactivated within a pH range of 0.25 units. Recently developed nanomaterials have been used to create pH nanoprobes, in addition to quantum dots and polymeric nanoparticles. Shi et al. used a ratiometric pH probe using carbon nanodots (CDs) to accurately track the intracellular pH throughout the entire cell. The surfaces were coated with different molar ratios of FITC, a pH-sensitive compound, and another pH-insensitive molecule. The pH response range can be effectively modified by the dual labeling of the CDs. In addition, the materials showed positive biocompatibility and were able to disperse within cells. The pH nanoprobes show promising potential in precisely measuring and visualizing acidity levels in the tumor microenvironment within living organisms. The combination of nanoparticles and small fluorescent probes led to improved compatibility with biological systems and more efficient transportation, while producing emissions within an appropriate range. Hence, using nanoprobes that are linked to pH-sensitive small molecule dyes enables the optical analysis of the tumor microenvironment. Target groups can be bound to the surface of nanoprobes to achieve specificity. These probes have certain limitations, including a restricted pH range and a tendency to be absorbed by kidney and liver cells during in vivo imaging. To address these concerns, it is crucial to advance the development of biocompatible nanocarriers and other pH nanoprobes. Gold nanoparticles are being used as effective contrast agents in cancer therapy due to their high atomic number and biocompatibility. Enhanced secondary electron generation can enable particles with a size below 100 nm to get through human cell membranes and concentrate in cancer cells. A recent study found that the application of gold nanoparticles, along with kilovoltage radiation, led to a notable increase in the survival rate of mice with EMT-6 mammary carcinoma cell line. According to a study, the survival rate increased significantly to 86% when radiotherapy was combined with another treatment, in contrast to the mere 20% survival rate observed when radiotherapy was used as the sole treatment. Gold-iron oxide nanoparticles were demonstrated to be effective for both therapeutic and diagnostic applications. Research findings demonstrated the successful targeting of nanoparticle deposition in SW1222 xenograft tumors using laser-assisted treatment and MRI-based imaging. Researchers were able to achieve both the eradication and detection of tumors. Gold nanoparticles alloyed with copper-64 and other similar alloy-based nanoparticles have been used in cancer imaging. Precursor $CuCl_2$ is added to achieve precise control over the specific radioactivity of the alloyed gold nanoparticles, enabling exceedingly sensitive detection. The incorporation of Cu into the gold nanoparticle framework ensured the durability of the radiolabel for precise localization within our body. A study was conducted to develop Au-Fe alloy nanoparticles for use as multimodal contrast agents. A compound known as iron carbide $Fe5C_2$ was synthesized and used as a contrast probe for magnetic resonance imaging (MRI). The magnetization of the sample approached its maximum capacity. It possessed a compact and modifiable size, measuring less than 25 nm. The range of sizes was limited, and it showed exceptional stability in colloidal form. It has been found that they tend to accumulate in tumors, resulting in a more pronounced change in signal [82–85].

6.5.3 Theragnostic Nanoprobes in Atherosclerosis

Molecular imaging plays an essential role in applying nanoprobes for the specific targeting of plaques. Molecular imaging is a non-invasive approach that focuses on specific molecules at the tissue and cell levels. It particularly highlights changes in these molecules during pathological conditions. The purpose of molecular imaging is to gain a comprehensive understanding of disease mechanisms, identify new targets for pharmacological interventions, and discover potential drug candidates. Molecular imaging is an interdisciplinary field that includes several areas such as medicine, radiology, materials science, chemistry, and mathematics. Molecular imaging has significant potential to provide an in-depth understanding of cardiovascular inflammation and its progression over time in the context of atherosclerosis. Furthermore, the use of cutting-edge imaging technology, including CT, MRI, and positron emission tomography (PET), is complemented by the development of secure contrast agents. Efficient imaging probes, such as formed nanoprobes, are of utmost importance. Therefore, considering the potential of nanoprobes in the early detection and diagnosis of atherosclerosis, as well as the significance of targeting first plaques, it is recommended that researchers concentrate on enhancing the sensitivity and specificity of nanoprobes. These nanoprobes can be used to create targeted contrast agents for imaging thrombosis and plaques. The proposed uses of engineering nano-probes in atherosclerosis can be categorized into two basic groups. Preliminary investigations have demonstrated that constructed nanoprobes have the ability to selectively identify early-stage plaques by targeting chemicals that are particular to plaques. Nanoprobes can be detected using several ways. The effective visualization of monocytes, macrophages, foam cells, and other constituents of plaques has rendered these nanoprobes exceedingly promising for the timely identification of atherosclerosis [87]. In addition, nanoprobes can serve as highly effective vehicles for delivering drugs that target inflammation and lipid metabolism, thereby aiding in the achievement of therapeutic goals. Organic nanoparticles are frequently used to improve the identification and management of atherosclerosis. They possess physical properties such as excellent biocompatibility and the ability to carry drugs, making them effective in molecular imaging and drug delivery for this condition. These engineering nanoprobes can function as carriers for both imaging and therapeutic medications for atherosclerotic plaques. This broadens their traditional clinical applicability within this specific discipline. The combination of multiple imaging techniques, such as optical/MR dual-model imaging, optical/ultrasound dual-modality imaging, and photoacoustic/ultrasound imaging, has gained significant interest and has been tested on atherosclerotic animal models. This is because single-mode imaging is insufficient to gather precise imaging data. Multi-mode imaging surpasses the limitations of single-mode imaging and enhances imaging outcomes by integrating the strengths of different imaging modalities. This enables the early detection of atherosclerosis. It is worth mentioning that recently developed nanoparticles for imaging have the potential to scavenge reactive oxygen species (ROS). These nanoparticles have demonstrated efficacy in the diagnosis and treatment of susceptible plaques, and they offer a new approach for managing atherosclerosis. This development represents a revolutionary nanoplatform for both therapy and diagnosis of the condition. The recent progress in imaging and treating atherosclerosis using different nanoprobes has several promising prospects for the future [88].

The following Fig. 6.4 illustrates an intravascular imaging method for detecting atherosclerosis with the help of nanomedicine.

6.5.4 *Nanoimaging to Diagnose Pulmonary Diseases*

Respiratory diseases together refer to conditions that impact both the upper and lower respiratory systems. This category contains a diverse range of diseases. Nanomedicine has demonstrated its efficacy in treating several hereditary diseases, including cystic fibrosis and chronic obstructive lung diseases such as asthma. Nanoplatforms can be used in the detection and management of lung cancer, as well as pulmonary tuberculosis. Studies have shown that the lung can be effectively targeted, especially when using inhaled aerosols. This is because these nanosystems are rapidly transported to the airways. Discovering imaging nanoplatforms with the ability to diagnose lung diseases is a challenging endeavor. Numerous diverse systems have been created in recent times. Aillon and colleagues discovered that iodine nanoclusters have the potential to serve as a distinct form of contrast agent for lung imaging. Positron emission tomography (PET) and magnetic resonance imaging (MRI) are the two most frequently used imaging techniques for lung imaging of nanoparticles (NPs). Currently, there is limited availability of nanosystems that

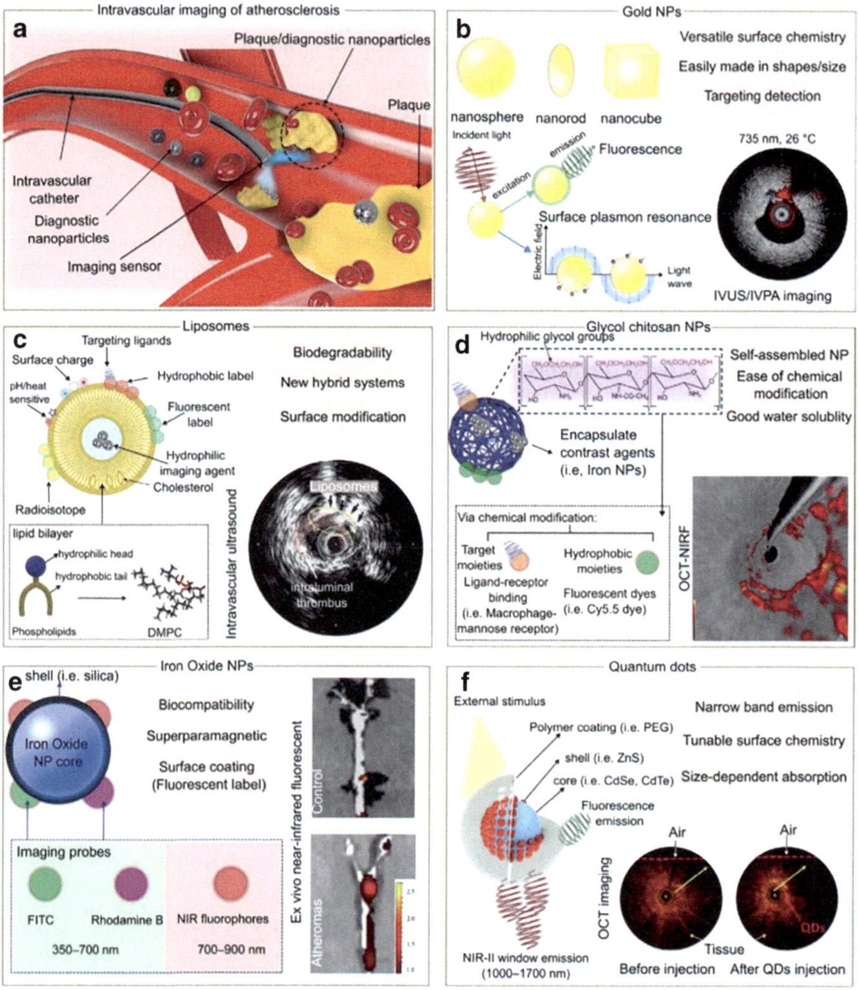

Fig. 6.4 An intravascular imaging method for atherosclerosis using nanomedicine. (**a**) A schematic illustration of how intravascular imaging uses nanoparticles. Comparing the advantages of different nanoparticle (NP) probes for intravascular imaging (**b**–**f**). (Reprinted from [89], Copyright, MDPI, 2023, This Open Access Article is licensed under a Creative Commons Attribution 4.0 International License)

integrate both imaging and therapeutic functionalities. Lanza et al. developed lipase-sensitive phospholipid prodrugs of fumagillin or docetaxel that were loaded into lipid-based micelles. The effectiveness of αv β3-targeted micelles, which are present on lung endothelial cells, in inhibiting the growth of new blood vessels was investigated in asthma using magnetic resonance imaging that simultaneously detects both 19F and 1H signals. Following a pulmonary injection, superparamagnetic iron oxide nanoparticles (NPs) were paired with a biocompatible antibody to evaluate their effects on living beings. Advanced technology allows for the precise targeting and scanning of a specific subset of macrophages in a mouse model with chronic obstructive lung disease induced by lipopolysaccharide [90, 91].

6.5.5 Nanoimaging for Diagnosing Neurological Conditions

Neurodegenerative disorders including Alzheimer's (AD), Parkinson's (PD), and Huntington's (HD), as well as other neurological diseases, have a profound global impact, affecting millions of individuals. The therapy remains unfinished due to the inadequate presence of active molecules with limited therapeutic efficacy, their limited ability to cross the targeted tissue due to the presence of the blood-brain barrier (BBB), and the incomplete understanding of their pathophysiological mechanisms. As a result, more and more researchers are focusing on the development of drug-delivery devices and therapeutic compounds that can effectively penetrate the blood-brain barrier (BBB) and reach the brain. In addition, the detection of these diseases primarily revolved around the use of PET, SPECT, MRI, and X-ray CT. PET provides enhanced imaging capabilities compared to SPECT due to its high sensitivity and superior resolution. Magnetic Resonance Imaging (MRI) and Computed Tomography (CT) are imaging techniques that can effectively visualize structural changes in affected brain regions without the need for invasive procedures. To improve drug absorption in the brain, nanocarriers can be modified with biologically active molecules that selectively attach to receptors found on brain endothelial cells. A new nanosystem was developed for use as an AD nanotheranostics. The process involved the application of ceria and iron oxide nanocrystals onto mesoporous silica nanoparticles (MSN). The MSNs were further modified with amino-T807, a positron emission tomography (PET) tracer for tau protein, as well as methylene blue. Birgitte and her colleagues synthesized manganese oxide nanoparticles (NPs) that were modified with L-dopa. The nanoparticles (NPs) can concurrently release both Mn2+ ions and L-dopa in water as a result of the NPs' degradation. The nanosystem served as an MRI agent for imaging, diagnosis, and therapy of Parkinson's disease (PD) [92].

6.5.6 Infectious Disease Nanodiagnostics

Nanodiagnostics refers to the application of nanotechnology in diagnostic processes. It has undergone thorough research to fulfill the demands of clinical diagnostics, specifically in terms of achieving increased sensitivity and early diagnosis of different disorders. The nanostructures' high surface-to-volume ratio makes them ideal for attaching several targeted molecules, hence enhancing the sensitivity of the detection results. Nanomaterials or nanostructures provide distinct characteristics that enable nanodiagnostics platforms to swiftly and instantaneously identify samples from patients, using only minuscule amounts. Therefore, nanodiagnostic techniques possess significant promise to be cost-effective, easy to use, and resilient devices. Presently, the primary emphasis of nanodiagnostic applications lies in identifying pathogens in infectious diseases and detecting cancer biomarkers in cancer therapies. Nanodiagnostic platforms offer a reliable and speedy means of obtaining conclusive results for infectious disorders. These platforms use simple and portable instruments that only require blood, sputum, or urine samples from patients. The highly responsive nanodiagnostics platforms, which have significant promise to be durable, cost-effective, and easily replicated, may be well-suited for use in diagnosing infectious diseases, especially in economically disadvantaged regions of developing nations. Multiple kinds of nanoparticles, including fluorescent, magnetic, and metallic nanoparticles, have been successfully used for diagnosing infectious diseases. Fluorescent nanoparticles are extremely sensitive and resilient markers that can be used to label a wide range of biological targets. Recent advancements in bioimaging and sensing techniques have demonstrated novel approaches for real-time disease detection. Quantum dots are fluorescent nanostructures composed of semiconducting materials, typically with dimensions ranging from 1 nm to 10 nm. They possess unique characteristics, including photostability, high quantum yield, and brightness. Quantum dots may readily adjust their fluorescence properties by modifying their size and composition. HBV (hepatitis B virus) has been effectively diagnosed using the dot immunoassay technique with the use of quantum dots nanobeads (QDNBs). The fluorescence emitted by the quantum dot nanobeads (QDNBs) can be enhanced due to the inclusion of several quantum dot within a single nanoparticle. The hepatitis B surface antigens were immobilized on the porous polyvinylidene difluoride. The QDNBs, which were coupled with antibodies, were used as molecular probes and subsequently exposed to the antigens. The luminous dots obtained were recorded using a charge-coupled device (CCD) camera, which was irradiated by a UV (ultraviolet) lamp. The effectiveness of this straightforward diagnostic system, based on quantum dot nanobeads (QDNBs), has been proven in detecting as little as 78 picograms of hepatitis B surface antigen. This demonstrates the high sensitivity of the QDNBs method in diagnosing infectious diseases and suggests its potential utility in detecting other biomarkers in complex biological environments [93].

6.6 Clinical Translations of Nanodiagnostics

The field of nanodiagnostics has advanced from its early stages in the laboratory, where it could detect biomolecules in controlled environments, to a collection of prototypes that are currently being validated in laboratory settings. Nevertheless, the quantity of validated systems is considerably lower in comparison to the number of reports found in the literature. It is worth noting that only a small subset of these systems has advanced to the preclinical or clinical stage. Converting the achievements of nanotechnology research into healthcare services can pose a substantial challenge. Translational research is the process of transforming scientific knowledge into practical applications that can be used in therapeutic settings. Efforts must be made to connect the findings of laboratory research with practical applications in clinical settings, ensuring a seamless translation of ideas from the research stage to the direct benefit of patients. Translating the promising results of fundamental research into therapeutic procedures is a challenging task that requires careful evaluation and critique. Many systems attempt this challenging endeavor, but only a few manage to successfully reach the bedside [94]. To effectively implement a conventional, traditional technology in clinical settings, it is essential to consider not only the technology itself, including its benefits, effectiveness, and worth but also the need for innovative teamwork and sufficient financial resources. In the field of nanodiagnostics, it is important to consider specific parameters because it relies on nanotechnology and the use of technologies at the nanoscale. At present, there are no regulations in place on either side of the Atlantic that specifically address the use of nanodiagnostics characteristics. One reason for this is the absence of well-defined and universally accepted techniques for characterizing nanoscale goods and products that are compatible with sensing platforms. It is necessary to improve our understanding of the interactions between nanoscale materials and biological systems. When considering different biological levels, it is important to consider factors like size, composition, structure, and aggregation rate. These factors are essential for understanding the intricate interactions between cells and macromolecules. Researchers have a limited understanding of the features and mechanisms that contribute to the effectiveness of nanodiagnostics systems in detecting biological substances. The majority of these approaches have not been verified in fundamental biological sample environments, let alone in clinical testing. To enhance or substitute traditional detection and biosensing technologies, it is crucial to strictly follow specific rules and requirements tailored to the desired objective. For example, the Organisation for Economic Cooperation and Development (OECD) recommends that laboratories offering genetic diagnostics should acquire accreditation or a similar form of recognition to ensure compliance with best practices. In the field of nanodiagnostics platforms, particularly those focused on molecular detection and characterization like genetic diagnosis, it is of utmost importance for the laboratory responsible for implementation to ensure the dependability, security, and flawless nature of the service or product. Usually, this task is accomplished using robust and widely accepted methods that are considered the most dependable way to identify a particular item. Initially, this should not create a problem. Nevertheless, nanodiagnostics techniques are continuously enhancing their sensitivity, occasionally resulting in "false positives" in comparison to the established standard. What is the most effective way to circumvent this obstacle? What is the clinical relevance of a decrease in the observed amount of a specific analyte? How can one obtain accurate validation for a system or platform? These concerns are currently occupying the attention of individuals responsible for draughting and proposing recommendations for nanodevices and diagnostic devices based on nanotechnology. Nanodiagnostics technology has made significant progress and is now well-suited for use in clinical settings. Transitioning these promising platforms from laboratory research to clinical settings is now imperative. A few of them have already taken measures. As an illustration, Nanosphere™ is a United States-based company that possesses multiple diagnostic devices that have been approved by the Food and Drug Administration (FDA). The products use gold nanoparticles to label probes for molecular recognition. The company offers a product called Verigene®, which uses a parallel technique that relies on gold nanoprobes to detect multiple pathogens in a single stage of the assay. There are various cartridges available to accurately detect infections and genetic diseases. The system uses the microarray technology as outlined by Storhoff and colleagues, which eliminates the need for DNA amplification beforehand. The system uses automated machinery for preparing and handling samples, which is smoothly integrated with the array and readout system for the interpretation of data. Their product range includes clinical microbiology tests for respiratory viruses, Gram-positive blood cultures, and Clostridium difficile. Researchers offer thrombophilia testing for F5, F2, and MTHFR (methylenetetrahydrofolate reductase), as well as drug metabolism tests for Warfarin and CYP2C19. The system has an impressively low detection limit of 50 fM of DNA. It is highly capable of identifying single base mismatches, making it ideal for mutation and SNP discrimination. The degree of the system's sensitivity and specificity may vary among different products but generally exceeds 90% when compared to the gold standard techniques. Another example is the Magtration® technology, which has been successfully commercialized by Precision System Science Co., Ltd. This platform uses magnetic nanoparticles for the extraction of specific biomolecules from intricate media. Chemicell GmbH offers highly purified products for the identification and isolation of nucleic acids from biological fluids and media. The purpose of these products is to improve downstream applications by using traditional molecular biology techniques [95].

6.7 Challenges and Future Perspectives

The following sections and Table 6.2 describe the challenges and the scope of diagnostic nanoprobes in modern healthcare systems.

6.7.1 Technical Challenges

6.7.1.1 Synthesis and Scalability

Challenges in the manufacture and scalability of diagnostic nanoprobes and imaging agents hinder them from unlocking their full potential in the field of biomedicine. Precise management of the production processes is essential to guarantee consistency and replicability, both of which are critical for clinical applications. Commonly used methods for synthesizing nanoparticles, including chemical vapor

Table 6.2 Challenges and future trends in nanoprobe development for diagnostics and therapy

SL No.	Challenges	Current solutions	Future directions	Reference
1.	Biocompatibility and toxicity	Surface functionalization with biocompatible materials	Development of wearable technologies and precision therapy	[105]
2.	High production cost and scalability issue	Introduction of hybrid technologies	Use of AI to design cost-effective manufacturing process	[105]
3.	Stability and degradation	Surface modification with biocompatible ligands and use of biodegradable materials in diagnostic probes	Development of smart and multifunctional nanoprobes	[106]
4.	Limited specificity to target tissues	Use of tissue-specific targeting ligands through surface functionalization	Introduction of personalized medicine	[106]
5.	Limited sensitivity in imaging	Introduction of hybrid modalities	Use of smart nanomaterials and targeted nanotheranostics	[106]
6.	Regulatory barriers	Establishment of regulatory guidelines by FDA, EMA, and other regulatory bodies	Application of AI to create a more efficient approval process and uniform regulatory rules	[105]

deposition, sol-gel procedures, and hydrothermal methods, typically encounter restrictions of limited batch prediction capacity, high production costs, and slow production rates. Transitioning from the laboratory to the industrial-scale manufacturing process, while preserving the physicochemical qualities and performance of the nanoprobes, is a major roadblock. The intricate nature of nanoparticle design adds another layer of complexity to the manufacturing process. To tackle these issues, it is necessary to make progress in manufacturing technology and establish robust protocols that guarantee consistency and quality on a greater scale [96].

6.7.1.2 Stability and Storage

Ensuring the stability and proper storage of diagnostic nanoprobes and imaging agents poses additional technological difficulties. Environmental conditions including temperature, light, and pH, can influence the stability and efficacy of the nanoparticles. To ensure long-term stability, it is essential to create appropriate storage solutions and packaging materials that safeguard the nanoprobes and prevent their rapid degradation. In addition, the accumulation of nanoparticles over time can hinder their effectiveness, requiring measures to retain their ability to disperse and function properly. Researching stabilizing agents, optimizing storage conditions, and developing new packaging techniques are crucial for addressing these limitations and guaranteeing that the nanoprobes maintain their desired qualities until they are used in clinical applications [97, 98].

6.7.2 Regulatory and Ethical Issues

6.7.2.1 Approval Processes

The regulatory framework governing diagnostic nanoprobes and imaging agents is complex and varies substantially across different regions. Acquiring regulatory approval is a demanding process that requires extensive preclinical and clinical testing to ensure the safety, effectiveness, and quality of the nanoprobes, making the procedure labor-intensive and expensive. It also requires strict documentation and validation requirements. To successfully navigate the regulatory routes, one must possess a thorough understanding of the norms and standards established by regulatory authorities such as the FDA (Food and Drug Administration), EMA (European Medicines Agency), and other national agencies. Moreover, the lack of standardized assessment methods for nanomaterials makes the process more complex and delays the approval process. Effective collaboration among researchers, manufacturers, and regulatory agencies is key to making the approval process streamlined and enabling a smooth transition of diagnostic nanoprobes from the laboratory to clinical use [98, 99].

6.7.2.2 Ethical Considerations in Clinical Use

Several ethical considerations must be addressed to ensure patient safety and maintain public trust in the clinical use of diagnostic nanoprobes and imaging agents. Important ethical concerns entail obtaining informed consent, safeguarding privacy, and the possibility of unforeseen repercussions. Before giving consent, patients must be well-informed on the properties of nanoprobes, the procedures, and any potential dangers or side effects involved. In addition, nanoprobes in imaging and diagnostics can produce very sensitive health information, which requires the implementation of stringent rules and regulations to safeguard patient privacy and maintain confidentiality. Furthermore, the improper disposal and possible accumulation of nanomaterials in living organisms may jeopardize ecosystems. So, the environmental impact of these substances must be taken into consideration. It is imperative to establish ethical rules and frameworks that specifically tackle these challenges so that the responsible use of nanotechnology in healthcare can be achieved [100].

6.7.3 Future Trends

6.7.3.1 Innovations in Nanoprobe Technology

The future of diagnostic nanoprobes and imaging agents is expected to witness significant developments due to the improvement in nanoprobe technology. Emerging trends involving theragnostic agents by which assess therapeutic effectiveness can be evaluated in real-time and specific medications can be administered concurrently. This novel approach is a valuable tool for improving personalized medicine strategies in the current healthcare sector. In addition, the progress in nanomaterials, particularly the use of biocompatible and biodegradable polymers, is improving the safety and effectiveness of nanoprobes. The integration of artificial intelligence (AI) and machine learning (ML) with nanoprobe technology is very promising as it allows for the analysis of complex imaging data and the generation of predictive diagnostic tools. Further investigation and collaboration with other scientific fields will propel these advancements, hence creating new doors for the developing novel tools to achieve timely identification and management of diseases [101, 102].

6.7.3.2 Integration with Digital Healthcare Systems

The incorporation of diagnostic nanoprobes and imaging agents into digital healthcare systems is a growing area that is expected to shift the paradigm of the traditional healthcare system. The integration of nanotechnology with digital health tools, such as electronic health records (EHRs), telemedicine, and wearable devices, presents novel opportunities for the remote monitoring and management of health issues. Nanoprobes with advanced intelligence, including biosensors and wireless connectivity, can provide real-time data to healthcare specialists, facilitating patient-specific treatment regimens. This further helps in the collection and examination of extensive health data, aiding in the management of population health and epidemiological research. As these technologies progress, they will have a crucial impact on the advancement of precision medicine, resulting in improved patient outcomes [103, 104].

6.8 Conclusion

Incorporating diagnostic nanoprobes and imaging agents into digital healthcare and theranostics is a substantial advancement in the fast detection, monitoring, and management of many medical conditions. The various ways that nanotechnology can improve the sensitivity, specificity, and effectiveness of diagnostic modalities have been explored in this chapter. Using nanoprobes and imaging agents has unparalleled prospects for accurate and immediate imaging at the molecular and cellular scales, enabling early detection and tailored therapy approaches. Notable advancements in the field have been achieved by developing nanoparticles with distinct properties that enhance image visibility in medical imaging techniques such as MRI, CT, PET, and optical imaging. Nanomaterials such as quantum dots, gold nanoparticles, and magnetic nanoparticles have been designed to specifically detect certain biomarkers. This allows for the creation of detailed images and improves the accuracy of identifying different disease conditions. Furthermore, the ability of these nanoprobes to perform several functions, such as diagnosing and delivering therapeutic chemicals at the same time, demonstrates the theranostic capabilities of nanotechnology. Although there have been some positive advancements, there are still some obstacles that need to be addressed to fully achieve the clinical use of diagnostic nanoprobes and imaging agents. It is crucial to thoroughly examine issues like biocompatibility, toxicity, long-term stability, and targeted distribution. The presence of regulatory obstacles and the requirement for uniform protocols add more complexity to the process of implementing clinical applications. Nevertheless, continuous research and technical progress are gradually overcoming these obstacles, thereby facilitating the wider implementation of these groundbreaking tools in clinical environments. The prospective impacts of diagnostic nanoprobes and imaging agents on numerous fields of healthcare are anticipated to have revolutionary effects in the years to come. To fully exploit the potential of nanotechnology for digital healthcare and theranostics, it is imperative to maintain ongoing interdisciplinary collaboration and allocate resources for research. Incorporating intelligent and eco-friendly nanomaterials will ultimately result in an enhanced, efficient, and customized healthcare system that will completely transform the field of disease control and enhance positive outcomes for patients.

Acknowledgments Not Applicable.

Data Availability Statement Data sharing is not applicablė to this chapter as no datasets were generated or analyzed during the current study period.

Ethics Statement Not Applicable.

Conflict of Interest The authors declare no conflict of interest.

Author Contributions *CRediT author statement*: Conceptualization: *Tanvir Ahmed*, Writing—Original Draft: *Tanvir Ahmed, Kazi Tasnuva Alam*, Writing—Review & Editing: *Tanvir Ahmed, Kazi Tasnuva Alam*, Visualization: *Tanvir Ahmed.*

FundingThis research did not receive any specific grant from funding agencies in the public, commercial, or not-for-profit centers.

References

1. Malik S, Waheed Y. Emerging applications of nanotechnology in dentistry. Dent J. 2023;11:1–30.
2. Bayda S, Adeel M, Tuccinardi T, Cordani M, Rizzolio F. The history of nanoscience and nanotechnology: from chemical-physical applications to nanomedicine. Molecules. 2020;25:1–15.
3. Iqbal P, Preece JA, Mendes PM. Nanotechnology: the "top-down" and "bottom-up" approaches. Supramol Chem. 2012.
4. Baker SN, Baker GA. Luminescent carbon nanodots: emergent nanolights. Angew Chem Int Ed. 2010;49:6726–44.

5. Thwala LN, Ndlovu SC, Mpofu KT, Lugongolo MY, Mthunzi-Kufa P. Nanotechnology-based diagnostics for diseases prevalent in developing countries: current advances in point-of-care tests. Nanomaterials. 2023;13:1–19.
6. Patra JK, Das G, Fraceto LF, Campos EVR, del Rodriguez-Torres MP, Acosta-Torres LS, et al. Nano based drug delivery systems: recent developments and future prospects. J Nanobiotechnol. 2018;16:71. https://doi.org/10.1186/s12951-018-0392-8.
7. Wang Z, Agrawal P, Zhang YS. Nanotechnologies and nanomaterials in 3D (Bio)printing toward bone regeneration. Adv NanoBiomed Res. 2021;1:1.
8. Vahedifard F, Chakravarthy K. Nanomedicine for COVID-19: the role of nanotechnology in the treatment and diagnosis of COVID-19. Emerg Mater. 2021;4:75–99.
9. Chi X, Huang D, Zhao Z, Zhou Z, Yin Z, Gao J. Nanoprobes for in vitro diagnostics of cancer and infectious diseases. Biomaterials. Elsevier Ltd. 2012;33:189–206.
10. Shahbazi-Gahrouei D, Khaniabadi PM, Khaniabadi BM, Shahbazi-Gahrouei S. Medical imaging modalities using nanoprobes for cancer diagnosis: a literature review on recent findings. J Res Med Sci. 2019;24.
11. Zhang Q, Hou K, Chen H, Zeng N, Wu Y. Nanotech probes: a revolution in cancer diagnosis. Front Oncol. 2022;12:1–6.
12. Burlec AF, Corciova A, Boev M, Batir-Marin D, Mircea C, Cioanca O, et al. Current overview of metal nanoparticles' synthesis, characterization, and biomedical applications, with a focus on silver and gold nanoparticles. Pharmaceuticals. 2023;16.
13. Ielo I, Rando G, Giacobello F, Sfameni S, Castellano A, Galletta M, et al. Applications of functional gold nanoparticles: a review. Molecules. 2021;26:1–40.
14. Xiao L, Yeung ES. Optical imaging of individual plasmonic nanoparticles in biological samples. Annu Rev Anal Chem. 2014;7:89–111.
15. Zhang XF, Liu ZG, Shen W, Gurunathan S. Silver nanoparticles: synthesis, characterization, properties, applications, and therapeutic approaches. Int J Mol Sci. 2016;17.
16. Takáč P, Michalková R, Čižmáriková M, Bedlovičová Z, Balážová Ľ, Takáčová G. The role of silver nanoparticles in the diagnosis and treatment of cancer: are there any perspectives for the future? Life. 2023;13.
17. Abdulsahib SS. Synthesis, characterization and biomedical applications of silver nanoparticles. Biomed. 2021;41:458–64.
18. Singh S, Dhawan A, Karhana S, Bhat M, Dinda AK. Quantum dots: an emerging tool for point-of-care testing. Micromachines. 2020;11:1–23.
19. Abdellatif AAH, Tawfeek HM, Younis MA, Alsharidah M, Al Rugaie O. Biomedical applications of quantum dots: overview, challenges, and clinical potential. Int J Nanomed. 2022;17:1951–70.
20. Zielińska A, Carreiró F, Oliveira AM, Neves A, Pires B, Venkatesh DN, Durazzo A, Lucarini M, Eder P, Silva AM, Santini A, et al. Polymeric nanoparticles: production, characterization, toxicology and ecotoxicology. Molecules. 2020;25:3731.
21. Aziz R, Falanga M, Purenovic J, Mancini S, Lamberti P, Guida M. A review on the applications of natural biodegradable nano polymers in cardiac tissue engineering. Nano. 2023;13:1–28.
22. Iron toxicity in the retina requires Alu RNA and the NLRP3 inflammasome. 乳鼠心肌提取 HHS Public Access. Physiol Behav. 2016;176:139–48.
23. Gunatillake PA, Adhikari R. Nondegradable synthetic polymers for medical devices and implants. Biosynthetic Polym Med Appl. Elsevier Ltd; 2016.
24. Mirahadi M, Ghanbarzadeh S, Ghorbani M, Gholizadeh A, Hamishehkar H. A review on the role of lipid-based nanoparticles in medical diagnosis and imaging. Ther Deliv. 2018;9:557–69.
25. Yingchoncharoen P, Kalinowski DS, Richardson DR. Lipid-based drug delivery systems in cancer therapy: what is available and what is yet to come. Pharmacol Rev. 2016;68:701–87.
26. Li X, Anton N, Zuber G, Vandamme T. Contrast agents for preclinical targeted X-ray imaging. Adv Drug Deliv Rev Elsevier BV. 2014;76:116–33.

27. Xie J, Lee S, Chen X. Nanoparticle-based theranostic agents. Adv Drug Deliv Rev. 2010;62:1064–79.
28. Bae KH, Lee JY, Lee SH, Park TG, Nam YS. Optically traceable solid lipid nanoparticles loaded with sirna and paclitaxel for synergistic chemotherapy with in situ imaging. Adv Healthc Mater. 2013;2:576–84.
29. Albuquerque J, Moura CC, Sarmento B, Reis S. Solid lipid nanoparticles: a potential multifunctional approach towards rheumatoid arthritis theranostics. Molecules. 2015;20:11103–18.
30. Speranza G. Carbon nanomaterials: synthesis, functionalization and sensing applications. Nano. 2021;11:11.
31. Gupta N, Gupta SM, Sharma SK. Carbon nanotubes: synthesis, properties and engineering applications. Carbon Lett. Springer Singapore. 2019;29:419–47.
32. Simon J, Flahaut E, Golzio M. Overview of carbon nanotubes for biomedical applications. Materials (Basel). 2019;12:1–21.
33. Maiti D, Tong X, Mou X, Yang K. Carbon-based nanomaterials for biomedical applications: a recent study. Front Pharmacol. 2019;9:1–16.
34. Bellier N, Baipaywad P, Ryu N, Lee JY, Park H. Recent biomedical advancements in graphene oxide- and reduced graphene oxide-based nanocomposite nanocarriers. Biomater Res. BioMed Central. 2022;26:1–23.
35. Bailey J, Oliveri A, Levin E. 基因的改变NIH public access. Bone. 2013;23:1–7.
36. Holmannova D, Borsky P, Svadlakova T, Borska L, Fiala Z. Carbon nanoparticles and their biomedical applications. Appl Sci. 2022;12:1–21.
37. Konnova S, Rozhina E. Magnetic nanoparticles for biomedical and imaging applications. Int J Mol Sci. 2024;25:10–1.
38. Brokowski CAM. 乳鼠心肌提取 HHS public access. Physiol Behav. 2019;176:139–48.
39. Dhawan AP, D'Alessandro B, Fu X. Optical imaging modalities for biomedical applications. IEEE Rev Biomed Eng. 2010;3:69–92.
40. Yoon S, Cheon SY, Park S, Lee D, Lee Y, Han S, et al. Recent advances in optical imaging through deep tissue: imaging probes and techniques. Biomater Res. BioMed Central. 2022;26:1–27.
41. Zambito G, Chawda C, Mezzanotte L. Emerging tools for bioluminescence imaging. Curr Opin Chem Biol. 2021;63:86–94.
42. Acharya G, Mitra AK, Cholkar K. Nanosystems for diagnostic imaging, biodetectors, and biosensors. In: Emerging nanotechnologies for diagnostics, drug delivery and medical devices. Elsevier; 2017.
43. Blasiak B, Van Veggel FCJM, Tomanek B. Applications of nanoparticles for MRI cancer diagnosis and therapy. J Nanomater. 2013;2013
44. Yang Y, Yue S, Qiao Y, Zhang P, Jiang N, Ning Z, et al. Activable multi-modal nanoprobes for imaging diagnosis and therapy of tumors. Front Chem. 2021;8:1–23.
45. Estelrich J, Sánchez-Martín MJ, Busquets MA. Nanoparticles in magnetic resonance imaging: from simple to dual contrast agents. Int J Nanomedicine. 2015;10:1727–41.
46. Lee N, Hyeon T. Designed synthesis of uniformly sized iron oxide nanoparticles for efficient magnetic resonance imaging contrast agents. Chem Soc Rev. 2012;41:2575–89.
47. Narayana A. Applications of nanotechnology in cancer: a literature review of imaging and treatment. J Nucl Med Radiat Ther. 2014;05:05.
48. Preslar AT, Parigi G, MT MC, Sefick SS, Moyer TJ, Haney CR, et al. Gd(III)-labeled peptide nanofibers for reporting on biomaterial localization in vivo. ACS Nano. 2014;8:7325–32.
49. X-ray-Computed Tomography Contrast Agents-Lusic 2013.pdf.
50. Ma X, Figl M, Unger E, Buschmann M, Homolka P. X-ray attenuation of bone, soft and adipose tissue in CT from 70 to 140 kV and comparison with 3D printable additive manufacturing materials. Sci Rep. Nature Publishing Group UK. 2022;12:1–13.
51. Stringer KL, Turan B, McCormick L, Durojaiye M, Nyblade L, Kempf M-C, Lichtenstein B. 乳鼠心肌提取 HHS public access. Physiol Behav. 2017;176:139–48.

52. Cruje C, Dunmore-Buyze PJ, Grolman E, Holdsworth DW, Gillies ER, Drangova M. PEG-modified gadolinium nanoparticles as contrast agents for in vivo micro-CT. Sci Rep. Nature Publishing Group UK. 2021;11:1–11.
53. Poggi C, Palavecino M. Ultrasound principles and instrumentation. Surg Open Sci. Elsevier Inc.; 2024;18:123–128.
54. Endo-Takahashi Y, Negishi Y. Microbubbles and nanobubbles with ultrasound for systemic gene delivery. Pharmaceutics. 2020;12:1–14.
55. Abeylath SC, Ganta S, Iyer AK, Amiji M. Combinatorial-designed multifunctional polymeric nanosystems for tumor-targeted therapeutic delivery. Acc Chem Res. 2011;44:1009–17.
56. Batchelor DVB, Armistead FJ, Ingram N, Peyman SA, McLaughlan JR, Coletta PL, et al. The influence of Nanobubble size and stability on ultrasound enhanced drug delivery. Langmuir. 2022;38:13943–54.
57. Berger A. Positron emission tomography. Br Med J. 2003;326:1449.
58. Bouchareb Y, AlSaadi A, Zabah J, Jain A, Al-Jabri A, Phiri P, et al. Technological advances in SPECT and SPECT/CT imaging. Diagnostics. 2024;14.
59. Pijeira MSO, Viltres H, Kozempel J, Sakmár M, Vlk M, İlem-Özdemir D, et al. Radiolabeled nanomaterials for biomedical applications: radiopharmacy in the era of nanotechnology. EJNMMI Radiopharm Chem. 2022;7.
60. Alqahtani FF. SPECT/CT and PET/CT, related radiopharmaceuticals, and areas of application and comparison. Saudi Pharm J. 2023;31:312–28.
61. Rizvi M, Gerengi H, Gupta P. Functionalization of nanomaterials: synthesis and characterization. ACS Symp Ser. American Chemical Society. 2022;1418:1–26.
62. Thiruppathi R, Mishra S, Ganapathy M, Padmanabhan P, Gulyás B. Nanoparticle functionalization and its potentials for molecular imaging. Adv Sci. 2017;4.
63. Konstantinos Avgoustakis. Pegylated poly(Lactide) and poly(Lactide-Co-Glycolide) nanoparticles: preparation, properties and possible applications in drug delivery. Curr Drug Deliv. 2004;1:13.
64. Parmar K, Patel J, Pathak Y. Factors affecting the clearance and biodistribution of polymeric nanoparticles. Pharmacokinet Pharmacodyn Nanoparticulate Drug Deliv Syst. 2022;5:261–72.
65. Lin B, Xiao F, Jiang J, Zhao Z, Zhou X. Engineered aptamers for molecular imaging. Chem Sci Royal Society of Chemistry. 2023;14:14039–61.
66. Li J, Wang Q, Xia G, Adilijiang N, Li Y, Hou Z, et al. Recent advances in targeted drug delivery strategy for enhancing oncotherapy. Pharmaceutics. 2023;15:1025.
67. Dmitrieva MD, Voitova AA, Dymova MA, Richter VA, Kuligina EV. Tumor-targeting peptides search strategy for the delivery of therapeutic and diagnostic molecules to tumor cells. Int J Mol Sci. 2021;22:1–10.
68. Kyriakides TR, Raj A, Tseng TH, Xiao H, Nguyen R, Mohammed FS, et al. Biocompatibility of nanomaterials and their immunological properties. Biomed Mater. 2021;16:1–49.
69. Bastús NG, Sánchez-Tilló E, Pujals S, Farrera C, López C, Giralt E, et al. Homogeneous conjugation of peptides onto gold nanoparticles enhances macrophage response. ACS Nano. 2009;3:1335–44.
70. Yang W, Wang L, Mettenbrink EM, Deangelis PL, Wilhelm S. Nanoparticle toxicology. Annu Rev Pharmacol Toxicol. 2021;61:269–89.
71. Xuan L, Ju Z, Skonieczna M, Zhou PK, Huang R. Nanoparticles-induced potential toxicity on human health: applications, toxicity mechanisms, and evaluation models. MedComm. 2023;4:1–39.
72. Azzawi M, Seifalian A, Ahmed W. Nanotechnology for the diagnosis and treatment of diseases. Nanomedicine. Taylor & Francis. 2016;11:2025–7.
73. Siegel RL, Miller KD, Jemal A. Cancer statistics, 2018. CA Cancer J Clin. 2018;68:7–30.
74. Siafaka PI, Okur NÜ, Karantas ID, Okur ME, Gündoğdu EA. Current update on nanoplatforms as therapeutic and diagnostic tools: a review for the materials used as nanotheranostics and imaging modalities. Asian J Pharm Sci. 2021;16:24–46.

75. Ahmed AA, Abedalthagafi M. Cancer diagnostics: the journey from histomorphology to molecular profiling. Oncotarget. 2016;7:58696–708.
76. Xu C, Chen F, Valdovinos HF, Jiang D, Goel S, Yu B, et al. Bacteria-like mesoporous silica-coated gold nanorods for positron emission tomography and photoacoustic imaging-guided chemo-photothermal combined therapy. Biomaterials. 2018;165:56–65.
77. Li A, Zhao J, Fu J, Cai J, Zhang P. Recent advances of biomimetic nano-systems in the diagnosis and treatment of tumor. Asian J Pharm Sci Elsevier BV. 2021;16:161–74.
78. Bardhan N. Nanomaterials in diagnostics, imaging and delivery: applications from COVID-19 to cancer. MRS Commun. Springer International Publishing. 2022;12:1119–39.
79. He X, Gao J, Gambhir SS, Cheng Z. Near-infrared fluorescent nanoprobes for cancer molecular imaging: status and challenges. Trends Mol Med Elsevier Ltd. 2010;16:574–83.
80. Bogdanov A, Bogdanov A, Chubenko V, Volkov N, Moiseenko F, Moiseyenko V. Tumor acidity: From hallmark of cancer to target of treatment. Front Oncol. 2022;12.
81. Wang L, Li C. pH responsive fluorescence nanoprobe imaging of tumors by sensing the acidic microenvironment. J Mater Chem. The Royal Society of Chemistry. 2011;21:15862–71.
82. Zhou K, Liu H, Zhang S, Huang X, Wang Y, Huang G, et al. Multicolored pH-tunable and activatable fluorescence nanoplatform responsive to physiologic pH stimuli. J Am Chem Soc. American Chemical Society; 2012;134:7803–11.
83. Zhao Y, Sultan D, Detering L, Cho S, Sun G, Pierce R, et al. Copper-64-alloyed gold nanoparticles for cancer imaging: improved radiolabel stability and diagnostic accuracy. Angew Chem Int Ed. John Wiley & Sons, Ltd. 2014;53:156–9.
84. Leung MKK, Chow JCL, Chithrani BD, Lee MJG, Oms B, Jaffray DA. Irradiation of gold nanoparticles by x-rays: Monte Carlo simulation of dose enhancements and the spatial properties of the secondary electrons production. Med Phys. John Wiley & Sons, Ltd. 2011;38:624–31.
85. Anshup, Venkataraman JS, Subramaniam C, Kumar RR, Priya S, Kumar TRS, et al. Growth of gold nanoparticles in human cells. Langmuir American Chemical Society. 2005;21:11562–7.
86. Kantamneni H, Barkund S, Donzanti M, Martin D, Zhao X, He S, et al. Shortwave infrared emitting multicolored nanoprobes for biomarker-specific cancer imaging in vivo. BMC Cancer. 2020;20:1–12.
87. Tu S, He W, Han J, Wu A, Ren W. Advances in imaging and treatment of atherosclerosis based on organic nanoparticles. APL Bioeng. 2022;6:41501.
88. Dai Y, Sha X, Song X, Zhang X, Xing M, Liu S, et al. Targeted therapy of atherosclerosis vulnerable plaque by ROS-scavenging nanoparticles and MR/fluorescence dual-modality imaging tracing. Int J Nanomedicine. 2022;17:5413–29.
89. Li J, Centurion F, Chen R, Gu Z. Intravascular imaging of atherosclerosis by using engineered nanoparticles. Biosensors. 2023;13:1–17.
90. Durham AL, Caramori G, Chung KF, Adcock IM. Targeted anti-inflammatory therapeutics in asthma and chronic obstructive lung disease. Transl Res. 2016;167:192–203.
91. Lanza GM, Jenkins J, Schmieder AH, Moldobaeva A, Cui G, Zhang H, et al. Anti-angiogenic nanotherapy inhibits airway remodeling and hyper-responsiveness of dust mite triggered asthma in the brown Norway rat. Theranostics. 2017;7:377–89.
92. Durães F, Pinto M, Sousa E. Old drugs as new treatments for neurodegenerative diseases. Pharmaceuticals. 2018;11:1–21.
93. Wang Y, Yu L, Kong X, Sun L. Application of nanodiagnostics in point-of-care tests for infectious diseases. Int J Nanomedicine. 2017;12:4789–803.
94. Mankoff SP, Brander C, Ferrone S, Marincola FM. Lost in translation: obstacles to translational medicine. J Transl Med. 2004;2:14.
95. Storhoff JJ, Marla SS, Bao P, Hagenow S, Mehta H, Lucas A, et al. Gold nanoparticle-based detection of genomic DNA targets on microarrays using a novel optical detection system. Biosens Bioelectron. 2004;19:875–83.
96. Veigas B, Portugal C, Valério R, Fortunato E, Crespo JG, Baptista PV. Scalable approach for the production of functional DNA based gold nanoprobes. J Memb Sci. 2015;492:528–35.

97. Jones E, He J, VanBrocklin H, Franc B, Seo Y. Nanoprobes for medical diagnosis: current status of nanotechnology in molecular imaging. Curr Nanosci. 2008;4:17–29.
98. Zhang P, Cui Y, Anderson CF, Zhang C, Li Y, Wang R, et al. Peptide-based nanoprobes for molecular imaging and disease diagnostics. Chem Soc Rev. Royal Society of Chemistry. 2018;47:3490–529.
99. Jain KK. Applications of Nanobiotechnology in clinical diagnostics. Clin Chem. 2007;53:2002–9.
100. Alharbi KK, Al-sheikh YA. Role and implications of nanodiagnostics in the changing trends of clinical diagnosis. Saudi J Biol Sci. 2014;21:109–17.
101. Wang Z, Song Y. Nanomedicine for bio-imaging and disease diagnosis. In: Nanomedicine; 2024. p. 207–26.
102. Fan Z, Liu Y, Ye Y, Liao Y. Functional probes for the diagnosis and treatment of infectious diseases. Aggregate. John Wiley & Sons, Ltd; 2024:e620.
103. Mishra A, Singh PK, Chauhan N, Roy S, Tiwari A, Gupta S, et al. Emergence of integrated biosensing-enabled digital healthcare devices. Sens Diagn. Royal Society of Chemistry. 2024;3:718–44.
104. Boukherroub R, Szunerits S. The future of nanotechnology-driven electrochemical and electrical point-of-care devices and diagnostic tests. Annu Rev Anal Chem (Palo Alto, Calif). 2024;17:173–95.
105. Schrader M, Fricker LD. Current challenges and future directions in peptidomics. Methods Mol Biol. 2024;2758:485–98.
106. Alrushaid N, Khan FA, Al-Suhaimi EA, Elaissari A. Nanotechnology in cancer diagnosis and treatment. Pharmaceutics. 2023;15:1025.

Chapter 7
Nanomaterials for Regenerative Medicine

Tanvir Ahmed and Kazi Tasnuva Alam

Abstract Nanomaterials have emerged as a promising type of material in regenerative medicine, providing novel ways to repair, replace, and regenerate damaged tissues and organs. This chapter discusses the diverse applications of nanomaterials in regenerative medicine, concentrating on their ability to improve biological responses, stimulate tissue regeneration, and facilitate drug administration. Key breakthroughs in the design and implementation of nanomaterials, including nanoparticles, nanofibers, and nanocomposites, are explored concerning bone, neural, and cardiovascular tissue engineering. Additionally, the chapter looks at how nanoparticles might alter the immune system, enhancing the functionality and integration of implanted materials. Furthermore, their integration with digital healthcare platforms emphasizes the importance of smart nanomaterials in personalized therapy and real-time monitoring. We conducted a thorough analysis of the sustainability of nanomaterials, accounting for the biocompatibility concerns and environmental effects related to their development and use. The chapter offers insights into the future of nanomaterials in regenerative medicine, where the combination of digital healthcare and nanotechnology can potentially improve treatment outcomes by addressing these problems.

Keywords Nanomaterials · Regenerative Medicine · Tissue Engineering · Scaffold

---

T. Ahmed (✉) · K. T. Alam
Department of Pharmaceutical Sciences, School of Health and Life Sciences, North South University, Dhaka, Bangladesh
e-mail: tanvir.ahmed111@northsouth.edu

S. Mondal et al. (eds.), *Smart and Sustainable Nanomaterials in Digital Healthcare and Theranostic*, https://doi.org/10.1007/978-981-95-9386-6_7

7.1 Introduction

The inception of regenerative medicine in human history dates back to 600 BC when the term regenerative medicine was first coined. The earliest known surgical textbook documents an Indian physician's instructions on repairing torn earlobes using skin from the cheeks and reconstructing a nose using a forehead flap, thus marking the emergence of regenerative medicine in the world. Regenerative medicine is an interdisciplinary field that integrates engineering and cell biology concepts to promote the regrowth of injured tissues and organs and restore, maintain, and enhance their natural function. The fundamental basis of this fascinating discipline relies on three pillars: tissue engineering, biomaterials, and cell therapy. Regenerative operations are performed by integrating stem cell infusion, biomaterials, grafts, scaffolds, and manipulation of cell sources. This leads to the efficient restoration and substitution of the impaired tissue, including its structural and functional aspects. During the late 2000s, the integration of stem cells into the field of tissue regeneration resulted in the development of a novel interdisciplinary field called regenerative medicine. Adult stem cells, embryonic stem cells, mesenchymal stem cells (MSCs), and induced pluripotent stem cells (iPSCs) play a vital role in the regeneration and repair of damaged tissues or organs. Stem cells are unique cells that have the ability to transform into many specialized cell types within our body through a process called differentiation [1]. Stem cells require a biomaterial-based structural framework that supports cell adhesion, migration, and the formation of functioning tissues that mimic the damaged organs in our body. The term used to refer to these frameworks in tissue engineering is 'scaffolds.' Tissue scaffolds are matrices that have a high level of porosity and well-defined features. They must possess biocompatibility, meaning they should not provoke any immune response within the body. Implanting these scaffolds successfully in our body can restore normal function in a diseased part, thereby assisting in wound healing. Due to its distinct ability to control the tumor environment, regenerative medicine has emerged as a fascinating area of research in the field of biomedicine. Currently, regenerative medicine uses stem cell therapy, immune cell therapy, and the development of three-dimensional (3D) tissue-engineered constructions as effective methods to address orthopedic problems, organ transplantations, inflammatory diseases, specific types of cancer, cardiac disorders, and other medical conditions [2]. Although this emerging discipline has great potential, several obstacles limit its widespread application in clinical settings. The problems are linked to the absence of an effective biomaterial-based delivery system, the complexity of navigating the scaffold framework, inadequate understanding of stem cell function, high costs of production, and ethical considerations.

Nevertheless, since the emergence of this field nearly two decades ago, several FDA-approved products have been available on the market. Biologics, such as Carticel and LaViv, use autologous fibroblasts and chondrocytes extracted from articular cartilage, cultured in a lab, and subsequently applied to the site of cartilage damage or injury. Furthermore, medical devices that are derived from cells, commonly referred to as 'dermagrafts' are specifically designed to address the issue of diabetic foot ulcers. In addition, there are a limited number of commercially accessible biopharmaceuticals, including GEM 125 and infused bone transplants used for treating periodontal abnormalities. Hemacord is a marketplace-available product that contains both hematopoietic stem cells and progenitor stem cells, commonly used for the treatment of several hematological disorders [2].

Scientists have long been studying methods to optimize the field of regenerative medicine to overcome its numerous limitations and enable its extensive application in clinical settings. Since its conceptualization by Richard P. Feynman in 1959, nanotechnology has progressively integrated with biomedicine in the twentieth century, offering immense potential to transform the domains of medicine and healthcare. This innovative technology has made significant milestones in the development of biosensors, diagnostic probes, drug delivery systems based on nanotechnology, nanobiopharmaceuticals, and personalized medicine. In more recent times, integrating engineering techniques with biology has led to various groundbreaking nanoengineering initiatives aimed at repairing and regenerating tissues and organs, reshaping the field of nanobiotechnology. Nanotechnology is an effective approach to tissue regeneration that aims to replicate the intricate characteristics of tissues at the nanoscale level, facilitating cellular attachment, migration, and cellular differentiation. Nanostructures possess distinctive chemical, physical, optical, electrical, and magnetic characteristics, with the added benefit of surface functionalization [3]. They offer precise manipulation of tissue scaffolds by adjusting their properties and creating scaffolds with improved biochemical, mechanical, optical, and electrical characteristics. In addition, nanomaterials regulate the release of certain bioactive substances to control the development of stem cells, reduce harmful effects, and enhance compatibility with living tissue by delivering them in a target-specific manner. As a result, the incorporation of nanoscience in regenerative medicine boosts its capacity for effective biomolecule transportation, use as scaffolds for tissue regeneration, in vivo cell tracking, and stem cell therapy [4].

7.2 Types of Nanomaterials Used in Regenerative Medicine

Nanoscale materials applied in regenerative medicine includes a wide range of entities, such as nanoparticles, nanodevices, nanofibers, nanoparticle scaffolds, nanocomposites, and more, which serve as carriers for various biomolecules and as biomaterials for enhancing the physiochemical properties of the tissue scaffolds used for regenerative purposes.

The following sections elaborate on the nanoparticles currently used in regenerative medicine.

7.2.1 Nanoparticles

Nanoparticles can be generated from several materials, including metals, ceramics, and polymers. Due to their nano size, ability to modify surface properties, high penetrability, enhanced biocompatibility, and targeted bioactive agent delivery, nanoparticles are considered highly suitable for use in regenerative medicine [5]. Figure 7.1 illustrates different types of nanoparticles along with their synthesis, characterization, functionalization, and use in tissue engineering.

This chapter explores metallic, ceramic, and polymeric nanoparticles in particular, which are outlined in Table 7.1 below.

7.2.1.1 Metallic Nanoparticles

Due to their ability to be synthesized and optimized through the attachment of several kinds of ligands with the help of functional groups, metallic nanoparticles like gold and silver find their applicability in regenerative medicine.

Gold nanoparticles (AuNPs) are used and widely investigated in bone regeneration procedures. Conjugating their surface with PEG, gold nanostructures are used to replace malignant tissue with implanted tissue following surgical resection. This type of functionalized nanomaterial also finds its use in cancer nanomedicine, where AuNPs help to disrupt the cancer cell division process by targeting the affected cells and inducing cytokine arrest. This eventually leads to a reduced possibility of tumor recurrence. Besides, AuNPs enhance the functionality of scaffolds used in bone tissue regeneration. Heo et al. developed a scaffold model combining gold nanoparticles and gelatin. When used, it increased the process of bone cell formation and was more readily taken up by mesenchymal stem cells (MSCs). Gold nanoparticles significantly influence vascular tissue engineering by improving the elasticity and thermal stability of the scaffold when they are incorporated into the coating material. In the research studies, AuNPs have shown notable efficacy in promoting wound healing and enhancing the development of new blood vessels, surpassing the control groups [8].

Silver nanoparticles (AgNPs) are well-known for their antimicrobial properties and ability to maintain colloidal stability. As a result, they are used in engineered tissues to reduce the probability of bacterial infection risks. Silver nanoparticles are predominantly used in wound dressing and therapeutic applications. The incorporation of nanoparticles into the composite material of scaffolds can be achieved by using reducing agents, resulting in the formation of antimicrobial scaffolds. Consequently, these scaffolds, composed of gelatin, cellulose, chitosan, alginate, and PVA (polyvinyl alcohol), show antibacterial properties. Research has demonstrated that the use of silver in wound therapy not only has antimicrobial effects but also accelerates the healing process. In certain cases, these particles can regulate the cytokines that are involved in the healing of burn wounds. The presence of silver has an impact on blood clotting as it alters the coagulation route through the denaturation of

Table 7.1 Types of nanomaterials and their application in regenerative medicine

SL No.	Type of nanomaterial	Structure/ Composition	Applications	Advantages	References
1.	Metallic nanoparticles	Gold, silver, iron oxide, zinc oxide	Drug delivery, molecular diagnostics, tissue engineering, wound healing	Enhanced antimicrobial and antitumor properties of tissue scaffolds, improved bioimaging and tissue targeting of diagnostic probes, enhanced optical response, and photostability	[4]
2.	Polymeric nanoparticles	PLGA (Poly (lactic-co-glycolic acid)), PEG (Polyethylene glycol), chitosan, gelatin, cellulose, alginate	Tissue engineering, drug delivery, gene delivery, diagnostic imaging	Improved bioimaging and tissue targeting of diagnostic probes, low cytotoxicity, good biocompatibility, and biodegradability	[4]
3.	Ceramic nanoparticles	Bioactive glass nanoceramics (hydroxyapatite, alumina, silica) Bioresorbable Nanoceramics (calcium carbonate, hydroxyapatite), bioinert Nanoceramics (titanium dioxide, zinc oxide)	Bone tissue engineering, dental implants, drug delivery	Enhanced biomechanical properties, good biocompatibility	[4]
4.	Carbon-based nanomaterials	Graphene, carbon nanotubes, fullerenes, and quantum dots (zinc sulfide and cadmium selenide)	Neural regeneration, bone regeneration, photodynamic therapy, drug delivery	Enhanced diagnostic imaging, unique optical properties, exceptional mechanical and electrical properties	[6]
5.	Lipid-based nanomaterials	Liposomes, phospholipids, solid-lipid nanoparticles, cholesterol	Tissue regeneration, drug delivery, wound healing, diagnostic imaging	Sustained release of bioactive agent, improved molecular imaging, low toxicity, excellent biocompatibility	[7]

anticoagulant proteins. This enhances blood clotting efficiency in chitosan/alginate antimicrobial scaffolds used in bone regeneration and skin repair [9].

7.2.1.2 Ceramic Nanoparticles

Ceramics are inorganic compounds that can be manipulated to form nanoscale particles. These materials are used in bone regeneration, wound healing, and delivery of bioactive substances. Depending on tissue response, nanoceramics can be classified into three types.

Bioactive glass nanoceramics were developed in 1969 using elements such as silicon, oxygen, sodium, potassium, phosphorus, and others. nBGCs (bioactive glass nanoceramics) show greater specific surface area and bioactivity in comparison to their larger counterparts. The antibacterial and angiogenic capabilities, as well as the outstanding bioactivity, of nBGCs, have made them a highly appropriate option for the regeneration of dentin and bone. Several studies have demonstrated that the use of miRNA (microRNA) delivery with nBGCs has led to targeted delivery and stimulation of osteoblast development by adipose-derived stem cells [10]. Bioresorbable nanoceramics are another type of ceramic-based substance that is primarily derived from calcium phosphate. Due to their higher stability compared to other calcium-phosphate-based nanoceramics, tissue regeneration applications widely use hydroxyapatite nanoceramics. Hydroxyapatite (HAp) possesses the ability to mimic bone-like characteristics, promote bone growth, and show biocompatibility. Due to these qualities, they are a popular choice for tissue grafting and scaffolding in surgical procedures involving bone defects, bone tissue repair, natural mineralization processes, and dental enamel restoration. In addition, HAp the lattice can incorporate various ions to precisely modify the unique characteristics of the scaffold for specific tissue engineering purposes, such as regulating degradation and biological reactions. It is feasible to fabricate composite scaffolds by combining PEG with other biomaterials, which can include hydroxyapatite crystals. This approach enhances the administration of bioactive substances and promotes bone repair [11]. Finally, bioinert nanoceramics, such as titanium oxide and zinc oxide, have recently emerged as an innovative technology for application in regenerative therapies. These compounds show significant affinity for tissues and have minimal impact on the overall toxicity of the body. When inserted into living bone, they assimilate into the bone tissue through "contact osteogenesis" and assist in the formation of stable grafts. In addition, their exceptional biocompatibility ensures that bone tissue does not elicit any immunological rejections [12].

7.2.1.3 Polymeric Nanoparticles

Polymer-based nanoparticles are the most extensively used and studied nanomaterials in regenerative medicine due to their high biodegradability, excellent biocompatibility, increased penetration and retention (EPR) impact, minimal cytotoxicity, and the ability to deliver a wide range of bioactive chemicals to specified targets. With the virtue of the aforementioned properties, polymeric nanostructures are used in biomaterial matrices to stimulate cell growth, proliferation, and stem cell differentiation into different lineages (e.g., chondrocytes, adipocytes, and osteoblasts) in tissue regeneration applications. Polymers can create scaffolds that mimic the ECM crucial for mesenchymal stem cell development and bone regeneration. Osteoregeneration extensively uses biodegradable polymeric nanoparticles like chitosan, gelatin, elastin, and hyaluronic acid because they accurately mimic the body's environment without causing any adverse effects. Currently, the polymers frequently employed for tissue repair and regeneration include polyglycolic acid (PGA), polylactic acid (PLA), polyanhydrides, polysaccharides, polyester, protein, polyacetals, and polyethylene glycol (PEG). Polymeric nanostructures find their applicability in drug delivery since their use can enable sustained release of therapeutic cargo without eliciting any immune response in the body. Researchers use these nanomaterials as carriers for DNA and siRNA in cartilage tissue regeneration procedures and also as biocompatible probes for tracking stem cells or drug carriers in CNS repair due to their ability to cross the BBB. Polymeric NPs as drug transport vehicles enhance the efficacy of stem cell therapy since they deliver bioactive molecules to targeted cells for the growth, proliferation, and differentiation of stem cells required for tissue regeneration and repair. Recent studies highlight the effectiveness of polymeric nanomaterials in promoting wound healing as well [13] (Fig. 7.1).

7.2.2 Nanofibers

Nanofibers are unique materials characterized by their small, lightweight fibers, exceptional mechanical strength, high surface-to-volume ratio, and porosity. In the field of regenerative medicine, these structures are commonly used as scaffolds for culturing biological cells because they can mimic the porous structure of the extracellular matrix (ECM). In addition, they serve as vehicles for delivering drugs, enabling precise control over the release of the payload. Among the various fabrication methods, electrospinning is a technology used to manufacture nanofibers of exceptional purity. Nanofiber scaffolds are improved by the inclusion of biodegradable polymers and functionalized polymers, making them very suitable for the regeneration of several parts of our body, including bone, skin, cartilage, tendon, and ligament [15].

The following sections describe two of the most used nanofiber-based scaffolds in tissue regeneration.

7.2.2.1 Electrospun Nanofibers

A key challenge in regenerative medicine is developing appropriate scaffolds that can mimic the function of the replacement organ or tissue and induce a biological response from nearby organs. With innovative research and experimentation on

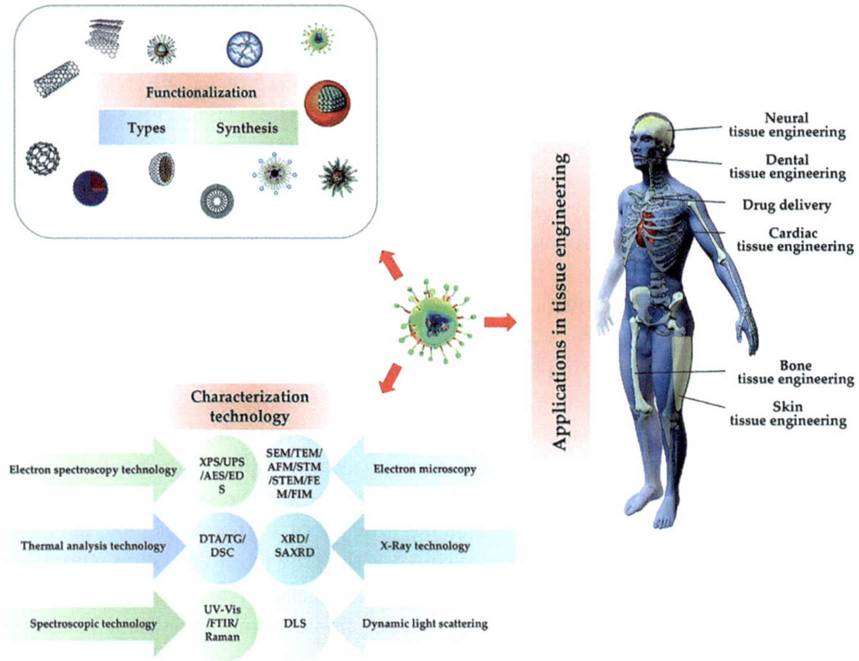

Fig. 7.1 Illustration of type, synthesis, characterization, and functionalization of nanoparticles (NPs) and their use in tissue engineering. (Reprinted from [14], Copyright, Royal Society of Chemistry, 2021, This Open Access Article is licensed under a Creative Commons Attribution 3.0 Unported Licence)

tissue scaffolding, biomedical engineers use advanced techniques like microfabrication to develop complex, 3D structures with cells. Their primary focus is on creating scaffolds that can imitate the significant features of the extracellular matrix (ECM), which are crucial in controlling cell division, migration, and differentiation. Currently, various methods are used to create fibrous scaffolds of such nature. Electrospinning is a reliable and uncomplicated technique that produces a highly porous nanomaterial known as 'Electrospun nanofibers.' The process of electrospinning is relatively straightforward and consists of a grounded fiber collector, a high--voltage source, a capillary tube, and a pipette. When a high voltage is applied, nanofibers that are randomly oriented are gathered on the static collector. At the same time, the revolving drum creates nanofibers that are aligned in a single direction. These aligned nanofibers are the electrospun fibers that are used as scaffolds for tissue regeneration. They possess an impressive ratio of surface area to volume and are well-suited for intercellular communication within a living organism. Their extensive surface area enables the incorporation of numerous bioactive components for scaffold grafting. Traditional methods cannot replicate the anisotropic features of the tendon, heart, and blood vessels in scaffolds. To overcome this limitation, a wide range of non-degradable and biodegradable polymers are utilized to coat electrospun nanofibers, resulting in the development of scaffolds that recapitulate the asymmetrical properties of these tissues. Currently, electrospun nanofiber scaffolds are most commonly applied in nerve injury repair, tendon regeneration, and tendon-to-bone insertion site repair. Therefore, scaffolds constructed from electrospun nanofibers with varying alignments have shown remarkable efficacy in shaping cells, guiding cell division, facilitating cell migration, and influencing cell differentiation, thus proving to be superior to the other forms in both laboratory experiments and living organisms [16, 17].

7.2.2.2 Self-Assembled Nanofibers

Self-assembly is the process of arranging the constituent components of a compound in a way that results in the formation of a higher-order structure. Self--assembling peptide (SAP) materials, among other gel delivery matrices, are the most frequently used nanofibers that utilize physical non-covalent bonding to self-assemble and create a supramolecular network structure of nanofibrous hydrogels. The stability of these structures can be enhanced by using hydrophobic packing in the core of the fiber. The release profile of the nanofibers and their cargo can be modified by adjusting the interactions between them. These nanofibers can mimic the three-dimensional microenvironment of the natural extracellular matrix (ECM) and influence the biological behavior of cells, including their growth, transport, and differentiation. This makes them highly suitable for tissue engineering purposes. In addition, these nanoscaffolds offer improved intercellular communication, more biodegradability, and enhanced cell proliferation. Currently, there are several techniques accessible for producing self-assembled peptide nanofibers, such as enzyme-catalyzed gel formation, solution mixing, and cross-linking methods. The applications of these techniques encompass the development of 3D tissue constructs, the regulated release of growth factors, the enhancement of wound healing and skin regeneration, and the facilitation of anti-tumor therapy [18].

7.2.3 Nanocomposites

Nanocomposites are created by incorporating suitable nanoparticles into a larger matrix. Some parts of the composite are highly concentrated and offer structural reinforcement, while others enhance the composite's performance by introducing additional characteristics like electrical conductivity, thermal conductivity, mechanical strength, optical clarity, magnetic attraction, and many more. These structures signify a compelling frontier in the field of biomedicine, providing solutions to ongoing obstacles. For instance, the field of biomedicine uses nanopolymers due to their exceptional biocompatibility and renewability. Nevertheless, the limited clinical application of these materials is due to their inferior mechanical qualities and quick deterioration. As a result, scientists have combined biopolymers, including cellulose, starch, and chitosan, with hydrogel matrices to address these constraints, leading to the creation of nanocomposite hydrogels. These novel materials demonstrate increased mechanical durability, enhanced compatibility with living organisms, and the capability to precisely adjust the release of drugs. By harnessing the distinctive properties of nanoparticles, various nanomaterials create nanocomposite frameworks currently used in diagnostics, drug administration, tissue engineering, medical implants, wound healing, bone restoration, and recovery. These biomaterials possess a distinct synergy of biocompatibility, tuneability, and multifunctionality, making them crucial contributors in the search for novel solutions to intricate biomedical problems [19, 20].

7.2.3.1 Advantages in Regenerative Applications

Nanoparticles show a wide range of distinctive characteristics that are used in scaffold generation in regeneration processes. Nanomaterials of various kinds can be cross-linked to create scaffolds based on hydrogel, fibers, and organic and inorganic nanomaterials that possess a meaningful synergy of essential properties in a nanocomposite, such as biocompatibility, efficient nutrient transport, biodegradability, strong tensile strength, appropriate pore size, surface area, and customizable surface topography. For instance, nanocomposite scaffolds prepared with nanoparticles like polymers offer better biocompatibility and bioactivity, which are used to demonstrate outstanding results in cell adhesion, proliferation, and differentiation. This is because polymer-based scaffolds can mimic the natural extracellular matrix (ECM) due to their physiochemical similarities. Researcher Liu et al. conducted an experiment where he and his team integrated hydroxyapatite (HAp) in the hydrogel matrix. This resulted in improving the hydrogel's stiffness and resilience. This addition significantly influences the differentiation patterns of MSCs. To enhance the mechanical and electrical properties of the hydrogel matrix, conductive nanomaterials such as carbon nanotubes, graphene, and metallic nanoparticles can be incorporated into the matrix system [21]. Nanostructures also allow for tissue-specific scaffold design since the selection of a nanocomposite scaffold relies on the particular tissue being treated. For example, to mimic the natural tissue arrangement, it is necessary to orient nanofiber scaffolds in a parallel manner for engineering tissues of the tendon. In cardiac tissue engineering, nanocomposite scaffold materials must possess specific electrical conductivity. These materials should assist in the gradual healing and renewal of tissue damaged by myocardial infarction while simultaneously supporting electrophysiological functions. This indicates an advance toward personalized medicine in tissue regeneration processes. However, nanocomposite scaffolds have some challenges and limitations, such as the potential for transmitting pathogens, causing allergic reactions, and having high production costs. Currently, researchers are actively working to construct scaffolds that are both potent and specifically designed for tissue regeneration, thereby paving the way for personalized medicine [22].

7.2.4 *Carbon-Based Nanomaterials*

Carbon, being one of the most abundant minerals on Earth, has been the subject of scientific investigation since its discovery, especially concerning its several allotropes. Consequently, carbon-based nanomaterials including carbon nanoparticles, fullerene, carbon dots, graphene and its derivatives, carbon nanotubes, and others have been discovered and are currently available for use in several industries. Solely composed of carbon, carbon-based nanostructures show exceptional stability, remarkable electrical and thermal conductivity, and impressive mechanical properties such as great strength and toughness. These nanostructures show high biocompatibility with low toxicity and can be readily modified to improve the behavior of specific cell types, including their shape, adhesion, growth, and division. Thus, carbon nanoparticles can be used as a coating material for tissue scaffolds. These scaffolds facilitate tissue development from stem cells, enabling their repair and healing. Therefore, carbon-based nanomaterials hold significant promise for application in tissue engineering and regenerative medicine [23].

7.2.4.1 Graphene and Its Derivatives

Graphene is one of the most extensively researched carbon nanomaterials and serves as the foundational structure for various carbon allotropes. Graphene, renowned for its remarkable mechanical strength, electrical conductivity, large surface area, and functionalizing ability, is considered one of the strongest materials in existence. These properties make an excellent choice for tissue regeneration, particularly in the context of bone tissue repair and regeneration. Multiple research investigations indicate that graphene shows improved cell adhesion due to its larger surface area, distinctive molecular structure, in vitro compatibility with living cells, and impressive mechanical strength. As a result, graphene can serve as a supportive material for scaffolds in developing three-dimensional bone structures. Graphene has also been used to treat neurological disorders. An experiment was recently performed in which an electrospun microfiber scaffold covered with self-assembled colloidal graphene was implanted into the striatum of adult rats. This resulted in a reduction in microglial and astrocyte activation following a brain lesion. Researchers use two-dimensional (2D) and three-dimensional (3D) scaffolds incorporating graphene oxide (GO) similarly for addressing several brain disorders. In cardiac tissue regeneration, studies that used a scaffold made of PEG and GO and newborn rat ventricular myocytes showed that cardiac cells grew faster, conducted electricity better, and contracted more than when PEG alone was used. Graphene and graphene oxide (GO) are used in wound healing and skin regeneration. Their ability to stimulate neoangiogenesis makes them suitable for repairing peripheral nerves. Hence, with its growing application, graphene and its derivatives have the potential to transform the use of carbon-based nanoparticles in regenerative medicine for the better [24].

7.2.4.2 Carbon Nanotubes

Among the conductive nanomaterials, carbon nanotubes have been extensively studied and designed. These nanostructures are characterized by cylindrical tubes with a diameter at the nanoscale dimensions. Their remarkable mechanical strength, large specific surface area, and exceptional thermal and electrical conductivity have made them a popular choice as a scaffolding material in various tissue engineering techniques presently. In bone tissue regeneration, carbon nanotubes (CNTs) serve as filler particles that improve the mechanical strength, elasticity, fatigue resistance, cell affinity, and structural integrity of the bone scaffolds or implants. Research indicates that when subjecting carbon nanotubes (CNTs) to different physical tests, the obtained Young's modulus and tensile strength demonstrate their highly rigid and durable structure. Both single-walled carbon nanotubes (SWCNT) and multi-walled carbon nanotubes (MWCNT) are used in nanocomposite frameworks with biodegradable or synthetic polymer scaffolds. The incorporation of carbon nanotubes into a nanocomposite structure enhances the structural integrity of the produced scaffold, enabling cell adhesion, growth, proliferation, and the controlled release of cytokines and growth factors to targeted regions. Using carbon nanotubes (CNTs) in the nanocomposite scaffold fabrication could effectively address many drawbacks associated with bone implants that use metal or ceramic nanomaterials. CNTs are also applied in retinal regeneration by facilitating the transformation of human embryonic stem cells into precursor cells for photoreceptors, particularly in cases of retinal damage. Besides these applications, CNTs contribute to multiple other fields, including cardiac tissue regeneration, neurological disorders, drug delivery, and therapies, positioning them as a versatile tool in regenerative medicine. Nevertheless, the biocompatibility of carbon nanotubes (CNTs) remains an issue due to their toxic properties and limited solubility in several cases. To address this challenge, scientists functionalize the surface of carbon nanoparticles by attaching antibodies, polymers, aptamers, or other ligands. This allows for the development of a biodegradable scaffold that has a higher biocompatibility, better targeting, cell adhesion, and proliferation abilities [25].

7.3 Mechanisms of Action of Nanomaterials in Tissue Regeneration

Nanotechnology has long been a crucial tool in regenerative medicine, providing substantial solutions to longstanding challenges in this field. With the virtue of their targeted and precise delivery of drugs and bioactive molecules and versatile physiochemical properties, researchers have made them ideal for use in tissue engineering applications. Hence, scientists and researchers have been investigating the underlying mechanisms by which these nanomaterials offer their capabilities to improve regenerative procedures. The subsequent sections discuss the mechanisms by which these nanostructures function to bestow various capabilities in the field of regenerative medicine.

7.3.1 Cellular Interactions

Cell-to-cell interactions are critical for any tissue regenerative process to be successful. This is because cellular interactions help cells to integrate structurally, aid in cell migration and survival, guide cell differentiation, and determine cell fate, potentially allowing the development of a scaffold that can mimic the natural biological environment of the ECM. Nanomaterials improve the overall functionality of the tissue scaffolds by serving as efficient carriers of drugs and bioactive molecules, biocompatible probes for cell tracking, or key components in biological matrices in scaffold fabrication. This results in improved cellular interactions, resulting in cell adhesion, migration, proliferation, and differentiation by the development of effective reconstituted tissues and organs for regeneration and healing that optimize tissue regeneration outcomes [26].

7.3.1.1 Cell Adhesion, Proliferation, and Differentiation

Tissue scaffolding is based on the principle of creating a structure that can recapitulate the natural environment of the extracellular matrix (ECM) in tissues. The ECM is composed of several biomolecules, including collagen, elastin, glycoproteins, and glycosaminoglycans. It also contains fibers and nanoscale pores, which contribute to its structural integrity. Therefore, to construct a scaffold that precisely resembles the ECM, the scaffold must demonstrate cellular behavior such as cell adhesion, migration, proliferation, and differentiation. A thorough understanding of the biological and physicochemical interactions that occur between cells and their surrounding environment is essential for achieving success in regenerative procedures. Nanomaterials are widely recognized for their ability to offer mechanical support, excellent thermal conductivity, and improved biocompatibility by virtue of their adjustable surface properties. Therefore, it is possible to produce scaffolds by using nanotechnology in tissue repair and regeneration for multiple conditions, such as bone defects, spinal injuries, cardiac problems, skin abnormalities, arthritis, digestive disorders, retinal damage, Parkinson's and Alzheimer's diseases, and aggressive cancers. Scaffolds are formed using nanoparticles made of metal, ceramic, polymer, magnet, and carbon. In addition, nanofibers and nanocomposites are commonly selected for such purposes. The nanoscale components serve as the mechanical support for the scaffold, allowing the biomaterials in the matrix to adhere together and form a 3D structure. Stem cells are crucial agents that facilitate the regeneration of tissues and organs by their potential to self-renew and differentiate into any kind of cell within our body. The nanoscale surfaces have been engineered to precisely align several types of stem cells, such as embryonic stem cells, mesenchymal stem cells (MSCs), and hematopoietic stem cells. Experiments with titanium dioxide nanotubes have demonstrated that these structures possess the ideal size for promoting integrin clustering, focal contact creation, and inducing cell migration, proliferation, and differentiation into osteogenic lineages, which are necessary for bone regeneration. Further, the scaffold must provide sufficient growth hormones, nutrition, pH levels, and temperature to stimulate cell division and differentiation of stem cells. Performing this procedure in an in vitro system using bioreactors is particularly challenging due to the inherent sensitivity of the process. The adoption of nano-based scaffolds facilitates the continuous and precise delivery of necessary biochemicals for cellular proliferation, hence enabling the regenerative process. Ongoing, extensive research is being conducted to thoroughly explain the effective methods of labeling, monitoring, and differentiating stem cells using nanomaterials. This research aims to facilitate the development of more optimal nanoscale scaffolds in the future [3, 27].

7.3.2 Molecular Pathways

Molecular pathways are a series of chemical reactions regulated by signaling molecules within a living organism that enable cells to communicate and perform their basic functions. Signaling molecules trigger a cascade of reactions within the cell, ultimately resulting in the generation of a biological response. This is the fundamental basis of all biological processes occurring within our body. It is well known that, without proper signaling, cells would not be able to differentiate and perform adequately in a tissue scaffold or construct. Therefore, to replace damaged cells and preserve the effectiveness of the regenerated tissue, it is crucial to have a comprehensive understanding of the molecular pathways influencing their growth and differentiation. Different growth factors and hormones are administered to the scaffold matrices to stimulate cell proliferation and differentiation. These include vascular endothelial growth factor (VEGF), which promotes the angiogenesis of vascular epithelial cells necessary for cell division and growth. Transforming growth factor (TGF) and bone morphometric proteins BMPs are involved in the BMP/TGFα signaling pathway that controls cell differentiation, migration, proliferation, and apoptosis, particularly in osteogenesis. In addition, Ca^{2+} signaling increases the activity of the transcription factor AP-1, resulting in the upregulation of many growth factors, including IGF1, VEGF, TGFα, and BMP, which are responsible for initiating cell division. Epidermal growth factor (EGF) and fibroblast growth factor (FGF) play a vital role in promoting cell development and specialization. Besides other signaling pathways, PDGF (platelet-derived growth factor), IGF (insulin-like growth factor), MAPK (mitogen-activated protein kinase), and the Notch pathway contribute to cell growth, division, and differentiation through the release of several growth factors and hormones. Several transcription factors play a vital role in controlling gene expression for tissue regeneration processes. Understanding cell signaling can help improve regenerative treatment modalities. As a result, several strategies are currently under study, including the integration of signaling molecules into nanocarriers, using cell-cell interactions, and enhancing material surface properties using nanocomposites or nanoparticles [28, 29].

7.3.2.1 Signaling Pathways Influenced by Nanomaterials

Nanomaterials have been recently developed that will accelerate the discovery of mechanisms driving stem cell fate. They not only contribute to in vivo stem cell tracking but also influence signaling mechanisms that are essential for cell growth and differentiation. Nanomaterials are well-known for their capacity to precisely transport payloads to a designated target. Regenerative medicine exploits this property to deliver several growth factors and hormones that trigger signaling cascades. Nanovesicles encapsulate these substances, enabling precise targeting of the stem cells. In addition, nanostructures can be enhanced with different ligands, which increases their biocompatibility, loading capacity, and targeting abilities. Nanocomposites incorporating biodegradable polymers or other nanoparticles have notable effects on the behavior of biomaterials and stem cells as they facilitate the activation of multiple biochemical pathways involved in tissue formation. In this scenario, scaffolds constructed using nanomaterials such as nanofibers (either self-assembled or electrospun) enhance the proliferation and differentiation of cells by expediting the activation of signaling pathways. This is because nanoscaffolds have a regulated release of biochemicals, unlike traditional scaffolds, and they can modify the scaffold's structural framework according to specific tissue regeneration techniques. Multiple studies have been undertaken to determine the signaling processes involved in tissue regeneration when nanomaterials are used. For example, when nanofiber scaffolds containing fibroblast growth factor are subjected to electrospinning, they activate skin stem cells and enhance the speed of wound healing. The integration of fibronectin-loaded gold nanoparticles into the tissue scaffold promotes the migration of mesenchymal stem cells through the VEGF signaling pathway. The use of PEG-coated dextran-based nanoparticles facilitates the activation of the Wnt and TGF signaling cascades in cardiac cell reprogramming and remodeling systems. Numerous nanosystems specifically focus on the EGFR pathway to promote the growth, specialization, and formation of new blood vessels in the context of regenerating cardiac tissue. Nevertheless, nanoparticles can function as extracellular signals, initiating many pathways and influencing cellular division. For example, aligned fiber structures containing multi-walled carbon nanotubes are used as extracellular signals to induce cell proliferation, differentiation, and collagen production, thereby promoting cytoskeletal activity in human umbilical cord cells [30, 31].

7.3.3 Bioactive Molecule Delivery

Tissue regeneration necessitates numerous compounds that stimulate cell growth, division, and proliferation to replace and repair damaged tissues or organs effectively. These compounds are commonly known as 'bioactive molecules.' Regenerative medicine uses growth factors, cytokines, hormones, chemokines, inhibitors, and nutrients as bioactive compounds in tissue scaffolds to control and enhance various regenerative and repair processes, including cellular survival, growth, adhesion, migration, proliferation, and differentiation. Ensuring precise and safe transportation of these substances is a significant issue in tissue regeneration technologies. Hence, it is imperative to have a specific carrier system that is biocompatible and shows minimal toxicity in vivo. To address the aforementioned issues, nanoparticles serve as appealing carriers to encapsulate and transport bioactive substances to specific locations. These advantages arise from their small size and unique properties, including biocompatibility, biodegradability, extended circulation time, reduced immunogenicity, and surface modification capabilities. Currently, the majority of drug delivery systems in biomedicine are moving toward the use of nanobased carriers to transport and deliver payloads [32].

7.3.3.1 Growth Factors and Cytokines

In order to achieve optimal results, the distribution of bioactive substances like growth factors and cytokines requires a nanoscale approach rather than a macroscopic one. Nanomaterial-based delivery helps to overcome the instability and short circulation lifetimes of bioactive substances in the system. Nanoscale compounds possess a large surface area and can have adjustable surface characteristics, in addition to their favorable size. Therefore, when nanoparticles or nanocomposites are incorporated into the tissue scaffold, they offer improved biocompatibility and reduced toxicity. Additionally, they can regulate the release of several bioactive molecules, including growth factors and cytokines, by delivering them specifically to their intended targets [5, 33]. Nanoparticles composed of gold, silver, ceramic, and carbon show favorable mechanical durability and enable surface customization, rendering them efficient vehicles for growth factors and cytokines. In addition, when these nanoparticles are combined with antibodies or polymers, they can carry a larger amount of cargo, remain in circulation for a longer time, and exhibit higher binding affinity to cell surface receptors. In the field of cancer medicine, nanocarriers are essential for the targeted delivery of bioactive substances to inhibit tumor growth. As an example, Epidermal growth factor receptor (EGFR) can be linked to gold nanoparticles (AuNPs) with the use of an antibody. This allows the nanocarrier to specifically target tumor cells and reduce the likelihood of tumor recurrence. Research indicates that the use of nanocarriers enhances the uptake of growth factors by MSCs. Polymer-based nanocarriers are widely used in regenerative procedures. This is due to their improved EPR effect, structural efficiency, and resistance to absorption by the reticuloendothelial system (RES). Synthetic and natural polymers are used to encapsulate cytokines and growth factors, enabling their controlled and targeted release within the body. Moreover, the customizable characteristics of polymeric nanoparticles offer flexible approaches for creating NPs by using chemical and physical methods to enhance controlled release. Plasma protein-based nanoparticles have recently become popular because they have high bioavailability, low toxicity, enhanced biodegradability, and longer half-lives in living organisms.

Similarly, by enclosing cytokines and growth factors such as VEGF, TGF, EFGR, BMP, etc. within nanomaterials, it becomes possible to produce the controlled and effective release of these molecules. This is not achievable with the conventional scaffolds that are typically used. Currently, nanomaterial-based delivery systems guide the differentiation of stem cells in bone regeneration, neurological diseases, wound healing, skin defects, cardiac tissue regeneration, and various other medical conditions. At present, scientists are researching the development of hybrid constructs using several types of polymeric nanoparticles to enhance the effectiveness of controlled release of bioactive agents in tissue regeneration [4, 34].

7.3.3.2 Gene Delivery Systems

Gene delivery is essential in regenerative medicine since it facilitates the use of cells to generate specific proteins, suppress excessive protein production, genetically modify and restore cell activities, and stimulate cell proliferation and differentiation. Currently, nanomaterials are being used to transport a therapeutic gene for a growth factor or cytokine into a specific tissue. This technique is used in the process of regenerating bone, cardiomyocytes, skin, nerve, tooth, and hair cells. Nanomaterials, specifically natural polymers and lipid-based nanosystems, are used to enclose siRNA, DNA, transcription factors, and other genes that encode various functions. These compounds have excellent biocompatibility, increased tissue permeability, and minimal toxicity. Studies indicate that these vectors at the nanoscale produce reduced amounts of inflammatory indicators, resulting in less absorption by macrophages and a longer duration of circulation within a living organism. In addition, PEGylated nanoparticles increased bone mineral density and promoted the development of new bone tissues in vivo for osteoporosis. But the processes of cellular uptake, accumulation in bodily fluids, escape from endosomes, and rapid breakdown through natural processes limit the practical use of nanomaterial-based gene therapy. Researchers are currently conducting ongoing research to develop improved nanodelivery techniques that can address the aforementioned limitations and enhance the potential use of nanomaterials in gene therapy and regenerative medicine [35].

7.4 Applications of Nanomaterials in Regenerative Medicine

7.4.1 Bone Tissue Regeneration

The scaffold is a crucial element in tissue engineering methods. It offers transient mechanical reinforcement at the region of the defect or injury and creates an optimal environment for cell growth. The importance of scaffolds in bone tissue engineering cannot be overstated. Bone is a very resilient load-carrying tissue in the human body, characterized by a significantly high Young's modulus of 17.5–18.9 GPa and requires scaffolds to support its regeneration. Therefore, the process of designing and selecting suitable materials to enhance tissue growth is challenging. An optimal scaffold should include the following key features: it must be three-dimensional, porous, capable of promoting biological conduction, compatible with living tissues, and capable of being naturally absorbed by the body. In addition, the material must show mechanical properties that are similar to those found in natural bone tissue, while featuring a surface that facilitates cell adhesion, proliferation, and differentiation. The material's characteristics, including its three-dimensionality and porosity, are critical for accurately reproducing the natural cell arrangement, promoting cell interaction and transport, and preventing tissue necrosis. In addition, it is worth noting that bioresorbable scaffolds have the potential to mimic the mechanical properties of natural tissue. These scaffolds can act as replacements for native extracellular matrix (ECM) molecules and may eventually be replaced by them. The use of bioresorbable and biocompatible scaffolds restricts the range of materials available for selection. Although polymers are useful, they may not possess the mechanical characteristics necessary for creating ideal bone tissue scaffolds. The advancements in nanomaterials have greatly contributed to the accomplishment of that goal. Incorporating nanoparticles as fillers into the matrix polymers can enhance the mechanical properties of the scaffolds [36]. As a result, researchers are investigating different nanomaterials to determine their impact on cells when used as fillers in scaffolds. A comprehensive investigation has been carried out on ceramic nanomaterials like hydroxyapatite (HAp) and bioactive glass; carbon-based materials such as carbon nanotubes (CNTs) and graphene; and metallic nanoparticles like gold and titanium oxide (TiO_2). These materials show promise as filling options in scaffolds.

Scaffolds benefit from nanoscale materials by improving their mechanical properties and influencing cell signaling pathways. Zhu et al. discovered that including magnetic nanoparticles in a scaffold led to a greater quantity and diversity of cytokines in the protein corona in comparison to a scaffold devoid of nanoparticles. The provided evidence suggests that these proteins augment the MAPK/ERK signaling pathway, leading to greater cellular proliferation. Liu et al. conducted a study to investigate the impact of hydroxyapatite nanoparticles (HApNPs) on electrospun chitosan matrix scaffolds. The study revealed that the nanoparticles stimulated the proliferation of bone marrow-derived mesenchymal stem cells (BM-MSCs) by activating the BMP/SMAD signaling cascade. HAp nanoparticles, known as hydroxyapatite nanoparticles, are the main inorganic component of bone tissue. As a result, they have significant appeal as a biomaterial for scaffold construction due to their ability to accurately mimic the natural inorganic phase of bone in comparison to organic polymeric nanoparticles. Considerable research has focused on incorporating HAp nanoparticle fillers into matrix materials to improve bone growth in composite scaffolds. Polymers including chitosan, gelatin, polycaprolactone (PCL), polylactic-co-glycolic acid (PLGA), and polyethylene glycol (PEG) are commonly used as matrix materials in conjunction with HAp nanoparticles. Maji et al. applied gelatin-carboxymethyl chitosan-integrated HAp nanoparticle scaffolds and grew spheroids of mesenchymal stem cells (MSCs) on them [37].

Foaming was achieved through the use of high-speed stirring, followed by freeze-drying to produce scaffolds with large pore diameters. The mechanical qualities demonstrated a significant improvement compared to the conventional freeze-drying method. Compared to the control culture conditions, researchers observed improved vitality, increased tissue penetration into the scaffolds, and elevated alkaline phosphatase (ALP) and osteocalcin (OCN) activities. These characteristics function as early and late indications for osteogenic activities, respectively. Achieving the objective of mimicking the inorganic component of bone, researchers have successfully developed scaffolds using hydroxyapatite nanoparticles (HApNPs) and nano-whitlockite particles (WHNP). Cheng et al. used a GelMA solution, HApNP, and WHNP that were dispersed using ultrasound. MSCs were cultured on scaffolds made of HApNP-WHNP-GelMA. The solution was exposed to UV light for 30 s to initiate crosslinking. The UV light intensity was precisely regulated to prevent any damage to the cells. Adding WHNP to HApNP caused a notable decrease in Young's modulus of the created scaffolds. The reduction, which varied based on the particle concentration, was approximately 20%. The results indicate that HApNP is more effective in giving mechanical support to the scaffold. The study found that the GelMA-100% WHNP scaffolds showed a significant increase in osteogenic activity relative to the GelMA-100% HApNP scaffolds. The most favorable outcomes were obtained by using a HApNP to WHNP ratio of 3:1, mirroring the ratio found in natural bone. It can be inferred that the combined impact of HApNP and WHNP is mutually beneficial. The GelMA-75% HApNP-25% WHNP exhibited higher ALP and OCN activities in both DMEM (Dulbecco's Modified Eagle's medium) and osteoinductive media, surpassing the levels observed in GelMA-100% HApNP and GelMA-100% WHNP. There has been a significant study undertaken on the integration of natural biopolymers with nanoparticles of bioactive glass-ceramic (nBGC). These nanomaterials have significant value due to their resemblance to the natural mineral composition of bone, in contrast to metallic nanoparticles. An example of combining materials is the use of silk fibroin and bioactive glass/polyvinyl alcohol (PVA) through electrospinning to produce a bilayer scaffold. Studies have discovered that the use of bioactive glass in this scaffold enhances the proliferation and differentiation of MSCs in comparison to scaffolds lacking bioactive glass [38].

The following diagram will help get a better insight into the potential of GelMA-based nanomaterials in bone regeneration (Fig. 7.2).

Carbon nanotubes (CNTs) have extraordinary mechanical qualities, defined by their high aspect ratios and high electrical and thermal conductivity. As a result, they have become highly sought-after for enhancing the properties of composite scaffolds. Jing et al. conducted a study where they integrated multiwall carbon nanotubes (MWCNT) with hydroxyapatite nanoparticles in a collagen matrix. The freeze-dried scaffolds showed enhanced mechanical characteristics, particularly a greater Young's modulus. In addition, researchers observed increased spreading and growth of rat BM-MSCs when the scaffolds were infused with 0.5% MWCNT. The

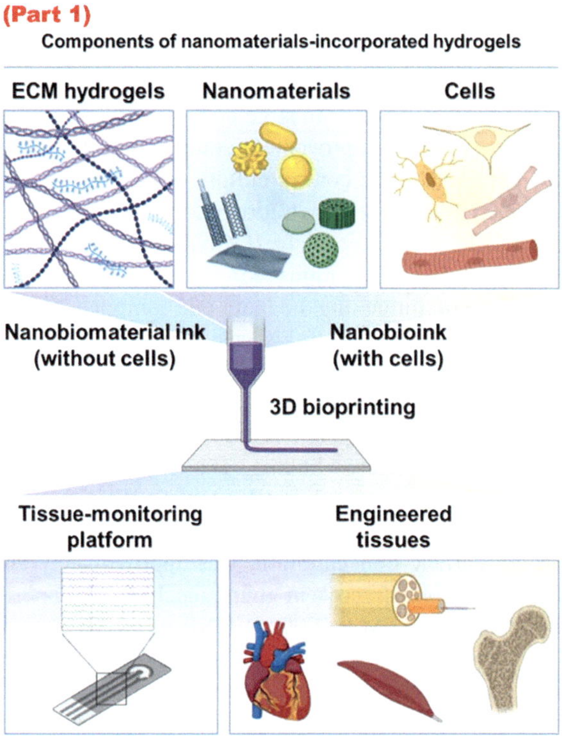

Fig. 7.2 (Part 1) The application of nanobioink and nanobiomaterial ink varies based on the cell component. (Reprinted from [39] Copyright, Springer Nature, 2023. This Open Access Article is licensed under a Creative Commons Attribution 4.0 International License). (Part 2) 3D bioprinted in vitro tissue structures made with nanobioinks based on GelMA. The development process of a customized GelMA bioink based on HAp nanoparticles for effective osseointegration and bone regeneration is shown in figure (**a**), which shows a schematic representation of HAp nanoparticle's surface modification and coupling with GelMA, and figure (**b**), which shows bone regeneration using a nanostructured 3D printed hydrogel scaffold. (**c**–**e**): Creation of a 3D vascularized bone--mimicking structure: c is a schematic representation of intricate natural bone architecture; (**d**) is for bioprinting, which creates bone tissue with perfusable vascular structure; and (**e**) is for 3D printing, which creates pyramidal structures out of cylindrical rods loaded with cells. (**f**, **g**) Heart tissue constructs with gold nanorod (GNR)-incorporated GelMA were created using the following bioprinting techniques: (**f**) lattice construct, created by stacking coaxially printed GNR-GelMA nanocomposite bioink layer by layer; (**g**) (i) embedded bioprinting, which created spiral constructs by printing spiral constructs (ii) in the support batch and (iii) in a culture medium. (Reprinted from [39], Copyright, Springer Nature, 2023, This Open Access Article is licensed under a Creative Commons Attribution 4.0 International License)

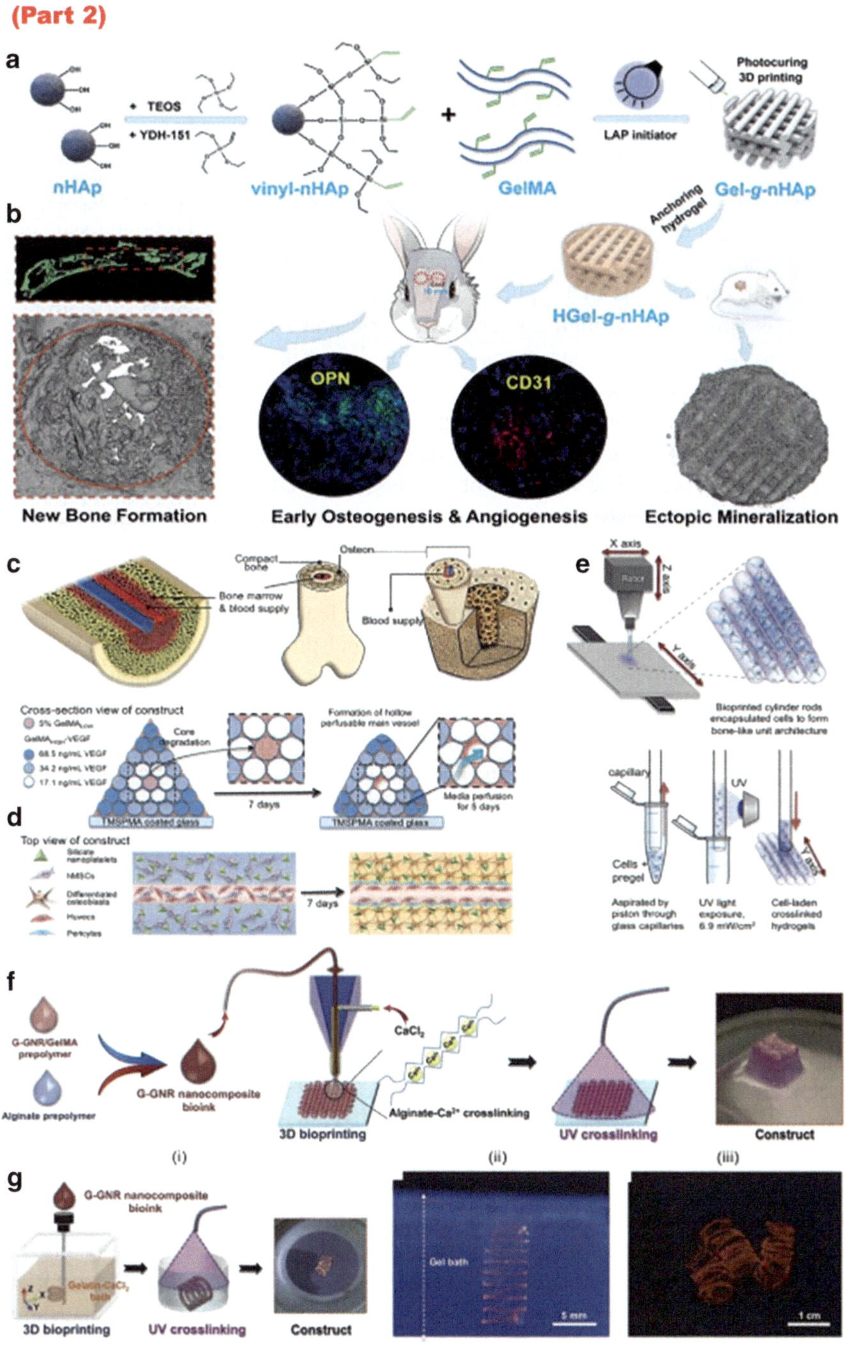

Fig. 7.2 (continued)

RT-PCR (reverse transcription polymerase chain reaction) findings revealed a noticeable increase in bone sialoprotein and OCN expression in all scaffolds containing MWCNT within the 0.25% to 2% range, with the most favorable result reported at 0.5%. Mesenchymal stem cells (MSCs) have been extensively used; however, induced pluripotent stem cells (iPSCs) have been used in conjunction with nanostructured scaffolds in bone tissue engineering. To minimize the likelihood of teratoma development, it is essential to commence the process of inducing iPSCs to grow into specialized cells before their use in cell therapy or the bone tissue engineering process. Wang et al. used a scaffold made out of the M12 phage, a benign virus with dimensions of roughly 880 nm in length and 6.6 nm in diameter. The phage is generated through bacterial infection and subsequently undergoes self-assembly to form various structural scaffolds. When investigating the effect of peptide recognition sequences compared to nanotopography, it was determined that the peptide sequence of the protein coating had a minimal effect on self-assembly. The achievement was made by genetically incorporating peptide recognition sequences into the coat protein. The side wall of the phage showed four peptides, consisting of two fibronectin adhesive domains, as well as a domain derived from osteogenic growth peptide and bone BMP-2. The recognition sequences did not have any impact on the adhesion qualities and structure of iPSCs. Instead, the organization of the fibers had a crucial role in determining these features. After converting induced pluripotent stem cells (iPSCs) into mesenchymal progenitor cells, the subsequent transformation into osteoblasts led to varying levels of alkaline phosphatase (ALP) activity, osteocalcin (OCN), and osteopontin (OPN) expression. The growth factor sequences resulted in higher levels of ALP activity, OCN expression, and OPN expression compared to fibronectin. The effects found on oriented fibers were markedly more pronounced than those observed on random fiber controls, indicating a substantial correlation between nanotopography and molecular identification in the progression of iPSC toward the osteogenic lineage [41].

Compared to small molecules, nanoparticles (NPs) possess the capacity to effectively traverse the cell membrane barrier by either specialized, receptor-mediated mechanisms or nonspecific processes. The choice between these mechanisms depends on the surface chemistry, shape, and size of the NP. Particle internalization, also known as endocytosis, involves mechanisms such as phagocytosis (cell eating) and pinocytosis (cell drinking). Phagocytosis primarily involves the engulfment of microparticles, whereas pinocytosis is the process by which nanoparticles are taken up. Following internalization, intracellular trafficking occurs; typically, particles are transported initially to endosomes and then to lysosomes, where the protein corona around the particle will be degraded. Afterward, the nanoparticles will have access to the cytoplasm. Nanoparticles can accumulate in different cellular organelles, based on their shape and surface properties. Nanoparticles have effectively aided the transfer of growth factors such as TGF-β, bFGF, BMP, IGF, VEGF, TNF, and PDGF [42]. BMPs are growth factors that are classified as part of the TGF-β superfamily. Bone morphogenetic proteins (BMPs) demonstrate notable abilities to promote the production of bone by stimulating the differentiation of mesenchymal stem cells (MSCs) into osteoblasts. For instance, research has demonstrated that BMP-2 is a powerful agent in promoting the growth of bones, and it is essential for initiating the process of bone production. The FDA has approved the utilization of BMP-2 and BMP-7 in spinal fusion surgeries for the treatment of long-bone fractures [43]. VEGF is crucial in the process of bone repair and in aiding the regeneration of damaged bone tissues. The significant influence of VEGF on osteoclastogenesis directly impacts the bone reconstructing process in the last stage of bone healing. Several research studies aim to ameliorate the defective vascularization and regeneration process in shattered bones by successfully delivering VEGF with optimal concentrations, despite its short half-life. Lu et al. performed an experiment in which they linked VEGF to PLGA nanofibers using biomimetic conjugation with heparin. As a consequence, VEGF was continuously released over 31 days [44]. In another investigation, the regulated release pattern of the vascular endothelial growth factor (VEGF) was achieved by developing a three-dimensional scaffold. This scaffold enables the controlled release of VEGF nanoparticles, which is reliant upon the contact between cells and the implant. The VEGF molecule was enclosed within chitosan NPs by using an inotropic gelling technique in this research. The nanoreservoirs containing VEGF NPs were formed using chitosan and then integrated into a 3D tissue construct composed of PCL through layer-by-layer electrospinning. Subsequently, the scaffold was seeded with osteoblasts and then with endothelial cells. Osteoblastic cells are used to promote the attachment of endothelial cells to the scaffold and the release of VEGF from the nanoreservoirs. As a result, the production of VEGF stimulates the development of new blood vessels by endothelial cells. Micro RNAs (miRNAs) are a set of short noncoding RNAs (20–24 nucleotides) that have a notable function in controlling gene expression following transcription. miRNAs commonly inhibit the expression of their specific target genes by either preventing the translation of mRNA or promoting the degradation of mRNA. This is achieved by binding to the 3-UTR of the mRNA. Approximately 3% of human genes are believed to encode for miRNAs, and miRNAs are predicted to influence the production of around 40–90% of proteins [45].

The following figure illustrates an example of the use of a nanoscale-based biomimetic scaffold in bone tissue regeneration (Fig. 7.3).

7.4.2 Cartilage Tissue Engineering

The primary techniques used for managing impaired cartilage tissue focus on symptom relief by mitigating discomfort and restoring functionality, without directly addressing the underlying tissue structures responsible for the issue. Regenerative therapies, on the other hand, aim to generate new cartilage tissue that is indistinguishable from the original one. Tissue engineering is a highly promising technique in the field of regenerative medicine where the collaboration of several scientific disciplines, including engineering, biology, material science, and chemistry, is necessary. Tissue engineering is currently founded upon three fundamental elements: cells, scaffolds, and signals, which collectively constitute the tissue engineering

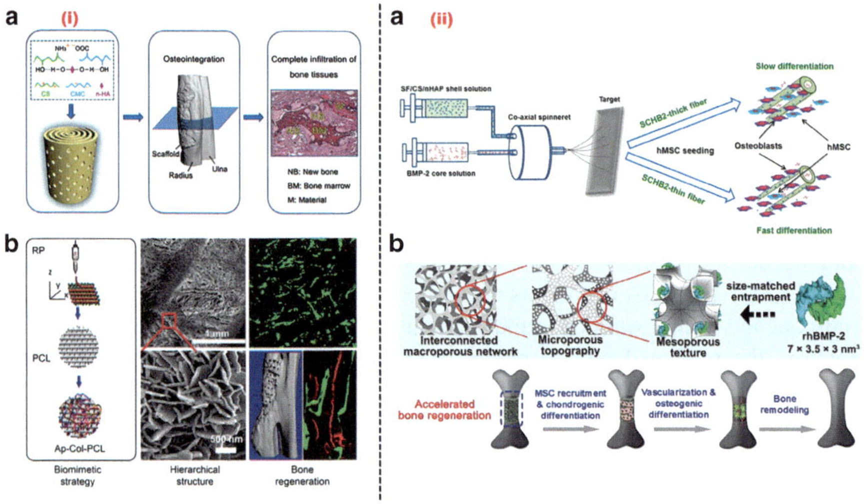

Fig. 7.3 (i) (**a**) Hybrid chitosan/cellulose/nano-hydroxyapatite membrane-based biomimetic spiral-cylindrical scaffold. (**b**) Using biomimetically embellished fast prototyping, an apatite--collagen-polycaprolactone composite material with a nano-micro-macro hierarchical structure was created. (Reprinted from [46], Copyright, Springer Nature, 2016, This Open Access Article is licensed under a Creative Commons Attribution 4.0 International License). (ii) (**a**) Using coaxial electrospinning to prepare Scheme B2-thick and Scheme B2-thin NFMs and their impact on hMSCs. (**b**) RhBMP-2-loaded tri-modal macro/micro/nanoporous scaffold for faster bone regeneration. (Reprinted from [46], Copyright, Springer Nature, 2016, This Open Access Article is licensed under a Creative Commons Attribution 4.0 International License)

trinity. Tissues have an intricate hierarchical organization spanning from the nanoscale to the macro scales. This has an impact on the biology of tissues, the process of shifting between layers, and controlling the interconnections between tissues. The macro level governs factors such as biocompatibility, biodegradability, and mechanical characteristics. On the other hand, the microscale regulates tissue structure, surface chemistry, surface rigidity, cell motility, nutrient delivery, and vascularization. The regulation of bioactive molecules, cell adhesion, gene expression, and mineralization is controlled on the nanoscale. Attaining a complex shape is critical for tissue engineering because natural tissues achieve balance through interactions at the nano- and micro-scales. Hence, nanomaterials, due to their remarkable physicochemical structures and biomimetic capabilities, have gained significant attention for enhancing cell growth and function, as well as for promoting and guiding tissue regeneration. In traditional tissue engineering, cells are initially grown in tissue scaffolds using static methods. Subsequently, they are transported to a bioreactor where they are cultured under conditions that mimic the tissue's physiological stresses. This developing tissue is expected to undergo restructuring after being implanted into the body. The current technique, however, aims to bypass the steps of cell seeding and differentiation that are involved in these procedures. By inserting just the scaffold and inducing microfractures to attract mesenchymal stem cells from tissues of the bone marrow, it is anticipated that this approach will effectively promote the development of mesenchymal stem cells. Nanomaterials provide novel opportunities for the manufacturing, delivery, discharge, and controlled activation of bioactive compounds. These offer a plethora of methodologies for cartilage regeneration, enabling researchers to experiment with novel combinations [47].

Novel techniques in nanomaterial science, such as electrospinning and 3D fiber deposition, have been devised to enhance the precision and excellence of nanoscale scaffolds. In the same manner, nanoparticles can be integrated into biomaterials. By including nanoscale characteristics, it is possible to develop scaffolds that mimic the extracellular matrix present in natural cartilage, as shown in Fig. 7.4. This is thought to strengthen the communication between cells and the scaffold, hence improving the performance of the engineered tissue construct. Nanoscale characteristics are widely regarded to have a significant influence on cell activity, resulting in alterations to the cytoskeleton, cell shape, focal adhesions, motility, and gene expression. Research has indicated that there might be a cell transduction process that is influenced by the topography of the environment, rather than biochemical signals. This phenomenon is connected to the arrangement and distance between sticky ligands. This form of cellular transduction has been discovered to have a resemblance to mechanotransduction.

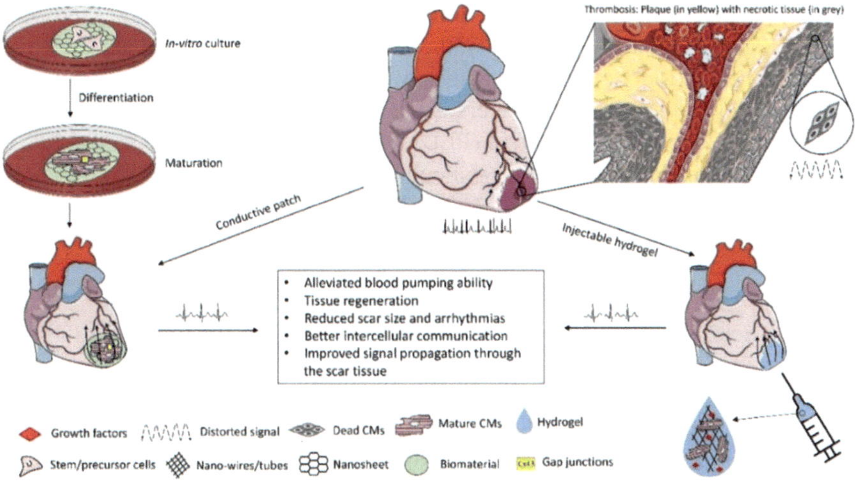

Fig. 7.4 Cardiac tissue engineering using conductive scaffolding. Collagen-rich scar tissue from the infarction severely reduces the myocardium's electrical conductivity. When implanted in vivo, conductive constructions containing cells and nanomaterials can reduce cardiac dysfunction and restore electrical activity. (Reprinted from [48], Copyright, MDPI, 2021, This Open Access Article is licensed under a Creative Commons Attribution 4.0 International License)

7.4.2.1 Biomaterials

Biomaterials primarily comprise ceramics, polymers, and metals, which can be obtained either naturally or through artificial production. Biomaterials intended for cartilage tissue engineering must possess biocompatibility, enabling cell retention, facilitating the transport of bioactive molecules, and supporting cell survival, proliferation, and secretory functions. Given that osteochondral tissues experience regular loads, it is necessary to utilize scaffolds constructed from materials that are capable of withstanding mechanical stress. Rigid polymers have been employed for imparting three-dimensional support to structures, but scaffolds made of hydrogel are better suited for facilitating cell transportation. Ongoing research is focused on creating composite biomaterials that replicate the complex structure of cartilage tissue, including the unique osteochondral interaction with bone tissue [49].

Cartilage scaffolds constructed from natural polymers are both biocompatible and safe. These scaffolds frequently have bioadhesive surfaces that facilitate the adhesion of cells. Nevertheless, they possess lower mechanical strength as a result of their quick deterioration characteristics. Several natural polymers that are currently under extensive study include polysaccharide structures such as chitosan, hyaluronan, alginate, agarose, chondroitin, and methylcellulose, as well as protein structures including collagen, gelatin, fibrin, silk, and keratin. Collagen and hyaluronan undergo higher facile adaptation and degradation due to their inherent presence in natural cartilage tissue. Synthetic polymers possess enhanced mechanical integrity, facilitate convenient processing, and may undergo sterilization. Unfortunately, they show reduced biological activity, have limited degradation capabilities, and may induce a more intense inflammatory reaction. Several synthetic polymers, such as polyethylene glycol (PEG), polylactide (PLA), poly(l-lactide) acid (PLLA), polylactic-co-glycolic acid (PLGA), polycaprolactone (PCL), polyvinyl alcohol (PVA), polyurethanes (PUR), polyglycolic acid (PGA), and PGA/PLA copolymers, have been used as scaffolds for cartilage [49, 50].

7.4.2.2 Scaffolds Based on Nanomaterials

Nanomaterials are becoming increasingly important in tissue engineering as they can control the structural, mechanical, and chemical aspects of conventional techniques at the nanoscale. This is accomplished by using nanofabrication technology. These materials can show a high degree of compliance and efficacy at the cellular level by facilitating molecular interactions with the cell. In addition, they possess distinct mechanical, optical, electrical, and magnetic properties that allow for improved control over cell processes. Nanomaterials can imitate the surface characteristics of the extracellular matrix, including energy and topography. Researchers are exploring the potential use of nanomaterials as tissue scaffolds, biomolecular transporters, and biosensor nanovehicles due to their versatile characteristics [51].

Cartilage tissue scaffolds are constructed using hydrogels, fibrous mesh structures, or foam depending on the methods used during their manufacture. Hydrogels are polymers or protein structures that swell in water and are cross-linked through physical, chemical, or hybrid means. Chemically interconnected hydrogels are bound by covalent bonds, while physically cross-linked ones are bonded by non-covalent weak molecular interactions such as hydrogen bonding, hydrophobic interactions, and electrostatic interactions. Currently, hydrogels are the most frequently used structures for cartilage scaffolding and are undergoing substantial research. The reason for their popularity lies in their ease of application and their ability to be administered via injection or minimally invasive procedures like arthroscopy. Hydrogels can efficiently occupy damaged areas in the joint and rapidly conform to the adjacent healthy tissue. Because of their abundant water content, they aid in the distribution of nutrients and waste. Cells within these gel structures can become fully surrounded by the gel rather than just sticking to it, and they can evolve in a way that resembles the characteristics of cartilage cells. PEG, agarose, alginate, hyaluronan, collagen, and chitosan are often used polymers that offer excellent biocompatibility and the possibility of biodegradability. Hydrogels have low mechanical strength, particularly when it comes to the cartilage surfaces of load-bearing joints. Therefore, ongoing research is focused on enhancing the mechanical strength of hydrogels [52]. Scaling down the gel to nano sizes is a crucial approach to enhance the reactivity of hydrogel dynamics towards stimuli. The incorporation of nanoparticles into the structure enhances both the mechanical properties and functional performance due to the significant increase in surface-to-volume ratios. Nevertheless, the range of nanostructuring techniques suitable for this objective is restricted because of the substantial water content present in hydrogels. The process of arranging hydrophobic sections of polymers together can still occur in water-based settings. Nanoparticle hydrogels, nanofiber hydrogels, and hybrid hydrogels are materials that are now under considerable development for this specific purpose. Researchers thoroughly evaluate molecular self-assembly and electrospinning strategies for the manufacture of nanofiber hydrogels. Self-assembled supramolecular materials with biomolecular structures that imitate the extracellular matrix can facilitate cell migration, growth, adhesion, and proliferation through their bioactive interactions. Peptide nanofiber gels are being recognized as a promising option for treating cartilage tissue in the field of self-assembling materials. Yaylacı et al. demonstrated that peptide nanofibers that mimic glycosaminoglycans can promote the development of cartilage cells in mesenchymal stem cells. Self-assembled peptide nanofiber gels that mimic hyaluronic acid may improve the process of cartilage regeneration. Scaffolds generated using electrospinning are derived from polymer-based solutions using high-voltage collectors, resulting in the formation of a non-woven fabric composed of fibers. These simple yet strong structures make it easier to explore new combinations of materials, as they can allow for the simultaneous rotation of different synthetic or natural substances. Electrospinning can be used to create scaffolds with customizable surface properties, including surface alterations, chemical modifications, and the addition of biologically active molecules. Growth factors and biologically active proteins can be used to produce composite materials. Electrospinning is an extensively researched subject for the creation of 3D scaffolds, with a specific focus on joint cartilage. A comprehensive investigation is currently underway on nano-level programmable composite tissue scaffolds in the field of cartilage tissue engineering. These composite materials provide new possibilities and promise, not only for cartilage but also for establishing a hierarchical connection between cartilage and bone. Nanomaterials are used in tissue engineering to manufacture and distribute tissue-stimulating compounds, such as growth factors and cytokines. Chahine et al. evaluated the suitability of single-wall carbon nanotubes (SWNTs) for articular cartilage tissue engineering by employing 2D and 3D composite tissue scaffolds. The study showed that the presence of SWNTs increased the amount of glycosaminoglycan (GAG) in nanocomposite scaffolds. The incorporation of SWNTs resulted in improved resistance to pressure and increased tensile modulus. The study showed that single-walled carbon nanotubes (SWNTs) possess the potential to improve the functionality of bioactive compounds and boost biomechanical properties [53].

7.4.3 *Neural Regeneration*

7.4.3.1 CNS Regenerative Applications

A potential method for repairing spinal cord injuries involves using collagen microchannel scaffolds to deliver paclitaxel-encapsulated liposomes. Neural stem cells (NSCs) showed a higher level of development into neurons after being treated with liposomes that included a chemotherapeutic drug that stabilizes microtubules. The microchannel scaffolding enabled a sustained release of paclitaxel from the liposomes, resulting in enhanced differentiation of both transplanted and natural neural stem cells (NSCs) into fully mature and functional sensory as well as motor neurons. This was assessed using a rat model in which a complete transection of the thoracic region was performed. Furthermore, it was shown that the collagen scaffolds, which included liposomes encapsulating paclitaxel, improved animal locomotion recovery as assessed over 8 weeks [54].

Adding growth factors (GFs) to nanomaterials, either through physical or chemical loading, is a versatile and efficient approach used in peripheral or central brain therapies for neuroregeneration or neuroprotection. Researchers have recently assessed the possibility of dextrin-GF conjugates as platforms for delivering bioactive proteins involved in neural regeneration processes in a local and sustained manner. The conjugates have demonstrated encouraging outcomes, such as increased and extended cell division, targeted development into nerve cells, and suppressed programmed cell death in neural stem cells produced from mice. The biopolymer-protein formulations, created by combining succinylated dextrin with epidermal growth factor (EGF) and basic fibroblast growth factor (bFGF), showed a sustained release of growth factors (GFs) when exposed to amylase at concentrations similar to those found in cerebrospinal fluid. In the study conducted on mouse NSC cultures, it was observed that dextrin-GF conjugates had a stimulating impact on the expression of nestin protein, which is linked to brain progenitor cells. In addition, these conjugates controlled the expression of brain differentiation indicators, which are related to neurons, oligodendrocytes, and astrocytes [55].

Immune-modifying nanoparticles (IMPs) have been a focal point in the field of immune nanoparticle-based pharmacology that promotes tolerance. These artificial nanoparticles possess a distinct capability to regulate the immune response by attaching to receptors on inflammatory monocytes. They possess a strong negative charge and are renowned for their exceptional efficacy in this domain. Administering commercial IMPs intravenously to mice with spinal cord injury, using carboxylated PLGA with a dimension of 500 nm, led to an immediate decrease in the local inflammatory response and eventually resulted in sustained decreases in fibrotic scarring and deposition of chondroitin sulfate proteoglycans, which were detected for 10 months. The utilization of PLGA in the treatment successfully conserved glial damage and demyelination levels. It resulted in enhanced densities of axons in both the regional and caudal areas, as observed for 6 months. This treatment demonstrated significant improvement in motor function [56].

Complex nanosystems were synthesized using a multi-step procedure that involved chitosan and branching polyethyleneimine (Chitosan-g-PEI). The nanosystems were modified by attaching polyethylene glycol (PEG) and forming covalent bonds with cyclic arginine-glycine-aspartate (cRGD) and twin-arginine translocation (TAT) peptides. The polyplexes obtained in this study were positively charged with a particle size below 150 nm. These polyplexes demonstrated outstanding biocompatibility and a high capacity for condensing DNA, as evidenced by the successful monitoring of a fluorescent plasmid reporter gene in NIH 3T3 and 293T normal cells, as well as HeLa tumoral cells. In addition, the transfection capacity was evaluated in all cultured cells. The 293T cells that were exposed to polymeric carriers containing the NT-3 gene exhibited differentiation into neurons and astrocytes, as well as stimulation of neurite growth in neural stem cells originating from mice. This study assessed the capacity of intricate polymeric carriers that contain the gene encoding the NT-3 protein. NT-3 is a neurotrophic factor that facilitates the survival, differentiation, and synaptogenesis of neurons. The study aimed to assess the effectiveness of these carriers as a stem cell-based approach for neural therapeutic systems. A strategy that has gained popularity in the development of neuroactive platforms is to enhance the reactivity of biomaterials towards particular receptors that play a role in chemokine-mediated regeneration mechanisms. This approach aims to promote cellular recruitment, improve cell survival, and increase cell retention. For example, biomaterials derived from hyaluronic acid (HA) have demonstrated significant effects on the upregulation of chemokine receptors in different stem cell types [57].

The figure below illustrates the role of biomaterials in enhancing the biocompatibility of the scaffold in nerve injuries (Fig. 7.5).

The porous composite hydrogels made from hyaluronic acid and laminin (HA-Lm) showed rigidity levels resembling that of natural neural tissue. These hydrogels possessed a microstructure that facilitated cellular migration, leading to improved

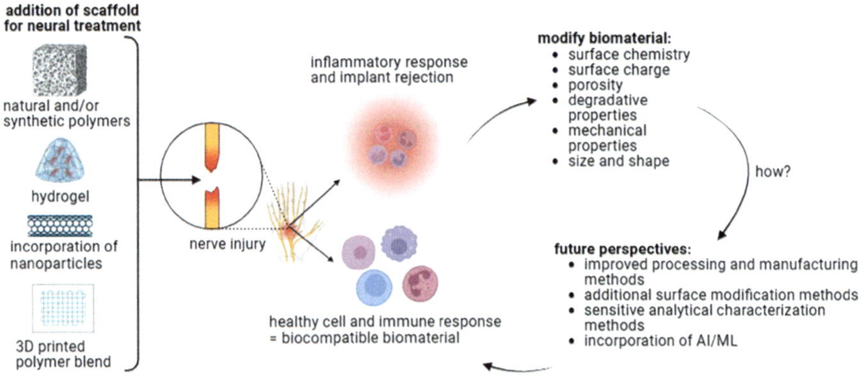

Fig. 7.5 The role of biomaterials in improving the biocompatibility of scaffolds for neural treatment and future developments. Biomaterial–cell interactions influence biocompatibility. The physical and chemical properties of biomaterials can be modified through the selection of polymers, production techniques, and further alterations. These characteristics affect the behavior of cells to establish both systemic and local immune responses. Future perspectives should be considered to provide treatment for neurological damage. (Reprinted from [58], Copyright, MDPI, 2023, This Open Access Article is licensed under a Creative Commons Attribution 4.0 International License)

survival and proliferation of neural progenitor stem cells (NPSCs). The composite hydrogels caused an increase in the expression of the CXCR4 receptor, which serves as the main receptor for the SDF-1α chemokine. This, in turn, facilitated the directed transport of NPSCs by responding to the SDF-1 gradients. Further, the administration of NPSCs solution along with HA-Lm gels into the cerebral tissues of adult mice led to a notable enhancement in the preservation of cellular transplants for 3 days. It was documented that transplanted NPSCs showed a greater tendency to go toward the location where exogenous SDF-1α was injected. The findings from additional research confirmed that the enhanced preservation of transplants was solely attributable to the HA-Lm composite gel. It was discovered that the movement of transplanted NPSCs in a living organism was a consequence of SDF-1α-induced chemotaxis [59].

A recent study presented the use of porous and aligned hydrogel tubes composed of PEG as a platform for regenerative therapy in spinal cord damage, due to their ability to solidify in the intended location. PEG tubes were acquired by using PEG microspheres and conducting an ultraviolet-initiated radical polymerization process in polydimethylsiloxane molds. The tubes have an inner diameter of 250 μm and an outside diameter of 450 μm. The PEG microspheres, synthesized through emulsification, have an average diameter of 45 μm. These microspheres show a macroporosity of 66.5%, which is conducive to cellular infiltration. A composite material composed of PEG tubes embedded in a fibrin matrix, comprising 5 tubes, was surgically implanted into mice that had been experimentally produced with thoracic spinal cord injury. The composite hydrogel led to a reduction in the inflammatory response duration and a decrease in the production of glial scars. In addition, the tubular structure has shown benefits in aiding the penetration of native cells, offering assistance and direction for the elongation of axons, and promoting improved re-myelination by oligodendrocytes, resulting in improved restoration of locomotor performance [60].

The researchers used electrospinning techniques to produce composites consisting of silk fibroin (SF) and naturally generated melanin. This process yielded nanofibrous meshes with either random or aligned orientations. These meshes provide exceptional hydrophilic characteristics and improved heat stability. Both SF materials containing melanin showed antioxidant activity, with superior outcomes reported when the nanofibers were randomly dispersed. All the composites demonstrated a higher proliferative capacity for neuron-like cells. Only the aligned distribution showed greater advantages in terms of cellular attachment and spreading. In addition, it was found that meshes stimulated the process of neural development in neuroblastoma cells taken from humans. The findings support the efficacy of melanin-containing SF nanofibrous scaffolds in regenerating and repairing CNS nerves [61].

In a recent development, the research group was able to successfully create a neural network using canine-derived bone marrow progenitor cells and sciatic nerve glial cells. This was achieved through the application of genetic engineering and GS co-culture standards, as mentioned earlier. The co-culture facilitated the transformation of MSCs into neuronal phenotypes, the formation of structures similar to synapses, and the display of electrophysiological properties. These functions were demonstrated through the assessment of voltage-gated ion channels, neurotransmitter synthesis potential, and synaptic current transmission. In addition, the three-dimensional GS scaffold served as a favorable template for the development of ECM. MSC-derived neural network tissues were implanted into Beagle dogs who had undergone full transection of the thoracic spinal cord. Following a comprehensive study lasting 6.5 months, there was significant regrowth of nerve fibers. There was a demonstrated enhancement in the recuperation of motor function in the paralyzed limbs observed throughout both open-field and submerged locomotion tests. Moreover, there was a notable improvement in the coordination between the front and pelvic limbs, as well as a better restoration of electrophysiological function [62].

A potential candidate for treating spinal cord injuries is a nanostructured substance called polysialic acid (PSA) polysaccharide. The expression level of PSA is closely related to the adhesion molecules on neural cell membranes, which indicates the potential to regulate interactions between cells and the extracellular matrix. Therefore, Zhang and colleagues created hybrid scaffolds using polycaprolactone (PCL) and PSA that contained methylprednisolone (MP) glucocorticoid. The electrospun nanofibrous scaffold displayed appropriate durability, deformability, and mobility. The hybrid PCL/PSA/MP scaffolds were tested with astrocytes and neuroblastoma cells to determine their compatibility as substrates for cellular attachment and proliferation. The findings indicated that the scaffolds exhibited no cytotoxicity and were appropriate for the intended objectives. The scientists noticed a reduction in the initial inflammatory response following the implantation of PCL/PSA/MP scaffolds in rats with thoracic spinal cord injury. This was accomplished by suppressing the localized amounts of pro-inflammatory cytokines and halting apoptosis. The hybrid scaffolds were subjected to long-term experiments lasting up to 7 weeks, which showed a notable effect in minimizing the formation of glial scars. In addition, they enhanced the process of axonal myelination and facilitated enhanced neuronal viability. The data suggest that there is an improved restoration of both the physical and functional aspects after treatment with PCL/PSA/MP scaffolds. Electroactive biomaterials have a multifunctional role in the field of smart biomedical materials and systems. These materials can easily modify their microstructure and electrical conductivity, which opens up exciting opportunities for externally controlling specific bioactivities. They also have great potential for creating innovative platforms for neuroregenerative applications [63].

7.4.3.2 PNS Regenerative Applications

Stimuli-responsive biopolymers are highly regarded in the field of smart biomaterials. These biopolymers provide therapy that is customized, targeted, and individualized to the patient's needs, making them a desirable component of healthcare solutions. Modifications in physicochemical properties, microstructure, and functionality can occur under specific external conditions, including variations in pH or temperature and the presence of electromagnetic or ultrasound fields. These modifications offer exciting possibilities for developing innovative therapies that improve performance and cater to the needs of patients [64]. The efficacy of thiolated trimethyl chitosan nanoparticles modified with tetanus neurotoxin (TMCSH-HC) and containing plasmid DNA encoding BDNF gene as non-viral carriers for peripheral nerve damage therapy was assessed. BDNF is essential in both the central nervous system (CNS) and peripheral nervous system (PNS). Its primary function is to ensure the viability and optimal maturation of sensory and motor neurons. BDNF stimulates the proliferation and specialization of newly formed neurons and synapses. The TMCSH-HC/BDNF platforms were observed to enhance the restoration of locomotor function and improve the recovery of thermal and mechanical sensory functions when injected into mice with sciatic nerve-induced damage via intramuscular administration. In addition, they promoted regeneration processes by increasing the production of growth-associated neural proteins, maintaining the density of unmyelinated axons, increasing the density of myelinated axons, and protecting muscles that have been injured and denervated [65]. In their study, Li and colleagues utilized a micromolding, lyophilization technique to create chitosan conduits. The conduits had a distinctive structure embedded within the walls, consisting of stiff patterns arranged lengthwise and strongly aligned. The walls had a porous microstructure with a porosity of around $88.19 \pm 0.75\%$. The micropatterned chitosan conduits exhibited mechanical characteristics comparable to a typical rat sciatic nerve, such as tensile strength, elasticity, folding, and knotting flexibility. The authors observed that after implanting micropatterned chitosan conduits in rats with sciatic nerve injuries, they found that the regenerative potential was similar to or slightly better than the autografted group. This included the restoration of neural connections to adjacent muscles, the infiltration of cells into the affected area, and the development of nerve tissue within the conduits, leading to the recovery of sciatic nerve myelination. The conduits made from polysaccharides and featuring a luminal in-wall pattern have shown great potential for long-term regenerative therapy in peripheral nerve damage. A study reported that the micropatterned chitosan conduits degraded slowly even after 3 months of implantation, making them a promising option for prolonged treatment [66].

Jing and colleagues introduced a novel approach for peripheral nerve regeneration by suggesting the use of composite conduits. The conduits consist of electrospun PLGA fiber-based meshes that are parallel aligned and coated with Ppy. The PLGA/Ppy fibrous mesh exhibited superior dimensional stability as compared to the electrospun PLGA mesh when subjected to physiologically simulated conditions but exhibited a slight decrease in both tensile strength and elasticity. In contrast, when evaluated with primary cells resembling neurons, the Ppy-coated PLGA fibrous meshes showed no toxicity, improved cell attachment, rapid cell proliferation, and a predominantly aligned cell structure. Following the application of inductive culture conditions, the PLGA/Ppy composite showed a notable ability to induce neurite outgrowth and spreading. This suggests that parallel-aligned conductive fibers have the potential to facilitate the differentiation of mature neural cells. The 12-week assessment was conducted under physiological settings and demonstrated that the PLGA/Ppy conduit produced showed prolonged and uniform deterioration, resulting in approximately 40% weight loss, while still preserving its tubular morphology. A study conducted on rats with transfected sciatic nerves compared the results of using PLGA/Ppy fibrous conduits to autografts. After 12 weeks, similar levels of functional and electrophysiological recovery were observed, along with regenerated axons [67].

Graphene and its derivatives have significant implications in neuroregenerative applications. These materials can be acquired via different physical or chemical procedures. The exceptional properties of these materials, such as their remarkable mechanical characteristics, unique optical properties, enhanced thermal stability, higher electrical conductivity, and excellent chemical stability, are determined by their atomic structure and electron distribution. Using single layers of hydrophilic graphene oxide (GO) and hydrophobic reduced graphene oxide (rGO) as substrates has proven to be beneficial in stimulating the differentiation of adipose-derived stem cells (ADSCs) into neurons, with a neurogenic differentiation rate over 90%. More precisely, mats made from graphene oxide (GO) have been discovered to enhance the speed at which adipose-derived stem cells (ADSCs) divide and transform into cells that resemble neurons [68].

The fabrication of hybrid scaffolds using electrospinning techniques has shown promising results for peripheral nerve regeneration. The scaffolds, composed of a blend of sodium alginate (SA), polyvinyl alcohol (PVA), and graphene nanosheets, demonstrate favorable microstructural characteristics, including a consistent and interconnected porosity arrangement. They show exceptional water-repellent properties and an extended rate of decomposition. These scaffolds demonstrate improved mechanical properties, including enhanced tensile strength, toughness, and elongation and favorable electrical properties. This study, referenced as [69], highlights the potential of these hybrid scaffolds for peripheral nerve regeneration.

7.4.4 Cardiac Tissue Regeneration

7.4.4.1 Scaffolds for Cardiac Tissue Engineering

The extracellular matrix (ECM) is an intricate fibrous network composed of structural and functional proteins that provide cells with both mechanical and biochemical signals necessary for their normal functioning. An optimal scaffold should be able to replicate the natural environment of ECM for the effective regeneration of tissues and organs. It should be a three-dimensional framework that facilitates efficient mass transfer, ideally degrades at a predetermined rate, and possesses the required surface chemistry to promote cell adhesion, proliferation, and differentiation along with possessing enhanced mechanical and electrical properties. The scaffolds should be easily moldable or adjustable according to specific use in tissue repair and regeneration. These scaffolds have been made using a wide variety of materials, both homogeneous and composite. Several of these materials incorporate nanoscale characteristics and nanomaterials to enhance their material qualities, including strength, biocompatibility, and functionality, and consequently optimize the regenerative process. Scientists are presently involved in the development of biomimetic scaffolds that function as both structural support and guiding tools for tissue regeneration. These bioinspired nanomaterials mimic the functional properties of ECM while supporting tissue regeneration. There is an increasing trend toward using electrically conductive substances, such as particular synthetic materials (carbon, gold), to assist in attaining desirable contraction-relaxation cycles in cardiac muscles (CMs) [70].

Synthetic Substances

Scaffolding often incorporates synthetic materials due to their ease of manufacturing and extensively studied mechanical characteristics. It is crucial to create scaffolds with a suitable elastic modulus to effectively support the contraction of cardiac muscle (CM) in the field of cardiac tissue engineering. Nonetheless, a disadvantage of using synthetic materials, particularly thermoplastic polymers derived from polyester, is their inclination to experience plastic deformation and ultimately collapse when subjected to prolonged cyclic load [71]. In addition, synthetic polymers exhibit limited hydrophilicity, resulting in the absence of surface cell recognition sites. Therefore, the cells' attraction to these materials decreases. Recent research suggests that the introduction of nanoscale topography on the material can greatly improve cell viability, offering a potential solution to this problem. Poly (ethylene glycol) (PEG) is a substance that is widely used in scaffolds due to its FDA approval and non-immunogenic properties. Kim et al. used PEG to fabricate a substrate featuring nanopillar morphology. On this substrate, a greater level of cell membrane adherence was observed in comparison to regular PEG substrates. The cellular modules displayed a spherical shape exclusively on the nanostructured surface, suggesting that the decreased stiffness of the nanopillars facilitated selective cell-cell communication. Another study investigated the potential influence of nanotopography on the direction of cardiac myocytes using a PEG hydrogel. This study examined the in vitro structure of cardiac tissue and its correlation with cell alignment and extracellular matrix (ECM) fiber alignment. On the PEG substrate with patterned nanotopography, a consistent alignment of cardiac myocytes was achieved, in contrast to the unpredictable alignment observed on substrates without nanotopography patterns. The research demonstrated that the use of patterned substrate resulted in a noticeable enhancement in cell diameters, indicating that nanotopographic patterns exerted a substantial impact on cell size.

Polyglycolic acid (PGA) is a substance that is both biocompatible and hydrophilic, making it ideal for use in biomedical applications. The degradation rates of this substance are favorable and it is non-toxic. PCL is a material with great potential for scaffolding purposes. It has been approved by the FDA, is cost-effective, and possesses desirable soft and flexible properties. In their study, Aghdam et al. used PCL and PGA materials to create a synthetic nanofibrous scaffold that was used for cultivating cardiac progenitor cells. Following 6 days, during which growth occurred on the artificial scaffold with a weight ratio of 65:35 PCL: PGA, the researchers observed the highest cell viability. This outcome is attributed to the scaffold's improved hydrophilic characteristics [72].

PLGA is a copolymer composed of polylactic acid (PLA) and polyglycolic acid (PGA). By combining these two elements, PLGA offers benefits such as the capacity to alter its mechanical features by adjusting the molecular weight of the polymer, a desirable rate of decomposition, and the capability to be molded and scaled according to necessity. Attributable to these features, PLGA has found extensive use in several biomedical applications. Simon-Yarza et al. used PLGA to fabricate a nanofibrous structure that encloses recombinant human neuregulin-1 beta isoform (Nrg), a growth factor for the cardiovascular system. This growth factor is widely recognized for its ability to enhance the recruitment of cells, blood vessel formation, and replication of cardiac muscle cells. The scaffold was successfully implanted into a rat model suffering from myocardial infarction and seamlessly integrated into the heart tissue. Simon-Yarza and colleagues observed a rise in the M2:M1 macrophage ratio, indicating a beneficial restructuring of the infarct region caused by the PLGA scaffold [73].

Polypyrrole (PPy) is an organic polymer that is also classified as a synthetic polymer. Polymers can be categorized according to their conductivity. PPy has been extensively studied and used to stimulate the process of neural differentiation in PC-12 cells and promote endothelial cell growth and is non-toxic, but because of its fragility and the difficulties involved in handling it, an additive is often used to enhance its potency and effectiveness for cardiac tissue engineering. Kai et al. used

PPy in conjunction with PCL and gelatin to create a scaffold that is strong both mechanically and electrically. The decision to use PCL as an additive was driven by its adaptable and durable properties. The authors suggest that the nanofibrous scaffold synthesized from these materials promotes cell growth and attachment by creating electrically charged binding sites that interact with the charged cell exterior, leading to enhanced adhesion points [74].

Natural Materials

Native ECM components are characterized by nanoscale dimensions. As a result, there is potential in using nanostructured components made from gelatin, collagen, or fibrin to develop an effective scaffold. It is crucial to incorporate nanofeatures as they enhance cellular adhesion and provide multiple focal attachment points. Given the high abundance of collagen as an extracardiac protein, using scaffolds made from this material would offer a physiologically relevant environment for conducting experiments with CMs. In addition, the formation of scar tissue following an infarction is predominantly made up of collagen types I and III. Gelatin is commonly used as a natural hydrogel component for cardiac tissue engineering. GelMA, a material derived from collagen, can undergo chemical cross-linking with methacrylamide to get a melting point that is capable of withstanding the temperature of the human body. Fibrin, a protein comparable to collagen, undergoes degradation and is subsequently substituted by the extracellular matrix (ECM) in the course of wound healing. Usually, these materials are subjected to electrospinning to produce nanofibers, which are then incorporated into the scaffold. It is vital to examine the constraints linked to these materials carefully. These scaffolds show significant promise for in vitro applications, but there are concerns about their contribution to fibrosis, rapid degradation, and potential immune response when used in vivo [75].

Nanoparticles & Nanotubes

Since the discovery of carbon nanotubes (CNTs), there has been a significant amount of study undertaken to investigate their potential uses in the biomedical domains. This material is acknowledged for its superior aspect ratio, robust mechanical strength, low weight, exceptional electrical qualities, and remarkable chemical and thermal stability. The tubes show a range of lengths, spanning from hundreds of nanometers to micrometers, and possess a diameter of 0.4–2 nm. In the field of cardiac tissue engineering, researchers frequently use single-walled carbon nanotubes (SWCNTs) and multi-walled carbon nanotubes (MWCNTs) to create scaffolds with a precise elastic modulus that enhances the electrical functions of cardiomyocytes [76].

Zhou et al. conducted a study in which they used single-walled carbon nanotubes (SWNTs) and gelatin to create a composite scaffold for implantation into Sprague-Dawley (SD) rats with severe cardiac infarction. The findings demonstrated a decrease in the size of the left ventricle after systole and a restriction in the advancement of left ventricle enlargement following the implantation of the graft for 4 weeks. The results suggest that SWNTs may have the ability to increase the occurrence of intercellular adhesive junctions and electrochemical junctions, particularly N-cadherin and connexin-43 (Cx43). This outcome is attributed to the electrical properties of the single-walled carbon nanotubes (SWCNTs) [77].

It is significant to mention that MWCNTs have been discovered to stimulate the proliferation of neonatal rat ventricular myocytes more effectively than fibroblasts in a laboratory setting. Recordings were obtained of the robust action potentials of individual ventricular myocytes that showed the ability to undergo proliferation. The study suggests that carbon nanotubes (CNTs) can prolong the time during which undifferentiated cells undergo cell proliferation and accelerate the maturation of differentiated cardiac muscle cells (CMs). The findings of this study provide valuable insights into the contribution of CNTs in facilitating the regeneration of cardiac tissue [78].

Gold has been discovered to improve the electrical connection between CMs. Prior research has shown that the use of gold nanoparticles on coiled electrospun PCL fibers can improve the conductivity of electrical signals in the scaffold. The findings demonstrate that the heart is composed of fibers that show the same stretching and recoiling properties as CMs. Following a week-long period of culturing, the application of gold nanoparticles to the PCL fibers led to an enhanced expression of α-sarcomeric actinin, a marker closely linked to the contraction of cardiac muscle. In addition, these fibers showed a considerably decreased response to electrical fields compared to the control group. These observations demonstrate significant potential as scaffolds need to generate sufficient contractile force for the treatment of cardiac dysfunction [79].

Electrospun Scaffolds

Electrospinning is an inexpensive technique used to produce materials consisting of extremely small fibers at the nanoscale diameter and interconnected pore structure. In addition, this method can work with a wide range of synthetic and biological materials, which makes it a highly appealing method for constructing scaffolds. Kai et al. fabricated a composite scaffold using electrospinning techniques, combining PCL and gelatin. This scaffold was designed to closely resemble the aligned nanofibrous extracellular matrix (ECM) found in the native heart muscle. The study revealed that composite scaffolds showed greater cell attachment in comparison to pure PCL scaffolds. In addition, it was observed that the CMs on the aligned nanofibers exhibited the same direction as the fibers, indicating a preference for anisotropic properties. Shin et al. devised a technique for enhancing the maturation of cultured cardiomyocytes before implantation. An electrospun PCL nanofibrous mesh was used and positioned on a wire ring to generate a passive load. This in vitro system aims to replicate the elongation and hypertrophy of native cardiac myocytes caused by mechanical loading. After 3 days of culture, the cardiac myocytes in this system showed contraction and expressed the regulatory proteins tropomyosin, actin, and cardiac troponin-I [80].

7.4.5 Skin Tissue Regeneration

Nanoparticles composed of a single chemical species, such as metals or metal oxides, have wide applicability in treating skin lesions and promoting wound healing as well as possess antimicrobial properties. In vitro tests using rat models demonstrate high efficiency, displaying enhanced cell uptake and improved cell proliferation of gold and silver nanoclusters, indicating their effectiveness in promoting skin repair. This may be attributed to their potential to enhance cell metabolism. In addition, they were able to enhance cell migration, which is an important aspect of skin repair, and exhibit anti-inflammatory properties by scavenging ROS. AuNPs contribute to the formation of granulation tissue and reduce inflammation owing to their anti-inflammatory properties. Gold nanostructures have high biocompatibility, ensuring that they are not rejected by skin tissues and result in adverse effects in the body. AuNPs can promote the growth of keratocytes and fibroblasts by inhibiting the respiratory pathways that sustain their survival. Nevertheless, they possess the capacity to suppress the innate immune system, resulting in faster wound healing and a reduced scarring process with enhanced skin repair outcomes [81].

Acticoat® is the pioneering wound dressing that incorporates silver nanoparticles, making it the first of its kind in the market. An illustrative case of the application of silver nanoparticles in skin regeneration can be found in clinical practice. Specifically, it was used to treat a patient with toxic epidermal necrolysis caused by carbamazepine administration. This resulted in the development of vesiculobullous lesions and erosions covering 70% of the patient's body surface. A nanosilver dressing, consisting of silver nanocrystals, was used exclusively to treat the skin lesions. It was applied and secured with cotton pads and crepe bandages, without the use of any conventional antibiotics. Re-epithelialization was observed after 5 days, with complete healing occurring after 9 days [82].

Nanofibers are characterized by their large surface area, low weight per unit area, minimum aspect ratio of 1000:1, great strength, and a high concentration of microscopic pores. These nanoparticles are intriguing due to their resemblance to the extracellular matrix and their ability to promote tissue regeneration. Nanofibers are well-recognized as very effective antibacterial materials that provide a protective layer for the skin. They are specifically designed to meet all safety regulations for medical use only 347, 348. Currently, nanofibers are used as scaffolding for skin regeneration and rejuvenation, as well as for drug administration. They can consist of natural, synthetic, or mixed polymers, each exhibiting distinct features [83]. Natural polymers offer strong biocompatibility, lack toxicity, are biodegradable, frequently possess inherent antibacterial properties, and can induce skin contraction to enhance wound healing, hence improving wound treatment. In contrast, synthetic polymers can be adjusted and altered throughout their production to fulfill specific criteria for each application. As a result, these materials exhibit precise control over their composition, molecular weight, crystalline structure, chemical properties, and mechanical characteristics, ensuring excellent reproducibility. Hybrid polymers combine these elements effectively, resulting in the highest documented results for nanofibers and scaffolds in terms of wound healing speed compared to other nanomaterials. The control of nanoporosity, along with other notable characteristics, can be achieved during the preparation process of nanofibers. Electrospinning is the predominant method used. Scaffolds can be created using various non-woven nanofibers, arranged in random orientations and with diverse shapes [84].

Presently, electrospun polycaprolactone (PCL) and polyvinyl alcohol (PVA) nanofibers have been characterized as secure, easily tolerated, and efficacious. These nanostructures can be used as a smart covering or dressing for the skin during the process of wound healing, either on their own or in conjunction with bioactive substances. Platelets have recently been used alongside nanofibers to construct a device that transports bioactive chemicals produced from platelets, which can enhance the growth of melanocytes. This finding is fascinating in the management of the skin vitiligo process, which involves melanocytes. PCL scaffolds with attached platelets possess the capability to enhance the proliferation of skin cells, hence facilitating the propagation of cells and metabolic activity in all types of skin-associated cells. In this particular context, nanofibers are increasingly being considered a promising option for treating diabetic foot ulcers [85]. The combination of PCL nanofibers and natural extracts can safeguard the skin's mesenchymal stem cells from aging caused by UV radiation, indicating its potential to revitalize the skin [84].

Electrospun wound dressings can be fabricated to incorporate various medicinal or antibacterial substances, thereby enhancing the process of wound healing. Regrettably, the wound dressings now on the market are unable to meet all expectations as they cannot fully restore the structural and functional characteristics of natural skin. Currently, nanofibers are being researched and enhanced for their use in tissue regeneration, specifically in the areas of wound healing and cosmetic treatment. In the first scenario, nanofibers are used to transport drugs or other biological substances (e.g., growth factors and stem cells) to the site of the wound [86].

7.5 Smart Nanomaterials in Regenerative Medicine

Regenerative medicine aims to restore by replacing, repairing, or growing damaged tissues and organs. Smart nanomaterials have been developed through the integration of nanotechnology into regenerative medicine that can self-heal, react to external stimuli, safely break down inside the body, and carry out several tasks at once [87].

7.5.1 Stimuli-Responsive Nanomaterials

The physical or chemical characteristics of stimuli-responsive nanomaterials can alter in response to various environmental stimuli, including light, pH, or temperature. These materials are specifically used in tissue engineering, regulated drug delivery, and diagnostics in the field of regenerative medicine [88].

7.5.1.1 Temperature-Responsive Systems

The characteristics of temperature-responsive nanomaterials, sometimes referred to as thermoresponsive materials, vary depending on the temperature to which they are exposed. These modifications may pertain to mechanical strength, form, or solubility. Poly(N-isopropylacrylamide) is a highly common kind of temperature-responsive polymer (PNIPAM). The lower critical solution temperature (LCST) for PNIPAM is around 32 °C, above which it becomes hydrophobic and separates from the solution. This characteristic can be used to administer drugs under control such that they are released at particular body locations when the temperature rises. Thermoresponsive hydrogels can be used in tissue engineering to build scaffolds that promote cell division and proliferation. For instance, a hydrogel based on PNIPAM can be injected while liquid, solidifying at body temperature to provide a scaffold that encourages tissue regeneration. Growth factors or other bioactive compounds can be encapsulated and released in temperature-responsive nanogels crosslinked polymer networks in response to temperature variations linked to tissue injury or healing processes. Further examples comprise liposomes and micelles that contain drugs and release them when heated; these can be especially helpful in addressing deep-seated malignancies when localized hyperthermia is applicable. To attain the intended temperature response and mechanical qualities, the crosslinking density, molecular weight, and polymer composition must all be carefully taken into account throughout the system's design [89].

7.5.1.2 pH-Responsive Systems

The pH of their surroundings affects the characteristics of pH-responsive nanomaterials. Targeting acidic microenvironments, like those present in cancers or inflammatory tissues, is one application for this. Since they are pH-sensitive, polymers like poly(2-(diisopropylamino)ethyl methacrylate) (PDPA) can be used to make drug delivery nanocarriers. PDPA is hydrophobic and capable of encasing drugs at neutral pH. PDPA turns hydrophilic in acidic environments, like those present in tumors, releasing the encapsulated drugs right at the site of action. The usage of poly(L-histidine) (PLH), whose solubility changes from hydrophobic to hydrophilic at acidic pH, is another illustration. This characteristic can be used to make drug administration more precise and effective by producing nanoparticles that release their cargo in the acidic environment of cancer cells. In tissue engineering, pH-responsive materials can be used to build scaffolds that break down in reaction to pH variations, enabling the slow release of growth hormones or other bioactive substances that support tissue regeneration. In reaction to the acidic milieu of wounded tissues, poly(β-amino ester) scaffolds disintegrate quickly in acidic environments, releasing encapsulated growth factors [90].

7.5.1.3 Light-Responsive Systems

Light-responsive nanomaterials alter when exposed to particular light wavelengths. Their ability to precisely control both spatial and temporal aspects of their activity makes them perfect for use in tissue engineering and drug delivery applications. Because gold nanoparticles have a strong plasmon resonance that can be controlled to absorb particular light wavelengths, they are frequently used in light-responsive devices. Gold nanoparticles can be utilized to ablate cancer cells or release drug by producing localized heat when exposed to near-infrared (NIR) light. This method, called photothermal therapy, offers a highly precise, least intrusive treatment alternative. Apart from gold nanoparticles, photochromic polymers and photosensitive hydrogels are among the other materials that react to light. When exposed to light, photochromic polymers alter their molecular makeup and mechanical characteristics, enabling the release of drugs under regulated conditions. However, when exposed to light, photosensitive hydrogels can gel or degrade, which makes them helpful for producing scaffolds that can be adjusted in real-time during tissue engineering techniques. For example, UV light can be applied to solidify a hydrogel containing a photosensitive crosslinker to create a scaffold that encourages cell development. It is possible to create light-responsive hydrogels that will release growth factors or drugs that have been encapsulated in them in reaction to light, offering a dynamic and controlled way to encourage tissue regeneration [91].

7.5.2 Self-Healing Materials

Materials with self-healing properties can repair themselves after injury, increasing their longevity and usefulness. In regenerative medicine, these structures are highly sought after because they may be used to make scaffolds and implants that are long-lasting and stable.

7.5.2.1 Mechanisms and Applications

In nanoscience, self-healing mechanisms are usually mediated by dynamic physical interactions or reversible chemical bonds. For instance, polymers with reversible chemical bonds like disulfide bonds break and reconstruct in reaction to environmental changes. Hydrogels with dynamic covalent connections, for example, can repair themselves and regain their mechanical characteristics and shape after sustaining an injury. Scaffolds that facilitate long-term tissue regeneration without the need for frequent replacements can be made using these self-healing hydrogels. Self-healing characteristics are added to scaffolds to increase their longevity and guarantee that tissues and cell growth will always have support. Another strategy could be the use of supramolecular interactions including metal-ligand coordination, host-guest interactions, and hydrogen bonding that allow material to self-repair after damage or injury. For example, reversible inclusion complexation enables self-healing in hydrogels, which relies on host-guest interactions between cyclodextrins and polymer chains. There are numerous applications for self-healing materials in regenerative medicine. Implants can be protected from deterioration by self-healing coatings in addition to hydrogels, which can repair small cracks and scratches, extending the implant's lifespan and reducing failure rates. For example, self-healing polymer coatings on cardiovascular stents can extend the device's life and shield it from mechanical stress-related damage. Wounds can be treated with injectable self-healing hydrogels, which take on the shape of the wound and create a moist environment that aids in healing. The hydrogel's ability to heal itself ensures that the wound site will always be covered and protected, even if mechanical force is applied [92].

7.5.3 Biodegradable and Biocompatible Nanomaterials

For applications in regenerative medicine, biodegradable and biocompatible nanomaterials are crucial because they can degrade within the body without triggering negative side effects. Scaffolds, drug delivery methods, and other devices that aid in tissue regeneration are made from these materials.

7.5.3.1 Design Principles and Examples

To create biodegradable nanoparticles, polymers that decompose gradually into non-toxic byproducts are chosen. Because of their well-established biocompatibility and degradation patterns, polymers including PLA, PGA, and their copolymer PLGA are frequently used. Because PLGA nanoparticles may encapsulate a variety of drugs and release them in a regulated manner when the polymer degrades, they are frequently used in drug delivery systems. This lessens the requirement for regular dosing by enabling sustained drug release over prolonged periods. Precise control over drug release kinetics is possible by varying the ratio of lactic acid to glycolic acid. This then alters the rate at which PLGA decomposes. Biodegradable PLA or PLGA scaffolds can be used in tissue engineering processes to temporarily support developing tissues. The scaffold does not need to be surgically removed because the newly produced tissue progressively replaces it as it deteriorates. To enhance tissue regeneration, these scaffolds can be designed with suitable pore sizes and structures that facilitate cell infiltration, nutrition transport, and waste elimination. Biodegradable nanoparticles can be natural polymers like gelatin, collagen, and chitosan. Derived from chitin, chitosan exhibits remarkable biodegradability, biocompatibility, and antibacterial characteristics, making it a valuable tool for wound healing applications. Naturally occurring proteins called collagen and gelatin can be combined to create hydrogels and scaffolds that have superior cell adhesion qualities and promote tissue regeneration. Biodegradable nanoparticles can be engineered to react with particular biological stimuli, such as enzymes. Specific enzymes can cause enzyme-responsive polymers to break down, enabling selective drug release or scaffold disintegration. For example, hydrogels that are responsive to matrix metalloproteinase (MMP) can break down in reaction to MMPs released by invasive cells, creating a dynamic environment that promotes tissue regeneration [93].

7.5.4 Multifunctional Nanomaterials

Multifunctional nanomaterials integrate several functions, such as therapeutic and diagnostic ones, onto one platform. With the promise to provide more personalized and effective treatments, these materials represent the cutting edge of regenerative medicine.

7.5.4.1 Combining Diagnostic and Therapeutic Functions

Nanomaterials are gaining attention in theranostics through the development of multifunctional nanomaterials that diagnose and treat diseases concurrently. Magnetic nanostructures are coated with a suitable drug or therapeutic agent that serves the dual purpose of diagnosis and therapy. These metallic nanomaterials can act as diagnostic probes in various imaging techniques like MRI. They can be used as transport vehicles to deliver drugs to targeted sites in the body. Metal nanoparticles, in particular gold, provide several benefits in diagnostics by enhancing the contrast of CT scans and imparting a dual therapeutic effect through the ablation of cancer cells by producing heat when exposed to near-infrared light. Multi-purpose scaffolds in tissue engineering contain growth factors responding to specific stimuli for the sustained release of diagnostic agents. For example, MRI tracking can be achieved with a scaffold that contains magnetic nanoparticles and delivers bioactive chemicals that encourage tissue growth. This makes it possible to evaluate tissue regeneration in real-time and modify the treatment plan promptly. Quantum dots (QDs) are another type of multifunctional nanomaterial that serves both imaging and therapeutic roles. Due to their unique optical properties, QDs can be used as fluorescent imaging probes for diagnostic purposes. These nanostructures can be functionalized with various biomolecules for integrated imaging and therapy. Multifunctional nanomaterials show promise for customized treatment. Through the combination of diagnostic and therapeutic features into a single platform, these materials are capable of delivering personalized therapies datable to individual patient profiles. To ensure accurate and efficient therapy, nanocarriers can be engineered to release drugs in response to particular biomarkers or physiological parameters that are distinct to each patient [94].

7.6 Challenges and Future Directions

Table 7.2 and the following sections provide a detailed account of the challenges and constraints associated with the use of nanomaterials in the field of regenerative medicine.

Table 7.2 Challenges and future trends in the use of nanotechnology for regenerative medicine

SL No.	Challenge	Description	Current solutions/ strategies	Future direction	References
1.	Biocompatibility and toxicity	Risk of systematic and cytotoxicity due to adverse immune response or nanoparticle degradation in vivo	Surface modification of nanomaterials with biocompatible ligands	Introduction of smart nanomaterials and personalized medicine to facilitate targeted therapy and reduce adverse effects	[99]
2.	Scalability and manufacturing	Large-scale production of nanomaterials to maintain consistent quality is challenging	Introduction of hybrid modalities and 3D bioprinting techniques	Integration of nanotechnology with digital health, AI, and use of nanorobotics to develop a robust and cost-effective manufacturing process	[99]
3.	Regulatory barriers	Lack of standardized regulatory framework for the development, approval, and implementation of nanomaterials in healthcare	Establishment of regulatory guidelines and collaboration with regulatory agencies such as FDA, EMA, ICH, etc.	Use of AI to develop a more streamlined approval process and standardized regulatory guidelines, redefined regulatory science, and innovation approaches	[99]
4.	Immunogenicity	Unwanted immune responses are triggered leading to inflammation, tissue rejection, and adverse effects	Use of surface modification techniques to improve biocompatibility and minimize immune reactions	Use of nanorobots for precise targeting of tissues, widespread use of biomimetic nanoparticles for drug delivery	[99]

7.6.1 *Biocompatibility and Toxicity*

7.6.1.1 Assessing Long-Term Safety

Biocompatibility and toxicity are two critical factors that need to be considered while integrating nanotechnology with regenerative medicine. This can be achieved through safety evaluation by in vitro studies followed by in vivo studies and adopting multidimensional approaches to assess the long-term safety of nanomaterials. The interactions of nanostructures used for generating scaffolds or drug carriers with biological tissues must be investigated to evaluate the compatibility of the nanostructure in the biological environment and be aware of any potential toxic effects. Studies should be conducted to determine the long-term effects such as tumorigenicity, fibrosis, or inflammation. Advanced tools like imaging and biomarker analysis can help to track the nanomaterials' biodistribution, degradation, and potential bioaccumulation within the body to assess their safety profile [95].

7.6.1.2 Strategies for Minimizing Adverse Effects

There are several ways to mitigate or reduce the negative impacts of nanomaterials. PEGylating or the use of PEG as a ligand on the surface of the nanoparticles reduces immunogenicity and enhances biocompatibility. Another way is to incorporate biodegradable components in their design that enable the structures to degrade into non-toxic metabolites. Also, natural substances can be used with nanomaterials to reduce any potential toxicity in the body. Lastly, by guaranteeing that the therapeutic drugs are administered in a way that is both safe and efficient, dose optimization and controlled release mechanisms can assist in reducing the possibility of negative side effects [96].

7.6.2 *Scalability and Manufacturing*

7.6.2.1 Challenges in Large-Scale Production

There are several challenges and limitations in moving from laboratory-scale production to large-scale production. For instance, nanoparticles must maintain consistent size, shape, and functionalization to ensure their reproducibility and efficacy. Acquiring exact control over the synthesis processes is necessary for this but is challenging on an industrial scale. The high cost and scalability of production are also issues that hinder large-scale production of these materials. Researchers, scientists, and industrialists need to find ways to overcome these roadblocks for the widespread application of nanomaterials in the future [97].

7.6.2.2 Solutions for Economic Viability

To create an economically viable manufacturing process, a cost-effective synthesis and purification method is necessary. Reducing labor costs and improving consistency in prediction will help to achieve process optimization, which will in turn reduce the costs of the whole process. The use of costly and dangerous reagents can be decreased, and the environmental effect can be minimized by putting green chemistry ideas into practice. Collaboration between research institutions, businesses, and government agencies can help standardize manufacturing processes, which will cut prices even more and hasten the transition of nanomaterials from laboratory settings to real-world medical applications [97, 98].

7.6.3 Regulatory and Ethical Considerations

7.6.3.1 Current Regulations and Standards

Strict regulatory oversight is essential to guarantee the safety and efficacy of nanomaterials used in regenerative medicine. Existing regional laws often contain directives on the toxicity, characterization, and clinical assessment of nanomaterials. Standards have been set by regulatory bodies like the FDA (Food and Drug Administration), EMA (European Medicines Agency), and ISO (International Organization for Standardization) for the evaluation and authorization of nanomaterials used in medical applications. According to these requirements, long-term safety data, biocompatibility, and material qualities must all be precisely documented to make sure that nanomaterials meet the stringent safety and efficacy benchmark before clinical application [100].

7.6.3.2 Ethical Implications in Clinical Use

Several ethical concerns are raised by the clinical application of nanomaterials. These issues must be addressed beforehand to promote the responsible use of nanomaterials in biomedicine. Patients must be fully informed about the potential dangers and advantages of therapy based on nanomaterials to give their informed consent. Constant patient monitoring and open communication are necessary to deal with any unanticipated long-term effects. To avoid gaps in healthcare access, the fair distribution of cutting-edge nanomaterial medicines must be taken into account, ensuring equitable access to all. Ethical norms governing the production, research, and clinical use of nanomaterials should be established to ensure patient safety and gain public trust [100].

7.6.4 Emerging Trends

7.6.4.1 Innovations in Nanomaterial Design

Nanomedicine is a rapidly advancing field where ongoing developments are improving the functioning and potential applications of nanomaterials in regenerative medicine. The development of smart stimuli-responsive nanomaterials that can react to particular physiological stimuli like pH, enzymes, temperatures, and heat activity is being facilitated by advancements in nanotechnology and is being incorporated into different areas of regenerative medicine. Research is focusing on designing multifunctional nanomaterials with simultaneous imaging, therapeutic, and monitoring capabilities. New directions in tissue engineering and personalized medicine are being made possible by the incorporation of nanomaterials with other innovative platforms such as organ-on-a-chip systems and 3D bioprinting [101].

7.6.4.2 Potential Future Applications

Nanomaterials possess a diverse array of promising applications in the field of regenerative medicine in the years to come. Nanomaterials improve cell survival, differentiation, and integration with host tissues and hence can be used to improve stem cell therapy outcomes. Nanomaterials can effectively deliver genetic materials, offering potential treatment for genetic problems at their root level. The development of bioactive nanoscaffolds holds the potential to revolutionize tissue engineering by providing an optimal environment for tissue growth and regeneration. Furthermore, nanomaterials provide precise and efficient therapeutic alternatives for cancer, cardiovascular diseases, and neurological disorders [102].

7.7 Conclusion

Nanomaterials have allowed regenerative medicine to enter into a new era of revolution in medical science through breakthroughs in repairing, regenerating, and replacing damaged or injured tissues and organs. This chapter explores a wide range of unique physiochemical properties of these nanomaterials that facilitate cellular adhesion, proliferation, and differentiation, all of which are essential for tissue engineering and regenerative processes. To improve the therapeutic outcomes of regeneration therapies, many nanomaterials, such as nanoparticles, nanofibers, and nanotubes, have been developed to be integrated with smart nanomaterials that respond to particular stimuli for transporting bioactive substances, such as growth factors and genes, directly to targeted sites. Furthermore, the development of 3D bioprinting technologies that use bioinks based on nanomaterials has opened up new doors for personalized tissue structures tailored to individual patients' needs.

Additionally, the ability of nanomaterials to seamlessly integrate with digital healthcare technology, such as wearables and biosensors, embodies the concepts of theranostics and enables real-time monitoring and improvement of regenerative processes. Despite the advancements, challenges including long-term biocompatibility, potential toxicity, and regulatory barriers hinder the implementation of these nanomaterials in clinical settings. To address these roadblocks effectively and standardize the use of nanomaterials in regenerative medicine, multidisciplinary research is required. The intersection of regenerative medicine and nanomaterials is paving the way for more efficient, personalized, and long-lasting healthcare solutions by uncovering the complexities of biological systems and developing highly efficacious treatment strategies. This could indicate a new era of treatment strategies aligned with smart and sustainable healthcare objectives.

Data Availability Statement Data sharing is not applicable to this chapter as no datasets were generated or analyzed during the current study period.

Conflict of Interest The authors declare no conflict of interest.

Funding This research did not receive any specific grant from funding agencies in the public, commercial, or not-for-profit centers.Author Contributions

CRediT Author Statement Conceptualization: TANVIR AHMED, Writing—Original Draft: TANVIR AHMED, KAZI TASNUVA ALAM, Writing—Review & Editing: TANVIR AHMED, KAZI TASNUVA ALAM, Visualization: TANVIR AHMED.

References

1. Tatullo M, Zavan B, Piattelli A. Critical overview on regenerative medicine: new insights into the role of stem cells and innovative biomaterials. Int J Mol Sci. 2023;24:7936.
2. Petrosyan A, Martins PN, Solez K, Uygun BE, Gorantla VS, Orlando G. Regenerative medicine applications: an overview of clinical trials. Front Bioeng Biotechnol. 2022;10:1–15.
3. Hasan A, Morshed M, Memic A, Hassan S, Webster TJ, Marei HES. Nanoparticles in tissue engineering: applications, challenges and prospects. Int J Nanomedicine. 2018;13:5637–55.
4. Fathi-Achachelouei M, Knopf-Marques H, Ribeiro da Silva CE, Barthès J, Bat E, Tezcaner A, et al. Use of nanoparticles in tissue engineering and regenerative medicine. Front Bioeng Biotechnol. 2019;7:1–22.
5. Colson YL, Grinstaff MW. Biologically responsive polymeric nanoparticles for drug delivery. Adv Mater. 2012;24:3878–86.
6. Ku SH, Lee M, Park CB. Carbon-based nanomaterials for tissue engineering. Adv Healthc Mater. 2013;2:244–60.
7. Filipczak N, Yalamarty SSK, Li X, Khan MM, Parveen F, Torchilin V. Lipid-based drug delivery systems in regenerative medicine. Materials (Basel). 2021;14:1–23.
8. Akturk O, Kismet K, Yasti AC, Kuru S, Duymus ME, Kaya F, et al. Wet electrospun silk fibroin/gold nanoparticle 3D matrices for wound healing applications. RSC Adv. 2016;6:13234–50.
9. Prabhu S, Poulose EK. Silver nanoparticles: mechanism of antimicrobial action, synthesis, medical applications, and toxicity effects. Int Nano Lett. 2012;2:1–10.

10. Guo Y, Xue Y, Niu W, Chen M, Wang M, Ma PX, et al. Monodispersed bioactive glass nanoparticles enhance the osteogenic differentiation of adipose-derived stem cells through activating TGF-Beta/Smad3 signaling pathway. Part Part Syst Charact. 2018;35:1–10.
11. Moreno-Vega AI, Gómez-Quintero T, Nuñez-Anita RE, Acosta-Torres LS, Castaño V. Polymeric and ceramic nanoparticles in biomedical applications. J Nanotechnol. 2012;2012 https://doi.org/10.1155/2012/936041.
12. Harini G, Bharathi R, Sankaranarayanan A, Shanmugavadivu A, Selvamurugan N. Nanoceramics-reinforced chitosan scaffolds in bone tissue engineering. Mater Adv R Soc Chem. 2023;4:3907–28.
13. Tang Z, He C, Tian H, Ding J, Hsiao BS, Chu B, et al. Polymeric nanostructured materials for biomedical applications. Prog Polym Sci (Elsevier Ltd). 2016;60:86–128.
14. Zheng X, Zhang P, Fu Z, Meng S, Dai L, Yang H. Applications of nanomaterials in tissue engineering. RSC Adv R Soc Chem. 2021;11:19041–58.
15. Phutane P, Telange D, Agrawal S, Gunde M, Kotkar K, Pethe A. Biofunctionalization and applications of polymeric nanofibers in tissue engineering and regenerative medicine. Polymers (Basel). 2023;15:1–38.
16. Avula. 基因的改变NIH public access. Bone. 2014;23:1–7.
17. Ogueri KS, Laurencin CT. Nanofiber technology for regenerative engineering. ACS Nano. 2020;14:9347–63.
18. Li S, Yu Q, Li H, Chen M, Jin Y, Liu D. Self-assembled peptide hydrogels in regenerative medicine. Gels. 2023;9:1–17.
19. Alshangiti DM, El-Damhougy TK, Zaher A, Madani M, Mohamady Ghobashy M. Revolutionizing biomedicine: advancements, applications, and prospects of nanocomposite macromolecular carbohydrate-based hydrogel biomaterials: a review. RSC Adv R Soc Chem. 2023;13:35251–91.
20. Shahbaz A, Hussain N, Mahmood T, Iqbal HMN, Bin Emran T, Show PL, et al. Polymer nanocomposites for biomedical applications. In: Smart polymer nanocomposites design, synthesis, functionalization, properties, and applications micro and nano technologies. Elsevier; 2022. p. 379–94.
21. Liu S, Li P, Liu X, Wang P, Xue W, Ren Y, et al. Bioinspired mineral-polymeric hybrid hyaluronic acid/poly (γ-glutamic acid) hydrogels as tunable scaffolds for stem cells differentiation. Carbohydr Polym (Elsevier Ltd). 2021;264:118048.
22. Yunus Basha R, Sampath SK, Doble M. Design of biocomposite materials for bone tissue regeneration. Mater Sci Eng C (Elsevier B.V.). 2015;57:452–63.
23. Holmannova D, Borsky P, Svadlakova T, Borska L, Fiala Z. Carbon nanoparticles and their biomedical applications. Appl Sci. 2022;12:1–21.
24. Cheng J, Liu J, Wu B, Liu Z, Li M, Wang X, et al. Graphene and its derivatives for bone tissue engineering: in vitro and in vivo evaluation of graphene-based scaffolds membranes and coatings. Front Bioeng Biotechnol. 2021;9:1–15.
25. Eivazzadeh-Keihan R, Maleki A, de la Guardia M, Bani MS, Chenab KK, Pashazadeh-Panahi P, et al. Carbon based nanomaterials for tissue engineering of bone: building new bone on small black scaffolds: a review. J Adv Res Cairo Univ. 2019;18:185–201.
26. Mitchell J, Lo KWH. The use of small-molecule compounds for cell adhesion and migration in regenerative medicine. Biomedicine. 2023;11:11.
27. Mimeault M, Hauke R, Batra SK. Stem cells: a revolution in therapeutics – recent advances in stem cell biology and their therapeutic applications in regenerative medicine and cancer therapies. Clin Pharmacol Ther. 2007;82:252–64.
28. Gonciar D, Mocan T, Agoston-Coldea L. Nanoparticles targeting the molecular pathways of heart remodeling and regeneration. Pharmaceutics. 2022;14:1–20.
29. Verma A, Verma M, Singh A. Animal tissue culture principles and applications. Anim Biotechnol (Elsevier). 2020:269–93. https://doi.org/10.1016/B978-0-12-811710-1.00012-4.

30. Ferreira MPA, Talman V, Torrieri G, Liu D, Marques G, Moslova K, et al. Dual-drug delivery using dextran-functionalized nanoparticles targeting cardiac fibroblasts for cellular reprogramming. Adv Funct Mater. 2018; https://doi.org/10.1002/adfm.201705134.
31. Nagel S, Papadakis M, Hoyte L, Buchan AM. Therapeutic hypothermia in experimental models of focal and global cerebral ischemia and intracerebral hemorrhage. Expert Review of Neurotherapeutics. 2008;8(8):1255–68. https://doi.org/10.1586/14737175.8.8.1255.
32. Li M, Fang F, Sun M, Zhang Y, Hu M, Zhang J. Extracellular vesicles as bioactive nanotherapeutics: an emerging paradigm for regenerative medicine. Theranostics. 2022;12:4879–903.
33. Shi J, Votruba AR, Farokhzad OC, Langer R. Nanotechnology in drug delivery and tissue engineering: from discovery to applications. Nano Lett. 2010;10:3223–30.
34. Idris DS, Roy A, Pandit S, Alghamdi S, Almehmadi M, Alsaiari AA, et al. Polymer-based nanocarriers for biomedical and environmental applications. E-Polymers. 2023;23:101174–4.
35. Hosseinkhani H, Domb AJ, Sharifzadeh G, Nahum V. Gene therapy for regenerative medicine. Pharmaceutics. 2023;15:856.
36. Hajiali F, Tajbakhsh S, Shojaei A. Fabrication and properties of polycaprolactone composites containing calcium phosphate-based ceramics and bioactive glasses in bone tissue engineering: a review. Polym Rev. 2018;58:164–207.
37. Mirza S, Zia I, Jolly R, Kazmi S, Owais M, Shakir M. Synergistic combination of natural bioadhesive bael fruit gum and chitosan/nano-hydroxyapatite: a ternary bioactive nanohybrid for bone tissue engineering. Int J Biol Macromol (Elsevier B.V). 2018;119:215–24.
38. Singh BN, Pramanik K. Development of novel silk fibroin/polyvinyl alcohol/sol-gel bioactive glass composite matrix by modified layer by layer electrospinning method for bone tissue construct generation. Biofabrication (IOP Publishing). 2017;9:015028.
39. Yoon J, Han H, Jang J. Nanomaterials-incorporated hydrogels for 3D bioprinting technology. Nano Converg (Springer Nature Singapore). 2023;10:52.
40. Tai I-C, Fu Y-C, Wang C-K, Chang J-K, Ho M-L. Local delivery of controlled-release simvastatin/PLGA/HAp microspheres enhances bone repair. Int J Nanomed (Dove Medical Press). 2013;8:3895–905.
41. Wang J, Wang L, Yang M, Zhu Y, Tomsia A, Mao C. Untangling the effects of peptide sequences and Nanotopographies in a biomimetic niche for directed differentiation of iPSCs by assemblies of genetically engineered viral nanofibers. Nano Lett (American Chemical Society). 2014;14:6850–6.
42. Wang F, Yu L, Monopoli MP, Sandin P, Mahon E, Salvati A, et al. The biomolecular corona is retained during nanoparticle uptake and protects the cells from the damage induced by cationic nanoparticles until degraded in the lysosomes. Nanomed Nanotechnol Biol Med. 2013;9:1159–68.
43. Begam H, Nandi SK, Kundu B, Chanda A. Strategies for delivering bone morphogenetic protein for bone healing. Mater Sci Eng C. 2017;70:856–69.
44. Lü L, Deegan A, Musa F, Xu T, Yang Y. The effects of biomimetically conjugated VEGF on osteogenesis and angiogenesis of MSCs (human and rat) and HUVECs co-culture models. Colloids Surfaces B Biointerfaces. 2018;167:550–9.
45. Bentwich I, Avniel A, Karov Y, Aharonov R, Gilad S, Barad O, et al. Identification of hundreds of conserved and nonconserved human microRNAs. Nat Genet. 2005;37:766–70.
46. Yi H, Ur Rehman F, Zhao C, Liu B, He N. Recent advances in nano scaffolds for bone repair. Bone Res (Nature Publishing Group). 2016;4:16050.
47. Armiento AR, Stoddart MJ, Alini M, Eglin D. Biomaterials for articular cartilage tissue engineering: learning from biology. Acta Biomater. 2018;65:1–20.
48. Ul Haq A, Carotenuto F, Di Nardo P, Francini R, Prosposito P, Pescosolido F, et al. Extrinsically conductive nanomaterials for cardiac tissue engineering applications. Micromachines. 2021;12:914.
49. Manoukian OS, Dieck C, Milne T, Dealy CN, Rudraiah S, Kumbar SG. Nanomaterials/nanocomposites for osteochondral tissue. Adv Exp Med Biol. 2018;1058:79–95.

50. Eslahi N, Abdorahim M, Simchi A. Smart polymeric hydrogels for cartilage tissue engineering: a review on the chemistry and biological functions. Biomacromolecules (American Chemical Society). 2016;17:3441–63.
51. Chen H, Zeng Y, Liu W, Zhao S, Wu J, Du Y. Multifaceted applications of nanomaterials in cell engineering and therapy. Biotechnol Adv. 2013;31:638–53.
52. Arslan E, Sardan Ekiz M, Eren Cimenci C, Can N, Gemci MH, Ozkan H, et al. Protective therapeutic effects of peptide nanofiber and hyaluronic acid hybrid membrane in in vivo osteoarthritis model. Acta Biomater. 2018;73:263–74.
53. Zhou Y, Chyu J, Zumwalt M. Recent progress of fabrication of cell scaffold by electrospinning technique for articular cartilage tissue engineering. Int J Biomater (John Wiley & Sons, Ltd). 2018;2018:1953636.
54. Li X, Fan C, Xiao Z, Zhao Y, Zhang H, Sun J, et al. A collagen microchannel scaffold carrying paclitaxel-liposomes induces neuronal differentiation of neural stem cells through Wnt/β--catenin signaling for spinal cord injury repair. Biomaterials. 2018;183:114–27.
55. Ferguson EL, Naseer S, Powell LC, Hardwicke J, Young FI, Zhu B, et al. Controlled release of dextrin-conjugated growth factors to support growth and differentiation of neural stem cells. Stem Cell Res. 2018;33:69–78.
56. Jeong SJ, Cooper JG, Ifergan I, McGuire TL, Xu D, Hunter Z, et al. Intravenous immune--modifying nanoparticles as a therapy for spinal cord injury in mice. Neurobiol Dis. 2017;108:73–82.
57. Agarwala S, Tamplin OJ. Neural crossroads in the hematopoietic stem cell niche. Trends Cell Biol (Elsevier). 2018;28:987–98.
58. Harley-Troxell ME, Steiner R, Advincula RC, Anderson DE, Dhar M. Interactions of cells and biomaterials for nerve tissue engineering: polymers and fabrication. Polymers (Basel). 2023;15(18):3685.
59. Addington CP, Dharmawaj S, Heffernan JM, Sirianni RW, Stabenfeldt SE. Hyaluronic acid--laminin hydrogels increase neural stem cell transplant retention and migratory response to SDF-1α. Matrix Biol. 2017;60–61:206–16.
60. Dumont CM, Carlson MA, Munsell MK, Ciciriello AJ, Strnadova K, Park J, et al. Aligned hydrogel tubes guide regeneration following spinal cord injury. Acta Biomater. 2019;86:312–22.
61. Nune M, Manchineella S, Govindaraju T, Narayan KS. Melanin incorporated electroactive and antioxidant silk fibroin nanofibrous scaffolds for nerve tissue engineering. Mater Sci Eng C. 2019;94:17–25.
62. Wu G-H, Shi H-J, Che M-T, Huang M-Y, Wei Q-S, Feng B, et al. Recovery of paralyzed limb motor function in canine with complete spinal cord injury following implantation of MSC--derived neural network tissue. Biomaterials. 2018;181:15–34.
63. Zhang S, Wang X-J, Li W-S, Xu X-L, Hu J-B, Kang X-Q, et al. Polycaprolactone/polysialic acid hybrid, multifunctional nanofiber scaffolds for treatment of spinal cord injury. Acta Biomater. 2018;77:15–27.
64. Manouras T, Vamvakaki M. Field responsive materials: photo-, electro-, magnetic- and ultrasound-sensitive polymers. Polym Chem R Soc Chem. 2017;8:74–96.
65. Pluchino N, Russo M, Santoro AN, Litta P, Cela V, Genazzani AR. Steroid hormones and BDNF. Neuroscience. 2013;239:271–9.
66. Li G, Xue C, Wang H, Yang X, Zhao Y, Zhang L, et al. Spatially featured porous chitosan conduits with micropatterned inner wall and seamless sidewall for bridging peripheral nerve regeneration. Carbohydr Polym. 2018;194:225–35.
67. Jing W, Ao Q, Wang L, Huang Z, Cai Q, Chen G, et al. Constructing conductive conduit with conductive fibrous infilling for peripheral nerve regeneration. Chem Eng J. 2018;345:566–77.
68. Feng Z-Q, Yan K, Shi C, Xu X, Wang T, Li R, et al. Neurogenic differentiation of adipose derived stem cells on graphene-based mat. Mater Sci Eng C. 2018;90:685–92.
69. Golafshan N, Kharaziha M, Fathi M. Tough and conductive hybrid graphene-PVA: alginate fibrous scaffolds for engineering neural construct. Carbon. 2017;111:752–63.

70. Amezcua R, Shirolkar A, Fraze C, Stout DA. Nanomaterials for cardiac myocyte tissue engineering. Nanomaterials. 2016;6:1–15.
71. Chen Q-Z, Bismarck A, Hansen U, Junaid S, Tran MQ, Harding SE, et al. Characterisation of a soft elastomer poly(glycerol sebacate) designed to match the mechanical properties of myocardial tissue. Biomaterials. 2008;29:47–57.
72. Aghdam RM, Shakhesi S, Najarian S, Mohammadi MM, Ahmadi Tafti SH, Mirzadeh H. Fabrication of a nanofibrous scaffold for the in vitro culture of cardiac progenitor cells for myocardial regeneration. Int J Polym Mater Polym Biomater (Taylor & Francis). 2014;63:229–39.
73. Simón-Yarza T, Rossi A, Heffels K-H, Prósper F, Groll J, Blanco-Prieto MJ. Polymeric electrospun scaffolds: neuregulin encapsulation and biocompatibility studies in a model of myocardial ischemia. Tissue Eng Part A (Mary Ann Liebert, Inc., publishers). 2015;21:1654–61.
74. Kai D, Prabhakaran MP, Jin G, Ramakrishna S. Polypyrrole-contained electrospun conductive nanofibrous membranes for cardiac tissue engineering. J Biomed Mater Res Part A (John Wiley & Sons, Ltd). 2011;99A:376–85.
75. Gasperini L, Mano JF, Reis RL. Natural polymers for the microencapsulation of cells. J R Soc Interface (Royal Society). 2014;11:20140817.
76. Bianco A, Kostarelos K, Partidos CD, Prato M. Biomedical applications of functionalised carbon nanotubes. Chem Commun (The Royal Society of Chemistry). 2005:571–7. https://doi.org/10.1039/b410943k.
77. Zhou J, Chen J, Sun H, Qiu X, Mou Y, Liu Z, et al. Engineering the heart: evaluation of conductive nanomaterials for improving implant integration and cardiac function. Sci Rep. 2014;4:3733.
78. Martinelli V, Cellot G, Toma FM, Long CS, Caldwell JH, Zentilin L, et al. Carbon nanotubes promote growth and spontaneous electrical activity in cultured cardiac myocytes. Nano Lett. 2012;12:1831–8.
79. Fleischer S, Shevach M, Feiner R, Dvir T. Coiled fiber scaffolds embedded with gold nanoparticles improve the performance of engineered cardiac tissues. Nanoscale (The Royal Society of Chemistry). 2014;6:9410–4.
80. Kai D, Prabhakaran MP, Jin G, Ramakrishna S. Guided orientation of cardiomyocytes on electrospun aligned nanofibers for cardiac tissue engineering. J Biomed Mater Res Part B Appl Biomater (John Wiley & Sons, Ltd). 2011;98B:379–86.
81. Lo S, Fauzi MB. Current update of collagen nanomaterials—fabrication, characterisation and its applications: a review. Pharmaceutics. 2021;13:1–18.
82. Bubna A. Iontophoresis with topical 0.05% tretinoin for the management of recalcitrant palmar psoriasis: a report of two cases. Indian J Dermatol Venereol Leprol. 2017;83:119–21.
83. Sylvester MA, Amini F, Tan CK. Electrospun nanofibers in wound healing. Mater Today Proc. 2020;29:1–6.
84. Bellu E, Garroni G, Cruciani S, Balzano F, Serra D, Satta R, et al. Smart nanofibers with natural extracts prevent senescence patterning in a dynamic cell culture model of human skin. Cells. 2020;9:9.
85. Beznoska J, Uhlík J, Kestlerová A, Královič M, Divín R, Fedačko J, et al. PVA and PCL nanofibers are suitable for tissue covering and regeneration. Kladno: Czech Technical University in Prague, Faculty of Biomedical Engineering; 2019. p. 68.
86. Graça MFP, de Melo-Diogo D, Correia IJ, Moreira AF. Electrospun asymmetric membranes as promising wound dressings: a review. Pharmaceutics. 2021;13:1–25.
87. Genchi GG, Marino A, Grillone A, Pezzini I, Ciofani G. Remote control of cellular functions: the role of smart nanomaterials in the medicine of the future. Adv Healthc Mater (John Wiley & Sons, Ltd). 2017;6:1700002.
88. Blum AP, Kammeyer JK, Rush AM, Callmann CE, Hahn ME, Gianneschi NC. Stimuli--responsive nanomaterials for biomedical applications. J Am Chem Soc (American Chemical Society). 2015;137:2140–54.

89. Shah RA, Frazar EM, Hilt JZ. Recent developments in stimuli responsive nanomaterials and their bionanotechnology applications. Curr Opin Chem Eng (Elsevier Ltd). 2020;30:103–11.
90. Tang H, Zhao W, Yu J, Li Y, Zhao C. Recent development of pH-responsive polymers for cancer nanomedicine. Molecules. 2019;24(1):4.
91. Zhang X, Wang S, Cheng G, Yu P, Chang J. Light-responsive nanomaterials for cancer therapy. Engineering. 2022;13:18–30.
92. Zhai L, Narkar A, Ahn K. Self-healing polymers with nanomaterials and nanostructures. Nano Today. 2020;30:100826.
93. Yan X, Zhou M, Yu S, Jin Z, Zhao K. An overview of biodegradable nanomaterials and applications in vaccines. Vaccine (Elsevier Ltd). 2020;38:1096–104.
94. Abd Elkodous M, El-Sayyad GS, Abdelrahman IY, El-Bastawisy HS, Mohamed AE, Mosallam FM, et al. Therapeutic and diagnostic potential of nanomaterials for enhanced biomedical applications. Colloids Surfaces B Biointerfaces (Elsevier). 2019;180:411–28.
95. Yoshioka Y, Higashisaka K, Tsutsumi Y. Nanomaterials in pharmacology. In: Biocompatibility of nanomaterials. Springer; 2016.
96. Yan L, Zhao F, Wang J, Zu Y, Gu Z, Zhao Y. A safe-by-design strategy towards safer nanomaterials in nanomedicines. Adv Mater (John Wiley & Sons, Ltd). 2019;31:1805391.
97. Charitidis CA, Georgiou P, Koklioti MA, Trompeta AF, Markakis V. Manufacturing nanomaterials: from research to industry. Manuf Rev. 2014;1:11.
98. González CMO, Kharissova OV, González LT, Méndez-Rojas MA, Quezada TS, Méndez YP. Scalable synthesis of nanomaterials. In: Kharissova OV, Torres-Martínez LM, Kharisov BI, editors. Handbook of nanomaterials and nanocomposites for energy and environmental applications. Cham: Springer International Publishing; 2021. p. 899–921.
99. Chaudhury K, Kumar V, Kandasamy J, RoyChoudhury S. Regenerative nanomedicine: current perspectives and future directions. Int J Nanomed. 2014;9:4153–67.
100. Sheikh FA, Majeed S, Beigh MA. Interaction of nanomaterials with living cells. In: Interact nanomater with living cells; 2023. p. 1–924.
101. Yao W, Ruan Y. Innovative Artistic design of nanomaterial products based on intelligent algorithm. J Nanomater (John Wiley & Sons, Ltd). 2022;2022:3019696.
102. Raju G, Nayak S, Acharya N, Sunder M, Kistenev Y, Mazumder N. Exploring the future of regenerative medicine: unveiling the potential of optical microscopy for structural and functional imaging of stem cells. J Biophotonics (John Wiley & Sons, Ltd). 2024;17:e202300360.

Chapter 8
Functionalization and Processing Approaches for the Production of Smart and Responsive Sustainable Nanomaterials

Swati Patel, Surbhi Sharma, Shivangi Verma, Prateek Mishra, and Shravan Kumar

Abstract A new era of innovation in digital healthcare has begun with the development of smart and sustainable nanomaterials, which provide game-changing solutions in various sectors. An overview of the main areas in which these nanoparticles are significantly advancing healthcare is given in this chapter. Because of their special physicochemical characteristics, nanomaterials are excellent choices for improving medical monitoring, therapy, and diagnostics. These materials can be precisely functionalized and characterized to fit specific needs, which makes it possible to construct extremely selective and sensitive biosensors for early disease detection. Furthermore, platforms based on nanomaterials show promise for targeted medication delivery, allowing for regulated release kinetics and reducing side effects. These platforms enable people to take proactive steps to maintain their wellbeing, ranging from implanted devices for intracellular monitoring to wearable sensors for continuous health tracking. Furthermore, the creation of affordable and ecologically friendly healthcare solutions is aided by the scalability and sustainability of nanomaterials. To guarantee the safe and successful integration of nanomaterial into clinical practice, we must address issues with biocompatibility, regulatory compliance, and scalability as we fully utilize their promise. We can create the foundation for a healthcare delivery system that is more easily accessible, effective, and individualized by utilizing the adaptability and inventiveness of nanotechnology.

S. Patel · S. Sharma · S. Verma · P. Mishra · S. Kumar (✉)
Department of Biochemical Engineering, Harcourt Butler Technical University, Uttar Pradesh, India

S. Mondal et al. (eds.), *Smart and Sustainable Nanomaterials in Digital Healthcare and Theranostic*, https://doi.org/10.1007/978-981-95-9386-6_8

Keywords Nanomaterial · Sustainable · Sensor · Nanomaterial platforms · Biocompatibility · Scalability

8.1 Introduction

The increasing world population has placed tremendous pressure and a socioeconomic burden on a better and more affordable healthcare system to protect people from diseases that can be life-threatening. In addition, the world is dealing with serious issues related to energy, climate, and environment. To address these issues, the United Nations (UN) established 17 SDGs (sustainable development goals) in 2015. One of these SDGs is to improve healthcare. UN has acknowledged that nanotechnology will help achieve 13 of the 17 SDGs by 2030. Since the late 1980s, applications of nanotechnology have drawn a lot of interest [168]. The scientific revolution of nanotechnology in the biomedical field has resulted in the development of wearable medical devices/sensors, wireless bandages that stimulate wound healing, and the discovery of mRNA-dependent vaccines for COVID-19 [62]. Numerous medical issues, including disease diagnosis, drug discovery, personalized medical procedures, cancer treatment, pharmaceutical discoveries, and the most recent medical tools and procedures, are now improving the uses of nanobiotechnology in everything from disease detection to treatment [107]. With time, nano-based medicine and nanovaccines are gaining regular medical approval, much like regular vaccination approval. For use in research and clinical settings, a range of diagnostic kits based on nanotechnology are being commercialized. These kits include nanosensors, nanoparticle-based imaging agents, nanoparticle-based Lab-on-a-Chip devices, PCR assays, and modern drugs and medicines such as polymeric nanoparticles, liposomal formulations, and nanomedicines, nanotechnology in nanoparticle-based vaccines, gene therapy, and antimicrobial agents, among others [34]. Graphene lattices and carbon nanotubes (CNTs) derived from nanoconfined graphite, ultra-strong composite materials, and high-performance transistors have been developed [100]. Businesses in the pharmaceutical industry are attempting to target cancer treatments with nanomaterials [47, 113].

The "morphology effect" of nanomaterial size and shape affects the materials' electrical conductivity, magnetic permeability, melting point, fluorescence, and chemical reactivity [68, 88]. Mechanical behavior, electrical and thermal transport, and "missing" atoms inside a lattice are all significantly impacted by vacancies [161]. Ensuring the sustainability of smart and responsive nanomaterials is one of the main objectives in their development. Functionalization and processing incorporate methods to improve the durability and responsiveness of these nanomaterials, including doping, surface modification, and hybridization with other materials [73, 133]. Sustainable nanomaterials with high efficiency and low toxicity can now be produced more easily, thanks to recent developments in green chemistry and environmentally friendly synthesis techniques [68]. Furthermore, the incorporation of intelligent features into environmentally friendly nanomaterials has created new opportunities for application in industries including smart textiles, medication delivery, and remediation of the environment. For example, it is possible to design stimuli-responsive nanoparticles that release therapeutic compounds at certain body locations, increasing treatment efficacy and minimizing side effects [59]. These materials can be made to selectively absorb and break down pollutants in environmental applications, resulting in more effective and focused cleanup procedures. Solid-phase, liquid-phase, and gas-phase techniques can all be used to create nanomaterials. Direct production of them as particles and their dispersion in liquids, glass, and gas are both possible. Liquid-phase techniques are comparatively inexpensive, adaptable, and easy to use. Low temperature and polar/nonpolar solvents are used. Through an improved understanding of nucleation and crystal growth, researchers continue to strive for synthesis innovation [86].

The first section of the chapter provides an overview of smart and sustainable nanomaterials and their types, emphasizing their importance in a range of fields including energy, biomedicine, and environmental remediation. Smart and responsive nanomaterials include stimuli-responsive nanomaterials, self-healing, self-assembling, biodegradable, and biocompatible nanomaterials. Furthermore, we discuss the definition, techniques, and types of functional groups used in functionalization. Processing approaches include various techniques used for the synthesis of nanomaterials such as top-down approaches, bottom-up approaches, green synthesis techniques, and scale-up techniques. The properties, mechanisms of responsiveness, and extensive applications of smart and responsive nanomaterials are covered in detail in a separate section. The chapter then turns to sustainability in the production of nanomaterials, the environmental impact, sustainable synthesis methods, and life cycle assessment. Lastly, the chapter discusses the market, technical, and regulatory aspects of the field's challenges and opportunities going forward.

8.2 Smart and Responsive Nanomaterials

Historically, smart and responsive nanomaterials were described as those capable of reacting promptly to their surrounding environment. The definition of smart and responsive nanomaterials has evolved to encompass materials that can be stimulated by external factors and exhibit new functional properties [163]. The responses of these materials can manifest as changes in color, heat, magnetic properties, deformation, and more. When exposed to specific stimuli, these materials can alter their properties, such as size, optical and mechanical properties, surface area, permeability, and solubility [20]. Smart and responsive nanomaterials generally exhibit five key characteristics: immediacy, transiency, self-actuation, directness, and selectivity [111]. Immediacy refers to the material's ability to respond quickly to stimuli. Transiency means the material can react to multiple environments, with its properties varying based on the specific conditions. Self-actuation describes materials that have intrinsic properties not induced by external actions. Directness implies that the response occurs at the point of input, making it a localized reaction. Lastly,

Table 8.1 List of sustainable nanomaterials, sources, and their application

Sustainable nanomaterial	Sustainable sources of nanomaterials	Biomedical application	References
Carbon dots (CDs)	Waste cooking oil plants (leaves, roots, seeds, and stem)	Drug delivery	[24]
		Biosensing (DNA, protein and disease-related biomolecules)	[18]
		Cellular bioimaging (bone regeneration monitoring)	[80]
Graphene oxide (GOX)	Plants, organic wastes (bone and bagasse newspapers), and natural waste	Biosensing (DNA, protein and disease-related biomolecules)	[66]
Graphene		Limited due to aggregation in tissue in drug delivery and transdermal drug delivery	[127]
		Drug delivery	[127]
		Microelectrodes	[101]
		Electromechanical actuators	[134]
		Cellular bioimaging	[50]
Graphene quantum dots (GDs)	Cotton, organic pollutants/ waste, vegetables, fruits, oysters, woods, and mushroom	Nano tweezers	[132]
		Cellular bioimaging	[144]
		Photothermal cancer therapy	[154]
		Drug delivery	[4]

selectivity ensures that the material's response is predictable and repeatable, with a single environmental state leading to a unique and consistent reaction. Their reactivity and interaction with the environment are greatly enhanced by their high surface-area-to-volume ratio and unique surface characteristics, which are a result of their nanoscale dimensions, which are typically between 1 and 100 nm. Certain nanomaterials can self-assemble into intricate structures in reaction to changes in their surroundings, creating novel functions [98]. Based on their composition, stimuli-responsiveness, and application domains, smart and responsive nanomaterials can be broadly categorized, demonstrating their adaptability and multifunctionality in a variety of sectors. They fall into two categories based on composition: inorganic nanomaterials, which include metal oxide and metallic nanoparticles like titanium dioxide and zinc oxide, metallic nanoparticles like gold and silver, quantum dots with size-dependent optical properties, and carbon-based nanomaterials like graphene and carbon nanotubes [158]. Biodegradable and biocompatible polymeric nanoparticles, highly branching dendrimers for gene therapy and medication administration, and lipid-based nanomaterials like liposomes for drug delivery are examples of organic nanomaterials as listed in Table 8.1. How these nanomaterials react to different stimuli can also be used to classify them. Physically stimuli-responsive nanomaterials can be used in targeted drug delivery, photothermal therapy, controlled drug release, and sensors because they respond. Chemically stimuli-responsive nanomaterials are helpful in targeted medication delivery, tissue engineering, and environmental monitoring because they react to changes in pH, oxidative or reductive conditions, or the presence of certain ions. When particular enzymes or antigen/antibody interactions are present, biological stimuli-responsive nanomaterials change their function, allowing for tailored therapy and diagnostics [95].

Nanomaterials can be classified on the basis of application areas. They are utilized in biomedical applications such as drug delivery systems, which transport and release therapeutic compounds in a regulated manner, imaging and diagnostics, which improve contrast or identify biomarkers, and theranostics, which diagnoses and treat diseases at the same time [39]. Smart and responsive nanomaterials are very adaptable in various applications due to their vast range of functions. Regarding medication delivery, these materials can contain therapeutic chemicals and release them at specified body areas, such as tumors, in response to particular stimuli like pH changes, guaranteeing a targeted and accurate course of therapy. Additionally, they provide gradual, regulated medication release, resulting in long-lasting therapeutic benefits [170]. Nanomaterials are used in energy harvesting and storage to improve solar cell efficiency by improving their response to light. They also improve charge/discharge rates and energy density of batteries and supercapacitors [67].

8.3 Functionalization Techniques

For the purpose of fully investigating their potential in the fields of biomedical, nanocomposite, imaging, sensing, energy, electronics, etc., it is essential to regulate how nanomaterials disperse across various matrices and interact with other molecules [133]. This is only possible by appropriately modifying the

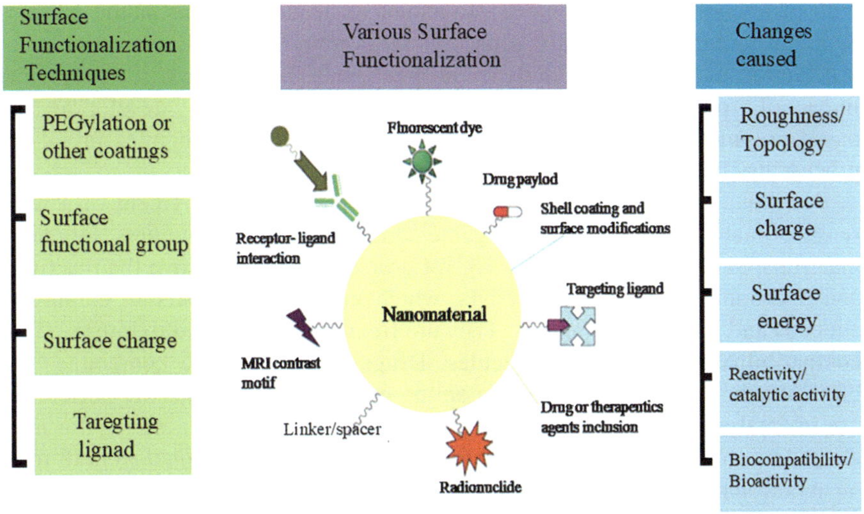

Fig. 8.1 Various types of surface functionalization of nanomaterial and its impact on the characteristics of the molecule

nanomaterials to functionalize their surface, which improves their ability to interact with their surroundings as shown in Fig. 8.1 [86]. The overall functionalization of nanomaterial affects regulated assembly, dispersion, and colloidal stability. The size, shape, and composition of nanomaterials can affect their plasmonic characteristics [166]. This procedure is essential for improving the compatibility, stability, and reactivity of nanomaterials by customizing them for particular uses [73]. Without any surface functionalization, the majority of nanomaterials often agglomerate or exhibit undesirable toxicity. The practice of adding appropriate elements to a nanomaterial's surface to increase its use and decrease its toxicity is known as surface functionalization [46]. Van der Waal's interaction, polymeric, and electrostatic double-layer forces are the main ones that govern nanomaterials generally. To display good stability, the nanomaterials in a colloidal condition should show minimal attractive forces that prevent the breaking of thermal motion. It is accomplished by adding ions or adjusting the pH of the solution to create an electric double layer at the solid-liquid interface. If it is insufficient, it is accomplished by stabilizing the surfactant or adding/functionalizing polymer [60].

There are two ways of functionalization: synthesis and postsynthesis. The intended functional materials are added straight to the process during the nanomaterial production in synthesis or in situ synthesis techniques. For instance, this technique is used in the reduction of auric chloride to create gold nanoparticles using cysteine and tyrosine [166]. Postsynthesis is used to accomplish the majority of surface functionalization. Generally speaking, these postsynthesis techniques fall into the following groups: physical adsorption techniques, grafting, covalent, and noncovalent functionalization [113]. Creating environmentally friendly nanomaterials requires integrating functionalization methods with sustainable practices. In order to reduce its negative effects on the environment, sustainable functionalization uses renewable resources, energy-efficient procedures, and environmentally friendly reagents. For instance, the ecological impact of producing nanomaterials can be greatly decreased by developing bio-based polymers for grafting and using green chemistry principles in sol-gel processing [65].

Functionalizing nanomaterial surfaces involves the employment of a wide range of materials, such as tiny organic compounds, dyes, polymers, inorganic materials, and biomolecules [73, 133]. Carboxyl groups improve the reactivity and hydrophilicity of nanomaterials, which makes them easier to employ in aqueous and biological contexts. They are frequently employed to improve biocompatibility and bind biomolecules. Drugs or other active compounds are often attached to nanomaterials via amino groups. Thiol groups are perfect for use in catalysis and sensor technologies because of their great affinity for metals. Additionally, they make it possible for self-assembled monolayers to form on metal surfaces. Metal oxides and other inorganic materials' surfaces are functionalized by silanes, which create a strong and stable bond for subsequent alterations. When developing hybrid materials with organic-inorganic interfaces, they are indispensable. For improving corrosion resistance and biocompatibility on metal surfaces, phosphate groups are especially helpful to enhance the way implants and bone tissue integrate [73]. For use in medical applications, functionalization of biomolecules can offer strong cellular internalization ability, effective intracellular distribution, stealth qualities, and general biocompatibility [115].

8.3.1 Techniques for Functionalization

8.3.1.1 Covalent Interactions

Covalent functionalization makes it possible to adhere to the surface of the nanomaterial and generate functional groups through covalent bonding. This method offers long-term stability and functionality by guaranteeing that the functional groups stay connected under diverse circumstances. These modifications allow materials to be optimized for a variety of uses, such as biosensors, bioimaging, environmental remediation, packaging, cosmetics, agriculture, and catalysis [86]. Covalent functionalization is frequently used to modify common nanomaterials such as metal oxide nanomaterials, 2D nanomaterials (like GO, CNTs, MoS2, and h-BN) and nanoclays. Organofunctional alkoxysilanes ((3-glycidoxypropyl)-dimethylethoxysilane, (3-aminopropyl)-triethoxysilane (APTES), (3-mercaptopropyl)-trimethoxysilane, etc.), 1-ethyl-3-(3-dimethylaminopropyl) carbodiimide, and glutaraldehyde, N-hydroxysuccinimide Cross linker are the most widely used techniques for covalent functionalization [157]. 2D nanomaterials have been created using a variety of synthetic techniques that focus on their point defects, edges, basal functions, and p-electron clouds, which change sp2 carbon into sp3 carbon [57, 118]. Using thiol chemicals as ligands, a simple method for creating organic functional group–adorned MoS_2 nanosheets was created [169]. By reacting with newly made $LixMoS_2$, thiol ligands such as 1-thioglycerol, mercaptopropionic acid, and L-cysteine were utilized to alter MoS_2. $AgNO_3$ was simply added to a solution of MPA-MoS2 and sodium borohydride to create a MoS_2-Ag nanocomposite. Because carboxylic groups are present, covalently functionalized MoS_2 nanosheets have a high density of nucleation sites [133].

8.3.1.2 Non-covalent Interactions

Numerous artificial and natural systems utilized for interaction, detection, and recognition can readily be shown to have non-covalent interactions [91]. P-P contacts, hydrogen bonding, polymer wrapping, electron donor-acceptor ligand systems, and weak interactions including hydrogen bonding, p-p interactions, and van der Waals interactions are a few examples of non-covalent interactions [21, 122]. Over vast interfaces, the overall effects of noncovalent interactions are similar to those of covalent bonds, even though their energies are lower. The kinetic lability or reversibility of noncovalent functionalization, which produces an auto-correcting system, is an interesting property. By utilizing these interactions, systems can be created that respond well to chemical and physical external stimuli, such as temperature and pH. This is now the basis for how drugs are delivered [36]. The hydrophilic and hydrophobic surface interactions as well as the solvation of nanoparticles are readily influenced by weak forces. Solvents like N-methylpyrrolidone (NMP), phenylethyl alcohol, and N, N-dimethylformamide can be used to create a high density of nanomaterials in the dispersion of 2D nanomaterials such as CNTs, graphene, and h-BN. NMP molecules can penetrate nanosheets during ultrasonication and adsorb to the surface. This adsorption can be readily removed by heating the sample to 340 °C because the NMP was physically adsorbed via van der Waals interactions on the surfaces [36].

8.3.1.3 Electrostatic Interactions

The attraction between functional groups with opposing charges and the surfaces of nanomaterials is known as electrostatic interaction. This method is very helpful for changing a nanomaterial's surface charge, which can affect the material's stability, dispersibility, and interactions with biological systems. Using electrostatic interactions, layer-by-layer assembly is a popular technique for creating multilayered coatings on nanomaterials.

8.3.1.4 Grafting Methods

Grafting is a covalent functionalization approach that is typically used to create polymer brush-coated nanoparticles for adsorption and sensing applications by introducing polymers onto the surface of nanomaterials [57]. Chemical grafting methods can be broadly divided into two categories: "grafting onto" and "grafting from." Attaching monomeric groups to the surface of the nanomaterial is the first step in the "grafting from" technique, which is then followed by in situ polymerization [14, 118]. Because they polymerize quickly, organo-functional silanes such as nipam are frequently utilized in "grafting from" procedures. Polymer chains have grown on nanomaterial surfaces using a range of polymerization processes, such as ring-opening, controlled radical, cationic, and free radical polymerizations [151].

8.3.1.5 Sol-Gel Processing

A flexible method for producing inorganic coatings on nanomaterials is sol-gel processing [71]. Using this technique, metal alkoxides are hydrolyzed and then condensed to create a gel-like network that can be utilized to coat or encapsulate nanoparticles. Sol-gel coatings can improve the optical qualities, chemical resistance, and thermal stability of nanomaterials [30].

8.3.1.6 Plasma Treatment

This method of surface modification involves applying functional groups to the surface of nanomaterials using ionized gases. This technique is beneficial for changing carbon-based and polymeric nanomaterials, offering a safe and efficient alternative to harsh chemicals for changing surface characteristics [28].

8.3.1.7 Self-Assembled Monolayers (SAMs)

Highly organized single level molecular structures known as self-assembled monolayers or SAMs are created when molecules spontaneously. These remarkably organized molecular assemblies are created when functional molecules spontaneously arrange themselves on the surface of nanomaterials. With the help of these monolayers, it is possible to precisely regulate the surface chemistry and design interfaces with certain chemical properties. Since the functionalized surface of SAMs may interact with target molecules in a targeted manner, they are widely used in sensor technology [15].

8.3.2 Impact of Functionalization

Carbon nanotubes are made more biocompatible and dispersible by functionalization so that they can be used in targeted medicine delivery. To add carboxyl groups to the surface of multi-walled carbon nanotubes, a solution of sulfuric and nitric acids is applied. The cytotoxicity of functionalized CNTs is decreased, and their compatibility with biological systems is improved. Drug compounds are conjugated using functionalized carbon nanotubes and then released in a controlled manner to target particular cells or tissues [105]. Gold nanoparticles (AuNPs) are made more stable through functionalization so that they can be used in diagnostic and biosensing applications. After being created, thiol-containing ligands like 11-mercaptoundecanoic acid are used to functionalize AuNPs. PEG chains are used in further modification to improve stability and biocompatibility. To create colorimetric biosensors that can identify biomarkers such as proteins and nucleic acids, functionalized AuNPs are employed [19]. Quantum dot surfaces are modified by functionalization in order to improve their optical characteristics for use in bioimaging. During synthesis, trioctylphosphine oxide is first used to cap QDs. Hydrophilic ligands such as polyethylene glycol or mercaptoundecanoic acid are substituted for these ligands. Biomolecules like peptides and antibodies are attached to ligands using their functional groups. Imaging precision is increased with the selective targeting of biological molecules or cells made possible by bioconjugation. Fluorescence imaging uses functionalized QDs to track biological activities, diagnose illnesses, and track the administration of drugs in real-time [115]. Magnetic nanoparticles (MNPs) to treat hyperthermia and enable targeted drug delivery. To increase MNP stability and biocompatibility, biocompatible polymers like PEG or dextran are coated on them. The polymer coating's functional groups are utilized to bind targeted ligands, like peptides or antibodies. MNPs' magnetic qualities enable the therapy of hyperthermia, which kills cancer cells by causing localized warmth to be generated by an alternating magnetic field. When paired with other therapies to treat cancer, functionalized MNPs have shown improved efficacy in identifying and eliminating tumor cells with no adverse effects [40].

8.4 Processing Approaches

Nanomaterials can be produced using two primary methods: top-down and bottom-up approaches. Additionally, green synthesis is another technique employed for creating nanomaterials. In top-down approaches, larger bulk materials are physically broken down into smaller, nano-sized particles. Conversely, in bottom-up approaches, nanomaterials are constructed by assembling smaller particles through processes such as self-assembly or co-precipitation [143].

8.4.1 Ball Milling

Ball milling is a mechanical technique (top-down approach) of processing nanomaterials. In this method, materials are placed in a sealed container and ground using small pebbles made of glass, ceramics, or stainless steel, which generate shear forces [32]. Factors that influence the dispersion of nanotubes include the size of the pebbles, the rotational speed, the duration of milling, and the quantity of nanotubes used. As a result, nanotubes smaller than 100 nm can be produced through grinding. This method transforms carbon nanotubes into fine carbon nanostructures while causing minimal damage to their surfaces [61]. Increasing the milling speed can be achieved by modifying the surface of single-walled carbon nanotubes (SWCNTs) with alkyl or aryl groups. High-energy ball milling can create metastable materials while maintaining thermal equilibrium. This technique differs from traditional ball milling methods, which do not generate enough energy for effective milling. This method can be used to create metallic hydrides and nitrides, which have crucial properties for various applications. Their hardness and stability make them suitable for cutting tools and tool coatings in microelectronics, such as titanium nitride (TiN) alloy [150]. In this technique, bulk metallic powder is placed in a sealed container filled with nitrogen gas and then subjected to high-energy ball milling that generates high pressure [13]. This process breaks down the metallic powders into tiny particles while creating oxygen-free active surfaces on the nanomaterials [124]. The ball-milling method offers several advantages: it can produce fine powders, is suitable for milling toxic materials, and can handle abrasive substances. However, it also has drawbacks, such as contamination from wear and tear of the milling balls, increased noise when the cylinder is metal (though this is reduced with a rubber cylinder), and a relatively long processing time [33].

8.4.2 *Physical Vapor Deposition (PVD)*

This process takes place in a vacuum chamber, maintained at approximately 10^{-6} Torr, using a cathodic-arc source [42]. Reactive PVD is a technique for depositing metal onto a surface while introducing reactive gases like oxygen, nitrogen, or methane into the vacuum chamber. A high-energy plasma beam then bombards the metal surface, resulting in a hard and dense coating. This method allows for the synthesis of nanoparticles and the fabrication of nanocomposites [141]. Thin film formation involves metal ions transitioning from the vapor phase to the condensed phase, where they then form the thin film. PVD involves both evaporation and sputtering techniques to create thin films. In this process, sputtering occurs in the vapor phase under conditions of super-saturation [3]. The benefits of PVD techniques include (i) enhanced properties of the deposited films compared to the substrate material and (ii) the use of inorganic and some organic materials, making it a more environmentally friendly option compared to electroplating [81]. This technique also has some challenges, difficulty in coating complex structures, high costs and low production efficiency, and overall complexity of the process [110].

8.4.3 *Lithography*

Lithography is a printing process where an image is created by applying ink to a stamp, which is then used to transfer the image onto a substrate [76]. The stamp used in lithography has both hydrophobic and hydrophilic areas. The hydrophobic regions attract and hold the ink, while the hydrophilic areas do not. This process typically reproduces a pattern that mirrors the pattern on the substrate [90]. There are two types of masks used for surface patterning: positive and negative. A positive photoresist becomes soluble when exposed to light, while a negative photoresist remains insoluble and hardens, making it more rigid [69, 70]. Various types of lithography are employed for surface patterning, including photolithography, UV-lithography, e-beam lithography, soft lithography, scanning probe lithography, and nanolithography [126]. Photolithography is a light-based method where an image is projected onto a photoresist layer coated on a substrate, such as a silicon wafer [121]. This technique is commonly used in the nano-electronics industry for patterning semiconductors. UV-lithography employs specific wavelengths of ultraviolet light to achieve sub-micron-level patterning in the photoresist [31]. When exposed to UV light, the solubility of the developer solution changes. The UV light causes photo-crosslinking in the photoresist, which leads to the hardening of the exposed areas. The unreacted parts of the photoresist are then removed through etching [160]. One of the drawbacks of this technique is the generation of free radicals during the photo-curing process, as well as potential DNA damage that can occur during photo-initiation. E-beam lithography is a technique that uses scanning electron beams to pattern a surface directly, without the need for a mask. This method can achieve accuracy levels of less than 1 nanometer [6]. The two main methods for scanning an electron beam are raster scanning and vector scanning. Raster scanning breaks an image into pixels and prints them in a sequence from left to right or top to bottom. In contrast, vector scanning involves the beam moving across the entire surface, including areas without features [41]. Soft lithography is a technique that employs an elastomeric stamp to transfer ink onto a substrate. It offers several benefits compared to other patterning methods, such as lower cost, easier setup, and higher throughput. This method can achieve a wide range of resolutions, from nanometers to micrometers, for patterning the substrate [162]. One drawback of the soft lithography method is that it necessitates the use of another lithography technique to create the stamp master. However, once the stamp is made, it can be used repeatedly to pattern surfaces [135]. Scanning probe lithography involves scanning the surface to create an image and then making modifications with atomic-level precision. This technique uses a probe similar to those used in atomic force microscopy (AFM) and scanning tunneling microscopy (STM) [129]. For instance, this technique can be used to create graphene nanoribbons by catalyzing graphene oxide with hydrogen, using a platinum-coated AFM tip. It achieves a resolution ranging from 20 to 80 nanometers [167]. One advantage of scanning probe lithography is its ability to create features of any shape or pattern on non-flat surfaces [85]. Additionally, this technique is straightforward to use in non-denaturing solution environments and allows for direct observation of protein binding events. Integrated circuits with nano-patterning have been created using micro and nano-lithography methods [103]. Lithography is followed by deposition and etching to achieve high-resolution patterns. There are two main types of lithography: masked and mask-less. Photolithography is an example of masked lithography, while e-beam lithography is a type of mask-less lithography.

8.4.4 Sol-Gel Method

Sol-gel is a common method for preparing nanoparticles, involving condensation and hydrolysis reactions. Heat treatment is applied during intermediate synthesis to ensure the nanoparticles become crystalline [131]. Alkoxides are used as precursors to create oxide nanoparticles. These nanoparticles interact through molecular forces like van der Waals forces or hydrogen bonding and are dispersed in a sol via evaporation or condensation [75]. The alkoxide precursor undergoes hydrolysis in the presence of a base or acid, forming a polymeric gel. The final product's characteristics depend on the rates of condensation and hydrolysis [58]. For instance, producing smaller nanoparticles requires a slower hydrolysis rate. This process is ideal for synthesizing composites, oxides, and ceramic nanoparticles, ensuring high purity and uniform distribution [130]. The sol-gel method has advantages over traditional oxide fusion methods. For example, xerogel nanocomposites of iron or silica can be produced by mixing iron (III) nitrate with TEOS in a sol-gel formulation. Ferric iron is then reduced to metallic iron using hydrogen gas at temperatures between 400 °C and 700 °C. Xerogel's applications include pressing the nanocomposite into pellets on glass slides for electrical or magnetic conductivity [87]. The sol-gel method offers the advantage of producing high-purity and uniformly nanostructured materials at low temperatures, with ligands acting as capping agents. However, a significant drawback is the high level of impurities from reaction by-products, which require post-treatment to remove [156].

8.4.5 Chemical Vapor Deposition Method (CVD)

Chemical vapor deposition (CVD) is a vacuum-based process used to produce high-quality, high-performance solid materials [152]. In this method, thin films are deposited on a substrate through chemical reactions between substances like organometallic compounds and other gases [82]. The uniqueness of CVD lies in its multidirectional deposition method to coat substrates, unlike PVD, which uses a line-of-sight impingement method [74]. CVD is widely used to deposit materials in various forms, including crystalline, amorphous, and epitaxial growth, during the micro-fabrication process [117]. In chemical vapor deposition (CVD), gases react chemically on the surface of a material, causing a chemical breakdown that results in a thick coating forming on the base of the material [112]. For instance, diamond crystals can be applied to silicon or molybdenum surfaces using the CVD method. Charged diamond nanoparticles can be created through the hot filament chemical vapor deposition (HFCVD) technique. These nanoparticles are then collected using floating and grounded substrates [89]. Substrates used include SiO, graphene membranes on copper TEM grids, and carbon. Various types of diamond allotropes are recognized, including hexagonal and cubic diamonds, i-carbon, and n-diamond particles [78]. Diamond nanoparticles can be analyzed using Raman spectroscopy, which reveals a distinct peak at approximately 1332 cm^{-1} [128]. The CVD process has the benefits of creating high-purity thin films and forming sharp junctions. However, its drawbacks include variability in the final product depending on the precursor properties and issues with uniformity [153].

8.4.6 Chemical Co-precipitation Method

The chemical co-precipitation method involves combining two different salts in an aqueous solution, typically a base, which leads to the formation of a precipitate [8]. For instance, magnetic nanoparticles (MNPs) are traditionally prepared using the

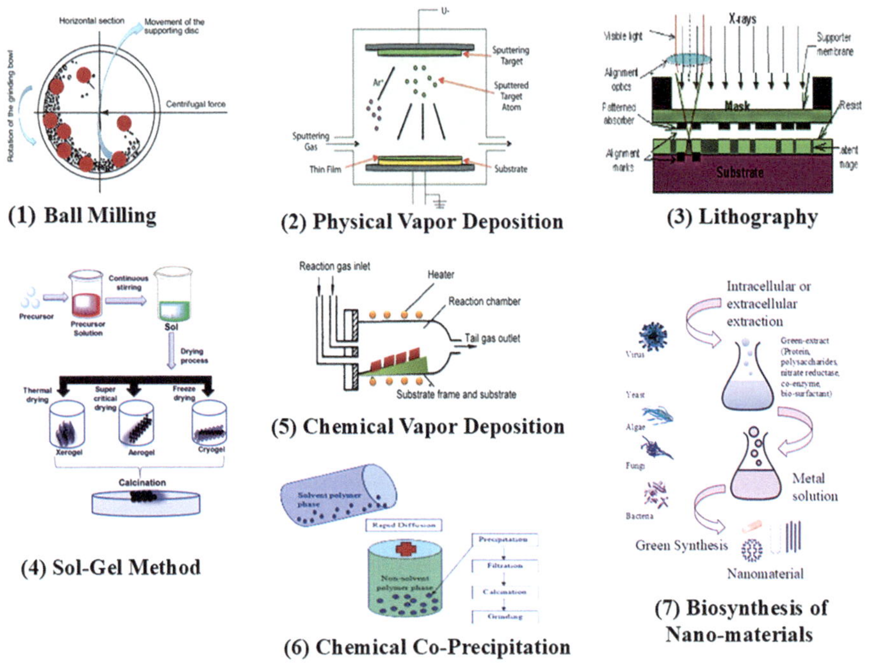

Fig. 8.2 Different approaches of nanomaterial processing

chemical co-precipitation method. This process involves mixing Fe^{2+} and Fe^{3+} salts in a NaOH solution [7]. Factors like morphology, size, and composition can be adjusted by modifying the pH, temperature, ligands, precursor salts, and chemical ratios [49]. The nanoparticles are stabilized by incorporating suitable stabilizers such as surfactants (e.g., oleic acid), ligands (e.g., aptamers), polymers (e.g., poly (ethylene glycol acrylate)) and inorganic molecules (e.g., NaOH) [16]. This method can be used to synthesize complex metals. For instance, iron-chromite is produced by mixing iron (III) salt with chromate. In an aqueous solution, these salts form metal ions, which are then precipitated using an ammonium base. The precipitate is subsequently heated to a high temperature to produce iron (III) chromite [155]. The chemical species produced by co-precipitation methods are typically insoluble and consist of small particles. Their insolubility results from the high level of supersaturation during the synthesis process [120]. Particle size can range from small to large. Larger particles typically form during the nucleation process. Factors influencing the size of the particles include aggregation and Ostwald ripening [63]. The co-precipitation method offers several advantages: it is straightforward, allows for control over particle size based on their composition, enables modification of particle surfaces with various functionalities, requires low temperatures for synthesis, avoids the use of organic solvents, and is energy-efficient [92]. The main drawbacks of this method include limitations on incorporating uncharged species, potential presence of impurities during precipitation, time consumption, inconsistent reproducibility, and sensitivity to the precipitation rate [106]. Figure 8.2 outlines various top-down and bottom-up approaches for synthesizing nanomaterials.

8.4.7 Biosynthesis of Nanomaterials

Biosynthesis of nanomaterials is an environmentally friendly, green, cost-effective, non-toxic, and efficient method for producing various nanoparticles. This approach uses biological systems such as yeast, bacteria, fungi, viruses, plant extracts, and actinomycetes to synthesize nanomaterials, including metal nanoparticles, metal sulfides, metal oxides, and carbon-based materials [44]. These nanomaterials are highly biocompatible, which is essential for their use in the biomedical industry. Plant biometabolites act as reducers and stabilizers and employ these in the production of nanoparticles [45]. Plant extracts contain various compounds such as amino acids, tannic acid, citric acid, tartaric acid, terpenoids, dehydrogenase, polyols, proteins, reducing sugars, and flavonoids. Shankar et al. reported using leaf extract from *Azadirachta indica* to synthesize silver (Ag), gold (Au), and core-shell gold-silver (Au–Ag) nanoparticles [140]. Seraphin et al. utilized *Aloe vera* extract to synthesize indium oxide (In_2O_3) nanoparticles with sizes ranging from 5 to 50 nm [125]. Other plant extracts have also been employed to produce nanoparticles of palladium (Pd) and platinum (Pt) [29, 138]. Significant research has been conducted to produce various nanoparticles by utilizing microorganisms as bioreactors. Microorganisms transform target ions into metal nanoparticles through enzymes produced during their cellular processes. *Lactobacillus* can serve as both a capping and reducing agent for the non-enzymatic synthesis of silver nanoparticles (AgNPs). Additionally, marine yeast (*Rhodosporidium diobovatum*) was used to biosynthesize lead sulfide nanoparticles (PbSNPs) [146]. Likewise, other researchers have reported the production of Fe_3O_4, SiO_2, and TiO_2 nanoparticles using different types of fungi [10, 12]. Biosynthesis is generally slower compared to other techniques and may not always produce nanoparticles with the exact shape, size, and morphology desired. Additionally, over time, biosynthesized nanoparticles may undergo decomposition.

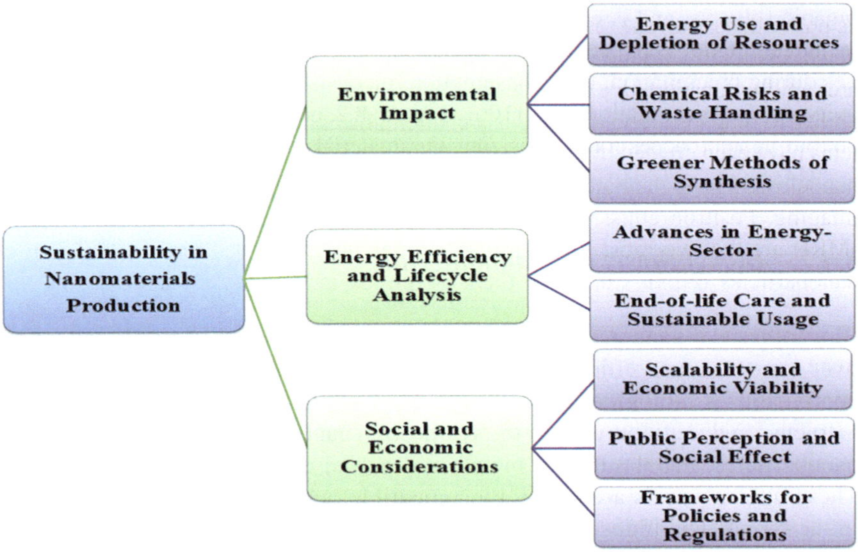

Fig. 8.3 Sustainability in nanomaterial production

8.5 Sustainability in Nanomaterials Production

The production of nanomaterials has significant environmental, social, and economic implications [109]. Conventional synthesis methods often require high energy and raw material inputs, leading to resource depletion, carbon emissions, and hazardous by-products that can contaminate ecosystems if not properly managed. To address these challenges, researchers are exploring eco-friendly synthesis techniques, such as biological processes using plant extracts, which minimize harmful chemicals and energy use as listed in Fig. 8.3. Recycling and reusing nanomaterials, coupled with advancements in energy-efficient methods like ultrasonic and microwave-aided synthesis, can further enhance sustainability [1]. Additionally, fostering fair labor practices, ensuring worker safety, and building public trust through transparent processes are critical for the broader acceptance and responsible development of nanomaterials [25].

8.5.1 Environmental Impact of Nanomaterials

The production of nanomaterials has significant environmental implications, primarily due to energy-intensive manufacturing processes, chemical risks, and waste generation. Conventional techniques like sol-gel processes, physical vapor deposition (PVD), and chemical vapor deposition (CVD) require substantial energy inputs, often derived from non-renewable sources, which increase carbon emissions and contribute to environmental degradation [35]. For example, the production of carbon nanotubes (CNTs) via CVD involves high temperatures and prolonged reaction times, leading to excessive energy consumption. Additionally, the extraction of raw materials, such as rare earth elements, exacerbates resource depletion and ecological disruption. The chemical processes involved in nanomaterial synthesis often utilize hazardous substances, generating toxic by-products and waste that, if improperly managed, can contaminate soil and water, threatening ecosystems and public health. For instance, heavy metals used in quantum dot synthesis result in difficult-to-handle hazardous effluents [145]. To mitigate these issues, sustainable practices such as improving process efficiency, using renewable energy, and adopting green chemistry principles—like non-toxic and biodegradable materials—are critical. Furthermore, efficient waste management and recycling strategies can reduce the ecological footprint of nanomaterials. Greener synthesis methods, including biological approaches that leverage fungi, bacteria, or plant extracts, offer a promising alternative. These methods not only minimize energy consumption and eliminate the need for toxic chemicals but also enhance the scalability and sustainability of nanomaterial production, presenting a holistic solution to reduce environmental impact.

8.5.2 Energy Efficiency and Lifecycle Analysis

Advances in nanomaterial synthesis and end-of-life management are crucial for enhancing their sustainability and minimizing environmental impact, particularly in the energy sector. Traditional synthesis methods often require high temperatures and prolonged reaction times, leading to excessive energy consumption. However, innovative techniques like microwave-assisted and ultrasonic-assisted synthesis offer energy-efficient alternatives. Microwave-assisted synthesis utilizes microwave radiation to uniformly heat reactants, reducing reaction times and energy needs, while ultrasonic-assisted synthesis employs high-frequency sound waves to accelerate chemical reactions with similar benefits [97]. These advanced methods not only improve energy efficiency but also enhance the quality and uniformity of nanomaterials, making them suitable for broader applications. To evaluate and optimize the sustainability of nanomaterials, a comprehensive life cycle assessment (LCA) is essential. LCA examines the environmental impact at every stage of a product's lifecycle, from raw material extraction to disposal, identifying areas for improvement such as resource usage, waste management, and recycling processes.

Equally important is the sustainable usage and end-of-life care of nanomaterials. Incorporating nanomaterials into products to enhance their performance and longevity, such as in renewable energy systems like solar cells and batteries, can contribute to overall energy sustainability. At the end of their lifecycle, effective recycling and disposal strategies are vital to prevent environmental contamination cycle [2]. Developing methods to extract valuable components from nanomaterials can reduce waste and the demand for virgin resources. Additionally, designing nanomaterials with biodegradability in mind can prevent their long-term persistence in the environment, further improving sustainability. Together, these advancements and practices can ensure that nanomaterials are utilized and managed in an environmentally responsible manner.

8.5.3 Social and Economic Considerations

Sustainable nanomaterial production requires addressing scalability, economic viability, public perception, social impact, and regulatory frameworks. Traditional manufacturing methods are often costly and difficult to scale, limiting accessibility and affordability [104]. Economies of scale in large-scale production facilities, combined with investments in research and development to optimize green synthesis techniques, can significantly reduce costs and enhance economic viability. Ensuring the affordability and scalability of sustainable nanomaterials is essential for broad adoption across industries, driving sustainability goals and promoting innovation [137]. Public perception and social impact also play a critical role in the acceptance of nanomaterials. Transparent safety evaluations, adherence to fair labor standards, and public education on the benefits and risks of nanomaterials are essential to building trust. Highlighting their environmental advantages, such as enhanced performance in renewable energy systems, can further improve public opinion [5]. Engaging stakeholders, including communities, regulators, and industries, is vital to addressing societal concerns and fostering an environment conducive to the sustainable development of nanomaterials [11].

Regulatory and policy frameworks are indispensable for promoting sustainable practices in nanomaterial production. Governments and regulatory agencies must establish standards to ensure the safe and environmentally friendly manufacturing of nanomaterials resources [148]. Regulations encouraging the use of biodegradable and non-toxic chemicals can incentivize the adoption of green synthesis methods, such as biological processes that utilize microbes or plant extracts. Policies that support sustainable practices through incentives for research and development can accelerate innovation and commercialization, reducing environmental impact while enhancing scalability and economic viability [43].

A holistic approach combining green synthesis innovations, lifecycle analyses, and robust policy frameworks is crucial for minimizing the environmental impact of nanomaterials while maximizing their societal benefits [149]. As the demand for nanomaterials grows, prioritizing sustainability will ensure their long-term viability, public acceptance, and performance in addressing global challenges. This integrated strategy underscores the importance of environmentally responsible production practices to achieve economic, social, and ecological goals in the evolving nanotechnology landscape [48].

Table 8.2 Nanomaterials and their functionalization with application in healthcare and diagnostics

S. No.	Nanomaterial	Functionalization	Elements	Absorption (nm)	Size (nm)	Application	References
1	Quantum dot	Protein (BSA)	CdTe, BSA CdS,	Nex = 450 nm Aem = 529 to 649 nm	~539	For long-term fluorescence monitoring, QD-BSA was used because exposure to 365 nm radiation caused an emission reduction of 4.06%	[165]
2	Quantum dot	Core/Shell-ZnS	ZnS, CdSe	580 nm	<10.1	Integrated Cd109-SPECT imaging agent for tumor identification through imaging and diagnosis	[22]
3	Carbon quantum dot	Amino groups, carboxy	Citric acid, tetraminoanthraquinone (TAAQ), and large amino acid mimicking (LAAM)	228 nm, 279 nm, 649 mm	~3.5	LAT-1-mediated tumor theranostics targeting	[96]
4	Quantum dot	Mercapto-succinic acid	P, Zn, P, In	646	15.2–20.4	This QD is based on non-cadmium and is used in diagnostic imaging to help spot cancer early	[159]
5	Quantum dot	Molic acid linked with chitosan biopolymer	ZnS, Mn	288	218	Diagnosis and management of 5-fluorouracil's anticancer efficacy in breast cancer therapy	[139]
6	Nanorod	CTAB, citrate	Au	780–810 nm	2.7–4	In the field of theranostics, lung cancer cells are treated with petawatt (PW) lasers as opposed to continuous wave (CW) lasers. A laser energy of 19 mJ/cm2 was employed	[27]

(continued)

Table 8.2 (continued)

S. No.	Nanomaterial	Functionalization	Elements	Absorption (nm)	Size (nm)	Application	References
7	Nanowire	Silicon nanowire adorned with gold nanoparticles	Si, Au	528 nm	–	When exposed to NIR radiation, AuNP@SiNW functions as a NIR hyperthermia agent and kills cancer cells in 3 min	[84]
8	Nanowire	Antibody, biotin	Magnetic polypyrrole, antibody, PEI		10.2	The recovery of uncommon circulating biomarkers using magnetic nanowires enhances cancer prognostic and diagnostic capabilities	[64]
9	Nanorod	Gd@AuNRs functionalized by PEG	Au, Gd	>748 nm	20.3–40.4	Gd@AuNRs functions as a potent theranostics agent for MIAPaCa-2 cell imaging and therapy regarding the utilization of NIR, 808 lasers with MRI T1 features at 7T	[9]
10	Nanorod	Functionalized AuNRs using nanoparticles of silica	Si, Au	AuNRs~589 nm Au@ SiNRs~728 nm Au-Janus~649 nm	3–4.4 aspect ratio	Drugs and imaging agents are delivered by Au@Si-Janus nanoparticles. Furthermore, it is helpful for combining photothermotherapy and chemotherapy for cancer	[56]
11	MXenes		Ti_3C_2	800.0	559	MXene has 100% efficiency in PTT as a material that converts light to heat	[93]

12	Nanosheets	PEG	Graphdiyne	700.0	355	In PAI and PTT for the treatment of cancer, GDY-PEG functions as a photothermal-acoustic wave transducer	[142]
13	Nanosheets	Tannic acid	Boron nitride	656	99.68	Theranostics with T1-weighted configuration based on the TA-Fe coordinated complex on a boron nitride nanosheet. Additionally, it helps with MRI-guided phototherapy	[94]
14	Nanosheets	PEG	Gd	709–849	100–150.6	MoSe2 functions as a photothermal agent in cancer therapy, whereas Gd offers T1-weighted MR-imaging	[53]
15	Nanosheets	PEG, DOX, BPEI	Graphene	–	50.2	In the context of UCL image-driven combinatorial PTT and chemotherapy for cancer treatment, graphene oxide nanocomposites function as theranostics agents. Using a 13.5 photothermal conversion efficiency NIR laser at 980 nm are used	[123]

8.6 Application of Smart Nanomaterials in Pharmaceuticals and Diagnosis

8.6.1 Multifunctional Drug Delivery System

Smart materials have emerged as a versatile and rapidly evolving field, especially in biological and medical applications. Recent advancements have significantly impacted medical research, particularly with stimuli-responsive nanoparticles (NPs). Nanoparticles show exceptional promise in diagnosing and treating various diseases as shown in Table 8.2 [119]. $CoFe_2O_4$-$BaTiO_3$ nanoparticles were used to treat Parkinson's disease [164]. Additionally, these nanoparticles have been applied in anti-HIV drug delivery and for paclitaxel delivery in ovarian cancer therapy. Lipid-assisted solid nanomaterials are gaining attention as a multifunctional drug delivery system. A recent study suggested that iron oxide nanoparticles encapsulated with the medication sorafenib in a lipid matrix demonstrated magnetically driven aggregation against hepatocarcinoma tissues in vitro, indicating a potential for localized treatment [52]. Similarly, a combination of inorganic and polymeric nanomaterials has been used for multimodal imaging of breast cancer tissues, enabling more precise imaging through magnetic resonance and luminescence [26]. The literature suggests that stimuli-responsive nanomaterials, such as $CoFe_2O_4$-$BaTiO_3$ and polymeric lipid matrices, have a significant impact on multifunctional drug delivery systems and the detection and treatment of various diseases.

8.6.2 Tissue Engineering

In recent developments, tissue engineering has seen a significant impact from advanced nanoparticles (NPs) at the nanoscale level. NPs are highly effective in regenerative medicine due to their low contrast behavior, minimal hazards, and stimuli-responsive properties. Modern technology leverages various NPs across a wide range of applications, including biological devices, photovoltaic devices, and sensors as shown in Fig. 8.4. Notably, gold nanoparticles (AuNPs) have shown great promise due to their exceptional light interaction properties. Monodisperse spherical gold NPs were first produced in 1951 [79]. In regenerative medicine, gold NPs can be used as an alternative when transplanted cells are rejected due to tumor progression. For instance, AuNPs can disrupt cancer cell division by delivering materials directly into the nucleus of affected cells. One such study demonstrated this by creating polyethylene glycol (PEG)-coated AuNPs, mixing nuclear localization signal peptides with arginine-glycine-aspartic acid [72]. Silver nanoparticles (AgNPs), colloids of nanometer-sized silver particles, are extensively used in the biomedical field due to their antibacterial properties. AgNPs with diameters of 1–10 nm could

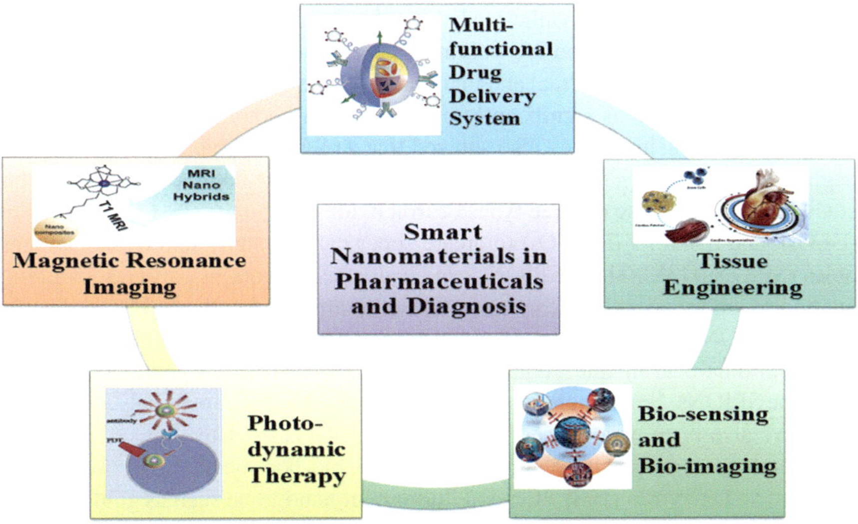

Fig. 8.4 Smart nanomaterials in pharmaceuticals and medicine

affect gram-negative bacteria by binding to cell membranes, altering respiration and permeability, entering the bacteria, causing damage, and releasing silver ions [114]. One study demonstrated that AgNPs with diameters around 5 nm exhibit antibacterial activity against both gram-positive and gram-negative microorganisms [54]. Recent research has also highlighted the use of poly (lactic-co-glycolic acid) (PLGA), an aliphatic polyester made of PGA and PLA with strong mechanical properties, variable degradation rates, and biocompatibility. PLGA-based composites are now employed in dental tissue engineering to suppress bacterial infection and guide tissue regeneration [55]. Additionally, a team of researchers developed a nondestructive technique for coating monodisperse silica nanoparticles on polyvinyl chloride, polyethylene, and polystyrene surfaces [17]. Their experimental results showed that silica NPs significantly reduced bacterial attachments and prevented biofilm formation, indicating enhanced surface roughness and antibacterial properties.

8.6.3 Bio-sensing and Bio-imaging

Bio-sensing and bio-imaging are crucial for studying molecular and pathological processes in living systems (Fig. 8.4). Recently, various nanomaterials and hybrid nanomaterials have shown significant potential in medical and biomedical applications by enhancing bio-sensing and bio-imaging devices for treating incurable diseases. A study developed an optical device using carboxy-methylcellulose (CMC) enhanced with ZnS fluorescent quantum dots (ZnS-QDs) [23]. The ZnS@CMC hybrid nanomaterial was synthesized through a one-step colloidal process, with CMC acting as a pH-responsive polymer. The cyto-compatibility of ZnS@CMC was tested in vitro using normal and malignant glioma cells, revealing that synthesis parameter modifications significantly influenced the photoluminescence emission energies and intensities. They also showed that ZnS@CMC nanohybrids exhibited negligible cytotoxicity, with a 90% cell survival rate for both cell types. Another study discussed the use of three types of iron oxides magnetite (Fe_3O_4), maghemite (Fe_2O_3), and hematite (α-Fe_2O_3) to create super-paramagnetic iron oxide nanoparticles (SPIONs) [38]. These SPIONs can be attached to various particles, including antibodies, and used as drug carriers in cancer treatment. Another explored the efficacy of SPIONs in stem cell tracking [77]. They used MRI to monitor labeled stem cells in glioma-bearing mice, confirming the successful tracking and low cytotoxicity of the SPIONs. Smart materials like photonic crystals, nanomaterials, and hydrogels have also been widely used for bio-sensing. Glucose detection systems often incorporate glucose-sensing elements such as phenyl-boronic acid, glucose-binding proteins, and enzymes [108]. Blended fluorescent nanoprobe such as gold nanoparticles (AuNPs) and quantum dots (QDs) can be used as a Forster resonance energy transfer pair to detect viral RNA in real-time. This construct shows significant quenching of QD emission due to the proximity of AuNPs to QDs, with a notable increase in fluorescence intensity when new viral RNA is present. This enabled the QD-AuNP probe to track viral RNA replication, crucial for understanding virus pathogenesis. In another study, Huang and coworkers designed a highly sensitive plasmonic biosensor for DNA detection. Using symmetrical DNA frames, they created pyramid formations that reconfigured or dissociated in the presence of target DNA, turning circular dichroism signals on or off. This allowed for the detection of target DNA at molar levels without amplification techniques. These studies demonstrate the significant impact of nanomaterials and hybrid nanoparticles, such as ZnS@CMC and SPIONs, in clinical applications. Future research should focus on developing new nanoparticles for detecting acute diseases, which could further advance bio-sensing and bio-imaging technologies.

8.6.4 Photodynamic Therapy

Photodynamic therapy (PDT) can greatly benefit from nanostructured delivery systems for photosensitizers. Firstly, these systems increase the amount of dye delivered to target cells due to their high surface-to-volume ratio. Secondly, they prevent premature release of the dyes before reaching the target, ensuring higher specific accumulation in target cells and thereby reducing side effects. Thirdly, the dyes, once bound to nanostructures, face minimal obstacles in the bloodstream and become amphiphilic, enhancing their ability to form tumors. The increased permeability and retention effect further promote the accumulation of nano-sized compounds in tumor tissues. Lastly, the surfaces of these nanostructures can be functionalized with various groups to tailor their surface chemistry, pharmacokinetics, cell absorption, and biodistribution for specific applications [102]. Quantum dots are another promising material for photodynamic therapy. For instance, the growth of tumor cells decreased from 35% to 20% with a 1.8 M concentration of graphene quantum dots, similar to results achieved with ZnO quantum dots illuminated with blue light. Silica nanoparticles are often used due to their non-toxic nature, optical transparency, and ease of surface functionalization. Silica can act as a carrier for photosensitizers, protecting them from enzymatic degradation and improving their penetration into tumors [83]. Recently, radio-sensitizers or scintillating materials have been used in X-ray-driven PDT. High-Z elements are particularly effective at capturing X-ray photons and converting them into visible light and electrons. Common scintillators include nanoparticles of high-Z elements doped with rare earth components, useful in clinical imaging and high-power physics. These materials can be found as metal-organic frameworks (MOFs), films, vitro-ceramics, coordination compounds, and hybrid organic-inorganic materials, with coatings, defects, media interaction, and nanometric size affecting their scintillation properties. MOFs consist of clusters or metallic ions and bridging linkers, mainly organic polydentate, that self-assemble into nanoscale structures. Depending on the application, MOFs can be decomposable, providing a significant advantage over other nanoparticles. The variety of available organic linkers and metallic elements allows nearly any structure to be created. However, selecting the elements according to the desired application is crucial for optimal results. The use of MOFs in medicine is still in its early stages, requiring further biological characterization, pharmacokinetics, and pharmacodynamics studies before clinical trials [99, 136]. To explore lanthanides as scintillators, Dou et al. [37] produced upconversion nanoparticles (UCNs) ($NaYF_4$, Yb, Tm) covalently coupled with chlorine to prevent premature release of the photosensitizer [37]. They tested these in vitro, finding that the nanoparticles outperformed the free photosensitizer even at low concentrations, with efficacy adjustable by changing the Ce-UCN dosage and light intensity. BaFBr: Barium Fluoride Bromide), generally impregnated with Europium is a generally used high-potential photostimulable storage phosphor, particularly in medical X-ray imaging plates (IPs) and computed radiography [147]. When exposed to 3 Gy of X-rays, the nanomaterials produced luminescence similar to the photosensitizer's irradiation wavelengths, resulting in a photodynamic effect that damaged mitochondrial DNA, killed prostate cancer cells, and caused high oxidative stress in vitro.

8.6.5 Magnetic Resonance Imaging

Nanomaterial-based MRI contrast agents have garnered significant attention in the past decade. These agents offer promising new platforms for enhancing the sensitivity and resolution of MRI in various biomedical applications due to their high payload capacity, enhanced accumulation at disease sites, and large surface area for further modification with targeting ligands. T1-based agents quickly became a prominent research topic in MRI due to their positive contrast, which mitigates issues related to signal decline. Super-paramagnetic iron oxide nanoparticles (SPIONs) were the first to demonstrate improved MRI sensitivity, sparking a surge of interest in developing finer nanoscale MRI contrast agents. Quantum dots (2–6 nm in diameter) are also of interest for imaging due to their strong phosphorescence, narrow emission spectrum, and fluorescence. Incorporating these semiconductor nanocrystals into the design of Gd-chelated nanomaterials achieves multimodal utility for both fluorescence microscopy and MRI. A team of researchers developed quantum dots with Gd chelates and a PEG-lipid coating (PQDs), transforming them into bimodal molecular imaging probes [116]. The PEGylated lipid coating protected the contrast compounds from interacting with plasma proteins, resulting in slower hepatic clearance. PQDs exhibited a T1 relaxivity of over 12 mM/s, three times greater than small molecular Gd chelates. Functionalizing PQDs with the RGD peptide sequence could create a cell adherence epitope, useful for identifying angiogenesis, a key pathological process in atherosclerosis and cancer [51]. These particles served as excellent drug carriers (with loading efficacies around 97.5% and 62.3%) and photothermal agents, and they had high relaxivity (7.43 m/s) in tumor sites at pH 5.0. These pH-sensitive nanoplatforms could deliver both Mn and doxorubicin (DOX) to the tumor simultaneously. The favorable correlation between DOX release and MRI intensity allowed for controlled drug release. Combining significant NIR absorbance with DOX treatment resulted in a synergistic chemo-thermal therapy that enhanced tumor therapeutic effectiveness. Feridex, with a diameter of 120–180 nm, was the first FDA-approved commercial product for detecting liver lesions and was administered intravenously via slow diffusion. Their results demonstrated the viability of using Feridex to track stem-cell engraftment and migration non-invasively via MRI. Studies suggest that various nanomaterials and hybrid materials, including SPIONs, Gd, and Feridex, have been successfully employed in human trials for detecting liver diseases and brain trauma. Future research should focus on discovering and developing new hybrid nanomaterials for diverse medical applications beyond the currently available options.

8.7 Challenges and Future Prospective

As discussed in the chapter, significant advancements have been made in synthesizing various smart materials in response to specific stimuli. However, several challenges remain that need to be addressed to improve their applications in the future. For instance, efforts must be made to develop thermosensitive smart nanomaterials for enhanced adaptability in cancer treatments and chronic diseases like diabetes, which require frequent dosing. The degradation of electric smart materials due to repetitive stresses is another significant issue. Therefore, the development of robust electro-responsive smart nanomaterials should be a priority for future applications. Additionally, pH-dependent nanostructures with programmable size variations could be highly beneficial for future biomedical applications, including diagnostics and tumor imaging. Developing photo-responsive smart nanomaterials for deep cancer treatments and fluorescence imaging also requires NIR-absorptive materials within a large biological window region. A critical issue in therapeutic investigations is the accumulation and aggregation of nanomaterials in non-targeted sites such as the kidney, liver, and spleen. This is mainly because most nanomaterials cannot effectively overcome biological barriers. Thus, more emphasis should be placed on creating smart nanomaterials that can bypass these barriers, reducing the negative effects of nanodrugs. Recently, dual or multi-responsive stimuli smart nanomaterials have garnered significant attention for their potential inefficient therapies. Compared to single-stimulus responsive materials, multi-stimulus nanomaterials offer more functionalities and allow for finer modulation through multiple parameters. Overall, smart, efficient, flexible, and multi-responsive stimuli at a single site hold great promise for the future.

8.8 Conclusion

The development of smart and responsive sustainable nanomaterials represents a significant breakthrough in the field of material science, offering a multitude of applications across diverse industries. The innovative functionalization techniques developed in recent years have enabled researchers to impart unique properties to nanomaterials, making them highly adaptable and efficient. These advanced functionalization methods, combined with sustainable processing approaches, have paved the way for creating materials that not only perform exceptionally but also adhere to environmental standards. The integration of green chemistry principles into the production processes has minimized the ecological footprint, promoting a more sustainable approach to nanomaterial fabrication. This alignment with environmental goals is crucial as industries seek to balance technological advancements with ecological responsibility. One of the most remarkable features of these nanomaterials is their multifunctionality and responsiveness. These characteristics allow nanomaterials to respond dynamically to external stimuli, such as changes in temperature, pH, or magnetic fields. This adaptability makes them particularly valuable in applications such as smart sensors, targeted drug delivery systems, and environmental monitoring tools. For instance, in the healthcare sector, responsive nanomaterials can revolutionize drug delivery by releasing therapeutic agents precisely at the target site, thereby maximizing efficacy and minimizing side effects. Furthermore, the potential applications of smart and responsive nanomaterials extend to energy storage, where they can enhance the performance and efficiency of batteries and supercapacitors. Looking ahead, researchers must focus on developing scalable and cost-effective production techniques that maintain the integrity and functionality of these advanced materials. Additionally, exploring the synergistic effects of combining different nanomaterials could lead to the discovery of new properties and applications, further expanding their utility. In conclusion, the advancements in the functionalization and processing of smart and responsive sustainable nanomaterials offer substantial economic and environmental benefits.

References

1. Abdelbasir SM, McCourt KM, Lee CM, Vanegas DC. Waste-derived nanoparticles: synthesis approaches, environmental applications, and sustainability considerations. Front Chem. 2020a;8:1–18. https://doi.org/10.3389/fchem.2020.00782.
2. Abdelbasir SM, McCourt KM, Lee CM, Vanegas DC. Waste-derived nanoparticles: synthesis approaches, environmental applications, and sustainability considerations. Front Chem. 2020b;8:1–18. https://doi.org/10.3389/fchem.2020.00782.
3. Abegunde OO, Akinlabi ET, Oladijo OP, Akinlabi S, Ude AU. Overview of thin film deposition techniques. AIMS Mater Sci. 2019;6(2):174–99. https://doi.org/10.3934/MATERSCI.2019.2.174.
4. Afzal O, Altamimi ASA, Nadeem MS, Alzarea SI, Almalki WH, Tariq A, Mubeen B, Murtaza BN, Iftikhar S, Riaz N, Kazmi I. Nanoparticles in drug delivery: from history to therapeutic applications. Nanomaterials (Basel). 2022;12(24) https://doi.org/10.3390/nano12244494.
5. Ahmed SF, Mofijur M, Rafa N, Chowdhury AT, Chowdhury S, Nahrin M, Islam ABMS, Ong HC. Green approaches in synthesising nanomaterials for environmental nanobioremediation: technological advancements, applications, benefits and challenges. Environ Res. 2022;204 https://doi.org/10.1016/j.envres.2021.111967.
6. Altissimo M. E-beam lithography for micro–/nanofabrication. Biomicrofluidics. 2010;4(2) https://doi.org/10.1063/1.3437589.
7. Anbarasu M, Anandan M, Chinnasamy E, Gopinath V, Balamurugan K. Synthesis and characterization of polyethylene glycol (PEG) coated Fe3O4 nanoparticles by chemical co-precipitation method for biomedical applications. Spectrochim Acta A Mol Biomol Spectrosc. 2015;135:536–9. https://doi.org/10.1016/J.SAA.2014.07.059.
8. Andhare DD, Jadhav SA, Khedkar MV, Somvanshi SB, More SD, Jadhav KM. Structural and chemical properties of ZnFe2O4 nanoparticles synthesised by chemical co-precipitation technique. J Phys Conf Ser. 2020;1644(1) https://doi.org/10.1088/1742-6596/1644/1/012014.
9. Anju S, Ashtami J, Mohanan PV. Black phosphorus, a prospective graphene substitute for biomedical applications. Mater Sci Eng C. 2019;97:978–93. https://doi.org/10.1016/J.MSEC.2018.12.146.
10. Bansal V, Rautaray D, Bharde A, Ahire K, Sanyal A, Ahmad A, Sastry M. Fungus-mediated biosynthesis of silica and Titania particles. J Mater Chem. 2005;15(26):2583–9. https://doi.org/10.1039/b503008k.
11. Barhoum A, García-Betancourt ML, Jeevanandam J, Hussien EA, Mekkawy SA, Mostafa M, Omran MM, Abdalla MS, Bechelany M. Review on natural, incidental, bioinspired, and engineered nanomaterials: history, definitions, classifications, synthesis, properties, market, toxicities, risks, and regulations. Nanomaterials. 2022;12(2) https://doi.org/10.3390/nano12020177.
12. Bharde A, Rautaray D, Bansal V, Ahmad A, Sarkar I, Yusuf SM, Sanyal M, Sastry M. Extracellular biosynthesis of magnetite using fungi. Small. 2006;2(1):135–41. https://doi.org/10.1002/smll.200500180.
13. Bi S, Xiao BL, Ji ZH, Liu BS, Liu ZY, Ma ZY. Dispersion and damage of carbon nanotubes in carbon nanotube/7055Al composites during high-energy ball milling process.

Acta Metallurgica Sinica (English Letters). 2021;34(2):196–204. https://doi.org/10.1007/s40195-020-01138-5.
14. Binder WH, Zirbs R, MacHl D, Gahleitner M. Grafting polyisobutylene from nanoparticle surfaces: concentration and surface effects on livingness. Macromolecules. 2009;42(19):7379–87. https://doi.org/10.1021/ma900535e.
15. Bishop AR, Nuzzo RG. Self-assembled monolayers: recent developments and applications. Curr Opin Colloid Interface Sci. 1996;1(1):127–36. https://doi.org/10.1016/S1359-0294(96)80053-7.
16. Bloemen M, Brullot W, Luong TT, Geukens N, Gils A, Verbiest T. Improved functionalization of oleic acid-coated iron oxide nanoparticles for biomedical applications. J Nanopart Res. 2012;14(9) https://doi.org/10.1007/s11051-012-1100-5.
17. Boguslavsky Y, Shemesh M, Friedlander A, Rutenberg R, Filossof AM, Buslovich A, Poverenov E. Eliminating the need for biocidal agents in anti-biofouling polymers by applying grafted nanosilica instead. ACS Omega. 2018;3(10):12437–45. https://doi.org/10.1021/acsomega.8b01438.
18. Boobalan T, Sethupathi M, Sengottuvelan N, Kumar P, Balaji P, Gulyás B, Padmanabhan P, Selvan ST, Arun A. Mushroom-derived carbon dots for toxic metal ion detection and as antibacterial and anticancer agents. ACS Appl Nano Mater. 2020;3(6):5910–9. https://doi.org/10.1021/acsanm.0c01058.
19. Borse V, Konwar AN. Synthesis and characterization of gold nanoparticles as a sensing tool for the lateral flow immunoassay development. Sens Int. 2020;1:100051. https://doi.org/10.1016/J.SINTL.2020.100051.
20. Bratek-Skicki A. Towards a new class of stimuli-responsive polymer-based materials – recent advances and challenges. Appl Surf Sci Adv. 2021;4:100068. https://doi.org/10.1016/J.APSADV.2021.100068.
21. Buitrón G, Carrillo-Reyes J, Morales M, Faraloni C, Torzillo G. Biohydrogen production from microalgae. In: Microalgae-based biofuels and bioproducts: from feedstock cultivation to end-products; 2017. p. 209–34. https://doi.org/10.1016/B978-0-08-101023-5.00009-1.
22. Bwatanglang IB, Mohammad F, Yusof NA, Abdullah J, Alitheen NB, Hussein MZ, Abu N, Mohammed NE, Nordin N, Zamberi NR, Yeap SK. In vivo tumor targeting and anti-tumor effects of 5-fluororacil loaded, folic acid targeted quantum dot system. J Colloid Interface Sci. 2016;480:146–58. https://doi.org/10.1016/J.JCIS.2016.07.011.
23. Caires AJ, Mansur AAP, Carvalho IC, Carvalho SM, Mansur HS. Green synthesis of ZnS quantum dot/biopolymer photoluminescent nanoprobes for bioimaging brain cancer cells. Mater Chem Phys. 2020;244:122716. https://doi.org/10.1016/j.matchemphys.2020.122716.
24. Calabrese G, De Luca G, Nocito G, Rizzo MG, Lombardo SP, Chisari G, Forte S, Sciuto EL, Conoci S. Carbon dots: an innovative tool for drug delivery in brain tumors. Int J Mol Sci. 2021;22(21) https://doi.org/10.3390/ijms222111783.
25. Chakrabartty I, Hakeem KR, Mohanta YK, Varma RS. Greener nanomaterials and their diverse applications in the energy sector. Clean Techn Environ Policy. 2022;24(10):3237–52. https://doi.org/10.1007/s10098-022-02368-0.
26. Cheng L, Yang K, Li Y, Zeng X, Shao M, Lee ST, Liu Z. Multifunctional nanoparticles for upconversion luminescence/MR multimodal imaging and magnetically targeted photothermal therapy. Biomaterials. 2012;33(7):2215–22. https://doi.org/10.1016/j.biomaterials.2011.11.069.
27. Cheng L, Wang X, Gong F, Liu T, Liu Z. 2D nanomaterials for cancer theranostic applications. Adv Mater. 2020;32(13):1–23. https://doi.org/10.1002/adma.201902333.
28. Chytrosz-Wrobel P, Golda-Cepa M, Stodolak-Zych E, Rysz J, Kotarba A. Effect of oxygen plasma-treatment on surface functional groups, wettability, and nanotopography features of medically relevant polymers with various crystallinities. Appl Surf Sci Adv. 2023;18:100497. https://doi.org/10.1016/J.APSADV.2023.100497.
29. Coccia F, Tonucci L, Bosco D, Bressan M, d'Alessandro N. One-pot synthesis of lignin-stabilised platinum and palladium nanoparticles and their catalytic behaviour in oxidation and reduction reactions. Green Chem. 2012;14(4):1073–8. https://doi.org/10.1039/c2gc16524d.

30. Danks AE, Hall SR, Schnepp Z. The evolution of "sol-gel" chemistry as a technique for materials synthesis. Mater Horiz. 2016;3(2):91–112. https://doi.org/10.1039/c5mh00260e.
31. del Barrio J, Sánchez-Somolinos C. Light to shape the future: from photolithography to 4D printing. Adv Opt Mater. 2019;7(16) https://doi.org/10.1002/adom.201900598.
32. Delogu F, Gorrasi G, Sorrentino A. Fabrication of polymer nanocomposites via ball milling: present status and future perspectives. Prog Mater Sci. 2017a;86:75–126. https://doi.org/10.1016/J.PMATSCI.2017.01.003.
33. Delogu F, Gorrasi G, Sorrentino A. Fabrication of polymer nanocomposites via ball milling: present status and future perspectives. Prog Mater Sci. 2017b;86:75–126. https://doi.org/10.1016/J.PMATSCI.2017.01.003.
34. Dessale M, Mengistu G. Nanotechnology: a promising approach for cancer diagnosis, therapeutics and theragnosis. Int J Nanomed. 2022;17:3735–49.
35. Devaray P, Hatta SFWM, Wong YH. An overview of conventional and new advancements in high kappa thin film deposition techniques in metal oxide semiconductor devices. J Mater Sci Mater Electron. 2022;33(10) https://doi.org/10.1007/s10854-022-07975-7.
36. Di Crescenzo A, Ettorre V, Fontana A. Non-covalent and reversible functionalization of carbon nanotubes. Beilstein J Nanotechnol. 2014;5(1):1675–90. https://doi.org/10.3762/bjnano.5.178.
37. Dou QQ, Teng CP, Ye E, Loh XJ. Effective near-infrared photodynamic therapy assisted by upconversion nanoparticles conjugated with photosensitizers. Int J Nanomedicine. 2015;10:419–32. https://doi.org/10.2147/IJN.S74891.
38. Dulińska-Litewka J, Łazarczyk A, Hałubiec P, Szafrański O, Karnas K, Karewicz A. Superparamagnetic iron oxide nanoparticles-current and prospective medical applications. Materials. 2019;12(4) https://doi.org/10.3390/ma12040617.
39. El-Kady MM, Ansari I, Arora C, Rai N, Soni S, Verma DK, Singh P, Mahmoud AED. Nanomaterials: a comprehensive review of applications, toxicity, impact, and fate to environment. J Mol Liq. 2023;370:121046. https://doi.org/10.1016/J.MOLLIQ.2022.121046.
40. Fatima H, Charinpanitkul T, Kim KS. Fundamentals to apply magnetic nanoparticles for hyperthermia therapy. Nanomaterials. 2021;11(5):1–20. https://doi.org/10.3390/nano11051203.
41. Carotta MC, Cervi A, di Natale V, Gherardi S, Giberti A, Guidi V, Puzzovio D, Vendemiati G, Martinelli Sacerdoti M, Calestani D, Zappettini A, Zha M, Zanotti. ZnO gas sensors: a comparison between nanoparticles and nanotetrapods-based thick films Sensors and Actuators B. Chemical. 2009;137(1):164–9.
42. Fox-Rabinovich GS, Gershman IS, Veldhuis S. Thin-film pvd coating metamaterials exhibiting similarities to natural processes under extreme tribological conditions. Nanomaterials. 2020;10(9):1–18. https://doi.org/10.3390/nano10091720.
43. Furxhi I, Costa A, Vázquez-Campos S, Fito-López C, Hristozov D, Tamayo Ramos JA, Resch S, Cioffi M, Friedrichs S, Rocca C, Valsami-Jones E, Lynch I, Araceli SJ, Farcal L. Status, implications and challenges of European safe and sustainable by design paradigms applicable to nanomaterials and advanced materials. RSC Sustain. 2023;1(2):234–50. https://doi.org/10.1039/d2su00101b.
44. Gahlawat G, Choudhury AR. A review on the biosynthesis of metal and metal salt nanoparticles by microbes. RSC Adv. 2019a;9(23):12944–67. https://doi.org/10.1039/c8ra10483b.
45. Gahlawat G, Choudhury AR. A review on the biosynthesis of metal and metal salt nanoparticles by microbes. RSC Adv. 2019b;9(23):12944–67. https://doi.org/10.1039/c8ra10483b.
46. Gao J, Gu H, Xu B. Multifunctional magnetic nanoparticles: design, synthesis, and biomedical applications. Acc Chem Res. 2009;42(8):1097.
47. Gelperina S, Kisich K, Iseman MD, Heifets L. Pulmonary perspective the potential advantages of nanoparticle drug delivery systems in chemotherapy of tuberculosis. Am J Respir Crit Care Med. 2005;172:1487–90. https://doi.org/10.1164/rccm.200504-613PP.
48. Giri VP, Shukla P, Tripathi A, Verma P, Kumar N, Pandey S, Dimkpa CO, Mishra A. A review of sustainable use of biogenic nanoscale agro-materials to enhance stress tolerance and nutritional value of plants. Plants. 2023;12(4) https://doi.org/10.3390/plants12040815.

49. Gnanaprakash G, Mahadevan S, Jayakumar T, Kalyanasundaram P, Philip J, Raj B. Effect of initial pH and temperature of iron salt solutions on formation of magnetite nanoparticles. Mater Chem Phys. 2007;103(1):168–75. https://doi.org/10.1016/J.MATCHEMPHYS.2007.02.011.
50. Gong L, Sun J, Zheng P, Liu Y, Yang G. Yellow fluorescent nitrogen and bromine co-doped graphene quantum dots for bioimaging. ACS Appl Nano Mater. 2021;4(8):8564–71. https://doi.org/10.1021/acsanm.1c02004.
51. Griffioen AW. Anti-angiogenesis: making the tumor vulnerable to the immune system. Cancer Immunol Immunother. 2008;57(10):1553–8. https://doi.org/10.1007/s00262-008-0524-3.
52. Grillone A, Riva ER, Mondini A, Forte C, Calucci L, Innocenti C, de Julian Fernandez C, Cappello V, Gemmi M, Moscato S, Ronca F, Sacco R, Mattoli V, Ciofani G. Active targeting of sorafenib: preparation, characterization, and in vitro testing of drug-loaded magnetic solid lipid nanoparticles. Adv Healthc Mater. 2015;4(11):1681–90. https://doi.org/10.1002/adhm.201500235.
53. Gulzar A, Xu J, Xu L, Yang P, He F, Yang D, An G, Ansari MB. Redox-responsive UCNPs-DPA conjugated NGO-PEG-BPEI-DOX for imaging-guided PTT and chemotherapy for cancer treatment. Dalton Trans. 2018;47(11):3921–30. https://doi.org/10.1039/c7dt04093h.
54. Gurunathan S, Han JW, Kwon DN, Kim JH. Enhanced antibacterial and anti-biofilm activities of silver nanoparticles against Gram-negative and Gram-positive bacteria. Nanoscale Res Lett. 2014a;9(1):1–17. https://doi.org/10.1186/1556-276X-9-373.
55. Gurunathan S, Han JW, Kwon DN, Kim JH. Enhanced antibacterial and anti-biofilm activities of silver nanoparticles against Gram-negative and Gram-positive bacteria. Nanoscale Res Lett. 2014b;9(1):1–17. https://doi.org/10.1186/1556-276X-9-373.
56. Gurunathan S, Kang MH, Qasim M, Kim JH. Nanoparticle-mediated combination therapy: two-in-one approach for cancer. Int J Mol Sci. 2018;19(10) https://doi.org/10.3390/ijms19103264.
57. Gusain R, Kumar P, Sharma OP, Jain SL, Khatri OP. Reduced graphene oxide–CuO nanocomposites for photocatalytic conversion of CO2 into methanol under visible light irradiation. Appl Catal B Environ. 2016;181:352–62. https://doi.org/10.1016/J.APCATB.2015.08.012.
58. Hakim SH, Shanks BH. A comparative study of macroporous metal oxides synthesized via a unified approach. Chem Mater. 2009;21(10):2027–38. https://doi.org/10.1021/cm801691g.
59. Haleem A, Javaid M, Pratap R, Rab S, Suman R. Applications of nanotechnology in medical field: a brief review. Glob Health J. 2023;7:70–7. https://doi.org/10.1016/j.glohj.2023.02.008.
60. Hamaker HC. The London—van der Waals attraction between spherical particles. Physica. 1937;4(10):1058–72. https://doi.org/10.1016/S0031-8914(37)80203-7.
61. Hecht DS, Hu L, Irvin G. Emerging transparent electrodes based on thin films of carbon nanotubes, graphene, and metallic nanostructures. Adv Mater. 2011;23(13):1482–513. https://doi.org/10.1002/adma.201003188.
62. Horejs C. Nebulized lipid nanoparticles. Nano Lett. 2021;6:41578. https://doi.org/10.1038/s41578-021-00392-y.
63. Hu Y, Li Q, Lee B, Jun Y. Aluminum affects heterogeneous Fe(III) (Hydr)oxide nucleation, growth, and ostwald ripening. Environ Sci Technol. 2014;48(1):299–306.
64. Huang Q, Wang Y, Chen X, Wang Y, Li Z, Du S, Wang L, Chen S. Nanotechnology-based strategies for early cancer diagnosis using circulating tumor cells as a liquid biopsy. Nanotheranostics. 2018;2(1):21–41). Ivyspring International Publisher. https://doi.org/10.7150/ntno.22091.
65. Hyeon J, Soo S, Min H, Gi S, Younggyun K, Sung C, Ahn H. Multi – functionalization strategies using nanomaterials: a review and case study in sensing applications. Int J Precis Eng Manuf-Green Technol. 2022;9(1):323–47. https://doi.org/10.1007/s40684-021-00356-1.
66. Iannazzo D, Espro C, Celesti C, Ferlazzo A, Neri G. Smart biosensors for cancer diagnosis based on graphene quantum dots. Cancer. 2021;13(13) https://doi.org/10.3390/cancers13133194.
67. İnada AA, Arman S, Safaei B. A novel review on the efficiency of nanomaterials for solar energy storage systems. J Energy Storage. 2022;55:105661. https://doi.org/10.1016/J.EST.2022.105661.

68. Ismagilov ZR, Shalagina AE, Podyacheva OY, Ischenko AV, Kibis LS, Boronin AI, Chesalov YA, Kochubey DI, Romanenko AI, Anikeeva OB, Buryakov TI, Tkachev EN. Structure and electrical conductivity of nitrogen-doped carbon nanofibers. Carbon. 2009;47(8):1922–9. https://doi.org/10.1016/J.CARBON.2009.02.034.
69. Jang JH, Ullal CK, Maldovan M, Gorishnyy T, Kooi S, Koh CY, Thomas EL. 3D micro – and nanostructures via interference lithography. Adv Funct Mater. 2007a;17(16):3027–41. https://doi.org/10.1002/adfm.200700140.
70. Jang JH, Ullal CK, Maldovan M, Gorishnyy T, Kooi S, Koh CY, Thomas EL. 3D micro – and nanostructures via interference lithography. Adv Funct Mater. 2007b;17(16):3027–41. https://doi.org/10.1002/adfm.200700140.
71. Kalidindi RSR, Subasri R. Sol-gel nanocomposite hard coatings. In: Anti-abrasive nanocoatings: current and future applications; 2015. p. 105–36. https://doi.org/10.1016/B978-0-85709-211-3.00005-4.
72. Kang B, Mackey MA, El-Sayed MA. Nuclear targeting of gold nanoparticles in cancer cells induces DNA damage, causing cytokinesis arrest and apoptosis. J Am Chem Soc. 2010;132(5):1517–9. https://doi.org/10.1021/ja9102698.
73. Kanth PC, Verma SK, Gour N. Functionalized nanomaterials for biomedical and agriculture industries. In: Handbook of functionalized nanomaterials for industrial applications. Elsevier; 2020. https://doi.org/10.1016/B978-0-12-816787-8.00010-7.
74. Kara F, Öztürk B. Comparison and optimization of PVD and CVD method on surface roughness and flank wear in hard-machining of DIN 1.2738 mold steel. Sens Rev. 2019;39(1):24–33. https://doi.org/10.1108/SR-12-2017-0266.
75. Kickelbick G. Introduction to hybrid materials. In: Hybrid materials: synthesis, characterization, and applications; 2007. p. 1–48. https://doi.org/10.1002/9783527610495.ch1.
76. Kim SJ, Lewis B, Steiner MS, Bissa UV, Dose C, Frank JA. Superparamagnetic iron oxide nanoparticles for direct labeling of stem cells and in vivo MRI tracking. Contrast Media Mol Imaging. 2016a;11(1):55–64. https://doi.org/10.1002/cmmi.1658.
77. Kim S, Sojoudi H, Zhao H, Mariappan D, McKinley GH, Gleason KK, Hart AJ. Ultrathin high-resolution flexographic printing using nanoporous stamps. Sci Adv. 2016b;2(12) https://doi.org/10.1126/sciadv.1601660.
78. Kim HY, Kim DS, Hwang NM. Comparison of diamond nanoparticles captured on the floating and grounded membranes in the hot filament chemical vapor deposition process. RSC Adv. 2021;11(10):5651–7. https://doi.org/10.1039/d0ra09649k.
79. Kimling J, Maier M, Okenve B, Kotaidis V, Ballot H, Plech A. Turkevich method for gold nanoparticle synthesis revisited. J Phys Chem B. 2006;110(32):15700–7. https://doi.org/10.1021/jp061667w.
80. Klosterhoff BS, Kaiser J, Nelson BD, Karipott SS, Ruehle MA, Hollister SJ, Weiss JA, Ong KG, Willett NJ, Guldberg RE. Wireless sensor enables longitudinal monitoring of regenerative niche mechanics during rehabilitation that enhance bone repair. Bone. 2020;135 https://doi.org/10.1016/j.bone.2020.115311.
81. Knotek O, Löffler F, Krämer G. Process and advantage of multicomponent and multilayer PVD coatings. Surf Coat Technol. 1993;59(1–3):14–20. https://doi.org/10.1016/0257-8972(93)90048-S.
82. Koponen SE, Gordon PG, Barry ST. Principles of precursor design for vapour deposition methods. Polyhedron. 2016;108:59–66. https://doi.org/10.1016/J.POLY.2015.08.024.
83. Krajczewski J, Rucińska K, Townley HE, Kudelski A. Role of various nanoparticles in photodynamic therapy and detection methods of singlet oxygen. Photodiagn Photodyn Ther. 2019;26:162–78. https://doi.org/10.1016/j.pdpdt.2019.03.016.
84. Kühne M, Börrnert F, Fecher S, Ghorbani-Asl M, Biskupek J, Samuelis D, Krasheninnikov AV, Kaiser U, Smet JH. Reversible superdense ordering of lithium between two graphene sheets. Nature. 2018;564(7735):234–9. https://doi.org/10.1038/s41586-018-0754-2.
85. Kühnel M, Fröhlich T, Füßl R, Hoffmann M, Manske E, Rangelow IW, Reger J, Schäffel C, Sinzinger S, Zöllner JP. Towards alternative 3D nanofabrication in macroscopic working volumes. Meas Sci Technol. 2018;29(11) https://doi.org/10.1088/1361-6501/aadb57.

86. Kumar N, Ray SS. Synthesis and functionalization of nanomaterials. Springer International Publishing; 2018. https://doi.org/10.1007/978-3-319-97779-9.
87. Kwiatkowski K, Lukehart C. Nanocomposites prepared by sol-gel methods: synthesis and characterization. In: Handbook of nanostructured materials and nanotechnology; 2000. p. 387–421. https://doi.org/10.1016/B978-012513760-7/50011-3.
88. Lee KT, Cho J. Roles of nanosize in lithium reactive nanomaterials for lithium ion batteries. Nano Today. 2011;6(1):28–41. https://doi.org/10.1016/J.NANTOD.2010.11.002.
89. Lee JI, Hwang NM. Generation of negative-charge carriers in the gas phase and their contribution to the growth of carbon nanotubes during hot-filament chemical vapor deposition. Carbon. 2008;46(12):1588–92. https://doi.org/10.1016/j.carbon.2008.07.006.
90. Lee KH, Kim SM, Jeong H, Jung GY. Spontaneous nanoscale polymer solution patterning using solvent evaporation driven double-dewetting edge lithography. Soft Matter. 2012;8(2):465–71. https://doi.org/10.1039/c1sm06431b.
91. Lehn JM. Towards complex matter: supramolecular chemistry and self-organization. Eur Rev. 2009;17(2):263–80. https://doi.org/10.1017/S1062798709000805.
92. Li J, Sun X, Liu S, Li X, Li JG, Huo D. A homogeneous co-precipitation method to synthesize highly sinterability YAG powders for transparent ceramics. Ceram Int. 2015;41(2):3283–7. https://doi.org/10.1016/j.ceramint.2014.10.076.
93. Li R, Zhang L, Shi L, Wang P. MXene Ti3C2: an effective 2D light-to-heat conversion material. ACS Nano. 2017a;11(4):3752–9. https://doi.org/10.1021/acsnano.6b08415.
94. Li S, Chen Y, Liu H, Wang Y, Liu L, Lv F, Li Y, Wang S. Graphdiyne materials as nanotransducer for in vivo photoacoustic imaging and photothermal therapy of tumor. Chem Mater. 2017b;29(14):6087–94. https://doi.org/10.1021/acs.chemmater.7b01965.
95. Li F, Qin Y, Lee J, Liao H, Wang N, Davis TP, Qiao R, Ling D. Stimuli-responsive nanoassemblies for remotely controlled drug delivery. J Control Release. 2020a;322:566–92. https://doi.org/10.1016/J.JCONREL.2020.03.051.
96. Li S, Su W, Wu H, Yuan T, Yuan C, Liu J, Deng G, Gao X, Chen Z, Bao Y, Yuan F, Zhou S, Tan H, Li Y, Li X, Fan L, Zhu J, Chen AT, Liu F, et al. Targeted tumour theranostics in mice via carbon quantum dots structurally mimicking large amino acids. Nat Biomed Eng. 2020b;4(7):704–16. https://doi.org/10.1038/s41551-020-0540-y.
97. Li Z, Dong J, Wang L, Zhang Y, Zhuang T, Wang H, Cui X, Wang Z. A power-triggered preparation strategy of nano-structured inorganics: sonosynthesis. Nanoscale Adv. 2021;3(9):2423–47. https://doi.org/10.1039/d1na00038a.
98. Li T, Lu XM, Zhang MR, Hu K, Li Z. Peptide-based nanomaterials: self-assembly, properties and applications. Bioact Mater. 2022;11:268–82. https://doi.org/10.1016/J.BIOACTMAT.2021.09.029.
99. Lismont M, Dreesen L, Wuttke S. Metal-organic framework nanoparticles in photodynamic therapy: current status and perspectives. Adv Funct Mater. 2017;27(14):1–16. https://doi.org/10.1002/adfm.201606314.
100. Liu Y, Wang F, Wang X, Wang X, Flahaut E, Liu X, Li Y, Wang X, Xu Y, Shi Y, Zhang R. Planar carbon nanotube–graphene hybrid films for high-performance broadband photodetectors. Nat Commun. 2015:1–7. https://doi.org/10.1038/ncomms9589.
101. Lu Y, Lyu H, Richardson AG, Lucas TH, Kuzum D. Flexible neural electrode array based-on porous graphene for cortical microstimulation and sensing. Sci Rep. 2016;6:1–9. https://doi.org/10.1038/srep33526.
102. Lucky SS, Soo KC, Zhang Y. Nanoparticles in photodynamic therapy. Chem Rev. 2015;115(4):1990–2042. https://doi.org/10.1021/cr5004198.
103. Lyles VD. Surface studies of organic thin films using scanning probe microscopy and nanofabrication. 2013. https://doi.org/10.31390/gradschool_dissertations.382
104. Mabrouk M, Das DB, Salem ZA, Beherei HH. Nanomaterials for biomedical applications: production, characterisations, recent trends and difficulties. Molecules. 2021;26(4):1–27. https://doi.org/10.3390/molecules26041077.
105. Maghimaa M, Sagadevan S, E B, Fatimah I, Lett JA, Moharana S, Garg S, Al-Anber MA. Enhancing biocompatibility and functionality: carbon nanotube-polymer nanocompos-

ites for improved biomedical applications. J Drug Delivery Sci Technol. 2024;99:105958. https://doi.org/10.1016/J.JDDST.2024.105958.
106. Maleki H, Haselpour M, Fathi R. The effect of calcination conditions on structural and magnetic behavior of bismuth ferrite synthesized by co-precipitation method. J Mater Sci Mater Electron. 2018;29(5):4320–6. https://doi.org/10.1007/s10854-017-8379-z.
107. Malik S, Muhammad K, Waheed Y. Emerging applications of nanotechnology in healthcare. Pharmaceuticals (Basel). 2023;14(8):707.
108. Maric T, Mikhaylov G, Khodakivskyi P, Bazhin A, Sinisi R, Bonhoure N, Yevtodiyenko A, Jones A, Muhunthan V, Abdelhady G, Shackelford D, Goun E. Bioluminescent-based imaging and quantification of glucose uptake in vivo. Nat Methods. 2019;16(6):526–32. https://doi.org/10.1038/s41592-019-0421-z.
109. Martínez G, Merinero M, Pérez-Aranda M, Pérez-Soriano EM, Ortiz T, Begines B, Alcudia A. Environmental impact of nanoparticles' application as an emerging technology: a review. Materials. 2021;14(1):1–26. https://doi.org/10.3390/ma14010166.
110. Mattox DM. Physical vapor deposition (PVD) processes. Met Finish. 2000;98(1):410–23. https://doi.org/10.1016/S0026-0576(00)80350-5.
111. Mekhzoum MEM, Qaiss A el Kacem, Bouhfid R. Introduction: different types of smart materials and their practical applications. In: Polymer nanocomposite-based smart materials: from synthesis to application; 2020. p. 1–19. https://doi.org/10.1016/B978-0-08-103013-4.00001-7.
112. Mochalov L, Logunov A, Kitnis A, Vorotyntsev V. Plasma-chemistry of arsenic selenide films: relationship between film properties and plasma power. Plasma Chem Plasma Process. 2020;40(1):407–21. https://doi.org/10.1007/s11090-019-10035-4.
113. Mody VV, Cox A, Shah S. Magnetic nanoparticle drug delivery systems for targeting tumor. Appl Nanosci. 2014:385–92. https://doi.org/10.1007/s13204-013-0216-y.
114. Morones JR, Elechiguerra JL, Camacho A, Holt K, Kouri JB, Ramírez JT, Yacaman MJ. The bactericidal effect of silver nanoparticles. Nanotechnology. 2005;16(10):2346–53. https://doi.org/10.1088/0957-4484/16/10/059.
115. Mout R, Moyano DF, Rana S, Rotello VM. Surface functionalization of nanoparticles for nanomedicine. Chem Soc Rev. 2012;41(7):2539–44. https://doi.org/10.1039/c2cs15294k.
116. Mulder WJM, Koole R, Brandwijk RJ, Storm G, Chin PTK, Strijkers GJ, De Mello Donegá C, Nicolay K, Griffioen AW. Quantum dots with a paramagnetic coating as a bimodal molecular imaging probe. Nano Lett. 2006;6(1):1–6. https://doi.org/10.1021/nl051935m.
117. Müller R, Gelme O, Scholz JP, Huber F, Mundszinger M, Li Y, Madel M, Minkow A, Kaiser U, Herr U, Thonke K. Epitaxial ZnO layer growth on Si(111) substrates with an intermediate AlN nucleation layer by methane-based chemical vapor deposition. Cryst Growth Des. 2020;20(9):6170–85. https://doi.org/10.1021/acs.cgd.0c00907.
118. Mungse HP, Verma S, Kumar N, Sain B, Khatri OP. Grafting of oxo-vanadium Schiff base on graphene nanosheets and its catalytic activity for the oxidation of alcohols. J Mater Chem. 2012;22(12):5427–33. https://doi.org/10.1039/c2jm15644j.
119. Mura S, Nicolas J, Couvreur P. Stimuli-responsive nanocarriers for drug delivery. Nat Mater. 2013;12(11):991–1003. https://doi.org/10.1038/nmat3776.
120. Othman MR, Helwani Z, Martunus, Fernando WJN. Synthetic hydrotalcites from different routes and their application as catalysts and gas adsorbents: a review. Appl Organomet Chem. 2009;23(9):335–46. https://doi.org/10.1002/aoc.1517.
121. Paik S, Kim G, Chang S, Lee S, Jin D, Jeong KY, Lee IS, Lee J, Moon H, Lee J, Chang K, Choi SS, Moon J, Jung S, Kang S, Lee W, Choi HJ, Choi H, Kim HJ, et al. Near-field subdiffraction photolithography with an elastomeric photomask. Nat Commun. 2020;11(1):1–13. https://doi.org/10.1038/s41467-020-14439-1.
122. Palit S, Hussain CM. Functionalization of nanomaterials for industrial applications: recent and future perspectives. In: Handbook of functionalized nanomaterials for industrial applications. INC; 2020. https://doi.org/10.1016/B978-0-12-816787-8.00001-6.
123. Pan J, Zhu X, Chen X, Zhao Y, Liu J. Gd3+-Doped MoSe2 nanosheets used as a theranostic agent for bimodal imaging and highly efficient photothermal cancer therapy. Biomater Sci. 2018;6(2):372–87. https://doi.org/10.1039/c7bm00894e.

124. Pentimalli M, Imperi E, Zaccagnini A, Padella F. Nanostructured metal hydride – polymer composite as fixed bed for sorption technologies. Advantages of an innovative combined approach by high-energy ball milling and extrusion techniques. Renew Energy. 2017;110:69–78. https://doi.org/10.1016/J.RENENE.2016.07.074.
125. Phokha S, Seraphin S, Maensiri S, Laokul P, Klinkaewnarong J, Phokha S, Seraphin S. Indium oxide (In_2O_3) nanoparticles using Aloe vera plant extract: synthesis and optical properties indium oxide (In_2O_3) nanoparticles using Aloe vera plant extract: synthesis and optical properties. Optoelectron Adv Mater Rapid Commun. 2008;2(3):161–5.
126. Pimpin A, Srituravanich W. Reviews on micro – and nanolithography techniques and their applications. Eng J. 2012;16(1):37–55. https://doi.org/10.4186/ej.2012.16.1.37.
127. Prabakaran S, Jeyaraj M, Nagaraj A, Sadasivuni KK, Rajan M. Polymethyl methacrylate–ovalbumin @ graphene oxide drug carrier system for high anti-proliferative cancer drug delivery. Appl Nanosci (Switzerland). 2019;9(7):1487–500. https://doi.org/10.1007/s13204-019-00950-5.
128. Prawer S, Nugent KW, Jamieson DN, Orwa JO, Bursill LA, Peng JL. The Raman spectrum of nanocrystalline diamond. Chem Phys Lett. 2000;332(1–2):93–7. https://doi.org/10.1016/S0009-2614(00)01236-7.
129. Quate CF. Scanning probes as a lithography tool for nanostructures. Surf Sci. 1997;386(1–3):259–64. https://doi.org/10.1016/S0039-6028(97)00305-1.
130. Rahman IA, Padavettan V. Synthesis of Silica nanoparticles by Sol-Gel: size-dependent properties, surface modification, and applications in silica-polymer nanocompositesa review. J Nanomater. 2012;2012 https://doi.org/10.1155/2012/132424.
131. Rane AV, Kanny K, Abitha VK, Thomas S. Methods for synthesis of nanoparticles and fabrication of nanocomposites. In: Synthesis of inorganic nanomaterials: advances and key technologies; 2018. p. 121–39. https://doi.org/10.1016/B978-0-08-101975-7.00005-1.
132. Raphey VR, Henna TK, Nivitha KP, Mufeedha P, Sabu C, Pramod K. Advanced biomedical applications of carbon nanotube. Mater Sci Eng C. 2019;100:616–30. https://doi.org/10.1016/J.MSEC.2019.03.043.
133. Rizvi M, Gerengi H, Gupta P. Functionalization of nanomaterials: synthesis and characterization. In: Functionalized nanomaterials for corrosion mitigation: synthesis, characterization, and applications, part 1 – functionalization of nanomaterials: synthesis and characterization; 2022. p. 1–26. https://doi.org/10.1021/bk-2022-1418.ch001.
134. Ru J, Bian C, Zhu Z, Wang Y, Zhang J, Horiuchi T, Sugino T, Liu X, Chen H, Asaka K. Controllable and durable ionic electroactive polymer actuator based on nanoporous carbon nanotube film electrode. Smart Mater Struct. 2019;28(8) https://doi.org/10.1088/1361-665X/ab2a28.
135. Sahin O, Ashokkumar M, Ajayan PM. Micro- and nanopatterning of biomaterial surfaces. In: Fundamental biomaterials: metals; 2018. p. 67–78. https://doi.org/10.1016/B978-0-08-102205-4.00003-9.
136. Samanta NS, Banerjee S, Mondal P, Anweshan, Bora U, Purkait MK. Preparation and characterization of zeolite from waste Linz-Donawitz (LD) process slag of steel industry for removal of Fe3+ from drinking water. Adv Powder Technol. 2021;32(9):3372–87. https://doi.org/10.1016/J.APT.2021.07.023.
137. Sartal A, Bellas R, Mejías AM, García-Collado A. The sustainable manufacturing concept, evolution and opportunities within Industry 4.0: a literature review. Adv Mech Eng. 2020;12(5) https://doi.org/10.1177/1687814020925232.
138. Sathishkumar M, Sneha K, Kwak IS, Mao J, Tripathy SJ, Yun YS. Phyto-crystallization of palladium through reduction process using Cinnamom zeylanicum bark extract. J Hazard Mater. 2009;171(1–3):400–4. https://doi.org/10.1016/J.JHAZMAT.2009.06.014.
139. Sethy C, Kundu CN. 5-Fluorouracil (5-FU) resistance and the new strategy to enhance the sensitivity against cancer: implication of DNA repair inhibition. Biomed Pharmacother. 2021;137 https://doi.org/10.1016/j.biopha.2021.111285.
140. Shankar SS, Rai A, Ahmad A, Sastry M. Rapid synthesis of Au, Ag, and bimetallic Au core–Ag shell nanoparticles using Neem (Azadirachta indica) leaf broth. J Colloid Interface Sci. 2004;275(2):496–502. https://doi.org/10.1016/J.JCIS.2004.03.003.

141. Sherif El-Eskandarany M, Al-Salem SM, Ali N. Top-down reactive approach for the synthesis of disordered zrn nanocrystalline bulk material from solid waste. Nanomaterials. 2020;10(9):1–11. https://doi.org/10.3390/nano10091826.
142. Shim G, Ko S, Park JY, Suh JH, Le QV, Kim D, Kim YB, Im GH, Kim HN, Choe YS, Cho J, Kim S, Oh YK. Tannic acid-functionalized boron nitride nanosheets for theranostics. J Control Release. 2020;327:616–26. https://doi.org/10.1016/J.JCONREL.2020.09.009.
143. Silvi S, Credi A. Nanotechnology for biology and medicine. Springer; 2011. p. 27–44. https://doi.org/10.1007/978-0-387-31296-5.
144. Singh V, Chatterjee S, Palecha M, Sen P, Ateeq B, Verma V. Chickpea peel waste as sustainable precursor for synthesis of fluorescent carbon nanotubes for bioimaging application. Carbon Lett. 2021;31(1):117–23. https://doi.org/10.1007/s42823-020-00156-8.
145. Singh P, Rani N, Kumar S, Kumar P, Mohan B, Pallavi, Bhankar V, Kataria N, Kumar R, Kumar K. Assessing the biomass-based carbon dots and their composites for photocatalytic treatment of wastewater. J Clean Prod. 2023;413:137474. https://doi.org/10.1016/J.JCLEPRO.2023.137474.
146. Sintubin L, De Windt W, Dick J, Mast J, Van Der Ha D, Verstraete W, Boon N. Lactic acid bacteria as reducing and capping agent for the fast and efficient production of silver nanoparticles. Appl Microbiol Biotechnol. 2009;84(4):741–9. https://doi.org/10.1007/s00253-009-2032-6.
147. Sivasubramanian M, Chuang YC, Lo LW. Evolution of nanoparticle-mediated photodynamic therapy: from superficial to deep-seated cancers. Molecules. 2019;24(3) https://doi.org/10.3390/molecules24030520.
148. Srivani Maddala VK, Sharma S, Chohan J, Kumar R, Singh S. Green mining techniques to curb environmental problems – a review. IOP Conf Ser: Earth Environ Sci. 2021;889(1) https://doi.org/10.1088/1755-1315/889/1/012026.
149. Stoycheva S, Zabeo A, Pizzol L, Hristozov D. Socio-economic life cycle-based framework for safe and sustainable design of engineered nanomaterials and nano-enabled products. Sustainability. 2022;14(9) https://doi.org/10.3390/su14095734.
150. Sun JF, Wang MZ, Zhao YC, Li XP, Liang BY. Synthesis of titanium nitride powders by reactive ball milling of titanium and urea. J Alloys Compd. 2009;482(1–2):L29–31. https://doi.org/10.1016/J.JALLCOM.2009.04.043.
151. Sun T, Zhang YS, Pang B, Hyun DC, Yang M, Xia Y. Engineered nanoparticles for drug delivery in cancer therapy. Angew Chem Int Ed Engl. 2014;53(46):12320–64. https://doi.org/10.1002/anie.201403036.
152. Sun L, Yuan G, Gao L, Yang J, Chhowalla M, Gharahcheshmeh MH, Gleason KK, Choi YS, Hong BH, Liu Z. Chemical vapour deposition. Nat Rev Methods Primers. 2021a;1(1) https://doi.org/10.1038/s43586-020-00005-y.
153. Sun L, Yuan G, Gao L, Yang J, Chhowalla M, Gharahcheshmeh MH, Gleason KK, Choi YS, Hong BH, Liu Z. Chemical vapour deposition. Nat Rev Methods Primers. 2021b;1(1) https://doi.org/10.1038/s43586-020-00005-y.
154. Suo X, Eldridge BN, Zhang H, Mao C, Min Y, Sun Y, Singh R, Ming X. P-glycoprotein-targeted Photothermal therapy of drug-resistant cancer cells using antibody-conjugated carbon nanotubes [Research-article]. ACS Appl Mater Interfaces. 2018;10(39):33464–73. https://doi.org/10.1021/acsami.8b11974.
155. Tang Y, Zhao J, Zhou J, Zeng Y, Zhang W, Shi B. Highly efficient removal of Cr(III)-poly(acrylic acid) complex by coprecipitation with polyvalent metal ions: performance, mechanism, and validation. Water Res. 2020;178:115807. https://doi.org/10.1016/J.WATRES.2020.115807.
156. Tillotson TM, Gash AE, Simpson RL, Hrubesh LW, Satcher JH, Poco JF. Nanostructured energetic materials using sol-gel methodologies. J Non-Cryst Solids. 2001;285(1–3):338–45. https://doi.org/10.1016/S0022-3093(01)00477-X.
157. Treccani L, Yvonne Klein T, Meder F, Pardun K, Rezwan K. Functionalized ceramics for biomedical, biotechnological and environmental applications. Acta Biomater. 2013;9(7):7115–50. https://doi.org/10.1016/J.ACTBIO.2013.03.036.

158. Truong TT, Mondal S, Doan VHM, Tak S, Choi J, Oh H, Nguyen TD, Misra M, Lee B, Oh J. Precision-engineered metal and metal-oxide nanoparticles for biomedical imaging and healthcare applications. Adv Colloid Interf Sci. 2024;332:103263. https://doi.org/10.1016/J.CIS.2024.103263.
159. Unnikrishnan B, Wu RS, Wei SC, Huang CC, Chang HT. Fluorescent carbon dots for selective labeling of subcellular organelles. ACS Omega. 2020;5(20):11248–61. https://doi.org/10.1021/acsomega.9b04301.
160. Vollenbroek FA, Spiertz EJ. Photoresist systems for microlithography. In: Electronic applications. Springer Nature; 2005. p. 85–111. https://doi.org/10.1007/bfb0025904.
161. Wang J, Chen R, Xiang L, Komarneni S. Synthesis, properties and applications of ZnO nanomaterials with oxygen vacancies: a review. Ceram Int. 2018;44(7):7357–77. https://doi.org/10.1016/J.CERAMINT.2018.02.013.
162. Whitesides GM, Ostuni E, Jiang X, Ingber DE. Soft lithography in biology. Annu Rev Biomed Eng. 2001;3:335–73.
163. Yildirim M, Candan Z. Smart materials: the next generation in science and engineering. Mater Today Proc. 2023; https://doi.org/10.1016/J.MATPR.2023.10.116.
164. Yue K, Guduru R, Hong J, Liang P, Nair M, Khizroev S. Magneto-electric nano-particles for non-invasive brain stimulation. PLoS One. 2012;7(9):1–5. https://doi.org/10.1371/journal.pone.0044040.
165. Zayed DG, Abdelhamid AS, Freag MS, Elzoghby AO. Hybrid quantum dot-based theranostic nanomedicines for tumor-Targeted drug delivery and cancer imaging. Nanomedicine. 2019;14(3):225–8. https://doi.org/10.2217/nnm-2018-0414.
166. Zeng S, Yong K, Roy I. A review on functionalized gold nanoparticles for biosensing applications. Plasmonics. 2011;6:491–506. https://doi.org/10.1007/s11468-011-9228-1.
167. Zhang K, Fu Q, Pan N, Yu X, Liu J, Luo Y, Wang X, Yang J, Hou J. Direct writing of electronic devices on graphene oxide by catalytic scanning probe lithography. Nat Commun. 2012;3(May):1–6. https://doi.org/10.1038/ncomms2200.
168. Zhang Y, Poon K, Masonsong GSP, Ramaswamy Y, Singh G. Sustainable nanomaterials for biomedical applications. Pharmaceutics. 2023;15(3):922.
169. Zhou L, He B, Yang Y, He Y. Facile approach to surface functionalized MoS2 nanosheets. RSC Adv. 2014;4(61):32570–8. https://doi.org/10.1039/c4ra04682j.
170. Zhu Q, Liu S, Sun J, Liu J, Kirubaharan CJ, Chen H, Xu W, Wang Q. Stimuli-responsive cellulose nanomaterials for smart applications. Carbohydr Polym. 2020;235:115933. https://doi.org/10.1016/J.CARBPOL.2020.115933.

Chapter 9
Biosensor for Disease Diagnosis

Umapada Pal

Abstract Healthcare is an important issue for human well-being. It involves the identification and treatment of diseases. Biosensors are devices capable of identifying chemical species in living organisms or biomolecules in a medium or environment. In this chapter, we explore the vital role of biosensors in healthcare, highlighting their roles in early diagnosis and treatment. In research and medical applications, biosensors provide exceptional value by enhancing disease detection and health monitoring. Integration of these devices into healthcare enables medical professionals to detect biomarker traces, facilitating timely interventions and improving diagnostic accuracy. In addition, this chapter highlights the fundamental concepts and operating principles of different biosensors and recent advances in the development of highly sensitive biosensors. These innovations employ advanced designs and innovative nanomaterials to detect viral and bacterial infections and to diagnose neurological and hormonal disorders.

Keywords Biosensing · Functional nanomaterials · Portable biosensors · Disease diagnosis

9.1 Introduction

Biosensors are analytical devices that detect chemical substances in living organisms or biological molecules. They are crucial in healthcare, ensuring the safety of food, water, and the environment. As prevention is better than cure, early detection of harmful biological molecules in the body or the environment is essential to improving healthcare. The idea of biosensing, or biosensors, dates back to 1906, when M. Cremer [1] reported that the acid concentration in a liquid is directly related to the electric potential difference between parts of the fluid on opposite

U. Pal (✉)
Institute of Physics, Autonomous University of Puebla, Puebla, Pue, Mexico
e-mail: upal@ifuap.buap.mx

S. Mondal et al. (eds.), *Smart and Sustainable Nanomaterials in Digital Healthcare and Theranostic*, https://doi.org/10.1007/978-981-95-9386-6_9

sides of a glass membrane. In the years that followed, Griffin and Nelson [2, 3] showed how the enzyme invertase could be immobilized on aluminum hydroxide and charcoal. However, it was Leland C. Clark, Jr, who developed the first true biosensor in 1956 for detecting oxygen [4]. The electrode developed for monitoring oxygen is named after the inventor as the "Clark electrode." In 1962, Leland Clark developed the amperometric enzyme electrode for glucose detection, followed by Guilbault and Montalvo, Jr's, introduction of the first potentiometric biosensor for urea detection in 1969 [5]. These advancements paved the way for Yellow Spring Instruments (YSI) to launch the first commercial biosensor in 1975. Biosensor development has primarily been driven by analytical needs. However, advances in other fields, such as communication, optics, and manufacturing, have significantly contributed to the current state of these devices [6]. For example, electrochemical biosensors are now relatively easy to miniaturize, greatly increasing their availability [7]. Most of the biosensors available in the market now are electrochemical ones, although the demand for biosensors based on optical and acoustic effects is also picking up.

Over the last century, advances in materials and technologies have enabled the development of a vast range of biosensors with enhanced sensitivity and specificity. These biosensors have found their utility in several fields, including healthcare monitoring, disease screening, clinical diagnostics, agriculture, and environmental monitoring. They offer cost-effective, user-friendly, sensitive, and accurate detection capabilities for a range of pathogens and biomolecules. The sensor technology transformed disease detection by enabling high-sensitivity identification of specific biomarkers even at the molecular level. In fact, modern sensors have redefined the way we interact with the environment. In this chapter, we explore different types of biosensors, their structures and functions, and their performance in disease diagnosis, with a focus on the use of innovative materials.

9.2 Working Principle of Biosensors

Biosensors contain a biological recognition element (e.g., an enzyme, antibody, nucleic acid, or nanoparticle) and a transducer that converts the biological response into a detectable electrical or optical signal. The recognition element ensures selective identification of the target, while the transducer enables precise detection of signals via readouts.

Different components of a biosensor are schematically depicted in Fig. 9.1. *Analytes* are the substances of interest that we desire to detect. The analyte may be glucose molecules, enzymes, antibodies, nucleic acids, or any other target for which the biosensor is designed to detect. On the other hand, the *bioreceptors* (biorecognition elements) are molecules that selectively recognize the analyte. Bioreceptors include cells, enzymes, aptamers, deoxyribonucleic acid (DNA), antibodies, and specially engineered nanoparticles. The process by which a bioreceptor interacts with an analyte and generates a measurable signal, such as heat, light, pH change,

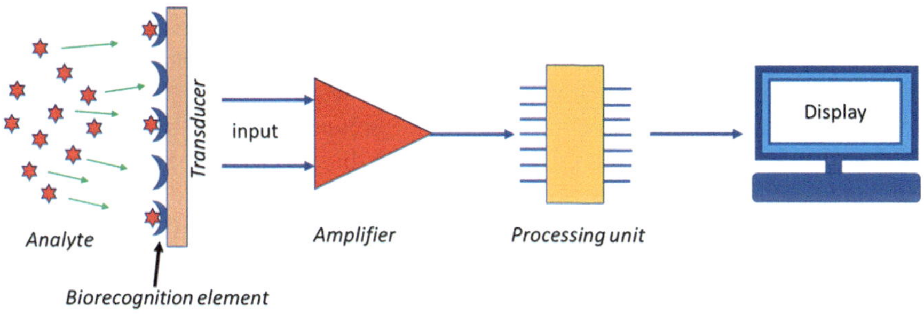

Fig. 9.1 Diagram illustrating different components of a typical biosensor

charge, or mass alteration, is known as bio-recognition. The *transducer* converts one form of signal to another, such as from optical to electrical, which is easily measurable. The electronic *processing unit* of a biosensor then processes the transduced signal to make it displayable. The processing unit contains a sophisticated electronic circuit that amplifies the signal and converts it from analog to digital. The *display* unit then presents the processed signals in a readable format. It typically includes a user interface, such as a liquid crystal display (LCD) or a printer, that generates numbers or curves that are easily interpretable by the user. This part of the system typically contains hardware and software. The output can be presented as numeric values, graphs, tables, or images, depending on users' specific needs. Calibration data or curves derived from standard samples are commonly used for quantitative estimation of the probe sample.

9.3 Classification of Biosensors

Biosensors are classified primarily by their sensing or transduction mechanisms, such as electrochemical, optical, or piezoelectric. They have also been classified by the type of analyte they detect, like enzymatic, immunological, or DNA-based sensors. While both classification criteria are well suited, classifying biosensors by their transduction mechanisms is more practical, considering the wide variety of analytes. Generally, biosensors fall into two broad categories: electrochemical and physical.

9.3.1 Electrochemical Biosensors

Electrochemical biosensors function as electrochemical cells and consist of electrodes, an electrolyte, a current or voltage source, and the analyte to be detected. These biosensors are frequently categorized into three primary types depending on the parameters they detect: amperometric biosensors, which measure current; potentiometric or voltammetric biosensors, which assess potential or charge buildup; and conductometric or impedimetric biosensors, which monitor conductivity or resistance. The latter two categories are often grouped together because of their similar measurement principles [7, 8]. Figure 9.2 illustrates schematic diagrams of each type of these sensors.

In electrochemical biosensors, the analytes interact with the surface of an active electrode, leading to a response that may involve electron transfer across the double-layer potential. In an amperometric biosensor, analytical information is obtained by changing the potential and measuring the current at the potential at which the reaction occurs on the active electrode surface. Amperometric biosensors are commonly employed to detect small molecules, using enzymes like peroxidase to catalyze a redox reaction [10]. The first biosensor principle was the amperometric biosensor for glucose detection using glucose oxidase [7]. Despite numerous improvements over the years, it remains the most widely used biosensor.

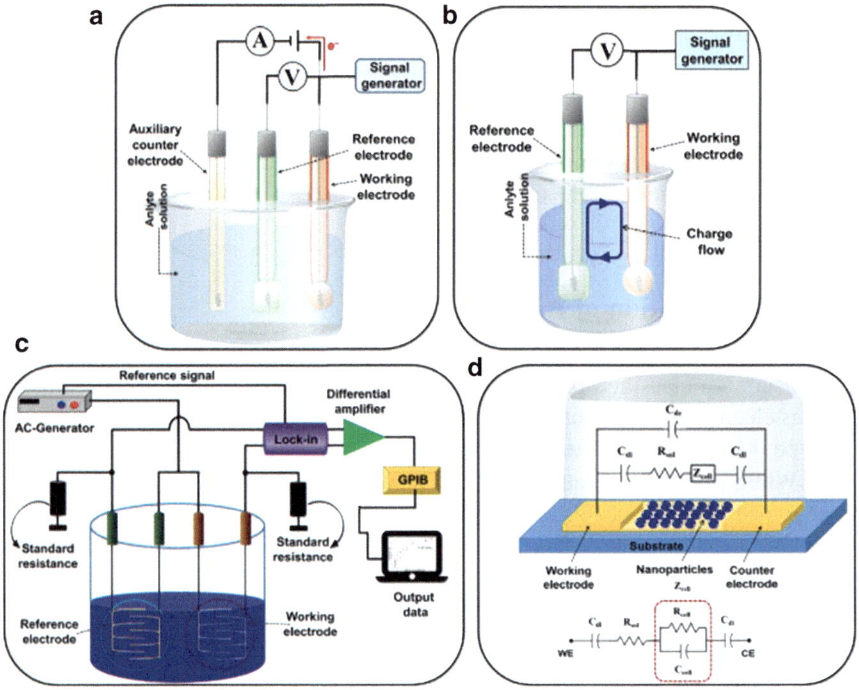

Fig. 9.2 Schematic representation of different types of electrochemical biosensors: (**a**) amperometric, (**b**) potentiometric, (**c**) conductometric, and (**d**) impedimetric. The diagrams in (**d**) illustrate the equivalent circuit components, where C_{dlC}_represents the double-layer capacitance of the electrodes, R_{sol}_is the solution resistance, C_{de} refers to the electrode capacitance, Z_{cell} indicates the impedance from the bound nanoparticles, and R_{cell} and C_{cell} represent the parallel resistance and capacitance, respectively. (Reproduced from Ref. [9], Copyright 2021, MDPI)

The voltammetric or potentiometric biosensors operate on a similar principle; in these systems, the target analyte concentration is determined by the change in potential (relative to the reference) required to initiate the reaction, which is reflected as a current peak during potential scanning. Like amperometric biosensors, potentiometric biosensors are particularly well suited for detecting small molecules [11]. Commonly used pH electrodes are the most primitive potentiometric biosensors. Potentiometric biosensors often employ field-effect transistor detectors, which have attracted considerable attention in recent years owing to advances in nanomaterials such as carbon quantum dots (CQDs), silicon nanotubes, and nanowires. These materials facilitate label-free detection, avoiding the need for enzyme or nanoparticle labeling to generate a signal, thereby reducing detection costs.

The conductometric or impedimetric biosensors rely on electrochemical impedance spectroscopy (EIS), a highly sensitive technique for assessing both the bulk and interfacial electrical properties of electrode systems. Impedimetric biosensors monitor interfacial changes associated with biorecognition events like enzyme-catalyzed reactions or the binding of specific biomolecules, including proteins, receptors, nucleic acids, lectins, cells, antibodies, and other related substances, that occur at the modified electrode surface. Immunosensors and aptasensors are two important examples of impedimetric biosensors. In impedimetric immunosensors, antibodies and antigens bind to form immunocomplexes on the working electrode, which is coated with a blocking layer. This binding increases the electron transfer (charge transfer) resistance (R_{ct}) at the electrolyte-electrode interface. Unlike amperometric and potentiometric systems, impedance biosensors operate without the need for labels or specific enzymes to detect analytes. Instead, they utilize a specialized bioreceptor that selectively binds to the target analyte, such as DNA [12], antibodies [13, 14], aptamers [15], or synthetic affinity proteins like Affimers [16]. Figure 9.3 illustrates the different steps of fabrication of impedimetric biosensors and how the impedance changes at each of the steps, bare electrode, electrode immobilized with bioreceptor, and analyte binding over the bioreceptor-immobilized electrode.

Research on impedimetric biosensors often centers around immunosensors and aptasensors. Immunosensors involve immobilizing antibodies or receptors on the electrode surface. When an immunological reaction occurs between an antibody and an antigen, or between a receptor and its target, the impedance changes. To improve the performance of label-free immunosensors, one approach is to increase the density of immobilized antibodies on the surface of the electrode. Another strategy involves the modification of electrodes with nanostructures such as gold or silver nanoparticles, carbon nanotubes, or polymers (e.g., chitosan, polyaniline). In impedimetric aptasensors, interactions such as probe-target DNA hybridization, conformational changes, or DNA damage cause impedance variations. Aptamer-based biosensors provide high binding specificity, greater stability, and long shelf life. Table 9.1 presents various types of electrochemical biosensors, providing information on their structures, functions, and applications.

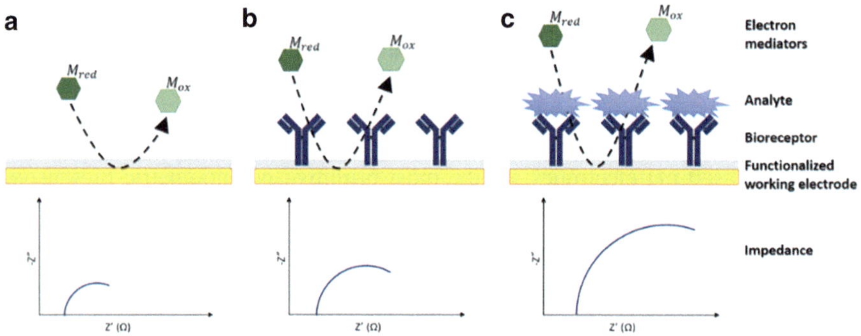

Fig. 9.3 Overview of impedance changes during the construction of a biosensor. As materials are layered onto the electrode surface, the impedance increases. The addition/deposition of material generally increases both resistance and capacitance, impeding electron transfer between solution-phase mediators and the electrode. The impedance sequentially rises from (**a**) the bare electrode to (**b**) post-bioreceptor immobilization and further to (**c**) after analyte binding. (Adapted from Ref. [17], Copyright 2020, Springer)

9.3.2 Physical Biosensors

Physical biosensors are the simplest and most common type. They are classified based on how human senses like hearing, sight, and touch respond to external physical stimuli. Similarly, physical biosensors detect physical properties of their environment. There are three primary types of physical biosensors: piezoelectric, thermometric or thermal, and optical.

9.3.2.1 Piezoelectric Biosensors

Piezoelectric biosensors utilize piezoelectric materials, such as quartz crystals, lead zirconate titanate, or poly(vinylidene fluoride). When mechanical stress is applied, these materials produce electric charges. The sensors operate based on "affinity interaction recording," where the sensor element detects changes in the electric field induced by a mass change on the piezoelectric crystal surface, following Eq. 9.1 (Sauerbrey equation).

$$\Delta f = \frac{-2 f_0^2 \Delta m}{A\sqrt{\rho_0 \mu_0}} \tag{9.1}$$

where f_0 is the resonant frequency (Hz), Δf is the frequency change (Hz), Δm is the change in mass (*g*), *A* is the active area (cm^2) of the crystal (oscillator), ρ_a is the density of piezoelectric crystal (2.648 g/cm^2 for quartz), and μ_a is the shear modulus of the piezoelectric crystal (2.947×10^{11} g/cm S^2 for quartz).

Table 9.1 Different types of electrochemical biosensors and their performances

Sensor type	Principal target	Detection strategy	Performance	Challenges	Integration in devices
Amperometric	Metabolites (e.g., amino acids, nucleotides, and vitamins)	Enzymatic reaction	High sensitivity (as high as 180 μAcm^{-2} $mmol^{-1}$ for glucose) [18] and moderate stability (about 1 month) [19]	Requires further improvement both in sensitivity and in stability	Can be integrated into portable and/or wearable devices
Voltammetric	Proteins and nucleic acids	Bio-affinity (biological binding interaction) recognition	High sensitivity and low detection limit (10 fM of insulin [20], 1 pg ml^{-1} glycoproteins, 100 fM of DNA [21, 22]	Simplification needed for automation of multistep affinity reactions	Portable
Potentiometric	Ionic electrolytes	Selective ion diffusion	Medium sensitivity (~60 mV per decade) and good stability (>1 month) [19]	Miniaturization and improvement in flexibility	Can be integrated into portable and wearable devices
Impedimetric	Immobilized biological recognition elements (unlabeled DNA and proteins) *targets* onto electrode surface	Hybridization between probe and target molecule and consequent change in electrical properties	High binding affinity, enhanced stability, and extended shelf life	Limitations to detect small molecules, reusability, and low selectivity	Can be miniaturized and integrated into portable devices

The piezoelectric sensor element is typically fabricated as a thin film, a plate, or a crystal. Metal electrodes, such as gold, silver, or platinum, are deposited onto the sensor element to collect the electrical signal generated by the piezoelectric effect. A biorecognition layer with specific biomolecules, such as antibodies or enzymes, is applied to the piezoelectric material. This layer selectively binds with the target analyte and is immobilized through chemical bonding or physical adsorption.

The entire setup is mounted on a substrate or housing that provides mechanical stability and protection. The module may include components for interfacing with external systems, such as fluidic channels or electrical connections. Upon binding the analyte to the biorecognition layer, the mass on the piezoelectric element changes. This change alters the resonant frequency of the piezoelectric element, which is monitored by the sensor. An increase in mass decreases the oscillation frequency. On the other hand, a decrease in mass increases the frequency shift (Eq. 9.1). The electrodes detect this shift and convert it into an electrical signal, which is processed by an electronic system and displayed as a quantitative output, indicating the analyte concentration.

Piezoelectric biosensors are very sensitive and can detect low analyte concentrations. They provide real-time monitoring without requiring chemical labels or dyes, simplifying the assay and minimizing potential interference. These sensors have been applied in clinical diagnostics, food safety testing, and environmental monitoring. The electrical signal generated by the oscillation of a piezoelectric crystal and its resonant frequency change due to changes in mass and in the anchoring of analyte molecules, as schematically illustrated in Fig. 9.4.

9.3.2.2 Thermoelectric Biosensors

The central component of a thermoelectric biosensor is its thermoelectric layer, which generates a voltage when a temperature difference exists. Common thermoelectric materials include bismuth telluride (Bi_2Te_3), lead telluride (PbTe), and silicon-germanium (SiGe) alloys, which are often assembled into thermocouples or thermopiles. A thermocouple is created by joining two different metals at one end, while a thermopile is made of multiple thermocouples connected in series to boost the voltage. Electrodes, usually made from conductive materials like gold or platinum, are attached to the thermoelectric material to collect the voltage generated by the thermoelectric effect.

A biorecognition layer is coated on the surface of the thermoelectric material. This layer contains biomolecules, such as antibodies, enzymes, or aptamers, which bind to the target analyte. The biorecognition layer is immobilized on the thermoelectric layer via chemical bonding or physisorption. The sensor assembly is supported by a substrate or housing that provides mechanical stability and allows for integration with external systems, including components for fluid handling or electrical connections.

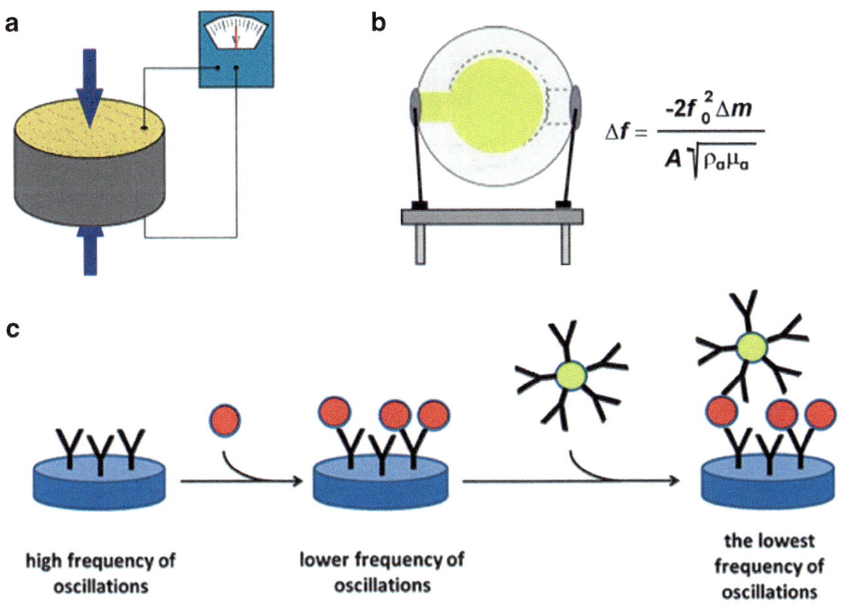

Fig. 9.4 (**a**) Schematic showing the generation of electrical signals in a piezoelectric crystal. (**b**) Illustration showing how resonant frequency changes due to the variations in mass. (**c**) Diagram of a piezoelectric immunosensor where immunoglobulins (Y-shaped) detect antigens (red spheres). The resonant frequency shift is enhanced by the addition of nanoparticles (yellow spheres). The blue disc represents the piezoelectric crystal. (Panel (**c**) is adapted from Ref. [23], Copyright 2018, MDPI)

When a sample containing the target interacts with the biorecognition layer, a biochemical reaction occurs. This reaction may produce heat or change the temperature of the biosensor, creating a thermal gradient across the thermoelectric material. This gradient is crucial for generating voltage through the thermoelectric (Seebeck) effect, where the material converts the thermal gradient into electrical voltage. The voltage, which is proportional to the temperature difference induced by the biochemical reaction, is measured at the electrodes. An external electronic system analyzes the electrical signal to estimate the concentration of the target analyte in the probed sample. The processed signal is then presented as a quantitative result, indicating the presence and concentration of the analyte. This data is used in numerous applications, such as clinical diagnostics and environmental monitoring.

Figure 9.5 shows the basic design of a thermocouple and a thermopile (Fig. 9.5a), along with the schematic of a thermoelectric generator (Fig. 9.5b). Sections (c) and (d) display schematics and a cross-sectional view of a wearable thermoelectric sensor. These sensors are very sensitive and can detect small temperature changes associated with biochemical reactions. They provide real-time feedback on the presence or concentration of target substances, making them well suited for real-time

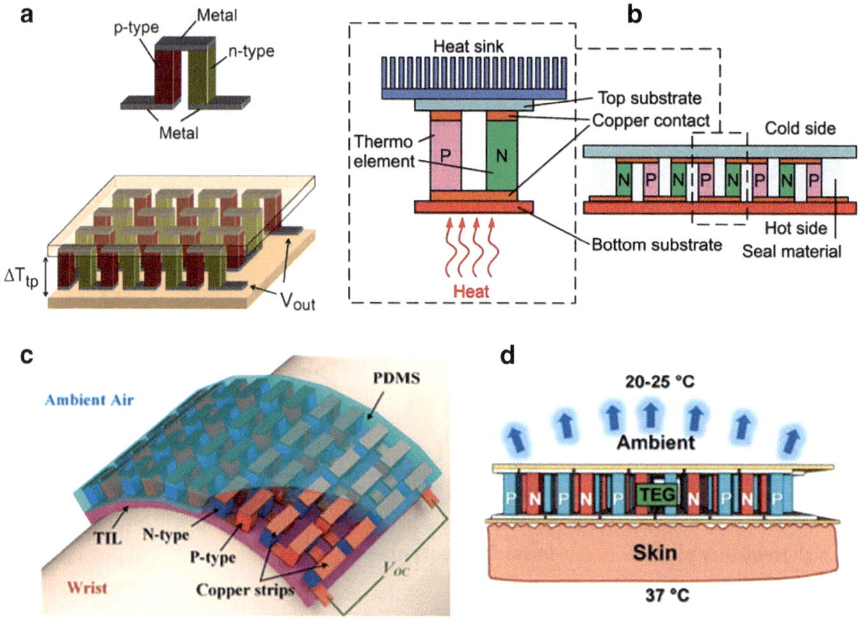

Fig. 9.5 (**a**) Basic design of (**a**) a thermocouple (top) and a thermopile (bottom). (**b**) Schematic presentation of a thermoelectric generator. Reproduced from Ref. [25], Copyright 2021, MDPI. (**c**) Schematic of a wearable thermoelectric generator on a human wrist. Reproduced from Ref. [26], Copyright 2017 Elsevier. (**d**) Cross-sectional view of the thermoelectric process in a wearable thermoelectric generator mounted over human skin. Reproduced from Ref. [27], Copyright 2019 Elsevier

monitoring. Thermoelectric biosensors are highly effective at detecting a wide range of analytes, including nucleic acids, proteins, and small molecules. In practice, they have been used to detect biomarkers or pathogens, measure environmental pollutants or toxins, and monitor spoilage in food packaging. For example, thermometric biosensors have been employed to estimate serum cholesterol levels [24] by measuring the heat generated by the enzyme cholesterol oxidase, which catalyzes the oxidation of cholesterol. They have also been used to assess the levels of glucose, urea, uric acid, and penicillin G in biological media.

Thermometric biosensors monitor temperature changes associated with biochemical reactions, enabling real-time tracking of target substances. These sensors are highly effective at detecting a broad spectrum of analytes, including proteins, nucleic acids, and other molecules. In medical diagnostics, biomarkers and pathogens are identified by measuring temperature changes related to biochemical activity. Additionally, these sensors are crucial for detecting contaminants and spoilage indicators by monitoring heat production or temperature variations.

9.3.2.3 Optical Biosensors

Optical biosensors use light-based measurement techniques, often incorporating optical fibers and optoelectronic transducers. The term "optrode" combines "optical" and "electrode" to describe these sensors. These sensors typically use antibodies and enzymes as key components. Optical biosensors can be divided into four main types based on their sensing mechanisms: surface plasmon resonance (SPR)-based, evanescent-wave fluorescence-based, luminescence-based (using bioluminescent materials), and surface-enhanced Raman scattering (SERS)-based.

A plasmon is the collective oscillation of electrons on the surface of a metal or conductive material. When this oscillation resonates with the frequency of incoming light, the phenomenon is called surface plasmon resonance (SPR). SPR takes place at the interface between a metal (or other conductive material) and a surrounding medium, typically glass and a liquid, by illuminating it with a polarized light at a specific angle. This effect permits a direct, label-free, real-time monitoring of changes in the refractive index at the sensor surface or shifts in the resonant frequency of biomolecules within the near field of the plasmonic substrate. To measure interactions between a ligand and an analyte, one of these molecules is immobilized on the surface of the sensor.

A typical SPR setup consists of an optical detector (used to measure peak shifts), a sensor chip with a gold-coated surface, a ligand-immobilization layer, and a fluidics system that enables continuous flow. The functional layer of the SPR chip, often composed of a self-assembled carboxymethylated dextran monolayer, facilitates molecular immobilization. The operating principle of a standard SPR instrument is depicted in Fig. 9.6. The setup enables effective protein immobilization via N-hydroxysuccinimide (NHS) chemistry. Optical biosensors are perfect for detecting a wide range of analytes, including antibodies, viruses, drugs, toxins, tumor biomarkers, and tumor cells. Localized surface plasmon resonance (LSPR) is an optical effect caused by the interaction of light with metallic nanoparticles (MNPs). In this process, the electromagnetic field of the incoming light induces collective oscillation of conduction electrons within the nanoparticles, leading to light absorption in the ultraviolet-visible (UV-VIS) spectrum (Fig. 9.6). Unlike traditional surface plasmon resonance, where plasmon oscillations happen at the metal dielectric interface, LSPR involves oscillations confined to the nanoparticles themselves. LSPR-based biosensing relies on detecting shifts in the absorption spectrum. These shifts arise from changes in the dielectric environment surrounding the nanoparticles during a binding event. The material, size, shape, and spacing between nanoparticles all influence LSPR characteristics, including sensitivity, as reflected in color changes and shifts in the absorption peak. By tuning these parameters during sensor fabrication, the performance of LSPR sensors can be optimized.

LSPR sensors offer greater fabrication flexibility compared to commercial SPR sensors. They can be constructed by attaching (immobilizing) MNPs on a substrate (e.g., a glass slide or optical fiber), or by dispersing the nanoparticles in a solution to create a solution-phase LSPR sensor. The two most common optical geometries for LSPR sensors are transmission mode and reflection mode.

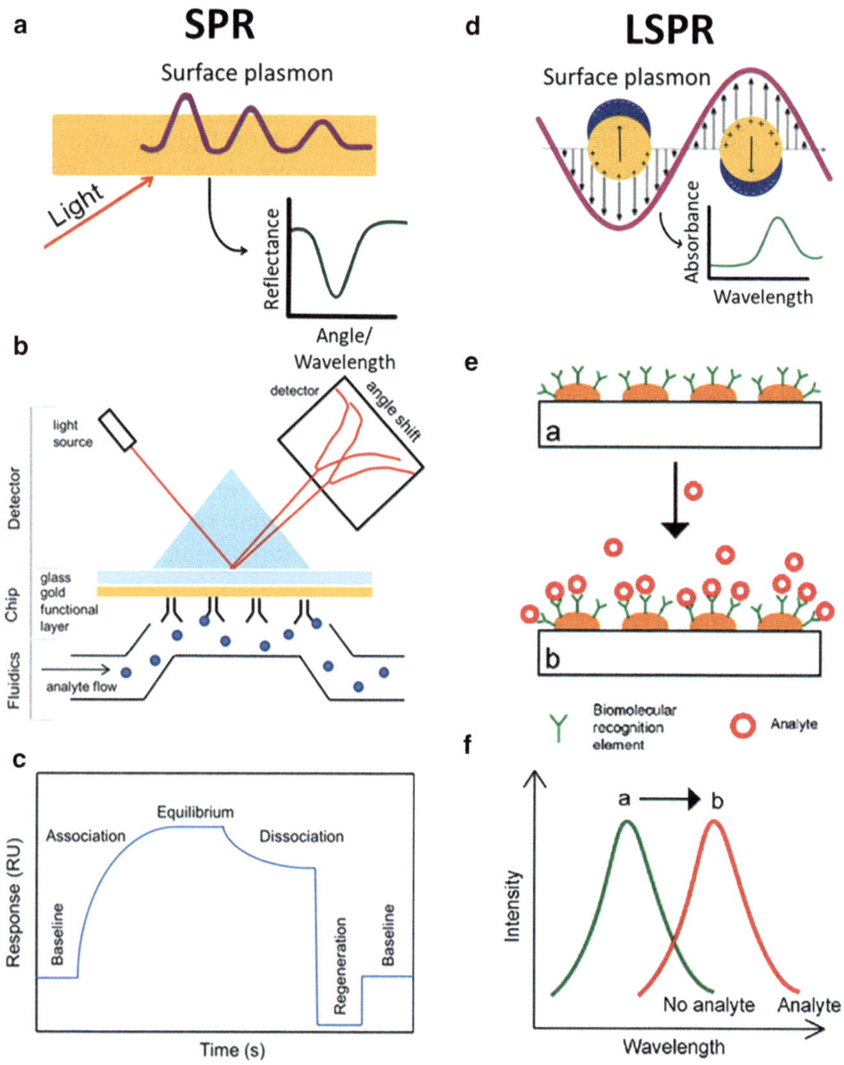

Fig. 9.6 Comparison of biomolecular detection methods using SPR (left column) and LSPR (right column). (**a**) Surface plasmon resonance generation at the metal surface. (**b**) Operational principle of an SPR instrument. (**c**) Example of an SPR sensorgram depicting the stages of an analytical cycle. Adapted from Ref. [28], Copyright 2016, Portland Press. (**d**) Localized surface plasmon resonance within a metal nanoparticle. (**e**) Biomolecular recognition elements (e.g., antibodies) on a metal nanoparticle surface, illustrating analyte capture (labeled as **a**) and the resulting local refractive index increase (labeled as **b**). (**f**) LSPR peak shift resulting from a local refractive index increase. Adapted from Ref. [29], Copyright 2018, Elsevier

The evanescent wave, introduced by Hirschfeld in 1966 [30], arises from light confined within an optical waveguide. When light reaches the interface between the waveguide and its surrounding medium with a lower refractive index, it undergoes total internal reflection (TIR). During this process, the Fresnel transmission coefficients for both transverse electric (TE) and transverse magnetic (TM) waves are non-zero. As a result, although the light is fully reflected, an electromagnetic field, known as an evanescent wave, extends from the interface into the lower refractive index medium. The wave propagates parallel to the surface in the plane of incidence and decays exponentially as it moves away from the surface, typically over a distance ranging from 100 nanometers to approximately one wavelength (Fig. 9.6a).

The intensity of the evanescent electric field decreases exponentially with distance from the interface. The penetration depth (*d*), or how far the evanescent field extends into the lower-index medium, can be calculated using the following equation, which depends on the incident wavelength (λ) and the angle of incidence:

$$d = \frac{\lambda}{2\pi}\left(n_1^2 \sin^2\theta - n_2^2\right)^{-1/2} \tag{9.2}$$

where n_1 and n_2 represent the refractive indices of the waveguide material (solid) and the surrounding medium (liquid or analyte solution), respectively. Figure 9.6 presents a schematic of a typical evanescent-wave planar optical waveguide chip. In this setup, a laser diode with a specified wavelength and power is attached to the slanted edge of the chip, where the light propagates along the chip's sensitive area via total internal reflection. The evanescent wave penetrates several tens of nanometers into the surrounding medium, making it suitable for studying turbid or strongly adsorbing media [31].

At the point of total internal reflection, the evanescent wave excites the fluorophores that are bound to the surface of fluorescence-labeled biomolecules. The resulting fluorescence emission is then captured by a high-numerical-aperture polymer optical fiber (e.g., NA = 0.46) placed beneath the biochip, on the opposite side of the biosensing layer. A high-pass filter is used to eliminate scattered or stray laser light from the collected signal, which is then detected by a photodiode and processed using a lock-in amplifier (Fig. 9.6b).

Because the evanescent wave is confined to the surface, biosensors that rely on this principle generate fluorescent signals exclusively from molecules attached to the sensor surface. This surface-specific nature minimizes background noise from the bulk sample and enhances detection of surface-bound fluorophores. Many biosensors have been developed using this approach. Since their introduction in 1985 [32], evanescent wave fluorescence biosensors have been widely employed in a range of applications, including environmental monitoring (e.g., water quality assessment), defense, security, food safety testing, and disease diagnosis. For more details on the development and application of these biosensors, readers can consult the review by Taitt et al. [33] (Fig. 9.7)

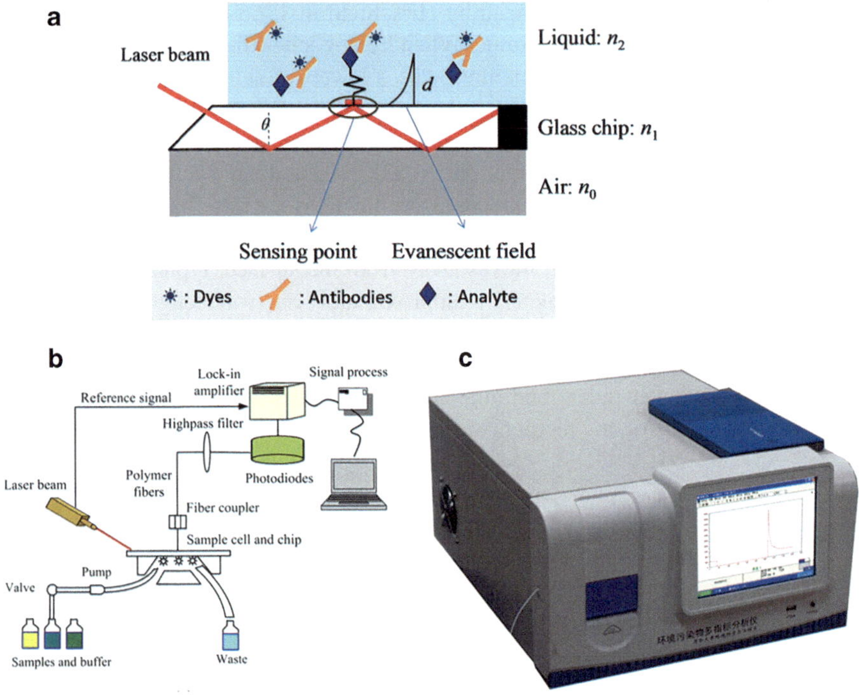

Fig. 9.7 (**a**) Diagram illustrating the working principle of a planar optical waveguide chip based on evanescence excitation. (**b**) Schematic of a planar-waveguide evanescent-wave immunosensing platform. (**c**) Photograph of a planar waveguide evanescent wave biosensing system designed for the detection of Bisphenol A. (Reproduced with permission from Ref. [31], Copyright 2014, Springer Nature)

9.3.2.4 Luminescence/Fluorescence Biosensors

The operating principle of luminescence- or fluorescence-based biosensors is similar to that of evanescent-wave fluorescence biosensors. However, in this case, a luminescent material, often in solution, is directly excited by a monochromatic light source (e.g., a laser beam), and the resulting change in emission intensity is measured upon interaction with the target analyte. Unlike evanescent wave fluorescence biosensors, this method does not require a specially designed biochip. However, it requires precise monochromatic excitation, a sensitive detection system, and a monochromator capable of operating within the wavelength range of the emitted signal.

Various mechanisms can influence the changes in fluorescence emission detected by luminescence-based biosensors. For bioluminescent analytes, changes in emission are typically due to variations in energy release (e.g., ATP) or charge transfer mediated by reactive oxygen species. For other analytes, the emission changes are often caused by charge transfer between analyte and probe molecules. In these cases, photosensitive polymers (PPs) or semiconductor materials, including their nanostructures, are commonly used in aqueous or buffer solutions. Upon illumination, excited electrons in the conduction band of PP or semiconductor nanostructures interact with analyte molecules, thereby facilitating charge transfer. This process reduces the recombination of excited electrons (with photo-generated holes), thereby decreasing the photoluminescence (PL) or fluorescence intensity of the nanostructures. Figure 9.8 illustrates the mechanism and performance of Ni- and Cd-doped CdTe nanoparticle-based luminescence quenching sensors used for detecting pyrazinamide (PZA) and diazinon (DZN), respectively.

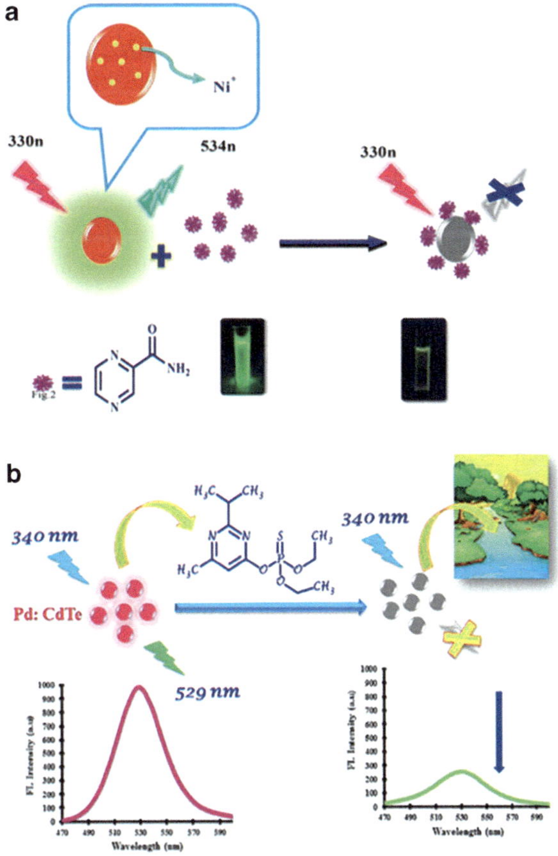

Fig. 9.8 (**a**) Diagram illustrating the detection of pyrazinamide (PZA) using Ni-doped CdTe quantum dots. Reprinted with permission from Ref. [34], Copyright 2019, Elsevier. (**b**) Schematic representation of diazinon (DZN) detection using Pd-doped CdTe quantum dots. Reprinted with permission from Ref. [35], Copyright 2019, Springer

9.3.3 SERS-Based Biosensors

Surface-enhanced Raman scattering (SERS) is a highly sensitive spectroscopic technique that can amplify Raman signals by up to a million times when using appropriate SERS substrates. First discovered on rough silver surfaces in the 1970s, SERS has since become a widely adopted tool in several fields like chemistry, materials science, biochemistry, and life science. SERS-based biosensors offer several key advantages in biomaterial analysis: (1) to detect molecular fingerprints with exceptional sensitivity (even at the single-molecule level); (2) durable with narrow peak bandwidths and resistance to photobleaching; (3) the availability of a diverse range of signal-enhancing substrates with different shapes and sizes for a variety of applications; and (4) greater laser penetration depth, suitable for both in vitro and in vivo diagnostics and imaging.

Raman scattering is the inelastic scattering of photons, in which energy is either lost (Stokes shift) or gained (anti-Stokes shift) due to molecular vibrations, thereby reflecting molecular structure and enabling real-time detection. SERS is a specialized form of Raman scattering that increases the Raman signal using plasmonic nanostructures, greatly boosting detection sensitivity to single molecules. This enhancement mainly occurs through two mechanisms: electromagnetic (EM) enhancement and chemical (CHEM) enhancement. EM enhancement occurs when incident light interacts with the localized surface plasmon resonances (LSPRs) of nanostructures, thereby concentrating the electromagnetic field and enhancing the SERS signal. Molecules within a sub-10-nanometer range of the nanostructures undergo this amplification, resulting in an enhancement factor between 10^4 and 10^7. Conversely, CHEM enhancement happens when analyte molecules bind directly to the plasmonic surface, forming a charge-transfer complex. Although CHEM enhancement depends on the molecule's chemical makeup and surface affinity, its overall contribution is generally small, with an enhancement factor of 10–100.

In recent years, SERS-based sensors have become widely used for detecting various biomolecules, including proteins, lipids, and nucleic acids, without requiring labels. This allows for detailed analysis of the molecular composition of samples. These sensors are also employed for imaging and detecting biological cells and tissues. Typically, such detections are label-free, meaning no receptor molecules need to be attached to the SERS surface. However, accurately determining protein structure and concentration using label-free methods remains challenging due to their low signal strength.

Indirect protein detection is often linked to enzyme-linked immunosorbent assays (ELISA), especially when SERS tags are used, forming SERS immunoassays [36]. ELISA is widely valued for its cost-effectiveness, simplicity, and high specificity, making it suitable for complex biological problems. When SERS tags are incorporated, these immunoassays achieve higher sensitivity, less spectral interference, and improved multiplexing capabilities. The most common method in SERS immunoassays is the sandwich assay, in which antibodies bind to antigens. For example, Yang et al. [37] fabricated an SERS immunoassay platform using alpha-fetoprotein (AFP) antibody-modified core-shell satellite nanostructures (acted as SERS tags), with a nitrocellulose membrane (acted as a solid substrate). The Au@Ag core-shell satellite nanostructures are notable for their strong SERS performance, with a thin silica layer that enhances long-range plasmon coupling and greatly boosts the signal. This sandwich-type SERS assay is very sensitive, detecting AFP up to 0.3 fg/mL concentration. Figure 9.9 shows a schematic of dual-reporter SERS immunoassays suitable for protein detection. Recent advances in this area have led to more sophisticated systems, evolving from the traditional sandwich assay to platforms that include test strips and microfluidic chips [38]. These dual-reporter systems have greatly improved the accuracy of parallel protein detection.

Cheng et al. [39] introduced a magnetic separation SERS immunoassay utilizing two distinct SERS tags to label two forms of prostate-specific antigen (PSA): complexed PSA (c-PSA) and free PSA (f-PSA). This dual-labeling technique allows simultaneous detection of both forms, providing a more precise determination of the free-to-total PSA ratio (f/t) in clinical samples (Fig. 9.9a). Building on this concept, Chuong et al. [40] further refined the dual-reporter approach (Fig. 9.9b) by using two affinity reagents, each labeled with a different Raman reporter, to reduce false positives. This enhanced approach is particularly effective at distinguishing true positives from false positives, even at low target protein concentrations, as demonstrated by the detection of alpha-thrombin and tumor necrosis factor-alpha in complex biological samples (Fig. 9.9b).

SERS-based biosensors are extensively used to detect biomolecules such as proteins, DNA, and microRNAs, as well as to monitor cellular conditions like temperature, pH, and ion concentrations. These biosensors have made notable progress in in vivo diagnostics, imaging, and therapeutic uses. Although challenges remain in in vitro applications, SERS assays and platforms are expected to impact point-of-care diagnostics significantly.

The most formidable challenge in SERS-based biosensing is improving the detection sensitivity of SERS substrates. Other challenges include enhancing specificity, reducing interference from surrounding molecules, and minimizing substrate photoluminescence. Overall, SERS biosensors hold great potential, but further refinements are needed for broader clinical adoption.

9.4 Integration of Electrochemical Biosensors into Portable and Wearable Devices

Electrochemical biosensors can be seamlessly integrated into a range of portable, wearable, and implantable devices, as listed in Table 9.1. These devices generally include components such as microfluidic systems, printed circuit boards (PCBs), software, signal processors, communication modules, and power sources. Among electrochemical biosensors, amperometric sensors are well advanced and widely used for metabolite detection. They achieve high selectivity through specific

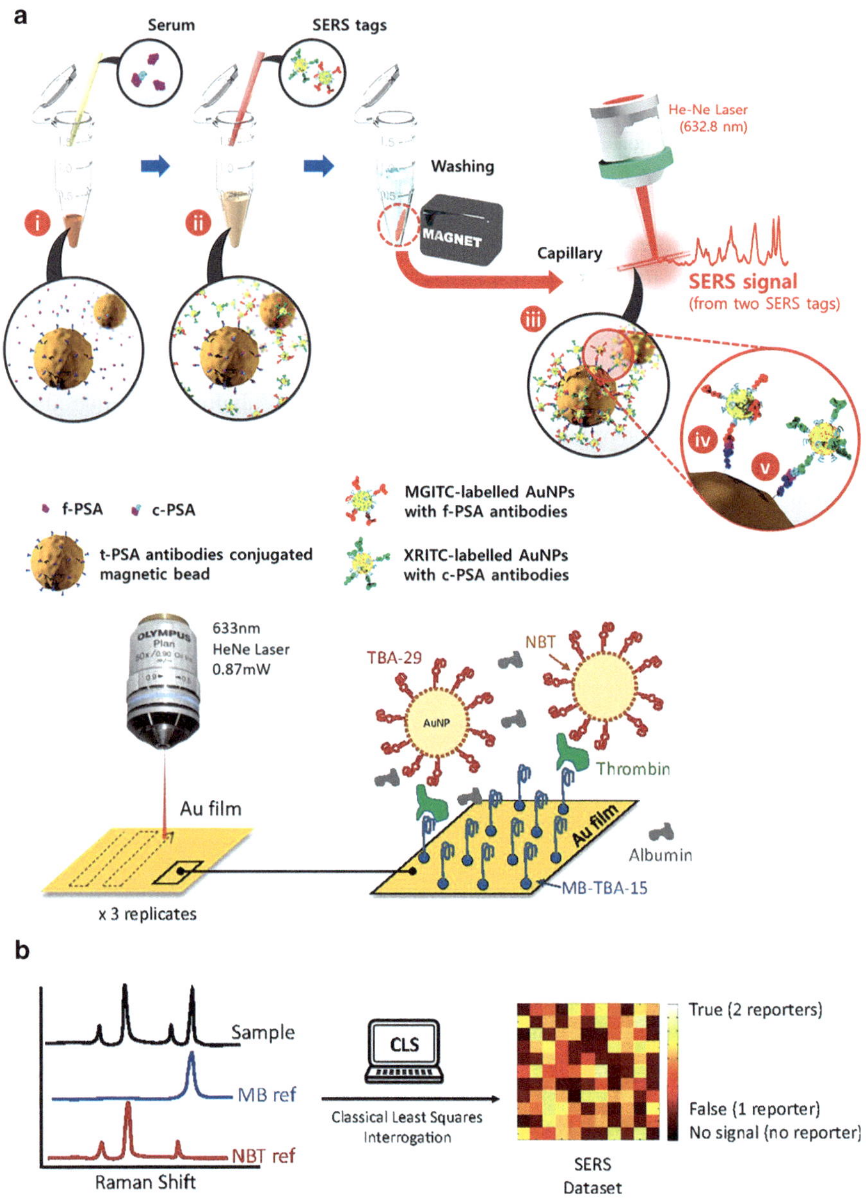

Fig. 9.9 Process for sequential SERS-based assay enabling the simultaneous detection of f-PSA (free prostate-specific antigen, not complexed or combined with other proteins) and c-PSA (prostate-specific antigen complexes, bound to the serum protease inhibitor α1-antichymotrypsin). (i) f-PSA, c-PSA, and t-PSA (total prostate-specific antigen) antibody-conjugated magnetic beads are mixed. (ii) SERS nanotags are introduced to form sandwich immunocomplexes. (iii) Magnetic immunocomplexes are separated using a magnetic bar. (iv) Simultaneous detection of f-PSA and (v) c-PSA. Adapted from Ref. [39], Copyright 2017, American Chemical Society. (**a**) Dual-reporter SERS immunoassays using gold nanoparticles labeled with two Raman reporters for sensing human α-thrombin. (**b**) SERS spectra are collected for each thrombi concentration, with analysis via the least-squares technique to distinguish actual binding events from false positives. True- and false-positive binding locations are shown in a heat map. Adapted from Ref. [40], Copyright 2017, National Academy of Science, USA. MB methylene blue, NBT 4-nitrobenzenethiol

enzymatic reactions, and their sensitivity can be enhanced by incorporating nanomaterials. While enzyme-based sensors are typically fabricated in batch with high reproducibility, environmental conditions can affect their performance.

Potentiometric biosensors are especially suitable for wearable uses, like sweat monitoring, because they measure electrolytes with ion-selective membranes. These sensors are known for their high selectivity, good reproducibility, and stability, although their sensitivity is usually lower than other sensor types. To enable continuous sweat monitoring, flexible, all-solid-state ion-selective electrodes are often employed. Additionally, other sensor types such as voltammetric, organic electrochemical transistors (OECT), photoelectrochemical, and electrochemiluminescent biosensors offer selective and sensitive detection of proteins and nucleic acids. However, these affinity-based sensors often require careful alignment of bioreceptors at the electrode surface, which makes their fabrication more intricate than of enzyme-based sensors. The following section highlights several examples of specific portable electrochemical biosensors.

9.4.1 Portable Glucose Meters

Portable electrochemical sensors were originally created to monitor glucose levels in the blood of diabetic patients. A typical personal glucose meter is an amperometric biosensor that quickly measures blood glucose concentrations. The system consists of a single-use test strip and a portable electrochemical reader (Fig. 9.10a). These test strips are affordable and made from materials such as plastics and conductive pastes, with screen-printing technology commonly used to produce thin-film electrodes at large scale. The test strip's sensing layer contains an enzyme and an electron mediator. When a blood sample is applied, glucose is oxidized by the redox mediator through catalysis by glucose oxidase (GOx), producing a measurable current. The handheld reader then converts this current into a glucose concentration value. Since the development of glucose enzyme electrodes in the 1960s, glucose meters have continued to improve in accuracy, reliability, ease of use, and cost. These devices have expanded their ability to detect various substances, including drugs, metal ions, organic metabolites, enzymes, proteins, DNA, and viruses, by linking target recognition with glucose production or usage. For example, personal glucose meters now can measure compounds like cocaine and uranium by triggering glucose release, or identify SARS-CoV-2 antigens in saliva for COVID-19 testing. This onsite testing method provides results within an hour and can detect concentrations as low as the picomolar level.

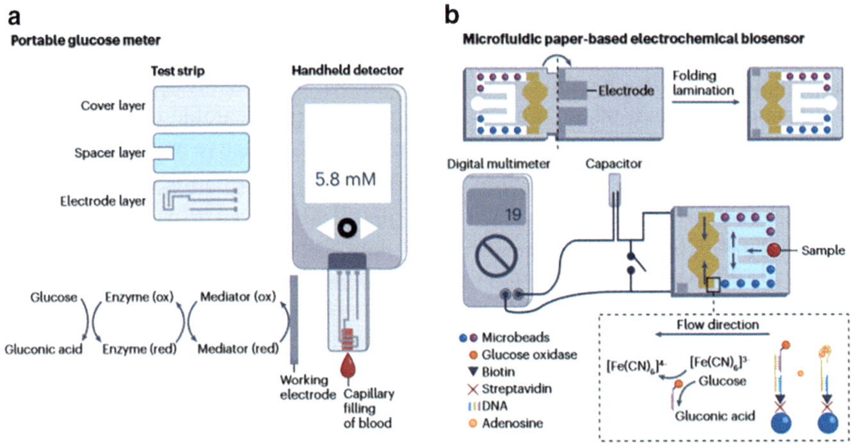

Fig. 9.10 Portable electrochemical biosensing devices. (**a**) A handheld blood glucose meter paired with a disposable test strip. The test strip includes a bottom electrode layer, an adhesive spacer, and a hydrophilic cover layer. The blood samples are drawn into the reaction chamber by capillary action. Adapted from Ref. [41]. Copyright 2023, Nature. (**b**) A paper-based microfluidic electrochemical biosensor for adenosine detection using aptamer-based affinity sensing. In one channel, adenosine is captured by aptamer-functionalized microbeads (blue), triggering the release of glucose oxidase-labeled DNA to catalyze glucose oxidation, converting $[Fe(CN)_6]^{3-}$ to $[Fe(CN)_6]^{4-}$. In the other channel, non-functionalized microbeads (purple) are used to measure adenosine concentration. The current signal from the discharging capacitor is recorded by a portable digital multimeter. Ox oxidation, red reduction. Reprinted with permission from Ref. [42]. Copyright 2012, Wiley

9.4.2 Biosensors Integrated with Microfluidics and Paper-Based Devices

To analyze complex samples that require pre-treatment and continuous monitoring, electrochemical biosensors can be integrated with microfluidic systems. For instance, a microfluidic device can detect SARS-CoV-2 RNA using an enzyme–DNA nanostructure with cascading molecular circuitry enhancement. This system automates assays using pressure-actuated microfluidics and embedded sensing electrodes. Additionally, paper-based microfluidic devices provide a low-cost, biodegradable, and easy-to-fabricate alternative that uses capillary action for fluid transport. Paper can be folded into 3D structures to control both fluidic and electrical connections. An example is a paper-based device for adenosine detection, where adenosine binds to an aptamer, causing measurable changes in redox concentrations (Fig. 9.10b). Miniaturized electrochemical analyzers can be paired with smartphones to process, store, and display data. The integration of a portable electrochemical detector with smartphone connectivity enables efficient data management and supports remote health monitoring.

9.5 Disease Detection Using Biosensors

9.5.1 Virus Detection

Early detection of viral infections is crucial for controlling their spread. Traditional methods, like plate culturing and quantitative RT-PCR, provide reliable results but are time-consuming, require specialized expertise, and involve costly equipment, making them inaccessible to many in low-income areas of developing countries. Moreover, mass testing during pandemics has led to shortages in testing kits and reagents, disrupting supply chains.

We urgently require high-sensitivity, low-cost biosensors that provide rapid results. For instance, while PCR tests can take 5–6 h, lateral flow immunoassays and other biosensors can provide results in about 20 min. A well-known example is the COVID-19 Rapid Point-of-Care (POC) test, which uses a lateral-flow immunoassay to detect IgM and IgG antibodies targeting the SARS-CoV-2 spike protein in capillary blood samples. This test has two parts: the IgM and IgG regions. When a sample is applied, it interacts with gold nanoparticle-coated SARS-CoV-2 antigens. If antibodies are present, they form complexes that move along the test strip. The presence of IgM antibodies shows a visible line at the M region, while IgG antibodies produce a line at the G region. A control line confirms the test worked correctly. If no antibodies are detected, no lines will appear, indicating a negative result. Regardless of the outcome, a control line will always appear to verify the test's function. Figure 9.11 shows the schematics of commercial COVID-19 detection kits and details of the test strip.

Various virus-related diseases, such as human immunodeficiency virus (HIV), Zika virus, and Ebola virus, have been monitored using highly sensitive biosensors made from innovative 2D materials. For example, graphene-based field-effect transistor (GFET) biosensors (Fig. 9.12a–d) have been employed for the precise

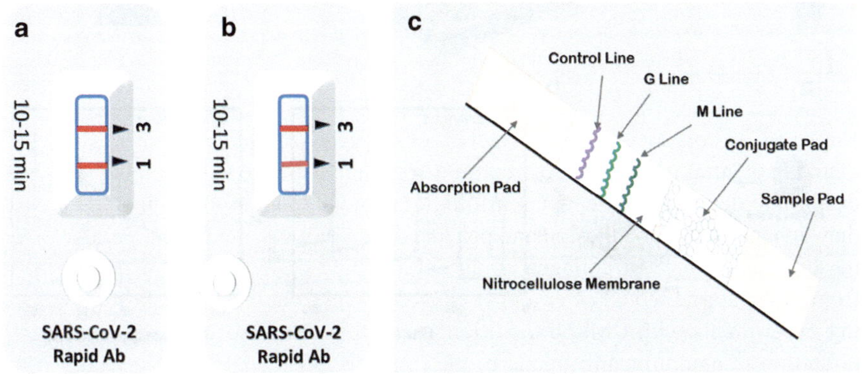

Fig. 9.11 Schematic representations of a commercial COVID-19 detection kit: (**a**) a positive test result, (**b**) a negative test result, and (**c**) an overview of a COVID-19 test strip, highlighting its key functional areas

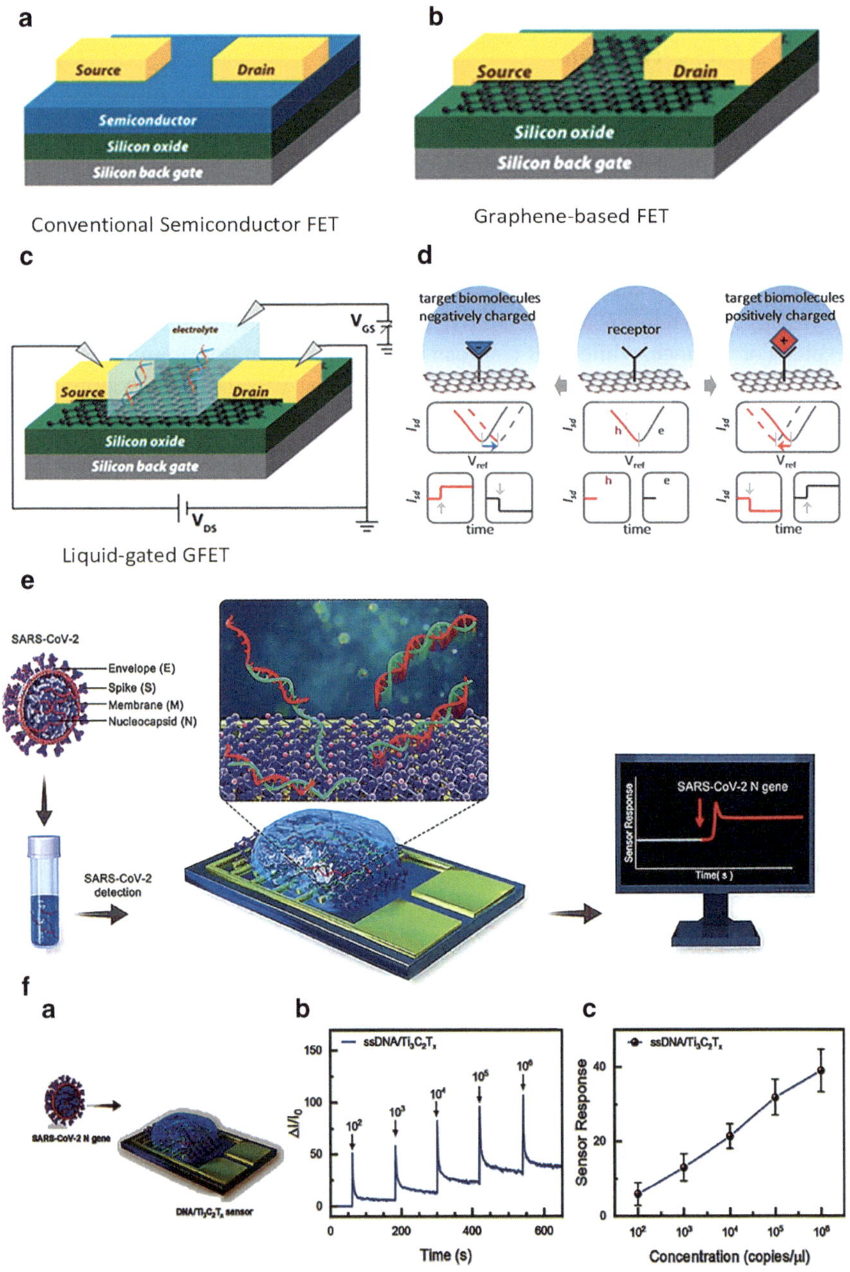
a
Source
Drain
Semiconductor
Silicon oxide
Silicon back gate
Conventional Semiconductor FET
b
Source
Drain
Silicon oxide
Silicon back gate
Graphene-based FET
c
electrolyte
V_{GS}
Source
Drain
Silicon oxide
Silicon back gate
V_{DS}
Liquid-gated GFET
d
target biomolecules negatively charged
receptor
target biomolecules positively charged
I_{sd}
V_{ref}
time
h
e
e
SARS-CoV-2
Envelope (E)
Spike (S)
Membrane (M)
Nucleocapsid (N)
SARS-CoV-2 detection
SARS-CoV-2 N gene
Sensor Response
Time(s)
f
a
SARS-CoV-2 N gene
DNA/Ti$_3$C$_2$T$_x$ sensor
b
ssDNA/Ti$_3$C$_2$T$_x$
ΔI/I$_0$
Time (s)
c
ssDNA/Ti$_3$C$_2$T$_x$
Sensor Response
Concentration (copies/μl)

Fig. 9.12 Schematic diagrams illustrating the structures of (**a**) a conventional semiconductor field-effect transistor (FET), (**b**) a graphene-based field effect transistor (GFET), and (**c**) a liquid-gated graphene-based field-effect transistor (LG-GFET). (**d**) Representation of sensing mechanism in LG-FET biosensors. The upper panel shows receptor molecules interacting with the graphene channel, while the lower panel displays the plots of source-drain current (I_{SD}) vs reference potential (V_{ref}) and I_{SD} vs time (t). Reprinted with permission from Ref. [49]. Copyright 2017, Wiley. (**e**) Schematic of the detection process for the SARS-CoV-2 nucleocapsid (N) gene using ssDNA/$Ti_3C_2T_x$ sensors. (**f**) Panel (**a**) presents the N gene from heat-inactivated SARS-CoV-2, panel (**b**) shows the real-time response, and panel (**c**) plots the sensor response against concentration. Reproduced from Ref. [46]. Copyright 2022, American Chemical Society

detection of these viruses. In 2013, Kwon et al. [43] used a GFET biosensor integrated with a microfluidic device for highly sensitive detection of HIV. The liquid-ion-gated GFET device was fabricated by combining a micropatterned graphene sheet with a densely packed array of carboxylated polypyrrole nanoparticles, which served as a flexible fluidic immunoassay platform. The large specific surface area of the graphene micropatterned channels offered a stable sensing platform in a liquid environment, enabling the immunosensor to detect HIV biomarkers at concentrations as low as 1 pM with remarkable sensitivity.

A GFET was developed by Kim et al. [44] on a flexible polyethylene terephthalate (PET) substrate for the detection of HIV-1 at the attomolar level. Antibodies (as probe molecules) were immobilized on the graphene gate surface using PBASE linker molecules. When the virus solution was introduced, the Dirac point voltage shifted downward due to the electrostatic gating effect of graphene in the virus-antibody complex. The sensor exhibited a remarkable limit of detection (LOD) of 47.8 aM for the HIV-1 virus.

On the other hand, MXenes are an advanced class of 2D materials known for their high surface area, large interlayer spacing, and easily modifiable structures. These materials feature excellent electrical conductivity, hydrophilicity, and thermal stability, making them ideal for creating advanced biosensors for virus detection. MXene-based electrochemical biosensors have shown significant potential in clinical applications due to their biocompatibility, high sensitivity, and selectivity. As a family of transition-metal carbides and nitrides, MXenes are easy to synthesize and modify, excelling at analyte detection. These biosensors offer many advantages, including low detection limits, strong stability, and quick response times. The surface properties of MXenes can be tailored to improve biocompatibility and support the immobilization of biological recognition elements, such as aptamers, enzymes, and antibodies. This capability simplifies the sensing process by eliminating the need for complex sample preparation, enabling direct detection of specific biomarkers in biological fluids. For example, an amperometric biosensor for SARS-CoV-2 used an MXene-based nanocomposite to amplify the signal for detecting the virus's antigens and antibodies [45, 46] (Fig. 9.12e, f). Additionally, a voltammetric biosensor was developed for rotavirus detection, using an Au/MXene/PPY nanocomposite with gold nanoparticles, which allows highly sensitive detection through DNA hybridization. This biosensor demonstrated a linear detection range from 0.1 fM to 10 nM, with a detection limit of 0.1 fM [47]. Further, an impedimetric biosensor based on an MXene nanocomposite was created for detecting influenza A virus [48].

The Zika virus, transmitted by mosquitoes, has been associated with severe neurological complications or disorders in adults, such as brain abnormalities and Guillain-Barré syndrome. While nucleic acid-based tests like RT-PCR are the primary methods for detecting the Zika virus, GFET biosensors have proven highly effective in detecting this virus, even at low concentrations. For instance, Asahi et al. [50] demonstrated the use of GFET devices functionalized with monoclonal antibodies to detect Zika virus antigens in real time, even at low concentrations. The GFET biosensor successfully detected Zika virus in both simulated human serum and real samples, demonstrating high sensitivity (LOD as low as 450 pM) and high selectivity. The above examples illustrate the versatility and efficacy of graphene- and MXene-based biosensors for viral detection and their potential to advance clinical diagnostics.

GFET biosensors have also shown promise in detecting the Ebola virus, which caused devastating outbreaks in West Africa from 2013 to 2016, resulting in over 11,000 deaths. Chen et al. [51] demonstrated that GFET devices could detect the Ebola glycoprotein (EPG) from the Zaire strain with a detection limit of 1 ng/mL. The GFET designed by Chen contained a reduced graphene oxide (rGO) channel, onto which anti-Ebola antibodies were immobilized via gold nanoparticles, which enabled selective capture of the EPG antigen. The binding of the Ebola antigen to these antibodies altered the conductance of rGO channel, which could be monitored by tracking variations in the device's ISD. This biosensor demonstrated significant potential for detecting Ebola antigens in real samples, including diluted human serum and plasma. Based on this concept, Maity et al. [52] developed an rGO-FET biosensor that enabled rapid and sensitive detection of Ebola glycoprotein within 1–2 min. The biosensor achieved an impressive LOD (0.001–3.401 mg/L) across both high and low frequencies, thereby reducing the detection limits of traditional GFET biosensors. By exploiting the electric field generated when the Ebola antigen binds to the antibody-functionalized rGO channel, the sensor modulated the channel's charge-carrier concentration, thereby enhancing its sensitivity and response time.

Several other nanostructures, including MoS_2 and carbon-based materials like carbon nanotubes, fullerenes, and carbon nanofibers, have been effectively used to develop biosensors for viral detection. One notable advancement by Zourob's research group involved creating a cost-effective cotton-tipped electrochemical immunosensor specifically designed to detect SARS-CoV-2. This sensor used a carbon nanofiber (CNF)-modified electrode [53]. The modification process included drop-casting CNF onto the surface of a carbon working electrode, followed by functionalization with carboxyphenyl groups through diazonium salt reduction (Fig. 9.13a). SARS-CoV-2 nucleocapsid (N) protein was immobilized on the CNF-modified electrode through electro-grafting, and viral antigens were detected using a competitive assay with a specific amount of N protein antibody. This immunosensor demonstrated exceptional sensitivity, detecting SARS-CoV-2 N protein with a limit of detection (LOD) of 0.8 pg/mL, and exhibited a wide linear response range from 1 to 1000 ng/mL. Additionally, it showed high selectivity against other viral antigens, such as influenza A and HCoV. In tests with patient samples, the

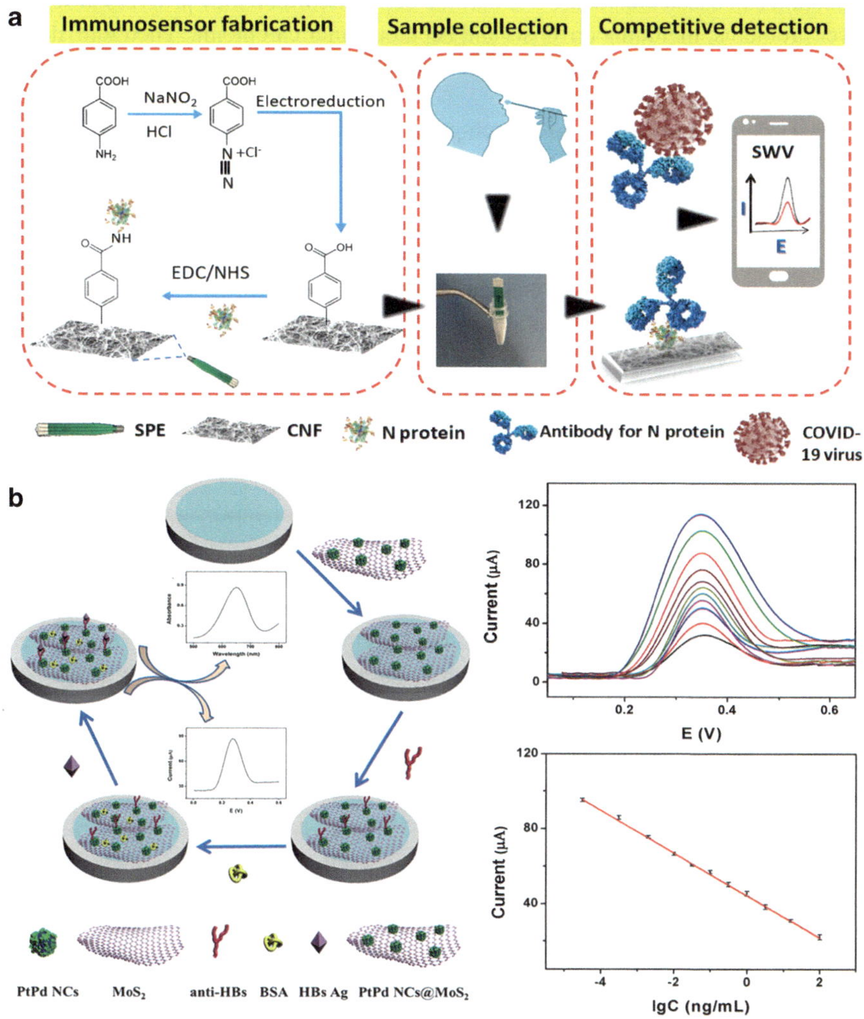

Fig. 9.13 (**a**) Diagram depicting an affordable cotton-tipped electrochemical immunosensor for SARS-CoV-2 detection, which uses a carbon nanofiber-modified electrode. It also shows the application of the immunosensor for COVID-19 detection through electrochemical analysis. Reproduced with permission from Ref. [53]. Copyright 2021, American Chemical Society. (**b**) Schematic illustration of a label-free immunosensor based on PtPd nanocube@MoS_2 nanoenzymes and its use in the detection of HBsAg (hepatitis B surface antigen). Reprinted with permission from Ref. [54]. Copyright 2019, Elsevier

immunosensor produced lower electrochemical signals compared to standard samples, aligning with its detection performance relative to PCR results.

Meanwhile, antibody-based immunosensors have gained attention for detecting hepatitis B virus (HBV) alongside coronaviruses. HBV, a small, enveloped DNA virus, primarily infects the liver and poses a significant global health threat. HBV infection can cause both acute and chronic hepatitis, which may progress to serious liver problems, including cirrhosis and hepatocellular carcinoma. Therefore, developing sensitive and selective detection methods for HBV biomarkers is crucial for effective diagnosis and monitoring.

In a related study, Dong's research group developed a label-free immunosensor using PtPd nanocube@MoS_2 nanoenzymes (PtPd NCs@MoS_2) to detect HBV antigens [54]. The synthesis of PtPd NCs@MoS_2 involved loading PtPd NCs onto MoS_2 nanosheets through in situ redox polymerization (Fig. 9.13b). The peroxidase-like activity of the PtPd NCs@MoS_2 was exploited for HBV antigen detection using both colorimetric and electrochemical methods. The colorimetric method achieved a detection limit of 3.3 pg/mL. In contrast, electrochemical detection, using the conductivity of PtPd NCs@MoS_2, yielded a high sensitivity of 10.2 fg/mL and a broad linear detection range from 32 fg/mL to 100 ng/mL.

9.5.2 Bacteria Detection

Biosensors are essential for detecting pathogenic bacteria, which pose a significant public health concern due to their widespread occurrence in food, water, and air, and their rapid proliferation. While traditional detection methods, such as biochemical tests and culturing, are effective, they are time-consuming and require specialized equipment and expertise. Alternative methods like PCR, mass spectrometry, ELISA, and lateral flow immunoassays (LFIA) are either slow or costly, highlighting the need for a faster, more precise, and easier detection approach.

In this context, MXene-based biosensors are emerging as promising tools, especially for detecting foodborne pathogens. For example, a highly sensitive electrochemical immunosensor was developed that combines MXene and graphene to detect *Listeria monocytogenes* (LM), a common foodborne pathogen. The sensor was designed by immobilizing a recognition element on the electrode surface, enabling the detection of antibody binding to specific antigens and producing measurable changes in current and/or voltage. The sensor incorporated carboxyl-functionalized $Ti_3C_2T_x$ MXene with a primary antibody to ensure selectivity, while Rhodamine B, Au nanoparticles, and rGO were used to amplify the signal. This immunosensor exhibited a detection limit as low as 2 CFU/mL, a linear range of $10–10^5$ CFU/mL, and a relative standard deviation of just 4.36% [55].

Another notable MXene-based sensor was developed for detecting *Mycobacterium tuberculosis* (M.tb). This genosensor combined $Ti_3C_2T_x$ MXene with polypyrrole (PPY) to target the IS6110 sequence of the M.tb genome. It achieved a detection limit of 11.24 fM, with a recovery rate of 90.52–100.8%, and a linear range of 100 fM–25 nM. The sensor exhibited strong selectivity for M.tb over other bacterial strains [56].

Furthermore, a dual-mode electroluminescent (ECL)-SERS immunosensor was developed to detect *Vibrio vulnificus* (VV), a pathogenic bacterium. This sensor utilized two detection modes: (i) Fe_3O_4 nanoparticles functionalized with antibody

1 (Ab1), which was immobilized on a magnetic glassy carbon electrode to capture VV and (ii) $Ti_3C_2T_x$ MXene modified with Rhodamine 6G and gold nanorods functionalized with antibody 2 (Ab2) for signal enhancement. The sensor (Fig. 9.14) demonstrated exceptional sensitivity, with detection limits of 1 CFU/mL for ECL and 102 CFU/mL for SERS, and strong selectivity for VV among other bacterial strains. The MXene surface enhances the sensitivity by providing ample space for functionalization and bacteria capturing [57].

GFETS have proven highly effective for virus detection applications. For example, Kim et al. [58] developed an advanced portable micropatterned GFET biosensor integrated with a microfluidic platform for early detection of both Gram-positive and Gram-negative bacteria. This device, designed with a two-layer structure, incorporates an antibiotic-functionalized surface and is equipped with components such as a SIM card slot, a microcontroller, a power supply, and a communication module, along with electronic inlets and outlets connected to a syringe pump. This unique chip allows for the selective detection of pathogenic bacteria in cultured samples, with a detection range of 10 to 10^3 CFU/mL, making it a promising tool for real-time, onsite bacterial monitoring in various environmental settings.

Using a different approach, Wu et al. [59] used a pyrene-tagged DNA aptamer as a sensing probe in GFET biosensors mounted on silicon chips, for selective detection of *E. coli.* Each silicon chip contained four individual GFET devices. The DNA aptamer was anchored to the graphene surface using pyrene phosphoramidite as a cross-linker, thereby ensuring stable attachment for specific detection of *E. coli.* When the aptamer binds to *E. coli*, it undergoes a conformational change that pulls the negatively charged bacteria closer to the graphene channel surface. This causes a specific p-doping effect, shifting the device's transfer characteristic curves. This aptamer-modified GFET biosensor can detect *E. coli* concentrations as low as 100 CFU/mL in about 72 s.

Chikungunya, an RNA virus in the genus *Alphavirus* within the family Togaviridae, was first identified in Tanzania in 1952. Despite its relatively low fatality rate, the virus has become a significant public health concern due to widespread outbreaks worldwide. The rapid spread of chikungunya poses substantial challenges for timely and accurate diagnosis, especially in resource-limited settings.

For addressing this challenge, several nanostructure-based biosensors have been developed for detecting the chikungunya virus. For example, Singhal et al. [60] fabricated a MoS_2 nanosheet biosensor for detecting chikungunya virus. The MoS_2 nanosheets were grown hydrothermally and then physically adsorbed onto screen-printed gold electrodes (SPGEs). This setup was used to electrochemically detect CHIGV DNA via voltammetry. The detection method took advantage of methylene blue, a redox indicator, which interacts differently with the guanine bases in single-stranded and double-stranded DNA, leading to measurable voltammetric signal changes. The sensor showed a broad, linear detection range of 0.1 nM to 100 μM for the DNA of chikungunya virus, demonstrating its potential for sensitive and effective virus detection.

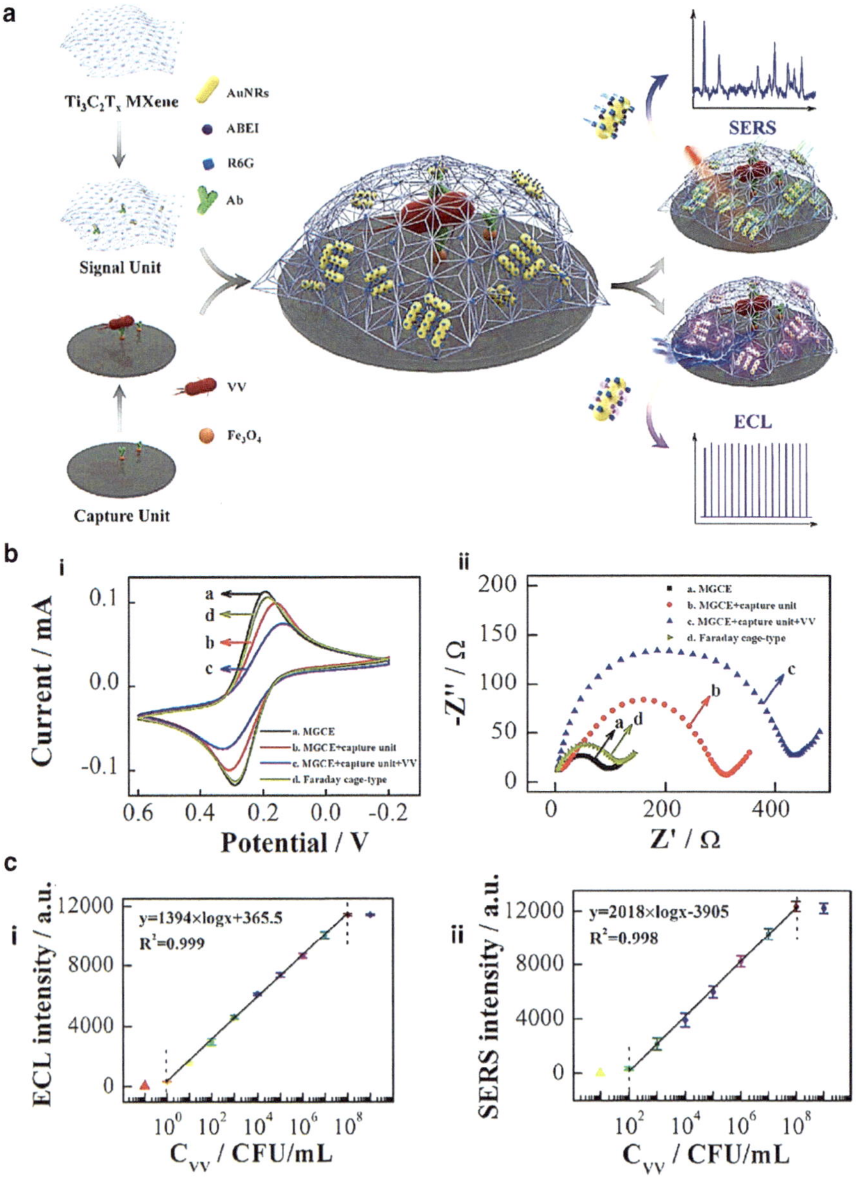

Fig. 9.14 (A) Diagram of an ECL/SERS immunosensor design. (B) Cyclic voltammetry (CV) (i) and EIS (ii) curves for (a) MGCE, (b) the MGCE with capture element, (c) the MGCE with capture element exposed to VV, and (d) a Faraday cage-type immunosensor. (**C**) Graph showing the correlation between the VV concentration and electrochemiluminescence (ECL) (i) and the SERS (ii) signals. (Reproduced with permission from Ref. [57]. Copyright 2021, Elsevier)

9.5.3 Other Disease Detection

As the global aging population continues to rise, efficient diagnosis and treatment of neurodegenerative diseases or disorders (NDDs) have gained paramount importance. Disorders like Alzheimer's, Parkinson's, motor neuron disease, and ataxia pose a significant public health challenge, affecting millions of people across the globe. These diseases are characterized by the gradual degeneration of the structure and function of nervous systems (central and peripheral), resulting in debilitating symptoms and diminished cognitive and motor abilities. Therefore, it is crucial to develop efficient diagnostic and therapeutic strategies to mitigate the adverse impact of NDDs.

Among the various materials studied for managing NDDs, two-dimensional (2D) nanostructures have shown exceptional promise. These materials provide unique opportunities to create highly sensitive, biocompatible theragnostic probes for NDD detection with high selectivity. Functionalized graphene, for instance, can interact specifically with biomolecules, facilitating the identification of markers associated with targeted NDDs. Graphene-based biosensors have been developed to detect amyloid-beta (Aβ) peptides, which are key biomarkers for Alzheimer's disease (AD) [61]. These biosensors deliver high sensitivity and specificity, enabling early and accurate diagnoses that facilitate prompt intervention and treatment. Additionally, the structural similarity of graphene to the extracellular matrix of tissues, combined with its outstanding mechanical properties, makes graphene an ideal material for biomedical applications.

Two-dimensional (2D) transition metal dichalcogenides (TMDs), such as MoS_2 and WS_2, have demonstrated significant potential for drug delivery and disease detection owing to their layered structures, high specific surface area, and ease of functionalization to enhance biocompatibility and targeting abilities. The remarkable surface-to-volume ratio and superior electronic properties of TMDs make them well suited for biosensing applications.

Dopamine (DPA), an essential catecholamine, plays vital roles in several physiological processes, including neurological signaling for movement, mood regulation, vasodilation outside the brain, and reward-related behaviors within the brain. An imbalance in dopamine release can contribute to a range of disorders, such as Alzheimer's disease, addiction, Parkinson's disease, schizophrenia, pheochromocytoma, and other psychiatric conditions. In this context, Abhilash et al. [62] proposed an innovative electrochemical sensing method for DPA by developing a unique electrode. The electrode, called WM-GP@NiMoP, consists of a composite material made from transition metal dichalcogenides (WS_2-MoS_2) supported on reduced graphene oxide (rGO) and polyaniline (PANI), fabricated through a simple electroless NiMoP plating technique (Fig. 9.15a). Cyclic voltammetry (CV) analysis conducted in a DPA containing phosphate buffer solution (PBS) revealed electrode's exceptional sensitivity for DPA oxidation, associated with the synergistic effects of PANI, rGO, and the mixed TMDs on the NiMoP-coated electrode surface. Figure 9.15 shows the electrode fabrication process for NiMoP, WM@NiMoP, and WM-GP@NiMoP, along with the molecular interactions of the WM-GP@NiMoP electrodes

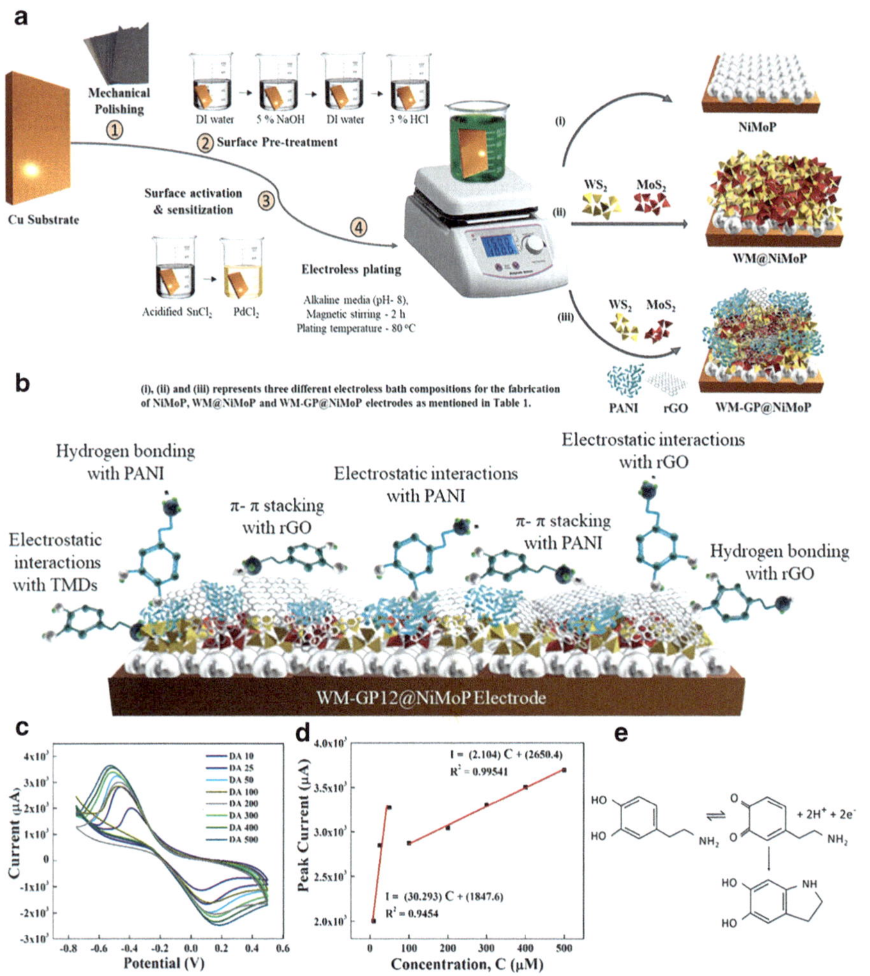

Fig. 9.15 (**a**) Schematic illustration showing the fabrication process of NiMoP, WM@NiMoP, and WM-GP@NiMoP electrodes. (**b**) Representation of the molecular interactions between WM-GP12@NiMoP electrodes and DPA. (**c**) Cyclic voltammetry curves for an optimized WM-GP@NiMoP electrode in DPA solutions with concentrations ranging from 10 μM to 500 μM in 0.1 M PBS solution (pH = 7), at a scan rate of 100 mV/s. (**d**) Peak current response for various DPA concentrations derived from corresponding CV curves. (**e**) Typical electrochemical redox reaction of DPA. (Reproduced with permission from Ref. [62], Copyright 2024, Elsevier)

with DPA and the current-voltage curves for various DPA concentrations (10 mM to 500 mM) in a 0.1 M PBS solution of pH 7.

Electrochemical biosensors fabricated using multi-walled carbon nanotubes (MWCNTs) have also shown great promise for detecting biomarkers and nucleoproteins. For instance, Yao and colleagues [63] developed a label-free electrochemical sensor using MWCNTs to detect miRNA-24, an endogenous, single-stranded

RNA molecule involved in regulating various health conditions, such as obesity, cellular apoptosis, and cardiovascular physiology. The sensor was fabricated by covalently immobilizing a probe on the electrode. The sensor's performance for miRNA-24 detection was evaluated using differential pulse voltammetry, yielding a sensitivity of 4.963 mA cm^{-2} $decade^{-1}$ and a detection limit of 1 pM.

9.6 Wearable Biosensors

Wearable biosensors (WBSs) are compact electronic devices designed for continuous monitoring of biological signals in the human body. By dynamically measuring biochemical markers in biofluids such as sweat, tears, saliva, and interstitial fluids, they offer real-time health insights in a noninvasive manner. To access interstitial fluids, which are found just below the skin, a microneedle structure is often used for sample collection and analysis. Each WBS comprises three components: a recognition region that detects the target signal, a transducer that converts this signal into measurable data, and an electronic processor that displays the results. These sensors can be worn in various forms, including tattoos, embedded in clothing, integrated into gloves and shoes, or implanted near the body, allowing for timely diagnosis, treatment, and health management. By comparing analyte levels in these biofluids to those in noninvasive fluids, WBSs improve our understanding of health conditions.

WBSs are primarily classified into two categories: physical sensors, which monitor parameters such as temperature, pressure, and strain, and chemical sensors, which detect specific analyte concentrations. Another critical category is self-powered sensors, which function without an external power source. To meet practical needs, wearable sensors are developed in various forms, such as patches, textiles, tattoos, microneedles, and contact lenses.

For instance, Park et al. [64] fabricated smart contact lenses with integrated wireless circuits for glucose sensing (Fig. 9.16a) using transparent and stretchable nanostructures. Those lenses can measure fasting glucose levels in the tears of diabetic patients and display the results. On the other hand, Jang et al. [65] fabricated a graphene-based field-effect transistor (GFET) biosensor and a skin-adherable therapeutic device for wireless monitoring of MNP-9 levels in tear fluids (Fig. 9.16b–e), which serves as a biomarker for ocular surface inflammation/injury (OSI) along with its treatment. The transparent, stress-tunable sensor incorporated a thin, photopatterned polymer to house sensitive components, including an NFC (near-field communication) chip, an MMP-9 sensor, a capacitor, and resistors, along with a soft matrix for positioning a silver nanowire antenna. The electronic components within this smart contact lens were interconnected using stretchable, printed interconnections fabricated from a liquid-metal alloy of gallium and indium. Moreover, the hybrid substrate with good refractive index matching exhibited high optical transparency without compromising visibility.

A variety of flexible WBSs have been designed and developed so far to monitor diverse biological indicators. For example, wearable pressure sensors are used to

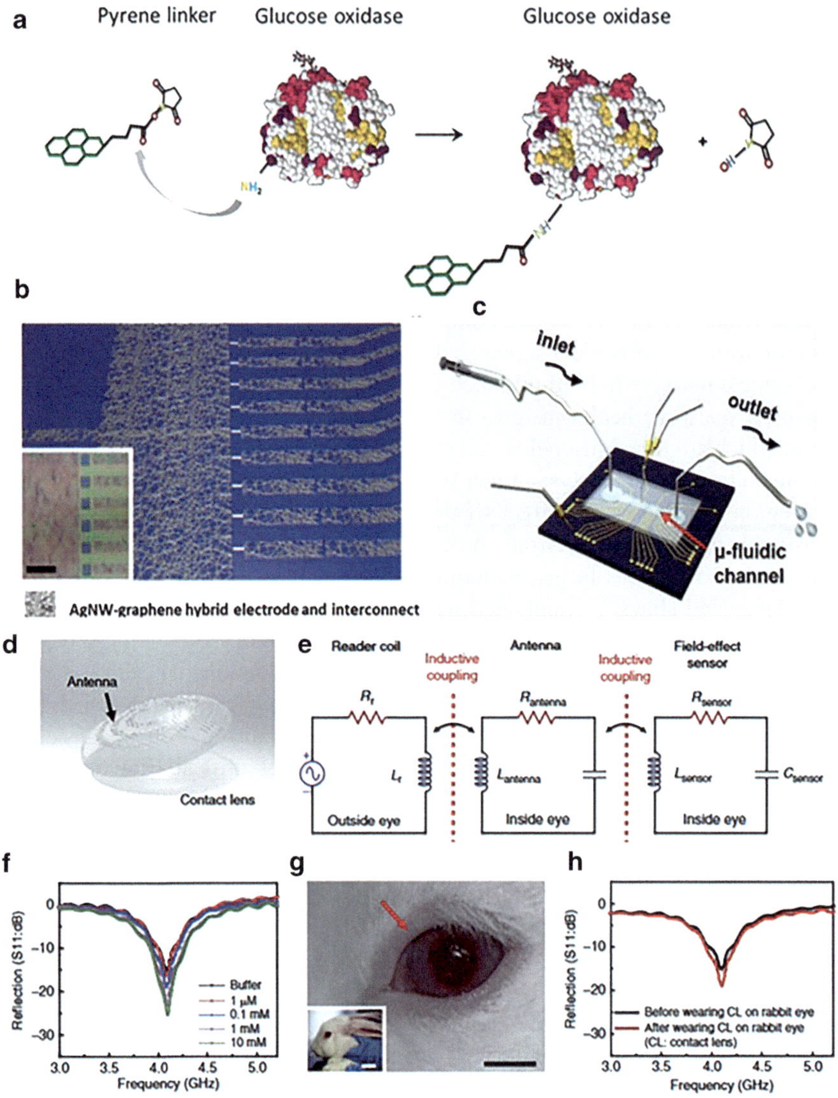

Fig. 9.16 (**a**) Schematic presentation of a graphene-based soft, smart contact lens for glucose detection. Reprinted with permission from Ref. [64]. Copyright 2018, AAAS. (**b**) Schematic illustrations of an integrated system for real-time monitoring and therapy of chronic operational stress injury (OSI). (**c**) Operation algorithms for an integrated system comprising a soft, smart contact lens (diagnostic device), an eyelid-attachable heat patch (therapeutic device), and the smartphone (wireless communication). (**d**) Photograph of the soft, smart contact lens. (**e**) Photograph of a rabbit wearing Ag nanofiber-based heat patches on its upper and lower eyelids. Scale bar = 2 cm. Reprinted with permission from Ref. [65]. Copyright 2021, AAAS

measure coronary pressure. In contrast, sweat sensors can track pH, glucose, urea, vitamin C, levodopa (a dopamine precursor), cortisol, along with K^+, Na^+, Ca^{2+}, and heavy metal ion levels in the body.

Advances in materials research, particularly the emergence of materials such as graphene, graphene oxide, MXenes, and other metallic and non-metallic nanostructures, have significantly advanced the field of WBSs. These advancements not only highlight the potential for fabricating new WBSs but also the potential for WBSs in point-of-care applications and wireless disease detection and monitoring. However, for widespread clinical application, further progress is needed to improve reliability, develop more detectable biomarkers, and conduct large-scale validation studies.

9.7 Prospects and Perspectives

At present, biosensors are widely used for diagnosing a range of diseases, including infectious diseases, cancer, cardiovascular conditions, diabetes, and neurological disorders. In the context of infectious disease diagnosis, biosensors provide rapid pathogen detection, which is crucial for the timely start of treatment and effective outbreak control. In cancer diagnosis, biosensors facilitate early identification of biomarkers, supporting personalized treatment approaches. Additionally, biosensors are essential for monitoring disease progression, evaluating treatment responses, and detecting recurrence.

Recent breakthroughs in biosensor technology have greatly transformed disease diagnosis. Advances in miniaturization and integration into portable devices have made these biosensors highly effective for point-of-care testing, allowing rapid results even in remote or resource-limited areas. The application of nanomaterials like nanoparticles and nanowires has further enhanced their sensitivity and selectivity. Additionally, advanced functionalization techniques have improved the stability and overall performance of biosensors. The combination of 1D and 0D nanomaterials with two-dimensional (2D) layered materials like TMDs, graphene, rGO, and MXenes, all of which have large surface areas and enhanced drug-loading capacities, has facilitated the development of modern biosensors, which are capable of detecting individual analyte molecules with exceptional sensitivity.

Although not all laboratory advancements have yet been turned into commercially available products or widely used at home, mostly due to regulatory hurdles and limited testing, there is growing confidence that these challenges will soon be resolved. Ongoing innovation in the design and synthesis of new functional composite materials, microfluidics, and artificial intelligence is anticipated to result in better biosensors with higher selectivity and sensitivity, allowing for more accurate detection of infectious diseases and neurological conditions. Additionally, the development of wearable biosensors will enable continuous health monitoring, ushering in an era of personalized and preventative medicine.

9.8 Conclusion

The future of biosensors for disease diagnosis is highly promising. Recent progress in nanotechnology, including designing and developing materials, functionalizing for conjugation with bioreceptors, and integrating devices, has greatly advanced the biosensing field. Improvements in the design and manufacturing of advanced microfluidic platforms, combined with artificial intelligence integration, are expected to further boost the sensitivity, specificity, and multiplexing abilities of biosensors. However, to accomplish these goals quickly, it is crucial to strengthen collaboration among research laboratories, industry, and governmental and non-governmental funding agencies.

References

1. Cremer M. Über Die Ursache Der Elektromotorischen Eigenschaften Der Gewebe, Zugleich Ein Beitrag Zur Lehre von Den Polyphasischen Elektrolytketten. Z Biol. 1906;47:562–608.
2. Griffin EG, Nelson JM. The influence of certain substances on the activity of Invertase. J Am Chem Soc. 1916;38:722–30. https://doi.org/10.1021/ja02260a027.
3. Nelson JM, Griffin EG. Adsorption of Invertase. J Am Chem Soc. 1916;38:1109–15. https://doi.org/10.1021/ja02262a018.
4. Heineman WR, Jensen WB. Leland C. Clark Jr. (1918–2005). Biosens Bioelectron. 2006;21:1403–4. https://doi.org/10.1016/j.bios.2005.12.005.
5. Guilbault GG, Montalvo JG Jr. Urea-specific enzyme electrode. J Am Chem Soc. 1969;91:2164–5. https://doi.org/10.1021/ja01036a083.
6. Renneberg R, Pfeiffer D, Lisdat F, Wilson G, Wollenberger U, Ligler F, Turner APF. Frieder Scheller and the short history of biosensors. Adv Biochem Eng Biotechnol. 2008;109:1–18. https://doi.org/10.1007/10_2007_086.
7. Grieshaber D, MacKenzie R, Vörös J, Reimhult E. Electrochemical biosensors—sensor principles and architectures. Sensors. 2008;8:1400–58. https://doi.org/10.3390/s80314000.
8. Pohanka M, Skládal P. Electrochemical biosensors—principles and applications. J Appl Biomed. 2008;6:57–64. https://doi.org/10.32725/jab.2008.008.
9. Naresh V, Lee N. A review on biosensors and recent development of nanostructured materials-enabled biosensors. Sensors. 2021;21:1109. https://doi.org/10.3390/s21041109.
10. Lojou É, Bianco P. Application of the electrochemical concepts and techniques to amperometric biosensor devices. J Electroceram. 2006;16:79–91. https://doi.org/10.1007/s10832-006-2365-9.
11. Koncki R. Recent developments in potentiometric biosensors for biomedical analysis. Anal Chim Acta. 2007;599:7–15. https://doi.org/10.1016/j.aca.2007.08.003.
12. Dinçkaya E, Kinik Ö, Sezgintürk MK, Altuĝ Ç, Akkoca A. Development of an Impedimetric aflatoxin M1 biosensor based on a DNA probe and gold nanoparticles. Biosens Bioelectron. 2011;26(9):3806–11. https://doi.org/10.1016/j.bios.2011.02.038.
13. Ahmed A, Rushworth JV, Wright JD, Millner PA. Novel Impedimetric Immunosensor for detection of pathogenic bacteria streptococcus Pyogenes in human saliva. Anal Chem. 2013;85(24):12118–25. https://doi.org/10.1021/ac403253j.
14. Conroy PJ, Hearty S, Leonard P, O'Kennedy RJ. Antibody production, design and use for biosensor-based applications. Semin Cell Dev Biol. 2009;20(1):20–6. https://doi.org/10.1016/j.semcdb.2009.01.010.

15. Song S, Wang L, Li J, Fan C, Zhao J. Aptamer-based biosensors. TrAC Trends Anal Chem. 2008;27(2):108–17. https://doi.org/10.1016/j.trac.2007.12.004.
16. Tiede C, Tang AST, Deacon SE, Mandal U, Nettleship JE, Owen RL, George SE, Harrison DJ, Owens RJ, Tomlinson DC, McPherson MJ. Adhiron: a stable and versatile peptide display scaffold for molecular recognition applications. Protein Eng Des Sel. 2014;27(5):145–55. https://doi.org/10.1093/protein/gzu007.
17. Leva-Bueno J, Peyman SA, Millner PA. A review on Impedimetric Immunosensors for pathogen and biomarker detection. Med Microbiol Immunol. 2020;209:343–62. https://doi.org/10.1007/s00430-020-00668-0.
18. Kim SK, et al. Bimetallic nanocatalysts immobilized in nanoporous hydrogels for long-term robust continuous glucose monitoring of smart contact lens. Adv Mater. 2022;34:2110536. https://doi.org/10.1002/adma.202110536.
19. Gao W, et al. Fully integrated wearable sensor arrays for multiplexed in situ perspiration analysis. Nature. 2016;529:509–14. https://doi.org/10.1038/nature16521.
20. Hu JM, et al. A reusable electrochemical proximity assay for highly selective, real-time protein quantitation in biological matrices. J Am Chem Soc. 2014;136:8467–74. https://doi.org/10.1021/ja503679q.
21. Ren KW, Wu J, Zhang Y, Yan F, Ju HX. Proximity hybridization regulated DNA biogate for sensitive electrochemical immunoassay. Anal Chem. 2014;86:7494–9. https://doi.org/10.1021/ac5012377.
22. Man Y, et al. An anchored monopodial DNA Walker triggered by proximity hybridization for amplified Amperometric biosensing of nucleic acid and protein. Anal Chim Acta. 2020;1107:48–54. https://doi.org/10.1016/j.aca.2020.02.013.
23. Pohanka M. Overview of piezoelectric biosensors, immunosensors and DNA sensors and their applications. Materials (Basel). 2018;11:448. https://doi.org/10.3390/ma11030448.
24. Qazi S, Raza K. Smart biosensors for an efficient Point of Care (PoC) health management. In: Chaki J, Dey N, De D, editors. Smart biosensors in medical care. Academic; 2020. p. 65.
25. Paterova T, Prauzek M, Konecny J, Ozana S, Zmij P, Stankus M, Weise D, Pierer A. Environment-monitoring IoT devices powered by a TEG which converts thermal flux between air and near-surface soil into electrical energy. Sensors. 2021;21:8098. https://doi.org/10.3390/s21.
26. Wang Y, Shi Y, Mei D, Chen Z. Wearable thermoelectric generator for harvesting heat on the curved human wrist. Appl Energy. 2017;205:710–9. https://doi.org/10.1016/j.apenergy.2017.08.117.
27. Nozariasbmarz A, Collins H, Dsouza K, Polash MH, Hosseini M, Hyland M, Liu J, Malhotra A, mateos Ortiz F, Mohaddes F, et al. Review of wearable thermoelectric energy harvesting: from body temperature to electronic systems. Appl Energy. 2019;258:114069. https://doi.org/10.1016/j.apenergy.2019.114069.
28. Damborský P, Švitel J, Katrlík J. Optical biosensors. Essays Biochem. 2016;60(1):91–100. https://doi.org/10.1042/EBC20150010.
29. Zhou J, Wang Y, Zhang L, Li X. Plasmonic biosensing based on non-noble-metal materials. Chin Chem Lett. 2018;29:54–60. https://doi.org/10.1016/j.cclet.2017.09.003.
30. Hirschdeld T. High-sensitivity attenuated total-reflection spectroscopy. Appl Spectrosc. 1996;20:336. https://doi.org/10.1366/000370266774385822.
31. Xiao-hong Z, Lan-hua L, Wei-qi X, et al. A reusable evanescent wave Immunosensor for highly sensitive detection of Bisphenol a in water samples. Sci Rep. 2014;4:4572. https://doi.org/10.1038/srep04572.
32. Hirschfeld TB, Block MJ. Assay apparatus and methods. 4558014. US patent. 1985.
33. Taitt CR, Anderson GP, Ligler FS. Evanescent wave fluorescence biosensors: advances of the last decade. Biosens Bioelectron. 2016;76:103–12. https://doi.org/10.1016/j.bios.2015.07.040.
34. Safari M, Najafi S, Akran E, Amani S, Shahlaei M. Facile aqueous synthesis of Ni-doped CdTe quantum dots as fluorescent probes for detecting pyrazinamide in plasma. Microchem J. 2019;146:293–9. https://doi.org/10.1016/j.microc.2019.01.019.

35. Najafi S, Safari M, Amani S, Mansouri K, Shahlaei M. Preparation, characterization and cell cytotoxicity of Pd-doped CdTe quantum dots and its application as a sensitive fluorescent Nanoprobe. J Mater Sci Mater Electron. 2019;30:14233–42. https://doi.org/10.1007/s10854-019-01792-1.
36. Lenzi E, Jimenez de Aberasturi D, Liz-Marzán L-M. Surface enhanced Raman scattering tags for three-dimensional bioimaging and biomarker detection. ACS Sens. 2019;4:1126–37. https://doi.org/10.1021/acssensors.9b00321.
37. Yang Y, Zhu J, Zhao J, Weng G-J, Li JJ, Zhau J-W. Growth of spherical gold satellites on the surface of Au@Ag@SiO_2 Core-Shell nanostructures used for an ultrasensitive SERS immunoassay of alpha-fetoprotein. ACS Appl Mater Interfaces. 2019;11:3617–26. https://doi.org/10.1021/acsami.8b21238.
38. Wang Z, Zong S, Wu L, Zhu D, Cui Y. SERS-activated platforms for immunoassay: probes, encoding methods, and applications. Chem Rev. 2017;117:7910–63. https://doi.org/10.1021/acs.chemrev.7b00027.
39. Cheng Z, Choi N, Wang R, Lee S, Moon KC, Yoon S-Y, Chen L, Choo J. Simultaneous detection of dual prostate specific antigens using surface-enhanced Raman scattering-based immunoassay for accurate diagnosis of prostate cancer. ACS Nano. 2017;11:4926–33. https://doi.org/10.1021/acsnano.7b01536.
40. Chuong TT, Pallaoro A, Chaves CA, Li Z, Lee J, Eisenstein M, Stucky GD, Moskovits M, Soh HT. Dual-reporter SERS-based biomolecular assay with reduced false-positive signals. Proc Natl Acad Sci. 2017;114:9056–61. https://doi.org/10.1073/pnas.170031711.
41. Wu J, Liu H, Chen W, Ma B, Ju H. Device integration of electrochemical biosensors. Nat Rev Bioeng. 2023;1:346–60. https://doi.org/10.1038/s44222-023-00032-w.
42. Liu H, Xiang Y, Lu Y, Crooks RM. Aptamer-based origami paper analytical device for electrochemical detection of adenosine. Angew Chem Int Ed. 2012;51:6925–8. https://doi.org/10.1002/anie.201202929.
43. Kwon OS, Lee SH, Park SJ, An JH, Song HS, Kim T, Oh JH, Bae J, Yoon H, Park TH, Jang J. Large-scale graphene micropattern Nano-biohybrids: high-performance transducers for FET-type flexible fluidic HIV immunoassays. Adv Mater. 2013;25:4177–85. https://doi.org/10.1002/adma.201301523.
44. Kim JW, Kim S, Jang Y-H, Lim K-I, Lee WH. Attomolar detection of virus by liquid coplanar-gate graphene transistor on plastic. Nanotechnology. 2019;30(34):345502. https://doi.org/10.1088/1361-6528/ab0f52.
45. Antiochia R. Electrochemical biosensors for SARS-CoV-2 detection: voltametric or impedimetric transduction? Bioelectrochemistry. 2022;147:108190. https://doi.org/10.1016/j.bioelechem.2022.108190.
46. Chen WY, Lin H, Barui AK, Gomez AMU, Wendt MK, Stanciu LA. DNA-functionalized Ti_3C_2T XMXenes for selective and rapid detection of SARS-CoV-2 Nucleocapsid gene. ACS Appl Nano Mater. 2022;5(2):1902–10. https://doi.org/10.1021/acsanm.1c03520.
47. Ketabi K, Soleimanjahi H, Teimoori A, Hatamluyi B, Rezayi M, Meshkat Z. Diagnostic Genosensor for detection of rotavirus based on HFGNs/MXene/PPY signal amplification. Microchim Acta. 2023;190(8):293. https://doi.org/10.1007/s00604-023-05871-3.
48. Li Y, Peng Z, Holl NJ, Hassan MR, Pappas JM, Wei C, Izadi OH, Wang Y, Dong X, Wang C, Huang YW, Kim D, Wu C. MXene-graphene field-effect transistor sensing of influenza virus and SARS-CoV-2. ACS Omega. 2021;6(10):6643–53. https://doi.org/10.1021/acsomega.0c05421.
49. Fu W, Jiang L, van Geest EP, Lima LMC, Schneider GF. Sensing at the surface of graphene field-effect transistors. Adv Mater. 2017;29(6):1603610. https://doi.org/10.1002/adma.201603610.
50. Afsahi S, Lerner MB, Goldstein JM, Lee J, Tang X, Bagarozzi DA, Pan D, Locascio L, Walker A, Barron F, Goldsmith BR. Novel graphene-based biosensor for early detection of Zika virus infection. Biosens Bioelectron. 2018;100:85–8. https://doi.org/10.1016/j.bios.2017.08.051.
51. Chen Y, Ren R, Pu H, Guo X, Chang J, Zhou G, Mao S, Kron M, Chen J. Field-effect transistor biosensor for rapid detection of Ebola antigen. Sci Rep. 2017;7:10974. https://doi.org/10.1038/s41598-017-11387-7.

52. Maity A, Sui X, Jin B, Pu H, Bottum KJ, Huang X, Chang J, Zhou G, Lu G, Chen J. Resonance-frequency modulation for rapid, point-of-care Ebola-glycoprotein diagnosis with a graphene-based field-effect biotransistor. Anal Chem. 2018;90(24):14230–8. https://doi.org/10.1021/acs.analchem.8b03226.
53. Eissa S, Zourob M. Development of a low-cost cotton-tipped electrochemical Immunosensor for the detection of SARS-CoV-2. Anal Chem. 2021;93(3):1826–33. https://doi.org/10.1021/acs.analchem.0c04719.
54. Tan Z, Dong H, Liu Q, Liu H, Zhao P, Wang P, Li Y, Zhang D, Zhao Z, Dong Y. A label-free Immunosensor based on PtPd NCs@MoS_2 nanoenzymes for hepatitis B surface antigen detection. Biosens Bioelectron. 2019;142:111556. https://doi.org/10.1016/j.bios.2019.111556.
55. Niu H, Cai S, Liu X, Huang X, Chen J, Wang S, Zhang S. A novel electrochemical Sandwich-like Immunosensor based on carboxyl $Ti_3C_2T_x$ MXene and Rhodamine b/gold/reduced graphene oxide for listeria monocytogenes. Anal Methods. 2022;14(8):843–9. https://doi.org/10.1039/d1ay02029c.
56. Salimiyan Rizi K, Hatamluyi B, Darroudi M, Meshkat Z, Aryan E, Soleimanpour S, Rezayi M. PCR-free electrochemical Genosensor for mycobacterium tuberculosis complex detection based on two-dimensional Ti_3C_2 Mxene-Polypyrrole signal amplification. Microchem J. 2022;179:107467. https://doi.org/10.1016/j.microc.2022.107467.
57. Wei W, Lin H, Hao T, Su X, Jiang X, Wang S, Hu Y, Guo Z. Dual-mode ECL/SERS immunoassay for ultrasensitive determination of vibrio Vulnificus based on multifunctional MXene. Sensors Actuators B Chem. 2021;332:129525. https://doi.org/10.1016/j.snb.2021.129525.
58. Kim KH, Park SJ, Park CS, Seo SE, Lee J, Kim J, Lee SH, Lee S, Kim JS, Ryu CM, Yong D, Yoon H, Song HS, Lee SH, Kwon OS. High-performance portable graphene field-effect transistor device for detecting gram-positive and -negative bacteria. Biosens Bioelectron. 2020;167:112514. https://doi.org/10.1016/j.bios.2020.112514.
59. Wu G, Dai Z, Tang X, Lin Z, Lo PK, Meyyappan M, Lai KWC. Graphene field-effect transistors for the sensitive and selective detection of Escherichia Coli using Pyrene-tagged DNA Aptamer. Adv Healthc Mater. 2017;6(19):1700736. https://doi.org/10.1002/adhm.201700736.
60. Singhal C, Khanuja M, Chaudhary N, Pundir CS, Narang J. Detection of chikungunya virus DNA using two-dimensional MoS_2 Nanosheets based disposable biosensor. Sci Rep. 2018;8(1):1–11. https://doi.org/10.1038/s41598-018-25824-8.
61. Sethi J, Van Bulck M, Suhail A, Safarzadeh M, Perez-Castillo A, Pan GA. Label-free biosensor based on graphene and reduced graphene oxide dual-layer for electrochemical determination of Beta-amyloid biomarkers. Microchim Acta. 2020;187(5) https://doi.org/10.1007/s00604-020-04267-x.
62. Abhilash S, Sarika S, Ambadi S, Akhila M, Sumi VS, Sreekala CO, Rijith S. Fabrication and performance evaluation of RGO-PANI supported NiP/TMD based biosensors for electrochemical detection of dopamine. Mater Today Commun. 2024;38:107946. https://doi.org/10.1016/j.mtcomm.2023.107946.
63. Li F, Peng J, Wang J, Tang H, Tan L, Xie Q, Yao S. Carbon nanotube-based label-free electrochemical biosensor for sensitive detection of MiRNA-24. Biosens Bioelectron. 2014;54:158–64. https://doi.org/10.1016/j.bios.2013.10.061.
64. Park J, Kim J, Kim S-Y, Cheong WH, Jang J, Park Y-G, Na K, Kim Y-T, Heo JH, Lee CY, Lee JH, Bien F, Park J-U. Soft, smart contact lenses with integrations of wireless circuits, glucose sensors, and displays. Sci Adv. 2018;4:1–12. https://doi.org/10.1126/sciadv.aap9841.
65. Jang J, Kim J, Shin H, Park Y-G, Joo BJ, Seo H, Won J-E, Kim DW, Lee CY, Kim HK, Park J-U. Smart contact lens and transparent heat patch for remote monitoring and therapy of chronic ocular surface inflammation using mobiles. Sci Adv. 2021;7:eabf7194. https://doi.org/10.1126/sciadv.abf7194.

Chapter 10
Point-of-Care Testing with Nanomaterials

Thenmozhi Rajarathinam, Sivaguru Jayaraman, and Seung-Cheol Chang

Abstract Nanomaterials have been widely employed in the fabrication of novel point-of-care testing (POCT) diagnostics for non-infectious and infectious diseases. Owing to their superior physical, chemical, optical, electrical, thermal, and mechanical properties, nanomaterial-customized POCTs are highly promising for rapid disease diagnosis. The transportation and processing of samples, their high cost, their duration, and the need for specialized personnel to operate them are the main constraints of conventional biochemical and immunological diagnostic techniques. Advanced POCT systems, which are more portable, quick, inexpensive, and automated with simpler detection procedures, overcome these limitations. Promising outcomes have been observed in these devices for the quick identification of various disease biomarkers, such as infectious (pathogen antigens and host antibodies), genomic (DNA, RNA, miRNA, and cancer cells), and proteomic (peptides and lipid metabolites) biomarkers. This chapter describes POCT immunoassays, specifically, the microfluidic, electrochemical, immunochromatographic, and enzyme-linked immunosorbent assays. The biosensing and related POCT utility is given a strong emphasis. In recent years, smart and sustainable nanomaterials, such as carbon nanomaterials (graphene, carbon nanotubes, carbon dots, and quantum dots), noble metal nanoparticles (NPs), mesoporous silica, and upconversion NPs, have been extensively used in POCT devices. The versatile physical and chemical properties of these smart nanomaterials bestow superior detection range, high sensitivity, selectivity, reproducibility, repeatability, and response time to POCT devices. This

T. Rajarathinam
Department of Cogno-Mechatronics Engineering, College of Nanoscience and Nanotechnology, Pusan National University, Busan, Republic of Korea

Engineering Research Center for Color-Modulated Extra-Sensory Perception Technology, Pusan National University, Busan, Republic of Korea

S. Jayaraman · S.-C. Chang (✉)
Department of Cogno-Mechatronics Engineering, College of Nanoscience and Nanotechnology, Pusan National University, Busan, Republic of Korea
e-mail: s.c.chang@pusan.ac.kr

S. Mondal et al. (eds.), *Smart and Sustainable Nanomaterials in Digital Healthcare and Theranostic*, https://doi.org/10.1007/978-981-95-9386-6_10

chapter will describe the recent advances in smart nanomaterial-based POCT devices for the analysis of various disease biomarkers. Existing challenges and future directions of these innovative POCT platforms are also discussed.

Keywords Point-of-care testing · Nanomaterials · Microfluidic · Electrochemical · Enzyme-linked immunosorbent assays

10.1 Introduction

Non-infectious diseases, such as cardiovascular diseases, cancer, diabetes mellitus, and respiratory diseases, contribute to global mortality issues. Of these, cancer is the deadliest disease, which is expected to increase more than 16.1 million by 2030 [7, 69]. Infectious diseases, caused by certain biological agents (bacteria, virus, and fungi), also inevitably interfere with human health. Because of the devastating consequences of these diseases, the healthcare system has tremendous difficulties, and early detection is becoming more and more important to enhance life expectancy and the prognosis of these diseases. Hence, there is a necessity for ubiquitous, cost-efficient, rapid, onsite, and portable detection of these biomarkers with high selectivity using advanced POCT devices [31].

Conventional assays require controlled biochemical conditions and specialized instruments, like high-performance liquid chromatography (HPLC) [18], mass spectrometry (MS) [4], HPLC-MS [86], and atomic absorption and emission spectroscopy [49]. Several conventional biological approaches have been developed for the early detection of cancer cells, including polymerase chain reaction (PCR) [16], genome sequencing [59], Raman flow cytometry [15], microarray analysis [1], immunohistochemistry [12], and fluorescence in situ hybridization [45]. While these approaches are unquestionably accurate, and dependable, most of them are expensive and labor-intensive, and need several hours of operation. Also, they are unsuitable for routine and rapid medical investigation due to the need for specialized equipment and several interwoven processing procedures.

In this decade, the conventional assays are expanding to POCT diagnostics, to realize bedside testing or home-testing based approaches to address these challenges [84]. With the help of integrated sensing systems, POCT diagnostics may automate many analytical steps, including target recognition, signal amplification, and sample preparation, into a single, automated unit. This method surpasses conventional diagnostic testing since it delivers results quickly, affordably, and practically without the need for specialized expertise. The POCT diagnostics are thus user-friendly, cost-effective, abundant, recyclable, and biosustainable. Also, selectivity and sensitivity are important parameters for successful POCT devices [52]. The low reagent and sample consumption, device compactness, and rapid analysis turnaround constitute several benefits to POCT devices. Rapid identification of the target enables early diagnosis of diseases, particularly those that are spreading quickly. To improve POCT's reliability and accuracy, new techniques seek to improve three factors: (1) a low limit of detection (LOD), which allows sensitive target detection in several sample matrixes; (2) sensitivity and specificity; and (3) integrated automation of the POCT instrument, which lowers labor costs, shortens the analysis time, and eliminates operation errors caused by operating personnels. With emphasis on POCT tests, the World Health Organization (WHO) has outlined certain vital elements as ASSURED criteria for evaluating these techniques: reasonably priced, sensitive, specific, easy to use (basic steps), reliable and quick (results within 30 min), equipment-free, and accessible to the end-users [3, 50]. To determine if the diagnostic tests meet the need for resource-constrained settings, these criteria act as a benchmark. It is impractical to fulfill all these requirements, though; therefore, creating top-notch POCT platforms that suit the needs is still difficult [68]. Till date, pregnancy test kits, glucometer, and viral and bacterial test kits are the popular optical and electrochemical-based POC devices available. These devices utilize the advantageous properties of nanomaterials by incorporating them into different parts of existing sensing platforms or by providing exceptionally creative detecting systems.

10.2 POCT Immunoassays

The basic concept of POCT immunoassays is the binding of antibody-antigen complexes. In clinical testing or disease diagnosis, and other biological applications, immunoassay is a highly beneficial technique. Two prominent immunoassay types are the sandwich and the competitive types. In a sandwich immunoassay, either a labeled molecule or an affixed antigen binds to the target in the sample to capture them. In this assay type, the number of labeled molecules is related to several targets in the sample. An unlabeled target in the test sample is assessed in a competitive immunoassay based on its binding capacity with a pre-labeled antibody. The labeled antibody concentration is assessed in the competitive format and is inversely linked to the amount of unlabeled antibody in the sample [6].

POCT immunoassays are classified into microfluidic immunoassays (MIAs), electrochemical assays (ELCAs), immunochromatographic assays (ICAs), enzyme-linked immunosorbent assays (ELISA), and microarrays. Microfluidic immunoassays involve complex channels, for example, lab on chip, while the ICAs involve paper strip-based lateral flow immunoassays in a single channel [65].

10.3 Types of POCT Immunoassays

10.3.1 MIAs

Microfluidic immunoassay devices are referred to as micro total analysis systems (μ-TAS) or lab-on-a-chip (LOC) devices. Microfluidic devices offer a collection of multifunctional fluidic units known as micro conduits, which facilitate

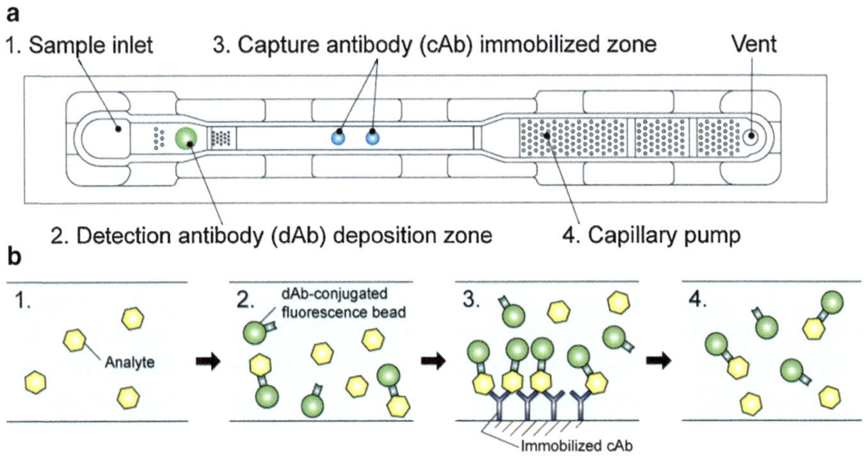

Fig. 10.1 Schematic of microfluidic immunoassay. (**a**) Microfluidic device and its elements; (**b**) antibody-target reactions. (Copyright (2020), with permission from Elsevier)

the convenient analysis of entire chemical or biological processes, such as the preparation, analysis, reaction, and collection of samples. Microfluidic platforms offer several benefits: (1) they exceptionally consume low fluid volume, < microliters, which reduces waste and reagent expenses; (2) because of the high surface-to-volume ratio and low diffusion distances of the nanomaterial, there is a rapid response of less than milliseconds and result output; (3) the safer and simpler functioning of the device enables in situ use by non-trained professionals; (4) examination of several samples is concurrently done through various routes. Capillary force or pressure facilitates efficient working of microfluidic platforms. The electrokinetic system and electrochemical test are closely related, and the lateral flow assay is based on capillary action. Pressure-driven laminar flow, segmented flow microfluidics, pressure-actuated devices, and microfluidic large-scale integration are a few examples of the various types of pressure-facilitated systems [39, 86]. The five areas of the microfluidic device shown in Fig. 10.1 are the sample input, capillary pump, detection antibody, capture antibody, and a vent. In microfabrication, thermoplastic substrates like poly (methyl methacrylate) are frequently utilized [32].

Nowadays, the biosensing field is seeing a rapid transition towards novel technical advancements such as organ-on-a-chip and human-on-a-chip. One illustration is digital microfluidics, which offers fluid control through discrete droplets, challenging conventional microchannels. Combining smart nanomaterials with microfluidics improves fluid manipulation accuracy, biological sample sensing and characterization precision, and overall automation and screening efficiency [84].

10.3.2 ELCAs

Due to the low cost, ease of use, and portability of electrochemical devices, electrochemical assays continue to get significant attention. Since nanomaterials enhance signals, they are a good choice for high-performance immunoassays on complicated samples containing low concentrations of targets. Specifically, noble metal NPs and carbon-based nanomaterials (CNMs) resemble enzymes and exhibit remarkable catalytic activity toward hydrogen peroxide (H_2O_2). For instance, the great surface area, ease of surface functionalization, outstanding conductivity, superior stability, and redox capacity of platinum (Pt), Au-, silver (Ag), and copper oxides (CuO) make them excellent catalysts/labels for immunoassays. It is feasible to detect multiple targets reliably, continuously, and simultaneously in complicated samples using the ELCA approach [34].

10.3.3 ICAs

Membrane or paper strips in ICAs clearly indicate protein biomarkers for infectious diseases, such as pathogen antigens and host antibodies. The fluid migration principle-based signal-generating system, antigens, and/or antibodies are all included in ICA devices, along with porous membranes. A well-known instance is the human chorionic gonadotropin (hCG) test strips, where the immune response is monitored via the color of the AuNPs is observed with the naked eye to determine the outcome. Numerous benefits come with immunochromatographic testing strips (ICTSs), including their low cost, easy operation, time-saving portability, and ability to be seen with the naked eye. The strips do have certain drawbacks, though, including low-viscosity liquid samples, qualitative or semi-quantitative detection, and false-positive or false-negative results [57].

10.3.4 ELISA

Although ELISA is an effective method for high-sensitivity and simultaneous target measurement, its cost makes it impractical for use in rapid clinical diagnosis. Before this approach is used as end-user POCT tests, more work need to be done on it. Comparing ELISA as a detection platform to real-time PCR tests reveals various advantages, such as reduced cost, less reagent use, and easier operation. It is commonly known that ELISA employs both catalyst-based signal transduction and an immunoassay for target detection based on the antibody-antigen interaction [72]. Several optical materials, such as AuNPs and organic dyes, have revolutionized conventional ELISA [26].

10.3.5 Microarrays

Sandwich immunoassays, which resemble the antigen–antibody interactions in ELISA, are also used in microarrays and microwells. Target detection using microarray techniques entails high throughput screening after amplification of the signal by PCR resulting from a fluorescent tag attached to the trace analyte. Microarray POCTs required less sample amount (5.0 μL), less reagent, and a shorter analysis time (1 h) as compared to ELISA. Using the camera on a smartphone, colorimetric (naked eye readable) signals can be produced via paper-based microarrays. In POCT microarray assays, multiplexed detection of several immunobinding responses is possible [8].

10.4 Smart Nanomaterials in POCT Immunoassays

Due to the varied sensitivity of the detecting systems, nanomaterial-incorporated POCT devices show varying detection limits. There are several reasons for the discrepancy, including the target analytes' validation, the signal processing or amplification mode, sample purification and integration protocols, the sensing interfaces, and the chemical modifications. This section discusses POCT systems based on various nanomaterial kinds, their importance, and their use in diagnostics [71].

POCT platforms, which are extensively employed in colorimetric [36], optical [51], electrochemical [65], and magnetic [25, 82] techniques, have advanced because of the development of novel nanomaterials and nanotechnology. For immunofluorescence labeling, dyes and microorganisms are also utilized; however, their fluorescence needs to be kept under tight storage conditions or is readily quenched. The safety risks and high cost of the devices make radioimmunoassay challenging to promote. Despite the widespread use of enzyme labeling technology, further research remains to be done to increase sensitivity. These shortcomings can be improved by using smart NPs [61] as they can offer an enormous active area for surface modification and dye loading, and different molecules can be connected to alter the chemical and physical properties of the particles. Because of their unique optical, magnetic, electrical, and thermal characteristics, they can function in a variety of ways in immunoassays, including as transporters, protective agents, fluorescence donators, and separation agents. Thus, the sensitivity and stability properties of the POCT platforms are improved.

A comparison between immunoassays that rely on smart nanomaterials is given in Table 10.1, in which the nanomaterials and their significance in sensing are described.

Table 10.1 POCT immunoassays utilizing smart nanomaterials and their significance in detecting the target

Type(s) of immunoassay	Smart nanomaterial	Significance of the assay	Target	LOD ($/mL^{-1}$)	Time	Ref
LFA & CMA	AuNPs	The multiplex test distinguishes the host's immunity from the target viral species. Identify cross-reactive immunity. The serological platform consists of capture ligands (with high specificity and sensitivity), in-house built strips, and a user-friendly smartphone.	Ebola virus IgG antibodies	200 ng	15 min	[6]
LFA & CMA	AuNPs	Combining the optical properties of AuNPs and the high efficiency of chromatographic separation, sandwich-type DNA hybridization occurs. Avoid multiple incubation times, separation, and washing steps in the well-established nucleic acid biosensors.	DNA	2.5 μg	15 min	[44]
SERS-LFA & Raman	AuNPs	Requires only 2–5 s for detection. Utilizes a fast and a SERS affordable reader.	hCG	1.6 mIU		[70]
LFA & Fluorescence	AuNPs-Cy5	Reverse fluorescence enhancement with a bimodal signal readout for ultrasensitive and fast estimation of CEA. Allowing on-the-spot spectrum screening by naked eye. Suitable for large-scale screening in both resource-abundant and resource-limited settings.	CEA	5.89 pg	10 min	[80]
Microfluidic assay	AgNCs	Three features: (i) a microfluidic multiantibody-array biosensing chip; (ii) a sensitive nanoplasmonic imaging technology with AgNCs for signal transduction; (iii) a rapid and precise machine-learning-based image processing method for signal analysis. Allows simultaneous analysis of six cytokines in a single run with wide working ranges of 1.0–10,000 pg mL^{-1}. Requires only a 3.0 μL sample volume.	Cytokine	0.46–1.36 pg	<100 min	[17]

(continued)

Table 10.1 (continued)

Type(s) of immunoassay	Smart nanomaterial	Significance of the assay	Target	LOD ($/mL^{-1}$)	Time	Ref
MagLISA	Fe_3O_4, AuNZs	Two essential strategies for sensitive sensing: facile target separation by magnetic beads and signal amplification by the AuNZs. Simple sample separation, enrichment, ultrasensitive readout, and anti-interference ability reduce the spread of viruses.	H1N1 virus	5.0×10^{-12} g	–	[47]
ECA and FET	Graphene	Coating graphene over the FET with a SARS-CoV-2 spike protein antibody forms a selective sensor. Requires no sample pretreatment or labeling.	SARS-CoV-2 spike protein	1.6×10^1 pfu; 2.42×10^2 copies	–	[63]
ULISA	UCNPs	Photon-UCNPs emit shorter wavelength light under near-infrared excitation and avoid optical background interference.	Pharmaceutical micropollutants of diclofenac	0.05 ng	>1 h	[21]
LFA & UC Fluorescence	UCNPs	Nanosized platform with high UC intensities. Simultaneous target detection feasible.	*Yersinia pestis*, *Burkholderia pseudomallei*	100 CFU per test	15 min	[39]
LFA & Fluorescence	Luminescent quantum dot beads	Sensitive than the conventional ELISA method.	Aflatoxin B1	0.42 pg	15 min	[57]
LFA & TRFIA	EuNSs	Can determine total aflatoxins in quality control.	Aflatoxin	0.16 μg kg^{-1}	12 min	[74]

LFA & Fluorescence	EuNSs	The LOD is approximately 185 times lower than that of the colloidal Au-strips. No cross-reactions with other interfering antigens.	Silk fibroin	8.09 ng	25 min	[83]
LFA & CA	Pt-AuNPs	The excellent peroxidase activity of Pt-AuNPs emits strong visible color in less than 1 min for visual observation even in low concentrations.	*E. coli* O157:H7	100 cells	20 min	[28]
Microfluidic assay	Semi-automatic platform	Can assess antibody reactivities against four SARS-CoV-2 antigens from up to 50 serum samples at the same time.	IgG and IgM levels against four SARS-CoV-2 proteins: the spike protein, the S1 subunit, the receptor-binding domain, and the nucleocapsid.	1.6 ng	–	[58]
Microarray	TiO_2	Simultaneous detection of a panel of EVs membrane proteins. The microarray platform consists of antibody arrays printed on a photonic crystal sensor with microscopic hyperspectral imaging technique that can rapidly detect EV binding to their respective antibodies. The assay requires only a 2.0 μL sample volume.	EVs	2.18×10^9	<2 h	[75]

LFA lateral flow assay, *CMA* colorimetric assay, *AuNPs* Au- nanoparticles, *IgG* immunoglobulin G, *DNA* deoxyribonucleic acid, *SERS* surface-enhanced Raman spectroscopy, *hCG* human chorionic gonadotropin, *Cy5* Cyanine5, *CEA* carcinoembryonic antigen, *AgNCs* silver nanocubes, *MagLISA* magnetic nano(e)zyme-linked immunosorbent assay, Fe_3O_4 Iron (III) chloride, *AuNZs* Au nanozymes, *H1N1* Influenza A virus subtype, *ECA* electrochemical assay, *FET* field effect transistor, *ULISA* upconversion-linked immunosorbent assay, *UCNPs* upconversion NPs, *TRFIA* time-resolved fluoroimmunoassay, *EuNSs* europium nanospheres, *CA* catalysis assay, *Pt* platinum, TiO_2, *EVs* extracellular vesicles

10.4.1 Carbon Nanomaterials (CNMs) and Their Allotropes

CNMs exist in a variety of allotropes and have garnered a lot of interest in recent years because of their inherent benefits, which include good biocompatibility, a high surface-to-volume ratio, high electrical conductivity, and chemical stability. One group recently published a study on the use of Au-graphene oxide (GO)-based electrochemical immunosensors for the detection of the CD44 biomarker for breast cancer [56]. Additionally, the same group developed dual-detection electrochemical immunosensor platforms based on antigen-antibody pairings and Au-functionalized GO for SARS-CoV-2 detection [60]. The smooth functionalization of carbon surfaces with organic or biomolecules is highly probable due to the covalent bonds between carbon and nitrogen, oxygen, and hydrogen. CNMs are divided into several allotropes according to their structures, as listed below [13].

(i) Zero-dimensional (0D) CNMs include carbon dots (CDs), graphene quantum dots (GQDs), and fullerene (C60).
(ii) One-dimensional (1D) CNMs consist of single-walled and multi-walled carbon nanotubes (SW- MW- CNTs).
(iii) Two-dimensional (2D) CNMs is composed of graphene and derivatives (GO) and reduced GO (rGO).

0D CNMs: Because of its electrical and optical properties, including fluorescence, chemiluminescence, and electrochemiluminescence, 0D CNMs are used in biosensors. The synthesis, combination, and functionalization of these materials are convenient and economical. It has been shown that carbon dots are both environmentally friendly and biocompatible. Compared to colloidal Au, CDs have demonstrated a twofold increase in sensitivity and a longer longevity due to their excellent quantum yields [2].

The optical properties of colloidal semiconductor nanocrystals, such as absorbance and photoluminescence, are exceptional. QDs are common semiconductors that are only a few nm in size. They are made from two or more heavy metals, CdTe and CdSe and InP, with core and core–shell arrangements. QDs generate electromagnetic radiation in the near-infrared or ultraviolet (NIR) regions of the electromagnetic spectrum when their high-energy electrons create holes. Because of this, electron bands in QDs exist as separate energy levels. The diameters of QDs are similar to the exciton Bohr radius. Because of their special optical characteristics, QDs are the best particles among the many fluorescence markers [20].

In core–shell QDs, the non-conductive inorganic core wrapped by a shell exhibits sufficient photochemical stability and significant molar extinction coefficient of up to 106.0 L (mol cm^{-1}). Additional features of QDs include their extended fluorescence lifetimes (20–50 ns), high-resolution threshold, broad excitation range, narrow emission, and exceptional resilience against photobleaching. The development of QDs in various fields, such as molecular or cellular biology, imaging, and medical diagnostics, has garnered substantial interest in recent decades (Fig. 10.2).

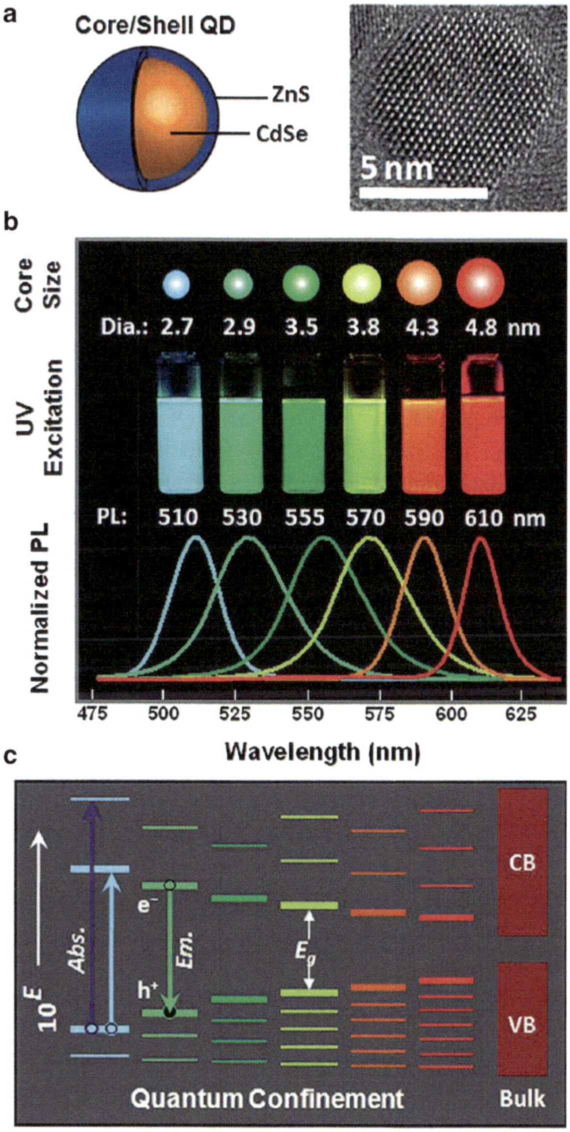

Fig. 10.2 (**a**) Diagram and TEM of a CdSe/ZnS QDs. (**b**) PL spectra showing color changes of QDs with increasing crystal size. (**c**) QD energy level variation with increasing sizes. Band gap energies (E_g), calculated from the PL spectra. Conduction (CB) and valence (VB) bands of CdSe. The energy scale expanded as 10_E. (Copyright (2011), with permission from ACS)

Owing to these benefits, QDs have been used as labels in lateral flow immunochromatographic tests (ICTS) to detect pesticides, bacteria, proteins, and even tiny drug molecules in addition to nucleic acids [87]. Protein detection has made extensive use of such QD-labeled ICTS devices. Nitrated ceruloplasmin has been measured using ICA with nanocrystal QDs that have been produced. With an LOD of 8.0 ng mL^{-1}, the biosensor showed a broad range and a quick response for 1.0 ng mL^{-1} target concentration. In another study, Cu:Zn–In–S/ZnS QDs have been used for the ICAs to find tetanus antibodies. This study offers a reference for antibody estimation, as the use of ICAs in antibody detection is uncommon. It is well established that ICST performance is significantly impacted by label size [38]. Nevertheless, QDs are also small; therefore, to maximize ICAs, the size must be improved. QD nanobeads (QBs) encasing several individual QDs in a polymer matrix show enhanced fluorescence intensity, environmental tolerance, sensitivity, and stability. To get rid of the drawbacks of low sensitivity and inadequate quantity, QBs and ICTS were merged. As previously mentioned, to create large QBs, the QDs were encapsulated in modified polymer matrix. Prostate-specific antigen (PSA) can be detected using the QBs-based ICTS system within 15 min. The developed fluorescent nanospheres that were larger than 200 nm, which was 380 times smaller than QDs. To detect CRP, fluorescent QDs were conjugated with monoclonal antibodies, which demonstrated a 257-fold increase in sensitivity over colloidal Au-based ICA [24]. Furthermore, UV light easily identified two test lines. Wang et al. reported highly fluorescent QBs by incorporating CdSe/ZnS QDs in copolymer matrixes. After surface blockage, these labeled QBs were employed as ICA signal amplification probes for aflatoxin B1 detection in maize [57]. A study showcased the synthesis of QBs of varied sizes (58, 124, 255, 365, and 598 nm), revealing that 124 nm QBs were the suitable detection platform for ochratoxin A working on competitive ICA. Furthermore, QBs demonstrated simultaneous estimation of neuron-specific enolase biomarkers and carcinoembryonic antigen (CEA) biomarkers. Small QBs exhibited lower fluorescence intensities compared to large QBs, making the latter more appropriate for ICA [76].

1D CNMs: CNTs consists of one or more graphene sheets wrapped into cylindrical tubes. Both SWCNTs and MWCNTs have been utilized as electrode modifiers for the detection of neurotransmitters, such as dopamine, norepinephrine, epinephrine, and cancer biomarkers [53, 55]. CNTs are modifiable with receptors like glutaraldehyde, ethyl(dimethylaminopropyl)carbodiimide (EDC) with N-hydroxysuccinimide (NHS), and cysteamine. Since CNTs are such adaptable nanomaterials, their sensing properties can be significantly changed by chemical functionalization. Carbonylated CNTs may generate sensors by combining them with proteins or viruses. These CNTs have superior electrochemical stability and increase electron transport by forming amide bonds with amine moieties. In immunosensors, aminated CNTs enhance charge transfer and offer a robust antigen immobilization platform. Because of their large surface area and ease of functionalization, CNT-based biosensors demonstrate high sensitivity [78]. To improve selectivity and sensitivity, for example, a modified electrode was built of MWCNTs, polypyrrole nanowires, and AuNPs. This electrode offered strong electrocatalytic activity, electrical conductivity, and a porous architecture with a wide active area. As a result, the accessibility of the target was preserved while the quantity of DNA aptamers fixed on the electrode was enhanced. Using metallic NPs for decorations is another method of adjusting the properties of CNTs. On MWCNTs, AuNPs have been scattered to add peroxidase-like activity [42].

Because of the special arrangement of the electrical bands, 2D graphene exhibits outstanding qualities such strong mechanical strength, rapid electron transport, and good chemical stability. Typical two-dimensional materials used in electrochemical experiments are graphene and graphene oxide. AuNPs were applied on cysteine (Cys)-rGOs, and these AuNPs were then conjugated with antibodies using EDC-NHS chemistry. The working electrode can be adjusted more easily attributable to the covalent interaction of S–Au between Cys-rGO and AuNPs. Mesoporous Cys-rGO hydrogel's high surface area, biocompatibility, and abundance of functional groups had allowed for the loading of several antibodies, which enhances sensitivity, selectivity, and binding kinetics. A signal generator with discrete Au-coated chips and a metal oxide semiconductor field-effect transistors (FET) constitutes the potentiometric sensor's enhanced signal. Real sample cardiac myoglobin (cMb) is detectable using this immunosensor. To optimize advantages of electrochemical sensing, the performance was improved by combining carbon materials with noble metal NPs [66].

Rapid and precise detection of CRP was achieved through the integration of rGO/Ni/PtNPs micromotors with an Au electrode [46]. To improve electrocatalytic performance, an in situ preparation of the AuNP/rGO nanocomposite was performed. With a low LOD and a dynamic linear range, the sensor was utilized to identify the endometriosis biomarker CA125 in endometriosis clients [62]. The biosensing device based on FETs based on rGO was developed to identify the harmful rotavirus quickly and accurately. Large, single-layered GO sheets with a thickness higher than 50.0 μm were produced using photolithography or micropatterning and reduction techniques in addition to a modified Hummers' approach. Certain rotavirus antibodies were covalently bonded to the graphene channels and were used to identify the rotavirus antigens [41].

10.4.2 Metallic NPs

Noble metal NPs binding principle: Noble metal NPs, including AuNPs and AgNPs, exhibit many interactions with proteins, including hydrophobic, electrostatic, and dative bonding. EDC and NHS activate carboxyl-group-containing NPs, which are subsequently joined with protein or other biomolecule amino groups. NPs containing amino groups are joined via glutaraldehyde linkages with the amino groups of proteins or other biomolecules. NPs with macropores, example, inorganic SiNPs can pass the biomolecules right through the pores and shield them from damage by electrostatic forces. NPs with great absorption capacities, such as, GO and CNTs easily adsorb biomolecules [54, 55].

10.4.2.1 AuNPs

Due to their distinct optical and electrocatalytic characteristics over other NPs, AuNPs are excellent labels for signal amplification in immunoassays. The synthesis hinges on the various reductants (sodium citrate, hydroxylamine, citric acid, tannin, and oxalic acid) chemically reducing Au salts. By varying the ratio of reductants,

AuNPs' particle size, shape, aggregation state, and surface characteristics can be tuned. The unique characteristics and uses of AuNPs are significantly influenced by their sizes and forms [19]. Because of their size variety, AuNPs have distinct LSPR features, high molar extinction coefficients, and chromogenic changes based on aggregation or disaggregation while the targeted analytes are present. From wine red (<100 nm) to brown (bigger particles), AuNPs can create a variety of colors. A substantial LSPR shift is strongly associated with the red-to-blue (or purple) color change that the colloidal Au solution exhibits. This color change also offers a straightforward platform for visual detection. Because AuNPs provide a microenvironment that is conducive to biomolecules, they continue to function even when immobilized. Lastly, AuNPs have superior biocompatibility and biosafety compared to other inorganic materials, and they may be used on most platforms for immunoassay applications [30]. While AuNPs are dispersed in liquids, stable colloidal Au formation is influenced by the shape, concentration, surface ligand, pH, and ionic strength of the solution. The typical process involves reducing chloroauric acid with citrate, which gives AuNPs with a negative surface zeta potential. The negatively charged shells of AuNPs could withstand aggregation. By coulombic repulsion, the carboxyl groups can prevent NPs aggregation once they have deprotonated. This probably maintains the NPs surface's zeta potential constant. Particle instability results from the substitution of monovalent mercaptan ions for trivalent citrate ions, which also promotes further aggregation and increases particle size. Because sulfide has a significant propensity for forming stable metal–sulfides (M–S) bonds and amine groups without the need for additional reagents to aid in surface modification, AuNPs are readily combined with biological receptors or ligands. Consequently, the surface of the AuNPs develops an electrical double layer after the immunological Au formation. The stern layer, the top layer is consistently positively charged. The second layer is diffusive in nature and is consistently negatively charged [11]. AuNPs and proteins typically interact by ionic, dative covalent, hydrophobic, and other link types. Furthermore, without the citrates being displaced, interlayer interactions such as hydrophobic effects, electrostatic, and hydrogen bonding may cause interparticle attraction. The generated structure may be disturbed, and the stability is significantly impacted by external variables, solvent effects, and substrate effects [48].

When the incident light stimulates noble metal NPs, LSPR is generated at their interfaces. The environment around a certain nanostructure, such as AgNPs or AuNPs, as well as the NPs' size, shape, and surface coating, might affect the frequency and intensity of LSPR absorption. Additionally, the LSPR generated several optical characteristics that have been applied to the detection of nucleic acids and proteins. These hierarchical AuNP-incorporated ICAs have shown great sensitivity for *E. coli* detection. In comparison to the visual-antibody-macroarray, the innovative AuNPs and ICAs increased the color intensity over twofold. These studies confirm that the morphology of AuNPs has a significant impact on ICA sensitivity [29]. Nucleic acid detection has also been accomplished with ICA systems. It has been reported that AuNPs were used as the label for an African swine fever virus DNA sensor. With a minimum detection limit of 200 copies, the ICAs quickly identified the African swine fever virus without any cross-reactivity to other viruses. Although miRNA is crucial to many biological processes, the conventional sandwich approaches might not be appropriate. Consequently, the development of AuNPs-labeled ICTSs for miRNA identification was required. An avidin-biotin-AuNPs complex was formed with AuNPs coupled with the thiol-DNA (detection probe) and biotin-single strand DNA (capture probe). It offered a technique for finding short oligonucleotides like siRNA and miRNA [23]. To identify Ebola virus–specific IgG antibodies in human serum, the researchers developed a point-of-care diagnostic method by combining ICTSs with a smartphone reader. The platform allowed for naked eye detection, expanding the potential applications of POCT [6].

10.4.2.2 AgNPs

Of all the metals, AgNPs have the highest conductivity, reflectivity, and size-dependent catalytic activity. Under incoming light, AgNPs exhibit strong surface plasmon resonance (SPR). Compared to AuNPs of the same size, AgNPs have higher extinction coefficients, making them useful for a range of colorimetric and optical sensors. Furthermore, the surfaces of different silver nanostructures exhibit considerable enhancements in fluorescence and Raman scattering signals, making them suitable as ultrasensitive optical sensing probes. Numerous tests utilizing AgNPs have been developed, such as chemiluminescence, surface-enhanced Raman scattering (SERS), electrochemistry, and Ag-enhanced fluorescence [37]. Because of their instability and complex modification, AgNPs are less used than the AuNPs. Contrarily, the biomedical applications of AgNPs have been sprouting via alternate synthesis and functionalization methods [77]. A new device fabrication method, successive ionic layer absorption and reaction (SILAR), was discovered for AgNPs, in which thin NPs films were self-assembled on a solid substrate without the requirement of further tag or chemical modifications for the early clinical diagnosis of HPV infection [35]. Modified Ag and Au nanomaterials have a stronger surface plasmon resonance than those of other metals, which makes them popular choices for SERS applications. To overcome surface oxidation of Ag and to maximize the SERS enhancement factor, many studies have been centered on the structure of bimetallic NPs. After the discovery of SERS in 1970s, extension of conventional Raman spectroscopy, that is surface-sensitive resonance, occurred. The target specimen or molecules are positioned adjacent or directly deposited on semiconductor substrates or rough metals, primarily Au-, Ag-, or Zn-based NPs. The spectra become stronger after the molecule-substrate system interactions. SERS-based platforms identify structurally comparable compounds based on their unique vibrational spectra by primarily using Raman shifts arising from molecular vibrational energy levels. Au/Ag SERS tags are the foundation for most SERS tags and ICA strip combinations; yet, in complex samples, Au/Ag NPs are easily impacted by environmental variables [35]. To address this issue, multiple strategies are used to boost the effectiveness of SERS-based ICAs. These strategies include optimizing particle size and shape by electron beam radiolysis method to cut down on nonspecific signals, enhancing the stability of SERS tags to aid in the identification of actual samples, and enhancing the analyte capacity of SERS tags [9]. AuNPs covered in a silica shell and adsorbed with methylene blue were developed as an immunoassay platform for SARS-CoV-2 spike protein detection [5]. Wang et al. developed dual-dye-loaded Ag-coated Fe_3O_4 MNPs (Fe_3O_4@Ag tags) as magnetic SERS tags to identify respiratory viruses. With the introduction of Fe_3O_4@Ag SERS tags into ICA strips, biological samples can be used without the need for sample pre-treatment procedures [73]. AgNPs are commonly employed as electrodes in electrochemical devices due to their superior conductivity.

10.4.2.3 PtNPs

The Pt-group metals have greater efficiency than natural enzymes and contribute significantly to high catalytic activity and stability. These metals have been used over other NPs to create an electrode or a core-shell structure. For several decades, biomedical researchers have regarded porous bimetallic Pt-NPs as promising nanomaterials due to their enhanced area, chemical composition, and exceptional electron conductivity, which have all contributed to their superior catalytic performance. One of the most significant characteristics of noble metals is their catalytic activity, which can significantly accelerate certain chemical reactions. Natural enzymes, on the other hand, are delicate biomolecules that readily lose their catalytic activity even in typical testing conditions and are thus unsuitable for POC applications [40] (Fig. 10.3).

Nanozymes have been intrigued by noble metal NPs loaded with enzyme catalysts. Since these nanozymes demonstrate catalytic activity similar to those of enzymes without denaturation, they can be used and maintained at a wide pH and temperature range. Enzyme-catalyzed biochemical reactions are vital in some POCT diagnostic devices. Noble metals are essential to the catalytic process as well. Because of their enormous surface area and specialized catalytic potentials,

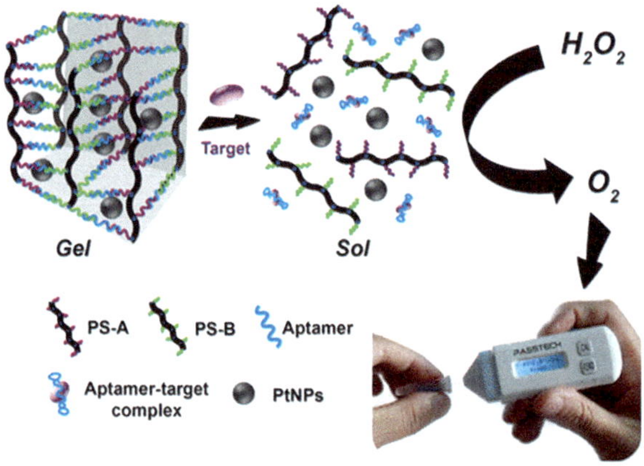

Fig. 10.3 The mechanism of the target-responsive hydrogel pressure-based assay. (Copyright (2017), with permission from ACS)

nanozymes are therefore easily generated on a wide scale and these properties have been utilized in POCTs. Jiang et al. emphasize Pt–Au bimetal NPs detect *E. coli* O157:H7. In addition to exhibiting strong electrocatalysis toward 3,3′,5,5′-tetramethylbenzidine (TMB) and producing a distinct blue color that was visible to the unaided eye, the nanoparticles aggregated on the test line. The blue color was visible in less than a minute due to the quick reaction and very low detection limit. The three orders of magnitude signal enhancement that Pt–Au bimetal NPs and the peroxidation catalysis process favors the sensitive detection of E. coli O157:H7 and other microorganisms. The p53 protein was then detected using the mesoporous Pt–Pd bimetallic NPs, extending the usage of this bimetallic NPs in POCTs. The peroxidase-like activity of Pt–Pd NPs catalyzed the reactions of TMB and o-phenylenediamine, produced the signal. The color was seen in 10 min. This assay was highly sensitive to electrochemiluminescence detection, although being less sensitive than the state-of-the-art fiber light-coupled optofluidic waveguide immunosensor. Nonetheless, the platform demonstrated robust stability throughout a broad pH and temperature range. Another fascinating example is the chemiluminescent and extremely sensitive visual detection of target biomarkers that was achieved by combining the HRP catalysis with the colloidal Au-lateral flow assay to generate a dual-readout [28].

Other NPs in addition to Pt-group metals have a significant impact on improving detection performance. Fe_3O_4 NPs have both peroxidase-like and magnetic properties. For instance, Fe_3O_4–Pt/core–shell NPs, synthesized by adding Pt to the outer layers of Fe_3O_4 NPs, showed increased catalytic activity. Using a heterogeneous nucleation and growth paradigm, Pt was decorated on the Fe_3O_4 NPs surface to create Pt NPs. It was demonstrated that the sensitivity of the novel bioassay platform was twofold greater than that of traditional AuNP-based ICA. Utilizing PtNPs' potent catalytic ability, a pressure-based test has been created to enable quantitative detection [34]. Pt nanoshells were made using a Pt-staining technique onto the AuNPs to combat the PtNPs' long-term instability. By employing this staining technique, PtNPs with catalytic activity were added as signal labels while maintaining the original benefits of AuNPs. Thus, the novel bioassay sensor's purpose of utilizing a core-shell Au@Pt NPs is to catalyze the breakdown of H_2O_2 and release O_2, which can be used to detect ractopamine and CEA [14].

Furthermore, PtNPs have been used to identify RNAs as significant biomarkers for cancer prognosis and diagnosis. PtNPs and magnetic beads worked together to make qualitative miRNA detection possible. miRNA 21 can be identified by a POCT utilizing the strand displacement reaction because PtNPs catalyze the breakdown of H_2O_2 [64]. Yin et al. reported a fluorescent/colorimetric dual-model biosensor for miRNA based on palladium nanoclusters (PdNCs). In this, PdNCs initiated a chromogenic reaction, which enabled to view the qualitative results. Signal amplification of the nucleic acid cycle was combined with graphitic carbon nitride's fluorescence quenching action on PdNCs to acquire precise results [81]. Thus, in the past decades, researchers have employed the remarkable catalytic properties of noble metals, specifically Pd, Pt, Au, and their alloys, to fabricate POCTs. This combines the ICA and catalysis of noble metals through signal magnitude, increasing the detection sensitivity for bacterial membrane proteins. This creates new avenues for biomolecule identification using POCT immunoassays.

10.4.3 Mesoporous SiNPs

Si is the most widely used material in target detection because it is cost-effective and non-toxic. Mesoporous SiNPs are the most prevalent type of Si-based NPs and are proven to be effective carriers of drug and protein molecules due to their wide pore channels and easily accessible interior surfaces. These NPs have been doped with different dyes or luminous rare earth complexes to expand their potential applications. SiNPs were typically made via a reverse microemulsion process and then functionalized with amino or carboxyl groups. By adding fluorescent dyes or NPs to functionalized SiNPs, fluorescent Si spheres were produced. Targets may be quantitatively detected using these fluorescent spheres. To create colored core–shell SiNPs, the SiNPs were loaded with Reactive Violet 5 dye encased in a silica shell. SiNPs were used to coat rare-earth complexes, namely Ru and Eu complexes to detect β-agonists [67]. An onsite detection technique using dual-color SiNPs@QDs nanotags could simultaneously detect procalcitonin (PCT) and CRP in serum. These nanotags demonstrated monodispersity and superior luminescence produced by electrostatically adsorbing dense red or green CdSe/ZnS–COOH QDs on SiNPs by PEI-mediated electrostatic adsorption. Later, these QDs nanotags were coupled with monoclonal antibodies against PCT and CRP to create stable, fluorescence-enriched QD nanotags in LFA. Thus, SiNPs@QDs with two varied fluorescence signals had contributed to the specificity of the LFA [79]. Dendritic Si spheres were used to create AuNPs, utilizing thiol-metal coordination to identify methamphetamine drug in urine. In comparison to Au, organic dye–doped SiNPs are substantially less expensive for sufficient signal amplification purposes. SiNPs can also be used to load a variety of small drug molecules, organic dyes, small QDs, and big enzymes [27].

10.4.4 Upconversion NPs (UCNPs)

Although optical ICAs have several benefits, their quantification and sensitivity are constraints. Large quantities of fluorescent NPs, especially UCNPs, have thus been used to replace conventional AuNPs. Also, to solve the shortcomings of traditional colorimetric ICTSs, a variety of fluorescent chemicals have been widely assembled into fluorescent ICTSs in recent decades. In sandwich-style ICTS, the label-reporters would be captured on both the test and control lines for a positive sample, and only on the control line for a negative sample. The occurrence and intensity of the immunological response are indicated by the optical signal. A lateral flow immunoassay platform based on NIR-to-NIR UCNPs has been developed for the quick and

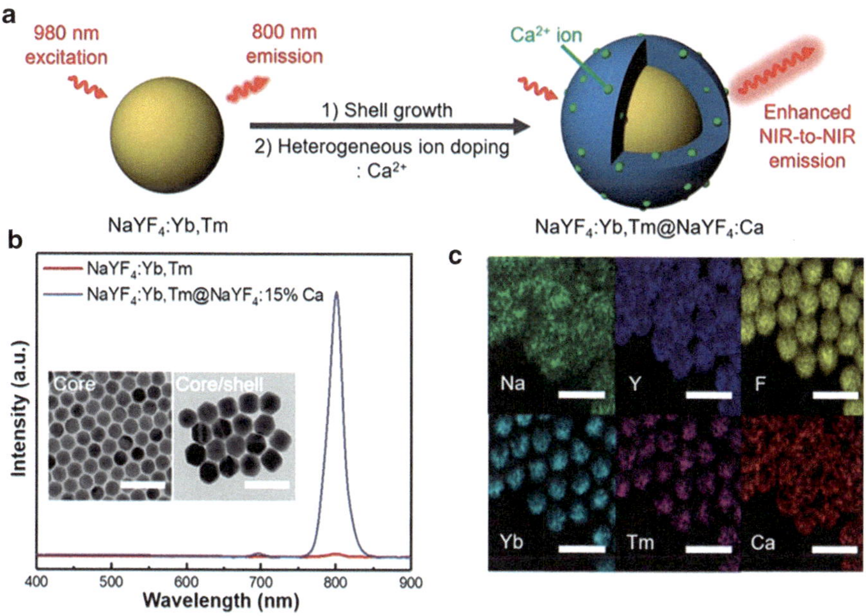

Fig. 10.4 (**a**) Schematic of synthesis of NIR core/shell UCNPs. (**b**) Emission spectra of the UCNPs, showing NIR emission after shell formation. Inset: TEM images. (**c**) Energy dispersive X-ray spectroscopy of the core/shell UCNPs. (Copyright (2018), with permission from Elsevier)

accurate onsite identification of avian influenza virus. Ca^{2+}-doped UCNPs were synthesized and following excitation at 980 nm, the researchers have demonstrated robust upconversion fluorescence emission centered at 800 nm, enabling background-free fluorescence signals. Thus, without interference from the unwanted signals, these UCNPs were employed to identify targets in opaque stool samples. In comparison to AuNPs, whose absorption was obscured by the brown backdrop, the LOD achieved using UCNPs was 10 times lower [33]. Another study employed ICA in conjunction with up-converting phosphor technology in a different investigation to profile antibodies toward *Yersinia pestis* demonstrating 10-channel determination [22] (Fig. 10.4).

10.4.5 Magnetic NPs (MNPs)

Iron oxide–based MNPs could function as complexing agents for magnetic enrichment, transducers, and catalysts. Since interferents in biological matrixes are nonmagnetic, magnetic sensor-based target detection is far more sensitive than optical and electrochemical methods. Magnetic NPs have been highly used in POCTs. To the best of our knowledge, because of their exceptional qualities, including a high surface-to-volume ratio, ease of production, an active surface, high chemical stability, modification possibilities, and quick reaction kinetics, iron oxides are considered outstanding magnetic NPs. Since iron oxides can be utilized directly for biomodification or as protective layer to the magnetic beads [43]. The avian influenza virus H5N1 was biosensitized by electrochemically converting MNPs to highly electroactive Prussian blue (PB). A sandwich immunosensor utilizing the ECC techniques quickly detected H_5N_1 avian influenza virus by producing PB using MNPs as self-sacrificial labels. By splitting H_2O to liberate Fe^{3+} from MNPs, a low-potential inducing the reduction of $K_3Fe(CN)_6$ and Fe^{3+} to $K_4Fe(CN)_6$ and Fe^{2+} to form PB [85].

Additionally, magnetic nanobeads are employed in conjunction with various NPs, including QDs and AuNPs. Magnetic nanobeads are used in the traditional assay to split and enrich targets from complicated samples. The AuNPs and magnetic nanobeads technology have been used to find malaria-related biomarkers. The applied magnetic field separate both the AuNPs conjugated to the target and the iron oxide NPs. As a result, big aggregates and bulk serum were effectively separated, generating an enhanced signal free from matrix interference. Based on immunomagnetic NPs and polystyrene spheres, a dual-enzyme-based bioluminescent sensor for adenosine triphosphate measurement was reported [10].

10.4.6 Conclusion and Future Perspectives

A comprehensive knowledge of the interactions between nanomaterials in these POCT systems may hasten the creation of highly reliable detection platforms. While there has been significant advancement in the POC assay using biosensors, there are still certain issues that need to be fixed in practical applications. For example, many platforms are employed in buffers and not in actual samples, and sophisticated equipment is needed for signal readout. Certain POCTs primarily concentrate on the sensors' sensitivity and accuracy. Few have advanced to the pre-clinical stage to examine actual samples, and even fewer are simple. For many platforms, sophisticated operators and intricate methods are also necessary. In addition, there are a lot of analysis objectives in complex matrices that are challenging to identify.

As is well known, some LFA findings can be read with naked eye based on the color of colloidal gold, which is easy to carry, conduct, and requires no additional equipment. These machines are essential for certain unique and sensitive essays. Maintaining a balance between sensitivity and equipment-free setting is challenging. Certain advanced devices can be employed in POCT tests, thanks to smartphones and wearable diagnostics. Due to their built-in sensors, high-resolution cameras, fast wireless connectivity, and numerous software and app options, smartphones allow for the quantification of sensitive data. For this reason, they can be used independently as mobile POCT sensors and detectors without needing professional training. The development of sensing and signal readout modes will hold promise for the future of NP-integrated biosensors for POCT. The development of new materials and sophisticated detection technologies are important components of biosensing, which promote considerable advancements in reliable, sensitive, and adaptable early detection systems.

Acknowledgments This research was supported by the Basic Science Research Program through the National Research Foundation of Korea (NRF), funded by the Ministry of Education (2022R1I1A3072535). This work was also supported by the National Research Foundation of Korea (NRF) grant funded by the Korean government (MSIT) (No. NRF-2021R1A5A1032937).

Declaration of Competing Interest The authors declare that they have no conflict of interest.

References

1. Al Madhoun A, Haddad D, Al Tarrah M, Jacob S, Al-Ali W, Nizam R, Miranda L, Al-Rashed F, Sindhu S, Ahmad R, Bitar MS, Al-Mulla F. Microarray analysis reveals ONC201 mediated differential mechanisms of CHOP gene regulation in metastatic and nonmetastatic colorectal cancer cells. Sci Rep. 2021;11(1):11893.
2. Alafeef M, Srivastava I, Aditya T, Pan D. Carbon dots: from synthesis to unraveling the fluorescence mechanism. Small. 2024;20(4):e2303937.
3. Baker AN, Hawker-Bond GW, Georgiou PG, Dedola S, Field RA, Gibson MI. Glycosylated gold nanoparticles in point of care diagnostics: from aggregation to lateral flow. Chem Soc Rev. 2022;51(16):7238–59.
4. Banerjee S. Empowering clinical diagnostics with mass spectrometry. ACS Omega. 2020;5(5):2041–8.
5. Bistaffa MJ, Camacho SA, Pazin WM, Constantino CJL, Oliveira ON Jr, Aoki PHB. Immunoassay platform with surface-enhanced resonance Raman scattering for detecting trace levels of SARS-CoV-2 spike protein. Talanta. 2022;244:123381.
6. Brangel P, Sobarzo A, Parolo C, Miller BS, Howes PD, Gelkop S, Lutwama JJ, Dye JM, McKendry RA, Lobel L, Stevens MM. A serological point-of-care test for the detection of IgG antibodies against Ebola virus in human survivors. ACS Nano. 2018;12(1):63–73.
7. Bray F, Laversanne M, Weiderpass E, Soerjomataram I. The ever-increasing importance of cancer as a leading cause of premature death worldwide. Cancer. 2021;127(16):3029–30.
8. Burrow DT, Heggestad JT, Kinnamon DS, Chilkoti A. Engineering innovative interfaces for point-of-care diagnostics. Curr Opin Colloid Interface Sci. 2023;66:101718.
9. Călinescu I, Martin D, Ighigeanu D, Gavrila A, Trifan A, Patrascu M, Munteanu C, Diacon A, Manaila E, Craciun G. Nanoparticles synthesis by electron beam radiolysis. Open Chem. 2014;12(7):774–81.
10. Chen Y, Xianyu Y, Wu J, Dong M, Zheng W, Sun J, Jiang X. Double-enzymes-mediated bioluminescent sensor for quantitative and ultrasensitive point-of-care testing. Anal Chem. 2017;89(10):5422–7.
11. Chou SF. Development of a manual self-assembled colloidal gold nanoparticle-immunochromatographic strip for rapid determination of human interferon-gamma. Analyst. 2013;138(9):2620–3.
12. Conde E, Hernandez S, Sanchez E, Regojo RM, Camacho C, Alonso M, Martinez R, Lopez-Rios F. Pan-TRK immunohistochemistry: an example-based practical approach to efficiently identify patients with NTRK fusion cancer. Arch Pathol Lab Med. 2021;145(8):1031–40.
13. Erol O, Uyan I, Hatip M, Yilmaz C, Tekinay AB, Guler MO. Recent advances in bioactive 1D and 2D carbon nanomaterials for biomedical applications. Nanomedicine. 2018;14(7):2433–54.

14. Fu Q, Wu Z, Du D, Zhu C, Lin Y, Tang Y. Versatile barometer biosensor based on Au@Pt Core/Shell nanoparticle probe. ACS Sens. 2017;2(6):789–95.
15. Gala de Pablo J, Lindley M, Hiramatsu K, Goda K. High-throughput Raman flow cytometry and beyond. Acc Chem Res. 2021;54(9):2132–43.
16. Ganova M, Zhang H, Zhu H, Korabecna M, Neuzil P. Multiplexed digital polymerase chain reaction as a powerful diagnostic tool. Biosens Bioelectron. 2021;181:113155.
17. Gao Z, Song Y, Hsiao TY, He J, Wang C, Shen J, MacLachlan A, Dai S, Singer BH, Kurabayashi K, Chen P. Machine-learning-assisted microfluidic nanoplasmonic digital immunoassay for cytokine storm profiling in COVID-19 patients. ACS Nano. 2021;15(11):18023–36.
18. Grant DA, Dunseath GJ, Churm R, Luzio SD. Comparison of a point-of-care analyser for the determination of HbA1c with HPLC method. Pract Lab Med. 2017;8:26–9.
19. Hammami I, Alabdallah NM, jomaa AA, kamoun M. Gold nanoparticles: synthesis properties and applications. J King Saud Univ Sci. 2021;33(7):101560.
20. Hildebrandt N, Spillmann CM, Algar WR, Pons T, Stewart MH, Oh E, Susumu K, Diaz SA, Delehanty JB, Medintz IL. Energy transfer with semiconductor quantum dot bioconjugates: a versatile platform for biosensing, energy harvesting, and other developing applications. Chem Rev. 2017;117(2):536–711.
21. Hlavacek A, Farka Z, Hubner M, Hornakova V, Nemecek D, Niessner R, Skladal P, Knopp D, Gorris HH. Competitive upconversion-linked immunosorbent assay for the sensitive detection of diclofenac. Anal Chem. 2016;88(11):6011–7.
22. Hong W, Huang L, Wang H, Qu J, Guo Z, Xie C, Zhu Z, Zhang Y, Du Z, Yan Y, Zheng Y, Huang H, Yang R, Zhou L. Development of an up-converting phosphor technology-based 10-channel lateral flow assay for profiling antibodies against Yersinia pestis. J Microbiol Methods. 2010;83(2):133–40.
23. Hou SY, Hsiao YL, Lin MS, Yen CC, Chang CS. MicroRNA detection using lateral flow nucleic acid strips with gold nanoparticles. Talanta. 2012;99:375–9.
24. Hu J, Zhang ZL, Wen CY, Tang M, Wu LL, Liu C, Zhu L, Pang DW. Sensitive and quantitative detection of C-reaction protein based on immunofluorescent nanospheres coupled with lateral flow test strip. Anal Chem. 2016;88(12):6577–84.
25. Hu X, Gao X, Chen S, Guo J, Zhang Y. DropLab: an automated magnetic digital microfluidic platform for sample-to-answer point-of-care testing-development and application to quantitative immunodiagnostics. Microsyst Nanoeng. 2023;9:10.
26. Huang JY, Lin HT, Chen TH, Chen CA, Chang HT, Chen CF. Signal amplified gold nanoparticles for cancer diagnosis on paper-based analytical devices. ACS Sens. 2018;3(1):174–82.
27. Huang L, Jin J, Wang J, Jiang C, Xu M, Wen H, Liao T, Hu J. Homogeneous and high-density gold unit implanted optical labels for robust and sensitive point-of-care drug detection. Nanoscale. 2019;11(34):16026–35.
28. Jiang T, Song Y, Wei T, Li H, Du D, Zhu MJ, Lin Y. Sensitive detection of Escherichia coli O157:H7 using Pt-Au bimetal nanoparticles with peroxidase-like amplification. Biosens Bioelectron. 2016;77:687–94.
29. Kelly KL, Coronado E, Zhao LL, Schatz GC. The optical properties of metal nanoparticles: the influence of size, shape, and dielectric environment. J Phys Chem B. 2002;107(3):668–77.
30. Khlebtsov N, Dykman L. Biodistribution and toxicity of engineered gold nanoparticles: a review of in vitro and in vivo studies. Chem Soc Rev. 2011;40(3):1647–71.
31. Kholafazad-Kordasht H, Hasanzadeh M, Seidi F. Smartphone based immunosensors as next generation of healthcare tools: technical and analytical overview towards improvement of personalized medicine. TrAC Trends Anal Chem. 2021;145:116455.
32. Kim J, Hong K, Kim H, Seo J, Jeong J, Bae PK, Shin YB, Lee JH, Oh HJ, Chung S. Microfluidic immunoassay for point-of-care testing using simple fluid vent control. Sensors Actuators B Chem. 2020;316:128094.
33. Kim J, Kwon JH, Jang J, Lee H, Kim S, Hahn YK, Kim SK, Lee KH, Lee S, Pyo H, Song CS, Lee J. Rapid and background-free detection of avian influenza virus in opaque sample using

NIR-to-NIR upconversion nanoparticle-based lateral flow immunoassay platform. Biosens Bioelectron. 2018;112:209–15.
34. Kim MS, Kweon SH, Cho S, An SSA, Kim MI, Doh J, Lee J. Pt-decorated magnetic nanozymes for facile and sensitive point-of-care bioassay. ACS Appl Mater Interfaces. 2017;9(40):35133–40.
35. Kim W, Kim YH, Park HK, Choi S. Facile fabrication of a silver nanoparticle immersed, surface-enhanced Raman scattering imposed paper platform through successive ionic layer absorption and reaction for on-site bioassays. ACS Appl Mater Interfaces. 2015;7(50):27910–7.
36. Ko A, Liao C. Paper-based colorimetric sensors for point-of-care testing. Anal Methods. 2023;15(35):4377–404.
37. Lee IH, Lee JM, Jung Y. Controlled protein embedment onto Au/Ag core-shell nanoparticles for immuno-labeling of nanosilver surface. ACS Appl Mater Interfaces. 2014;6(10):7659–64.
38. Li Z, Wang Y, Wang J, Tang Z, Pounds JG, Lin Y. Rapid and sensitive detection of protein biomarker using a portable fluorescence biosensor based on quantum dots and a lateral flow test strip. Anal Chem. 2010;82(16):7008–14.
39. Liang Z, Wang X, Zhu W, Zhang P, Yang Y, Sun C, Zhang J, Wang X, Xu Z, Zhao Y, Yang R, Zhao S, Zhou L. Upconversion nanocrystals mediated lateral-flow nanoplatform for in vitro detection. ACS Appl Mater Interfaces. 2017;9(4):3497–504.
40. Liu D, Jia S, Zhang H, Ma Y, Guan Z, Li J, Zhu Z, Ji T, Yang CJ. Integrating target-responsive hydrogel with pressuremeter readout enables simple, sensitive, user-friendly, quantitative point-of-care testing. ACS Appl Mater Interfaces. 2017;9(27):22252–8.
41. Liu F, Kim YH, Cheon DS, Seo TS. Micropatterned reduced graphene oxide based field-effect transistor for real-time virus detection. Sensors Actuators B Chem. 2013;186:252–7.
42. Liu X, Cheng Z, Fan H, Ai S, Han R. Electrochemical detection of avian influenza virus H5N1 gene sequence using a DNA aptamer immobilized onto a hybrid nanomaterial-modified electrode. Electrochim Acta. 2011;56(18):6266–70.
43. Ma T, Hou Y, Zeng J, Liu C, Zhang P, Jing L, Shangguan D, Gao M. Dual-ratiometric target-triggered fluorescent probe for simultaneous quantitative visualization of tumor microenvironment protease activity and pH in vivo. J Am Chem Soc. 2018;140(1):211–8.
44. Mao X, Ma Y, Zhang A, Zhang L, Zeng L, Liu G. Disposable nucleic acid biosensors based on gold nanoparticle probes and lateral flow strip. Anal Chem. 2009;81(4):1660–8.
45. Mok T, Peters S, Camidge DR, Noé J, Gadgeel S, Ou S-HI, Kim D-W, Konopa K, Pozzi E, Liu T, Loftin IR, Williams C, Shaw AT. Outcomes according to ALK status determined by central immunohistochemistry or fluorescence in situ hybridization in patients with ALK-positive NSCLC enrolled in the phase 3 ALEX study. J Thorac Oncol. 2021;16(2):259–68.
46. Molinero-Fernandez A, Lopez MA, Escarpa A. Electrochemical microfluidic micromotors-based immunoassay for C-reactive protein determination in preterm neonatal samples with sepsis suspicion. Anal Chem. 2020;92(7):5048–54.
47. Oh S, Kim J, Tran VT, Lee DK, Ahmed SR, Hong JC, Lee J, Park EY, Lee J. Magnetic nanozyme-linked immunosorbent assay for ultrasensitive influenza a virus detection. ACS Appl Mater Interfaces. 2018;10(15):12534–43.
48. Park JW, Shumaker-Parry JS. Strong resistance of citrate anions on metal nanoparticles to desorption under thiol functionalization. ACS Nano. 2015;9(2):1665–82.
49. Parsons PJ, Barbosa F. Atomic spectrometry and trends in clinical laboratory medicine. Spectrochim Acta B At Spectrosc. 2007;62(9):992–1003.
50. Pashchenko O, Shelby T, Banerjee T, Santra S. A comparison of optical, electrochemical, magnetic, and colorimetric point-of-care biosensors for infectious disease diagnosis. ACS Infect Dis. 2018;4(8):1162–78.
51. Pioz MJ, Espinosa RL, Laguna MF, Santamaria B, Murillo AMM, Hueros AL, Quintero S, Tramarin L, Valle LG, Herreros P, Bellido A, Casquel R, Holgado M. A review of optical point-of-care devices to estimate the technology transfer of these cutting-edge technologies. Biosensors (Basel). 2022;12(12):1091.

52. Quesada-Gonzalez D, Merkoci A. Nanomaterial-based devices for point-of-care diagnostic applications. Chem Soc Rev. 2018;47(13):4697–709.
53. Rajarathinam T, Jayaraman S, Seol J, Lee J, Chang SC. Utilizing a disposable sensor with polyaniline-doped multi-walled carbon nanotubes to enable dopamine detection in ex vivo mouse brain tissue homogenates. Biosensors (Basel). 2024;14(6):262.
54. Rajarathinam T, Kwon M, Thirumalai D, Kim S, Lee S, Yoon JH, Paik HJ, Kim S, Lee J, Ha HK, Chang SC. Polymer-dispersed reduced graphene oxide nanosheets and Prussian blue modified biosensor for amperometric detection of sarcosine. Anal Chim Acta. 2021;1175:338749.
55. Rajarathinam T, Thirumalai D, Kwon M, Lee S, Jayaraman S, Paik HJ, Lee J, Chang SC. Screen-printed carbon electrode modified with de-bundled single-walled carbon nanotubes for voltammetric determination of norepinephrine in ex vivo rat tissue. Bioelectrochemistry. 2022;146:108155.
56. Ranjan P, Abubakar Sadique M, Yadav S, Khan R. An electrochemical immunosensor based on gold-graphene oxide nanocomposites with ionic liquid for detecting the breast cancer CD44 biomarker. ACS Appl Mater Interfaces. 2022;14(18):20802–12.
57. Ren M, Xu H, Huang X, Kuang M, Xiong Y, Xu H, Xu Y, Chen H, Wang A. Immunochromatographic assay for ultrasensitive detection of aflatoxin B(1) in maize by highly luminescent quantum dot beads. ACS Appl Mater Interfaces. 2014;6(16):14215–22.
58. Rodriguez-Moncayo R, Cedillo-Alcantar DF, Guevara-Pantoja PE, Chavez-Pineda OG, Hernandez-Ortiz JA, Amador-Hernandez JU, Rojas-Velasco G, Sanchez-Munoz F, Manzur-Sandoval D, Patino-Lopez LD, May-Arrioja DA, Posadas-Sanchez R, Vargas-Alarcon G, Garcia-Cordero JL. A high-throughput multiplexed microfluidic device for COVID-19 serology assays. Lab Chip. 2021;21(1):93–104.
59. Roepman P, de Bruijn E, van Lieshout S, Schoenmaker L, Boelens MC, Dubbink HJ, Geurts-Giele WRR, Groenendijk FH, Huibers MMH, Kranendonk MEG, Roemer MGM, Samsom KG, Steehouwer M, de Leng WWJ, Hoischen A, Ylstra B, Monkhorst K, van der Hoeven JJM, Cuppen E. Clinical validation of whole genome sequencing for cancer diagnostics. J Mol Diagn. 2021;23(7):816–33.
60. Sadique MA, Yadav S, Ranjan P, Khan R, Khan F, Kumar A, Biswas D. Highly sensitive electrochemical immunosensor platforms for dual detection of SARS-CoV-2 antigen and antibody based on gold nanoparticle functionalized graphene oxide nanocomposites. ACS Appl Bio Mater. 2022;5(5):2421–30.
61. Saha K, Agasti SS, Kim C, Li X, Rotello VM. Gold nanoparticles in chemical and biological sensing. Chem Rev. 2012;112(5):2739–79.
62. Sangili A, Kalyani T, Chen SM, Nanda A, Jana SK. Label-free electrochemical immunosensor based on one-step electrochemical deposition of AuNP-RGO nanocomposites for detection of endometriosis marker CA 125. ACS Appl Bio Mater. 2020;3(11):7620–30.
63. Seo G, Lee G, Kim MJ, Baek SH, Choi M, Ku KB, Lee CS, Jun S, Park D, Kim HG, Kim SJ, Lee JO, Kim BT, Park EC, Kim SI. Rapid detection of COVID-19 causative virus (SARS-CoV-2) in human nasopharyngeal swab specimens using field-effect transistor-based biosensor. ACS Nano. 2020;14(4):5135–42.
64. Shi L, Lei J, Zhang B, Li B, Yang CJ, Jin Y. Ultrasensitive and facile detection of MicroRNA via a portable pressure meter. ACS Appl Mater Interfaces. 2018;10(15):12526–33.
65. Shi SS, Li XJ, Ma RN, Shang L, Zhang W, Zhao HQ, Jia LP, Wang HS. A smartphone-based electrochemical POCT for CEA based on signal amplification of Zr(6)MOFs. Lab Chip. 2024;24(2):367–74.
66. Singh N, Ali MA, Rai P, Ghori I, Sharma A, Malhotra BD, John R. Dual-modality microfluidic biosensor based on nanoengineered mesoporous graphene hydrogels. Lab Chip. 2020;20(4):760–77.
67. Song C, Zhi A, Liu Q, Yang J, Jia G, Shervin J, Tang L, Hu X, Deng R, Xu C, Zhang G. Rapid and sensitive detection of beta-agonists using a portable fluorescence biosensor based on fluorescent nanosilica and a lateral flow test strip. Biosens Bioelectron. 2013;50:62–5.

68. Tang L, Li J. Plasmon-based colorimetric nanosensors for ultrasensitive molecular diagnostics. ACS Sens. 2017;2(7):857–75.
69. Thun MJ, DeLancey JO, Center MM, Jemal A, Ward EM. The global burden of cancer: priorities for prevention. Carcinogenesis. 2010;31(1):100–10.
70. Tran V, Walkenfort B, Konig M, Salehi M, Schlucker S. Rapid, quantitative, and ultrasensitive point-of-care testing: a portable SERS reader for lateral flow assays in clinical chemistry. Angew Chem Int Ed Engl. 2019;58(2):442–6.
71. Tsai TT, Huang CY, Chen CA, Shen SW, Wang MC, Cheng CM, Chen CF. Diagnosis of tuberculosis using colorimetric gold nanoparticles on a paper-based analytical device. ACS Sens. 2017;2(9):1345–54.
72. Van Gool A, Corrales F, Colovic M, Krstic D, Oliver-Martos B, Martinez-Caceres E, Jakasa I, Gajski G, Brun V, Kyriacou K, Burzynska-Pedziwiatr I, Wozniak LA, Nierkens S, Pascual Garcia C, Katrlik J, Bojic-Trbojevic Z, Vacek J, Llorente A, Antohe F, Suica V, Suarez G, t'Kindt R, Martin P, Penque D, Martins IL, Bodoki E, Iacob BC, Aydindogan E, Timur S, Allinson J, Sutton C, Luider T, Wittfooth S, Sammar M. Analytical techniques for multiplex analysis of protein biomarkers. Expert Rev Proteomics. 2020;17(4):257–73.
73. Wang C, Wang C, Wang X, Wang K, Zhu Y, Rong Z, Wang W, Xiao R, Wang S. Magnetic SERS strip for sensitive and simultaneous detection of respiratory viruses. ACS Appl Mater Interfaces. 2019;11(21):19495–505.
74. Wang D, Zhang Z, Li P, Zhang Q, Ding X, Zhang W. Europium nanospheres-based time-resolved fluorescence for rapid and ultrasensitive determination of total aflatoxin in feed. J Agric Food Chem. 2015;63(47):10313–8.
75. Wang Y, Zhang Q, Yuan W, Wang Y, Loghry HJ, Zhao Z, Kimber MJ, Dong L, Lu M. Hyperspectral imaging-based exosome microarray for rapid molecular profiling of extracellular vesicles. Lab Chip. 2021;21(1):196–204.
76. Wu R, Zhou S, Chen T, Li J, Shen H, Chai Y, Li LS. Quantitative and rapid detection of C-reactive protein using quantum dot-based lateral flow test strip. Anal Chim Acta. 2018;1008:1–7.
77. Xu L, Wang YY, Huang J, Chen CY, Wang ZX, Xie H. Silver nanoparticles: synthesis, medical applications and biosafety. Theranostics. 2020;10(20):8996–9031.
78. Yang H, Xu W, Liang X, Yang Y, Zhou Y. Carbon nanotubes in electrochemical, colorimetric, and fluorimetric immunosensors and immunoassays: a review. Mikrochim Acta. 2020a;187(4):206.
79. Yang X, Liu X, Gu B, Liu H, Xiao R, Wang C, Wang S. Quantitative and simultaneous detection of two inflammation biomarkers via a fluorescent lateral flow immunoassay using dual-color SiO(2)@QD nanotags. Mikrochim Acta. 2020b;187(10):570.
80. Yao Y, Guo W, Zhang J, Wu Y, Fu W, Liu T, Wu X, Wang H, Gong X, Liang XJ, Chang J. Reverse fluorescence enhancement and colorimetric bimodal signal readout immunochromatography test strip for ultrasensitive large-scale screening and postoperative monitoring. ACS Appl Mater Interfaces. 2016;8(35):22963–70.
81. Yin X, Liang L, Zhao P, Lan F, Zhang L, Ge S, Yu J. Double signal amplification based on palladium nanoclusters and nucleic acid cycles on a muPAD for dual-model detection of microRNAs. J Mater Chem B. 2018;6(36):5795–801.
82. Yoon J, Kang Y, Kim H, Ali A, Kim K, Torati SR, Im MY, Jeon C, Lim B, Kim C. Tailored micromagnet sorting gate for simultaneous multiple cell screening in portable magnetophoretic cell-on-chip platforms. Adv Funct Mater. 2024;34:2312875.
83. You Q, Liu M, Liu Y, Zheng H, Hu Z, Zhou Y, Wang B. Lanthanide-labeled immunochromatographic strip assay for the on-site identification of ancient silk. ACS Sens. 2017;2(4):569–75.
84. Young N, Taegtmeyer M, Aol G, Bigogo GM, Phillips-Howard PA, Hill J, Laserson KF, Ter Kuile F, Desai M. Integrated point-of-care testing (POCT) of HIV, syphilis, malaria and anaemia in antenatal clinics in western Kenya: a longitudinal implementation study. PLoS One. 2018;13(7):e0198784.

85. Zhang Q, Li L, Qiao Z, Lei C, Fu Y, Xie Q, Yao S, Li Y, Ying Y. Electrochemical conversion of Fe(3)O(4) magnetic nanoparticles to electroactive prussian blue analogues for self-sacrificial label biosensing of avian influenza virus H5N1. Anal Chem. 2017;89(22):12145–51.
86. Zhou H, Xiang H, Cai J, Wang Y, Zhang M, Han Y, Zhang Y. Comparison of a point-of-care testing with enzyme-multiplied immunoassay technique and liquid chromatography combined with tandem mass spectrometry methods for therapeutic drug monitoring of mycophenolic acid: a preliminary study. Ther Drug Monit. 2021;43(5):630–6.
87. Zhou JW, Zou XM, Song SH, Chen GH. Quantum dots applied to methodology on detection of pesticide and veterinary drug residues. J Agric Food Chem. 2018;66(6):1307–19.

Chapter 11
Environmental and Food Safety Biosensors

Suman Saha

Abstract The indispensable use of nanomaterial-based biosensors has attained extreme importance across numerous domains including the discovery of supreme drugs, areas in biomedicine, observance of food safety values, security and defense zones, and ecological intensive care. Biosensors deliver a modest, instantaneous, delicate, sensitive and precise exposure method to analyze environmental impurities, mostly phenols and phenolic complexes, heavy metals such as chromium, mercury, lead, arsenic, etc., and toxic substances like insecticides, pesticides, and various natural organic matters. Whereas, food safety observation plays a critical role in protecting civic health, preserving consumer assurance, subsidiary economic firmness, and smoothing global trade. Thus, specific and controlling systematic measuring tools have been invented utilizing biological detection elements known as biosensors. The continuing research in emerging control systems to monitor food quality and safety aims to progress effectiveness, diminish the risks engrossment to control food quality, and boost customer assurance in the food stock chain. Nanomaterial-based biosensors and bio-diagnostic systems appear to complement traditional systematic methods to monitor environmental contaminants and control food quality significantly. This chapter deals with existing and forthcoming practices of different types of nanomaterial-based biosensors and bioanalytical methods in the field of environmental applications and food quality control systems.

Keywords Environment · Contaminants · Food safety · Nanomaterial-based biosensors · Food quality · Biosensing

S. Saha (✉)
Department of Chemical Engineering, Haldia Institute of Technology, Haldia, West Bengal, India

S. Mondal et al. (eds.), *Smart and Sustainable Nanomaterials in Digital Healthcare and Theranostic*, https://doi.org/10.1007/978-981-95-9386-6_11

11.1 Introduction

Authoritative application of biosensors has developed supreme importance in the area of drug delivery, biomedicine, food safety values, and also in the field of defense, security, and environmental observation [5]. Biosensors have commanded the creation of accurate and influential systematic tools using biological detection elements. Implausible advancement has been made equally in technology and utilization of biosensing elements with pioneering approaches in the field of electrochemistry, biochemistry, nanoscience, etc. [5, 51].

The use of biosensors in bioelectronics has also created emerging trends to detect various contaminations in food and monitor environmental quality as well [5]. At present, numerous research exertions are dedicated to emerging control schemes confirming food value and safety [62]. The consciousness of food regulator also improved freshly due to the significantly increased global population in the next years [17]. Revolution and expansion in the agricultural and food sectors and the current internationalization of agro-industrial markets enhance the requirement for food safety and food quality control, which have become of countless apprehension for human and ecological health [41].

The taste of food, its appearance, values of nutritional benefits, activities of ingredients, its impact on flavor and freshness, and chemical texture are associated with monitoring food quality [31]. Natural components such as amino acids, sugar contents, -OH functional groups, vitamins, and other additives are generally considered to characterize food materials with the help of different biosensors [14]. The requirement of food safety involves ensuring the production of food beverages free from pathogens and toxic organic compounds [41].

However, the food safety process also involves commercializing the food that contains allergens, pesticides, heavy metals, and toxins [89]. These impurities could extremely distress human health, leading to foodborne ailments with serious value for the healthcare scheme and commercial yield [5]. It is obligatory to recognize and to arrange promotive procedures, examinations, and control schemes to diminish the contaminants that originate from insecure and low-quality final products [5].

Biosensors deliver modest, hasty, delicate, and careful recognition techniques for the investigation of environmental impurities, mostly counting phenolic compounds, various heavy metals, different toxins, insecticides, and further organic contaminants [48, 72, 73]. Biosensors, which are typically characterized by affording the biorecognition compounds such as enzymatic components, antibodies, DNA samples, and whole-cell detection, are conversed correspondingly [72, 73]. With the volatile evolution of world inhabitants and the speedy expansion of industrialization, the quantity of noxious chemical compounds released into the atmosphere has grown extremely due to regular human action [64]. Toxic chemicals released from different industrial activities may cause environmental damage and health issues [16]. Environmental contamination has developed one of the furthermost critical complications and unsurprisingly apprehended the world's courtesies [97]. Studying on environmental impurities is a crucial step in understanding and dealing with risks to social health and the ecosystem [16, 47]. Hence, an imperative requirement to develop profligate and consistent environmental observation approaches [27].

The growing expanse of possibly critical impurities in the environment requires rapid and profitable analytical methods [10]. Though extremely sensitive, discerning and conservative analytical procedures, like chromatographic and spectroscopic tests, are inconvenient and laborious during the analysis of a huge number of samples significantly [8, 33].

Besides, they require affluent instruments, accomplished operatives, and complex preliminary processes. The requirement of expandable instruments for ecological monitoring boosts the progress of modest, hasty, incessant, profitable, and field-movable screening procedures for the investigation of ecological impurities [47].

Most of the biosensing elements described in the review are followed by the principle of electrochemical analysis and optical technology [8]. The different spectroscopic biosensors, like potentiometric, amperometric, and voltametric, generally follow the principle of electrochemical methodology where impact comes out during the specific interactions between targeted species and recognition components [81]. The electrical signal is developed by these interactions that are connected to the concentration of the targeted species which is going to be studied. Ecological challenges are becoming a crucial influence in the social and technical exertions to defend living society [5]. The rising world populace, inadequacy of water resources, air contamination, and toxic ingredients can contaminate the terrestrial, air, and aquatic as the foremost ecological encounters. An extensive variety of chemicals can pollute aquatic bases, air, and land-living which influence the atmosphere and human well-being [45]. The uninhibited release of poisonous heavy metals and their oxides, hydrocarbons and their derivative compounds, organophosphorus mixtures, insecticides, and pesticides in the environment is a thoughtful environmental apprehension recently [74]. The utmost sources of environmental pollution are the various activities of industries [45]. Outmoded sources of ecological impurities include oil processing industries, activities of refinery processes, petrochemical productions, chemical industries, agricultural actions, infirmary wastes counting biochemicals, microorganisms, and germs, wastewater treatment plants, and sewage schemes [63]. These sources contribute suggestively to the contamination of air, marine resources, and terrestrial. Most of the unconfined impurities are steady in the contaminated zones for centuries and remain to damage the ecosystem [45]. In addition, some contaminants like pesticide compounds and various herbicides oppose breakdown progressions in the ecosystem and lastly penetrate the food supply chain, which might be ingested by human beings [44]. Conversely, long-term contact with the toxins resulted in probable health issues, comprising numerous problems in the living society [63].

Nervous system failure, heart disease, cancer risk, complications in eyesight, liver problems, dermatitis issues, blood cholesterol increase, etc., are the major health issues identified due to environmental pollution [2]. In addition, the introduction of noxious industrial chemicals and biochemical compounds into the soil and sediments can influence coastal areas. These toxic elements portend the health of human beings and decrease the commercial stability of regions that depend on a healthy and nonviolent coastal ecosystem [97]. Chemical contaminants and biological impurities are the main classifications of environmental contaminants. Additionally, biological impurities pose substantial ecological hazards with significant impacts. These types of impurities can arise from different activities of living species; consequently, recognizing and understanding the biological contaminations is of great awareness recently [33].

With increasing concentrations of toxic compounds in the environment, it is essential to develop suitable methods for their detection and determination, given the nature of these pollutants [87]. Numerous approaches can be used to analyze the categories and doses of different contaminants coming from various activities of industries. Thus, significant exertions have been prepared to develop operative procedures for the determination of ecological contaminants [37]. A biosensing device is an analytical instrument that can perceive specific components or analytes in different phases, providing information about chemical structures and concentration in the fluid phases [21]. The purpose of designing a biosensing device is to generate advanced instruments proficient in sensing explicit analytes with accurate selectivity, sensitivity, duplicability, rapidity, cost-effectiveness, and ease of use [22].

Consequently, it is vital to design a contracted and computerized biosensing device. Among the countless approaches, electrochemical biosensing tools can be transportable to detect environmental contaminants significantly [30]. However, biosensing devices prepared by electrochemical processes have also exposed their ability to sense various impurities in food and beverages [37]. Presently, electrochemical biosensing devices are expansively researched. These sensing devices are acknowledged for their substantial sensitivity and stability. The following sections will explore the fundamentals and applications of electrochemical biosensing instruments in detail [22].

11.2 Principles of Biosensors

Biosensing instrument is a device that generates systematic responses based on the chemical evidence of a species, including the concentration of the specific sample compounds or the overall composition scrutiny [5, 21, 30].

11.2.1 Fundamentals of Biosensing Process

In general, a biosensing system encompasses three essential necessities. First, a recognition unit is designed to detect specific species in the liquid or gas phase [77, 83]. A signal transducer known as the second important element helps to translate the species recognition into a quantifiable response. The third component namely an electronic system assists in managing the data generation process [30]. Figure 11.1

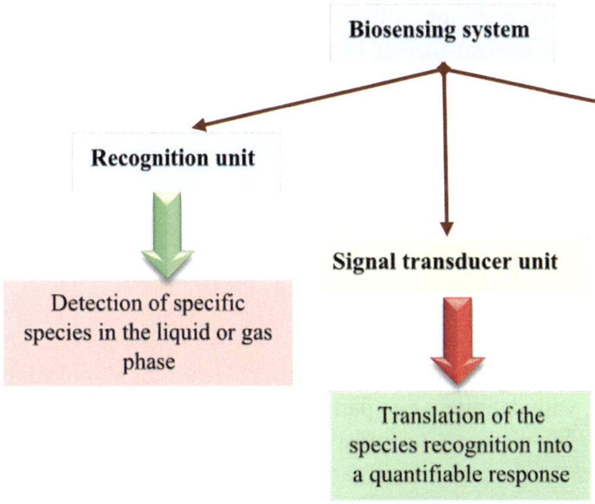

Fig. 11.1 The three essential requirements of a biosensing system

represents the pictorial explanation of three essential requirements of a biosensing system.

A biosensing system contains a biological section such as numerous enzymes, different antibodies, nucleic acid compounds, or various cells that precisely cooperate with the target chemical or biochemical species [65]. This constituent is crucial for the selective requisite or identification of the detected ingredient. A signal progression is engendered during the interactions between different analytes and the biorecognition materials [56]. The automated system produces and intensifies the quantifiable responses, converting them into a legible arrangement. This evidence can then be exhibited on several devices, like computer devices and digital screens, to analyze and interpret in the future [30].

The ultimate output is a vibrant signal. This clear signal indicates the final concentration or existence of the chemical species in the sample. This output permits the monitoring and investigation of biotic, chemical, and ecological circumstances [5]. The biosensing process applies several principles to sense and quantify the precise species [58]. Amperometry biosensing elements analyze the current generated during the oxidation or reduction processes of an electro-active constituent [4]. On the other side, potentiometric sensing devices also follow the principle of basic electrochemical process [55]. The ionic concentration difference is detected by the potentiometer by changing the voltage of these devices. The different electrical conductivities of the various solutions are also detected by another electrochemical device named the conductometric biosensing device [5]. The heat difference accompanying biochemical reactions is measured by the calorimetric biosensing device [55].

Whereas, absorbance and fluorescence-based biosensors act by following the principal operation of optical devices [30]. These systems measure the changes in the light absorbance and fluorescence intensities, respectively, during the interaction of different chemical or biological species in the fluids [5]. Each of these ideologies influences different physical, chemical, and biological properties to recognize and enumerate specific constituents. The selection of the working principle depends on issues like the nature of the chemical species, the essential sensitivity, and the explicit uses of the biosensing devices [88].

11.2.2 Biosensing Elements

Biosensing elements perform a crucial role in bio-detective processes by significantly identifying and cooperating with definite target particles, known as chemical or biological species [82]. These bio-elements comprise enzymatic compounds, several antibodies, amino and nucleic acids, and different active cells. These components are selected according to their abilities for the exact binding with species [88]. Enzymes help to catalyze different biochemical reactions with numerous substrates. Antibodies display high attraction in the presence of antigens. Amino and nucleic acids can configure exact base-pair relations with corresponding arrangements [79]. The selection of a suitable biosensing element depends on the appearance of the species and the detailed application, confirming accurate recognition competences across innumerable arenas like medicinal diagnostics, ecological monitoring, and food protection [7]. By interpreting biotic interactions into quantifiable signals, these biosensing elements permit detectors to execute qualitative and quantitative examinations of target chemical and biological species with sensitivity and dependability [5, 40].

11.2.3 Theory of Biosensing Process

The biosensing process is entrenched in the essential concept of detecting chemical and biological particles and species through exact communications that generate assessable signals [5]. Characteristically, this contains the usage of chemical and biological receptors such as organic compounds, enzymatic components, different antibodies, amino acids, and nucleic acids, which create bonds with exact species during the analysis [21]. The interaction between receptors and the species develops a signal process transduction mechanism renovating the molecular identification into a computable indication, repeatedly using different principal processes like optical, electrochemical, or mechanical approaches [38]. Figure 11.2 represents the schematic approach of the different steps of the biosensing process.

The meticulousness and sensitivity of biosensing schemes are censorious, confirming exact exposure even at very low concentrations of active species [30]. Sustainability in nanotechnology, material sciences, polymerization process, biochemistry, and biophysics have suggestively amended biosensing processes, intensifying their utilization across miscellaneous arenas, like pathology and diagnostics

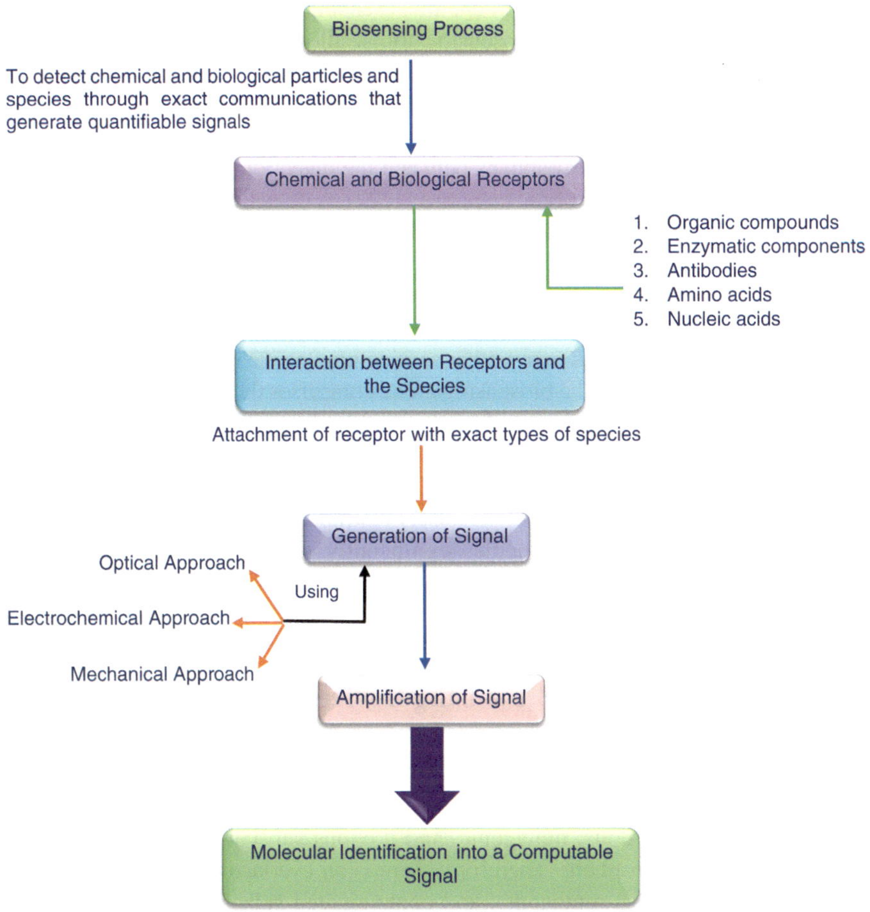

Fig. 11.2 The schematic approach of the different steps of the biosensing process

centers, detection of pollutants in the environment, food, and beverage protection fields, and around biodefence [43]. The continuing investigation aims to modernize by emerging a new class of chemical and biological receptors, enhancing signal intensification practices, and producing contracted devices, promising additional progressions in technical and applied fields [57].

11.2.4 Biomolecular Sensors

Electrochemical sensing devices are considered promising instruments for recognizing several biomolecules such as protein complexes, the structure of DNA, and lipids and phospholipids, which are decisive for the primary analysis of diseases and syndromes [22]. Evolution in electrochemical sensing stages has controlled the conception of a new category of biosensing tools, allowing label-free, non-invasive recognition of active cell feasibility, function, and genomic signatures [24, 46].

Conventionally, several electrochemical sensing devices have been advanced for the recognition of comprehensive kinds of components. In biochemical sensing devices, an electron transfer happens between the detection layer and the designed toxins, resulting in an electrolytic response [1, 22]. A detection regime is situated on the surface of a conductive subsurface to perceive exact chemical and biological species [22]. Various compounds have been engaged as detecting regimes in ecological applications, incorporating nanostructured metallic compounds, several carbon allotropes, complexes of metal-nanostructured constituents, encompassing boron-doped diamonds, and many other semiconductors [25].

An incipient frontier in the biosensing arena comprises the competence to exactly enumerate precise target biomolecules, attaining high enough accuracy to discriminate specific units within test models and to perceive the elusive characteristics of biomolecular relations at a discrete level [23]. Advanced strategies in biomolecular sensors have emerged, the policy of precisely restraining the active area of a sensing element to identify discrete molecules significantly, although this may not achieve ultrasensitive detection limits [1, 21].

11.3 Classification of Biosensing Devices

Modern developments and economic growth have made lifecycles more expedient; they have also led to substantial health complications [32, 88]. Every single year, large extents of hazardous, mutagenic, and noxious substances are produced and released into the atmosphere. Therefore, there is an everlasting necessity to detect and monitor poisonous, mutagenic, and contaminated substances. Alongside progressions in conventional approaches for observing these harmful ingredients, there remains an inevitability for bio-assays [8]. These bio-assays should not only perceive oncogenic and contaminated substances but also evaluate their bioavailability and estimate their impression on humanoid health [10].

Biosensing devices can be categorized according to numerous aspects, counting the type of bio-detection component, the theory and principle of transduction conditions, the target chemical and biological species, and the application extent [78]. The classification of biosensing devices is represented in Fig. 11.3.

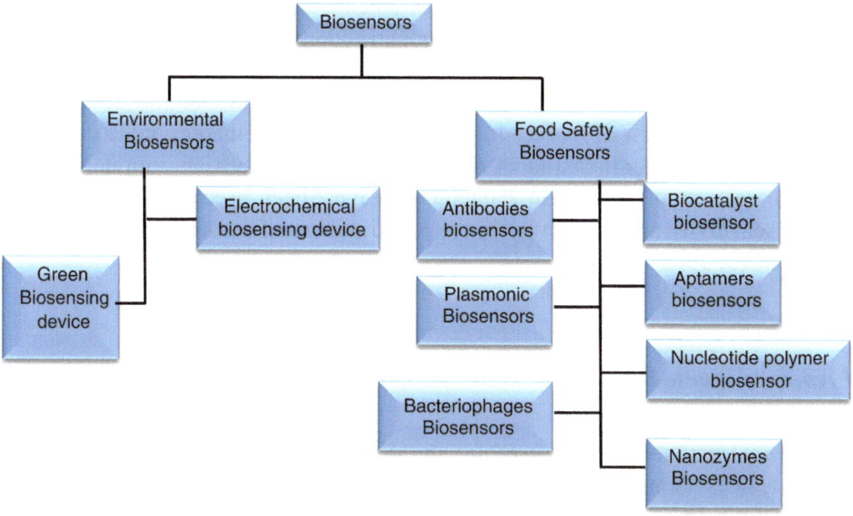

Fig. 11.3 Classification of biosensing devices

11.3.1 Electrochemical Biosensing Devices for Environmental Pollutants

Electrochemical biosensing devices offer abundant assistance, including transportability, effortlessness, comfort of use, cost-economic, and single-utilized ability in utmost cases [7, 8, 19]. The definite exposure abilities of biosensing tools are heightened by the affinity of the bio-detection components for their target chemical and biological species, which correspondingly improves discrimination [17]. Based on biosensing device design and the categories of biorecognition particles used, electrochemical biosensing tools are generally classified into various types including immunosensor electrochemical biosensing devices, aptasensor sensing tools, enzymatic biosensing instruments, and genosensor devices depending on nucleic acid biosensing methods ([8, 15, 52].

In immunosensors, a precise interface happens between an antibody and its consistent antigen. In electrolytic immunosensors, a specific antibody is restrained on the electrode superficial [12, 49, 90]. The interaction between the antibodies and antigens produces an electrolytic response. Due to the usage of antibodies in immunosensing instrument design, the desired compounds are inadequate to certain categories, for example, organophosphorus complexes. Subsequently, there are no provisions for markers in the design of the elementary antigen and antibody design approach as it is label-free [60, 79].

The recommended immunogen is added to the restrained immunoglobulin on the substrate's superficial in this recognition method. When the biosensor's external surface experiences an immunogen and immunoglobulin reaction, the antigen-antibody-assay exposure progression is finished [91]. The conception of the immunogen and immunoglobulin complex amends the electrical characteristics of electrode exteriors. As a result, the immunogen and immunoglobulin response modifies the electrochemical responses of redox elements formed during the reaction, which is directly associated with the aimed antigen concentration [5]. The sensitivity and exposure limit of marker-free immunosensors are inappropriate due to the nonappearance of significant label regime. The sandwich-variant immunoglobulin 1-immunogen-immunoglobulin 2 interactions have been used recently to achieve greater sensitivity and selectivity in the identification of numerous environmental pollutants [5, 99].

11.3.2 Green Biosensor Technology

Several instruments must be used for the detection of environmental toxins [5]. These devices should be inexpensive, sensitive, quick, durable, and able to automate and minimize processes. The researchers are searching for biorecognition molecules to satisfy these obstacles by achieving appropriate detection circumstances [8].

The researchers are searching for biorecognition molecules to attain appropriate detection settings to overcome these obstacles. Nucleic acids containing amino acid sequences are known as aptamers which are also called green biosensing elements. Because of their distinct binding sites, the aptamers may attach themselves to their targets with specificity. Furthermore, the specific aptamers may be produced in vast, pure, and high quantities using a repeatable synthesis process [11].

To progress both the compassion and discernment of the formed green biosensing element, numerous functional groups, such as fluorophores, nanoparticles, or enzymes, have been hired to amend the aptamers further while maintaining the affinity of the sensing element [13]. Lastly, the biosensing compounds are far more stable than the antibodies and can regain their active confirmation after usage [8].

However, to achieve a particular attachment to their targets, the green biosensing elements characteristically turn into an appropriate three-dimensional structure. For the electrolytic analysis of complex organic materials, a green electrochemical biosensing element has been developed [12, 90]. Immobilized aminated compounds are used to create green probes for the detection of organic compounds such as organophosphorus. Nanocomposite-based single-walled carbon tubes are the base constituent of the green biosensing probes which are also modified by copper oxide nanomaterials [5]. To detect toxic chemical species, an electrolytic green sensor has already been developed with high selectivity. These regenerative biosensors are produced by copper oxide nano complexes with high surface area, good chemical stability, and low financial cost for the detection of the chemical species [7].

11.3.3 Applications in Environmental Observation

This analysis precisely focuses on different green biosensing tools such as immunosensing method, aptasensing device, and genosensors utilized for detecting environmental contaminants [12, 90]. It delivers a brief synopsis of the assembly and design procedures for these categories of sensing devices. Immunosensing devices are a category of biosensing instruments that practice immunogens and immunoglobulins as the detecting materials to sense detailed characteristic features of a chemical or biological species, natural protein components, pathogenic complexes, and different biomolecules [78]. An immunosensing device with graphene quantum dots alteration has already been prepared and modified to detect highly toxic organophosphate insecticides namely parathion. Whereas, a low detection perimeter and perfect dynamic linear regimes have been conveyed to detect parathion compounds using immunosensing devices [12, 39, 90]. The recognition of parathion using the projected immunosensing device is not exaggerated by the existence of toxic paraoxon metabolite. The reproducibility and constancy reviews of the projected immunosensing devices display that these devices have probably applied pertinency. An electrolytic immunosensor has been employed to detect the sensitivity and toxicity of chlorpyrifos, applying ferric oxide (Fe_3O_4)-altered carbon nanotubes to enhance the multi-enzyme label composite, intended to improving insecticide exposure [70, 71, 101].

In this research, flake-like iron oxide (Fe_3O_4) nanocomposites were introduced to the surface of carbon nanotubes, forming a nanoscale structure that was then layered onto the biosensing probe. The exposure technique exhibited high sensitivity, principally due to the extensive surface area provided by the crumbly iron oxide (Fe_3O_4) morphology [71, 101].

11.4 Food Safety Biosensors

Food safety is a universal apprehension affecting the whole world and will endure to be a substantial encounter for human well-being. Confronting this matter demands the expansion of hasty, sensitive, effectual, and profitable approaches for sensing food impurities [17].

Bioanalytic sensors have been discovered as a significant constituent in resolving detection issues during the monitoring of food and beverages. Recent progressions in nano research and nanotechnology, attached with diminishment and connectivity developments through the Internet of Things, suggestively increase the proficiencies of bioreceptor-based sensors [85].

Consequently, they are composed to become a decisive component in addressing this global encounter. Having admittance to safe and beneficial food is crucial for sustaining the lifecycle and indorsing healthy strength, and it also acts as a serious role in supportable expansion by strengthening nationwide economic growth [20].

Ensuring food security remains an unceasing contest worldwide, not just in emerging countries. This requirement is emphasized by the persistent or even cumulative number of food memories seen in advanced republics over the previous era [17, 29].

A contaminant is demarcated as any constituent that is not deliberately supplied to the food chain or feedstuff but is extant due to several phases of production, like the manufacturing process, raw material preparation, and treatment, conveying the products and by-products, stuffing, wrapping, and storage of the final products, or because of ecological pollution [17]. The various biosensors are designed for the sensitive detection of food contaminants, with research interests closely aligning with market demand [14]. Most publications focus on detecting microorganisms, followed by mycotoxins, pesticides, and veterinary drugs. With the world population continuing to rise, the production of crops, food substances, and their safety must discourse the requirements of both existing and forthcoming generations [15]. Regrettably, modern commercial agronomy often proves unmanageable, triggering significant damage to natural properties and the environment [5]. This comprises widespread farmland deprivation, diminished inherent diversity in crops, and the alteration of woodlands for other drives [95].

Detection technology, including the bio-detection process, can be efficiently implemented to several critical extents [80]. These detection units provide capable explanations for undertaking food uncertainty, observing, and dealing with water and soil quality, which in turn can help minimize the excessive use of fertilizers and pesticides. Additionally, biosensors can enhance integrated pest management in both crops and livestock by enabling continuous monitoring and early disease detection, thereby preventing outbreaks [42].

11.4.1 Classification of Food Safety Biosensors

The extensively studied biological sensors for detecting impurities, food deception, or pathogens deploy immunoglobulins, nucleic acids and their ligands, and biocatalysts as their bio-detection components [35]. In some cases, biological sensors also employ other proteins, viruses, or various microorganisms such as bacteriophages [80].

11.4.1.1 Biocatalyst Biosensor

Biocatalysts are generally deployed as labels in immune-analyses, where chemical and biochemical reactions are catalyzed to produce colored or luminous dyes or electrolytically dynamic markers. Furthermore, biocatalysts can assist as biorecognition components [96]. They can be used precisely to recognize enzymatic elements directly or conversely, to display biocatalytic activity for the non-specific exposure of numerous inhibitory particles [42].

11.4.1.2 Nucleotide Polymer Biosensor

Nucleotide polymers are regularly employed as exact bio-detection components in conventional deoxyribonucleic acid hybridization evaluates, as demonstrated by their application in sensing microbes in the revised literature [17, 79].

In the dominion of food security, the limited applications of deoxyribonucleic acid-based analysis are moderately employed due to the requirement of extra sample preparation [86]. For sensitive exposure to agricultural disease-causing agents such as viral pathogens, fungi, and bacteriological organisms, and to identify foreign species in cases of food deception, deoxyribonucleic acid hybridization evaluates are more prevalent, particularly after deoxyribonucleic acid intensification [17, 18].

11.4.1.3 Antibody Biosensors

Immunoglobulins are often applied as detection components in immune analysis due to their capability to exactly bind and quarantine the object analyte from the sample medium [59]. The extremely high binding affinity of immunoglobulins, unparalleled by other detection components, creates them essential in many recognized analyses and decisive for the expansion of innovative responsive detection approaches.

11.4.1.4 Aptamer Biosensors

Synthetic oligonucleotides have expanded important appreciation as a substitute to immunoglobulins, progressively serving as biorecognition detection components in scientific exploration previously [96]. This growing attention is due to their invention process, which does not require any living cells, and the high reliability between consignments, making this sensing process profitable compared to immunoglobulins [84]. Oligonucleotides such as aptamers also propose prolonged ledge life, and steadiness under non-biological circumstances, and can be simply improved to boost their capabilities. The use of oligonucleotides is predominantly beneficial to recognize minor molecules, outclassing equivalent immunoglobulins in this respect [17].

The revised study highlights the dominance of synthetic oligonucleotides as bio-detection components, mostly for sensing fungal toxins. Furthermore, oligonucleotides are regularly active in analyses for classifying microbes, veterinary medications, and insecticides [96].

11.4.1.5 Bacteriophage Biosensors

Lysogenic viruses which contaminate and imitate inside microorganisms such as bacteria can assist as biosensing components for recognizing bacteriological cells due to their facility to attach explicitly to binding sites [68]. Beyond their high particularity for bacterial objects, bacterial viruses propose the supplementary benefit of discriminating among living and dead bacteriological cells. This detection technique provides an imperative feature often missing in immunoglobulin-based evaluation [17, 69].

11.4.1.6 Plasmonic Biosensors

The plasmonic sensor process follows the phenomena of surface plasmon resonance, localized surface plasmon resonance, fiber optic surface plasmon resonance, etc. [75]. Plasmonic sensors classically employ several noble metal thin films and nano-scale structures due to their robust photosensitive absorption in the visible to near-infrared array of the electromagnetic band, acknowledged as the plasmonic sensing band. The noble metals such as silver (Ag), gold (Au), and rare group of metals namely, rhodium (Rh), palladium (Pd), and platinum (Pt), are generally chosen to apply in plasmonic instruments due to their optimum properties to detect food impurities significantly [17, 67].

These noble and rare groups of metals display high electrical efficiency, transmissivity, reflectance, biological compatibility, non-toxicity, and durable to deterioration and oxidation, confirming reliability [67]. One of the noble metals, silver (Ag), is recognized for its excellent surface plasmon-based properties [6]. To protect from the speedy corrosion this noble metal can be layered with silicon oxide (SiO_2) and zirconium oxide (ZrO_2) thin film. Surface plasmon resonance (SPR) and localized surface plasmon resonance (LSPR) arise when the transient field of transverse magnetic differentiated light (TMDL) significantly pairs with an equivocating wave of delocalized electrons at the metal-dielectric boundary [6, 76]. Under resonance circumstances, the incident transverse magnetic differentiated light will experience diminution, which can be detected in the replicated light at definite resonance constraints, contingent upon whether pointed or spectrum-based approaches are applied [9].

11.4.1.7 Nanozymes Biosensors

Nanozymes are nanomaterials, encircling both metallic and non-metallic categories, that imitate the catalytic functions of natural biocatalysts [79]. Since their commencement in the previous era, these nanoscale enzymatic imitators have become essential in several biological detection applications [86]. Nanoscale enzymes suggest various assistances over natural biocatalysts, counting improved constancy, inferior cost, ease of alteration, and greater competence [59]. Investigation into their composition and high catalytic activities has led to notable progress in nanozyme-added biological detection [92].

This evaluation showcases numerous protruding nanozymes, predominantly those categorized as peroxide enzymes and oxidases [86]. It pronounces the enzyme-imitating processes of these nanoscale enzymes, which principally produce colorimetric indications, making biological detection forthright and reachable [67]. Superior consideration is prearranged to nanozyme-added biological detection to perceive chemical toxins such as ionic compounds and insecticides and residues of pesticides, in addition to inherent pollutants, for instance, diseases-causing microorganisms and toxic biological derivatives that distress food security and superiority [34]. The different portable biosensing devices to detect biological contaminants in various food items have been represented in Table 11.1. Forthcoming advances may emphasize enhancing the structure of nanoscale biocatalysts for the additional improvement of their biocatalytic activity and precision. Generally, nanozymes propose considerable capacity for bio-recognizing implementation across food security and non-food provinces [86, 100].

11.5 Conclusions

Environmental contamination control and food safety are both critical global issues, as the contaminated nutrients contribute suggestively to disease and mortalities worldwide each year, predominantly disturbing emerging nations. Hence, there is an imperative requirement to progress manageable, hasty, profitable, and online approaches for analyzing food toxins, specifically organic ones, to confirm food product security and quality. Portable biosensing elements are characterized as a capable solution for biorecognition of food and environment contamination due to their compactness, user-friendly, and mobile diagnostic tools that enable real-time screening for food and environment adulteration. Innovations in nanotechnology, microscale fluid mechanics, smartphone incorporation, and biotic design approaches, alongside improvements in wireless interaction, have simplified the expansion of these transportable biosensors. In recent years, several biosensing devices applying principles of electrolytic process, magnetic, and photosensitive properties have been engineered to perceive biological impurities in food items and the environment. These biorecognition systems deliver improved sensitivity and discernment toward specific organic toxins, and some can be altered to detect additional microorganisms through amendments in immunoglobulins and aptamer explicitness. However, the forthcoming investigation should concentrate on the supplementary characterization technique of these biorecognition elements, addressing factors such as extent, cost, duplicability, and accurateness during the detection of various contaminants in the environment and food materials.

Table 11.1 List of biosensors for monitoring biological contaminants in various food items

Biosensor type	Types of contaminants	Food items	Limit of detection	Functional benefits	References
Portable nuclear magnetic resonance-based bioreceptor (pNMR)	*E. coli O157:H7 (EHEC)*	Drinking water and milk sample	76 colony-forming units (CFU)/mL in drinking water and 92 colony-forming units (CFU)/mL in milk items	Compact, adjustable, and profitable on-site measurement Acts on the basis of the self-assembly of diffused magnetic nanoparticles into firm nano-conventions through affinity coordinating molecules	[94]
Fluorescence imaging scheme	*E. coli O157:H7 (EHEC)*	Yoghurt and egg	1 colony-forming unit (CFU)/mL and 10 colony-forming units (CFU)/mL	Excellent portable systems to detect contaminants, Informal analysis	[50]
Cyclic voltammetry system (CVS)	*E. coli O157:H7 (EHEC)*	Numerous food industries	5×10^8 colony-forming units (CFU)/mL	Use of Bluetooth connectivity via portable potentiostat for the data transfer Electrochemical detection process using linear voltage scanning inflammation	[98]
Portable quantum dot biosensor (PQdB)	*Salmonella: S. enteritidis,* *S. Typhimurium*	Eggs, meat, and dairy products	5×10^3 colony-forming units (CFU)/mL	Cost-effective, profligate rapidity High-throughput screen analysis and improved analytical presentation	[28, 36]
Impedimetric biosensor system (IBS) based on glucose oxidase	*E. coli O157:H7,* *S. Typhimurium*	Ground beef and poultry industries	*E. coli O157:H7:* 2.05×10^3 colony-forming units (CFU)/g1, *S. Typhimurium:* 1.04×10^3 colony-forming units (CFU)/mL,	Rapid reaction of glucose oxidase immunoglobulin conjugates with magnetic beads entrenched targeted bacteria complexes Fast increased ion concentration	[68]

Portable biosensor using colorimetric screening analysis	*Listeria* spp.: *L. monocytogenes*	Spiked milk and spiked meat.	Spiked milk: 11.7×10^2 colony-forming units (CFU)/mL spiked meat: 13.8×10 colony-forming units (CFU)//g	Modest and cost-operative screening analyses Magnetic nanoparticles conjugated with peptides such as d-amino acid	[66].
Magnetic tunneling junction biosensor system (MTIJBS)	*L. monocytogenes* genome	Multiplexed pathogens in foods	Below the nanomolar range	Scalability, low power ingesting and potentially unrestricted acceptance Ferromagnetic layers provide unchangeable magnetic induction	[53]
Portable bioelectric recognition assay (pBERA)	*L. monocytogenes*	Sterile saline solution	10^2 colony-forming units (CFU)/mL	Use of electroporation process to insert receptors into the targeted cells Endorses the high selectivity of the cell to identify the target components	[3]
Portable silver nanoparticle-based immunochromatographic (AuNP-ICT) band	*Staphylococcus aureus*	Meat, egg, milk-dairy products, salad items, bakery items	2.5 to 5 ng/mL	Detection of various enterotoxins in *Staphylococcal* strains simultaneously AuNP-ICT bands presented significant accuracy, duplicability, and longstanding steadiness	[87]

(continued)

Table 11.1 (continued)

Biosensor type	Types of contaminants	Food items	Limit of detection	Functional benefits	References
Label-free electrolytic DNA biosensor Sensing particle: CeO_2 nanoparticles	*Clostridium* spp.: *Clostridium perfringens and Cl. botulinum*	Milk-dairy products, meat and fish products, fresh and preserved fruits, and root vegetables	7.06×10^{-15} mol/L	Supplement the electrode surface, and improve microelectronic properties and electrocatalytic commotion to progress their rapidity, recognition competence, and specificity	[93]
DNA interbreeding-associated biosensor-linked with methylene blue	*Vibrio parahaemolyticus*	Various sea food: cockle samples	5.3×10^{-12} M	Polylactide-reinforced silver nanoparticles modulated DNA interbreeding probes provided significant detection criteria	[54]
Portable surface plasmon resonance (pSPR) sensor	*Mycotoxigenic fungi: Aspergillus, Fusarium*, and *Penicillium Aflatoxin:* *A. flavus, A. parasiticus*, and *A. nomius*	Preserved food items, wheat, barley, and corn	Limit of detection approximation: 2.51 ppb	High selectivity, significant accuracy, miniatured sensor system Rapid identification of polynucleotides, proteins, whole cells	[26, 61]

References

1. Dias AD, Kingsley DM, Corr DT. Recent advances in bioprinting and applications for biosensing. Biosensors (Basel). 2014;4:111–36.
2. Capodaglio AG. In-stream detection of waterborne priority pollutants, and applications in drinking water contaminant warning systems. Water Sci Technol Water Supply. 2017;17:707–25.
3. Hadjilouka A, Loizou K, Apostolou T, Dougiakis L, Inglezakis A, Tsaltas D. Newly developed system for the robust detection of Listeria monocytogenes based on a bioelectric cell biosensor. Biosensors. 2020;10:178.
4. Hulanicki A, Glab S, Ingman F. Chemical sensors: definitions and classification. Pure Appl Chem. 1991;63:1247–50.
5. Khanmohammadi A, Ghazizadeh AJ, Hashemi P, Afkhami A, Arduini F. An overview to electrochemical biosensors and sensors for the detection of environmental contaminants. J Iran Chem Soc. 2020;17:2429–47.
6. Sharma AK, Jha R, Gupta B. Fiber-optic sensors based on surface plasmon resonance: a comprehensive review. IEEE Sensors J. 2007;7:1118–29.
7. Kozitsina A, Svalova T, Malysheva N, Glazyrina Y, Matern A. A new enzyme-free electrochemical immunoassay for Escherichia coli detection using magnetic nanoparticles. Anal Lett. 2016;49:245–57.
8. Singh A, Sharma A, Ahmed A, Sundramoorthy AK, Furukawa H, Arya S, Khosla A. Recent advances in electrochemical biosensors: applications, challenges, and future scope. Biosensors. 2021;11:336–67.
9. Shalabney A, Abdulhalim I. Sensitivity-enhancement methods for surface plasmon sensors. Laser Photonics Rev. 2011;5:571–606.
10. Williams A, Keshani MRA, Arachchillage GGP, Chandra S, Rangan S, Gupta SG, Vivancos JMA. Biosensors for public health and environmental monitoring: the case for sustainable biosensing. ACS Sustain Chem Eng. 2024;12:10296–312.
11. Kaur B, Kumar S, Kaushik BK. Recent advancements in optical biosensors for cancer detection. Biosens Bioelectron. 2022;197:113805.
12. Wang B, Takahashi S, Du X, Anzai J. Electrochemical biosensors based on ferroceneboronic acid and its derivatives: a review. Biosensors (Basel). 2014a;4:243–56.
13. Chen C, Wang J. Optical biosensors: an exhaustive and comprehensive review. Analyst. 2020;145:1605–28.
14. Hermann CA, Duerkop A, Baeumner AJ. Food safety analysis enabled through biological and synthetic materials: a critical review of current trends. Anal Chem. 2019;91:569–87.
15. Flynn CD, Chang D, Mahmud A, Yousefi H, Das J, Riordan KT, Sargent EH, Kelley SO. Biomolecular sensors for advanced physiological monitoring. Nat Rev Bioeng. 2023;1:560.
16. Fang C, Dharmarajan R, Megharaj M, Naidu R. Gold nanoparticle- based optical sensors for selected anionic contaminants. TrAC Trends Anal Chem. 2017;86:143–54.
17. Griesche C, Baeumner AJ. Biosensors to support sustainable agriculture and food safety. Trends Anal Chem. 2020;128:115906–21.
18. Mateo C, Palomo JM, Lorente GF, Guisan JM, Lafuente RF. Improvement of enzyme activity, stability and selectivity via immobilization techniques. Enzym Microb Technol. 2007;40:1451–63.
19. Huang CW, Lin C, Nguyen MK, Hussain A, Bui XT, Ngo HH. A review of biosensor for environmental monitoring: principle, application, and corresponding achievement of sustainable development goals. Bioengineered. 2023;14:58–80.
20. Wang D, Hinkley T, Chen J, Talbert JN, Nugen SR. Phage based electrochemical detection of: Escherichia coli in drinking water using affinity reporter probes. Analyst. 2019;144:1345–52.
21. Bahadir EB, Sezginturk MK. Electrochemical biosensors for hormone analyses. Biosens Bioelectron. 2015;68:62–71.

22. Hamidi-Asl E, Palchetti I, Hasheminejad E, Mascini M. A review on the electrochemical biosensors for determination of microRNAs. Talanta. 2013;115:74–83.
23. Schneider E, Clark DS. Cytochrome P450 (CYP) enzymes and the development of CYP biosensors. Biosens Bioelectron. 2013;39:1–13.
24. Kong F, Xu M, Xu J, Chen H. A novel lable-free electrochemical immunosensor for carcinoembryonic antigen based on gold nanoparticles–thionine–reduced graphene oxide nanocomposite film modified glassy carbon electrode. Talanta. 2011;85:2620–5.
25. Scheller FW, Yarman A, Bachmann T, Hirsch T, Kubick S, Renneberg R, Schumacher S, Wollenberger U, Teller C, Bier FF. Future of biosensors: a personal view. In: Advances in biochemical engineering/biotechnology, vol. 140. Berlin, Heidelberg: Springer; 2014. p. 1–28.
26. Borile G, Rossi S, Filippi A, Gazzola E, Capaldo P, Tregnago C, Pigazzi M, Romanato F. Label-free, real-time on-chip sensing of living cells via grating-coupled surface plasmon resonance. Biophys Chem. 2019;254:106262.
27. Hernandez-Vargas G, Sosa-Hernández JE, Saldarriaga-Hernandez S, Villalba-Rodríguez AM, Parra-Saldivar R, Iqbal HMN. Electrochemical biosensors: a solution to pollution detection with reference to environmental contaminants. Biosensors. 2018;8:1–21.
28. Luka G, Ahmadi A, Najjaran H, Alocilja E, DeRosa M, Wolthers K, Malki A, Aziz H, Althani A, Hoorfar M. Microfluidics integrated biosensors: a leading technology towards lab-on-a-chip and sensing applications. Sensors. 2015;15:30011–31.
29. Kim H, Lee W, Yoon Y. Heavy metal(loid) biosensor based on split-enhanced green fluorescent protein: development and characterization. Appl Microbiol Biotechnol. 2019;103:6345–52.
30. Kumar H, Rani R. Development of biosensors for the detection of biological warfare agents: its issues and challenges. Sci Prog. 2013;96:294–308.
31. Yousefi H, Ali MM, Su HM, Filipe CDM, Didar TF. Sentinel wraps: real-time monitoring of food contamination by printing DNAzyme probes on food packaging. ACS Nano. 2018;12:3287–94.
32. Cho IH, Kim DH, Park S. Electrochemical biosensors: perspective on functional nanomaterials for on-site analysis. Biomater Res. 2020;24:6. https://doi.org/10.1186/s40824-019-0181-y.
33. Camilleri J, Baudot R, Wiest L, Vulliet E, Cren-Olivé C, Daniele G. Multiresidue fully automated online SPE-HPLC-MS/MS method for the quantification of endocrine-disrupting and pharmaceutical compounds at trace level in surface water. Int J Environ Anal Chem. 2015;95:67–81.
34. Wei J, Yang L, Luo M, Wang Y, Li P. Nanozyme-assisted technique for dual mode detection of organophosphorus pesticide. Ecotoxicol Environ Saf. 2019;179:17–23.
35. Moore JC, Spink J, Lipp M. Development and application of a database of food ingredient fraud and economically motivated adulteration from 1980 to 2010. J Food Sci. 2012;77:R118–26.
36. Hu J, Tang F, Jiang YZ, Liu C. Rapid screening and quantitative detection of Salmonella using a quantum dot nanobead-based biosensor. Analyst. 2020;145:2184–90.
37. Arlett JL, Myers EB, Roukes ML. Comparative advantages of mechanical biosensors. Nat Nanotechnol. 2011;6:203–15.
38. Wu J, Liu H, Chen W, Ma B, Ju H. Device integration of electrochemical biosensors. Nat Rev Bioeng. 2023;1:346–60.
39. Abe K, Yoshida W, Ikebukuro K. Electrochemical biosensors using aptamers for theranostics. In: Advances in Biochemical Engineering/Biotechnology, vol. 140. Berlin, Heidelberg: Springer; 2014. p. 183–202.
40. Cash KJ, Clark HA. Nanosensors and nanomaterials for monitoring glucose in diabetes. Trends Mol Med. 2010;16:584–93.
41. Biji KB, Ravishankar CN, Mohan CO, Srinivasa Gopal TK. Smart packaging systems for food applications: a review. J Food Sci Technol. 2015;52:6125–35.
42. Punakivi K, Smolander M, Niku-Paavola ML, Mattinen J, Buchert J. Enzymatic determination of biogenic amines with transglutaminase. Talanta. 2006;68:1040–5.

43. Ding L, Bond AM, Zhai J, Zhang J. Utilization of nanoparticle labels for signal amplification in ultrasensitive electrochemical affinity biosensors: a review. Anal Chim Acta. 2013;797:1–12.
44. Li L, Liang J, Hong W, Zhao Y, Sun S, Yang X, Xu A, Hang H, Wu L, Chen S. Evolved bacterial biosensor for arsenite detection in environmental water. Environ Sci Technol. 2015;49:6149–55.
45. Bilal M, Rasheed T, Sosa-Hernández J, Raza A, Nabeel F, Iqbal H. Biosorption: an interplay between marine algae and potentially toxic elements—a review. Mar Drugs. 2018;16:65–80.
46. Citartan M, Gopinath SC, Tominaga, Tang JTH. Label-free methods of reporting biomolecular interactions by optical biosensors. Analyst. 2013;138:3576–92.
47. Kibria MG, Masuk NI, Safayet R, Nguyen HQ, Mourshed M. Plastic waste: challenges and opportunities to mitigate pollution and effective management. Int J Environ Res. 2023;17:20.
48. Govindhan M, Lafleur T, Adhikari BR, Chen A. Electrochemical sensor based on carbon nanotubes for the simultaneous detection of phenolic pollutants. Electroanalysis. 2015;27:902–9.
49. Li M, Li R, Li CM, Wu N. Electrochemical and optical biosensors based on nanomaterials and nanostructures: a review. Front Biosci (Schol Ed). 2011;3:1308–31. https://doi.org/10.2741/228. PMID: 21622273.
50. Zeinhom MMA, Wang Y, Song Y, Zhu MJ, Lin Y, Du D. A portable smart-phone device for rapid and sensitive detection of E. coli O157: H7 in yoghurt and egg. Biosens Bioelectron. 2018;99:479–85.
51. Medina-Sánchez M, Mayorga-Martinez CC, Watanabe T, Ivandini TA, Honda Y, Pino F, Nakata K, Fujishima A, Einaga Y, Merkoçi A. Microfluidic platform for environmental contaminants sensing and degradation based on boron-doped diamond electrodes. Biosens Bioelectron. 2016;75:365–74.
52. Nejadmansouri M, Majdinasab M, Nunes GS, Marty JL. An overview of optical and electrochemical sensors and biosensors for analysis of antioxidants in food during the last 5 years. Sensors. 2021;21:1176–224.
53. Maciel N, Marques E, Naviner L, Zhou Y, Cai H. Magnetic tunnel junction applications. Sensors. 2020;20:121.
54. Nordin N, Yusof NA, Abdullah J, Radu S, Hushiarian R. A simple, portable, electrochemical biosensor to screen shellfish for Vibrio parahaemolyticus. AMB Express. 2017;7:1–9.
55. Reta N, Saint CP, Michelmore A, Prieto-Simon B, Voelcker NH. Nanostructured electrochemical biosensors for label-free detection of water- and food-borne pathogens. ACS Appl Mater Interfaces. 2018;10:6055–72.
56. Dardano P, Rea I, De Stefano L. Microneedles-based electrochemical sensors: new tools for advanced biosensing. Curr Opin Electrochem. 2019;17:121–7.
57. Erden PE, Kilic E. A review of enzymatic uric acid biosensors based on amperometric detection. Talanta. 2013;107:312–23.
58. Mehrotra P. Biosensors and their applications–a review. J Oral Biol Craniofac Res. 2016;6:153–9.
59. Wang Q, Wei H, Zhang Z, Wang E, Dong S. Nanozyme: an emerging alternative to natural enzyme for biosensing and immunoassay. TrAC Trends Anal Chem. 2018;105:218–24.
60. Akter R, Kyun C, Rahman A. A stable and sensitive voltametric immunosensor based on a new non-enzymatic label. Biosens Bioelectron. 2013;50:118–24.
61. Chauhan R, Singh J, Sachdev T, Basu T, Malhotra B. Recent advances in mycotoxins detection. Biosens Bioelectron. 2016;81:532–45.
62. Monosik R, Stredansky M, Tkac J, Sturdik E. Application of enzyme biosensors in analysis of food and beverages enzyme and microbial technology. Food Anal Methods. 2012;5:40–53.
63. Mendes RK, Arruda BS, De Souza EF, Nogueira AB, Teschke O, Bonugli LO, Etchegaray A. Determination of chlorophenol in environmental samples using a voltammetric biosensor based on hybrid nanocomposite. J Braz Chem Soc. 2017;28:1212–9.
64. Rapini R, Marrazza G. Electrochemical aptasensors for contaminants detection in food and environment: recent advances. Bioelectrochemistry. 2017;118:47–61.

65. Azimi S, Farahani A, Docoslis A, Vahdatifar S. Developing an integrated microfluidic and miniaturized electrochemical biosensor for point of care determination of glucose in human plasma samples. Anal Bioanal Chem. 2021;413:1441–52.
66. Alhogail S, Suaifan GA, Zourob M. Rapid colorimetric sensing platform for the detection of Listeria monocytogenes foodborne pathogen. Biosens Bioelectron. 2016;86:1061–6.
67. Balbinot S, Srivastav AM, Vidic J, Abdulhalim I. Plasmonic biosensors for food control. Trends Food Sci Technol. 2021;111:128–40.
68. Eyvazi S, Baradaran B, Mokhatrzadeh A, de la Guardia M. Recent advances on development of portable biosensors for monitoring of biological contaminants in foods. Trends Food Sci Technol. 2021;114:712–21.
69. Hameed S, Xie L, Ying Y. Conventional and emerging detection techniques for pathogenic bacteria in food science: a review. Trends Food Sci Technol. 2018;81:61–73.
70. Jahanbani S, Benvidi A. Comparison of two fabricated aptasensors based on modified carbon paste/oleic acid and magnetic bar carbon paste/Fe_3O_4@oleic acid nanoparticle electrodes for tetracycline detection. Biosens Bioelectron. 2016;85:553–62.
71. Erogul S, Bas SZ, Ozmen M, Yildiz S. A new electrochemical sensor based on Fe_3O_4 functionalized graphene oxide–gold nanoparticle composite film for simultaneous determination of catechol and hydroquinone. Electrochim Acta. 2015;186:302–13.
72. Lee S, Oh J, Kim D, Piao Y. A sensitive electrochemical sensor using an iron oxide/graphene composite for the simultaneous detection of heavy metal ions. Talanta. 2016a;160:528–36.
73. Lee S, Park S-K, Choi E, Piao Y. Voltammetric determination of trace heavy metals using an electrochemically deposited graphene/bismuth nanocomposite film-modified glassy carbon electrode. J Electroanal Chem. 2016b;766:120–7.
74. Mao S, Chang J, Zhou G, Chen J. Nanomaterial-enabled rapid detection of water contaminants. Small. 2015;11:5336–59.
75. Mittal S, Sharma T, Tiwari M. Surface plasmon resonance based photonic crystal fiber biosensors: a review. Mater Today Proc. 2021;43:3071–4.
76. Raz SR, Liu H, Norde W, Bremer MG. Food allergens profiling with an imaging surface plasmon resonance-based biosensor. Anal Chem. 2010;82:8485–91.
77. Singh S, Kumar V, Dhanjal DS, Datta S, Prasad R, Singh J. Biological biosensors for monitoring and diagnosis. In: Microbial biotechnology: basic research and applications. Singapore: Springer; 2020. p. 317–35.
78. Vigneshvar S, Sudhakumari C, Senthilkumaran B, Prakash H. Recent advances in biosensor technology for potential applications–an overview. Front Bioeng Biotechnol. 2016;4:11.
79. Yin S, Zhao L, Ma Z. Label-free electrochemical immunosensor for ultrasensitive detection of neuron-specific enolase based on enzyme-free catalytic amplification. Anal Bioanal Chem. 2018;410:1279–86.
80. Dodevska T, Lazarova Y, Shterev I. Amperometric biosensors for glucose and lactate with applications in food analysis: a brief review. Acta Chim Slov. 2019;66:762–76.
81. Chadha U, Bhardwaj P, Agarwal R, Rawat P, Agarwal R, Gupta I, Panjwani M, Singh S, Ahuja C, Selvaraj SK, Banavoth M, Sonar P, Badoni B, Chakravorty A. Recent progress and growth in biosensors technology: a critical review. J Ind Eng Chem. 2022;109:21–51.
82. Naresh V, Lee N. A review on biosensors and recent development of nanostructured materials-enabled biosensors. Sensors. 2021;21:1109–44.
83. Perumal V, Hashim U. Advances in biosensors: principle, architecture and applications. J Appl Biomed. 2014;12:1–15.
84. Singh V, Kumar V, Kashyap S, Singh AV, Kishore V, Sitti M, Saxena PS, Srivastava A. Graphene oxide synergistically enhances antibiotic efficacy in vancomycin-resistant staphylococcus aureus. ACS Appl Bio Mater. 2019;2(3):1148–57.
85. Scognamiglio V, Arduini F, Palleschi G, Rea G. Biosensing technology for sustainable food safety. TrAC Trends Anal Chem. 2014;64:1–10.
86. Wang W, Gunasekaran S. Nanozymes-based biosensors for food quality and safety. TrAC Trends Anal Chem. 2020;126:115841–56.

87. Wang W, Liu L, Xu L, Kuang H, Zhu J, Xu C. Gold-nanoparticle-based multiplexed immunochromatographic strip for simultaneous detection of staphylococcal enterotoxin A, B, C, D, and E. Part Part Syst Charact. 2016;33:388–95.
88. Huang X, Zhu Y, Kianfar E. Nano biosensors: properties, applications and electrochemical techniques. J Mater Res Technol. 2021;12:1649–72.
89. Zhu X, Wu G, Lu N, Yuan X, Li B. A miniaturized electrochemical toxicity biosensor based on graphene oxide quantum dots/carboxylated carbon nanotubes for assessment of priority pollutants. J Hazard Mater. 2017;324:272–80.
90. Wang X, Lu X, Chen J. Development of biosensor technologies for analysis of environmental contaminants. Trends Environ Anal Chem. 2014b;2:25–32.
91. Cao Y, Sun X, Guo Y, Zhao W, Wang X. An electrochemical immunosensor based on interdigitated array microelectrode for the detection of chlorpyrifos. Bioprocess Biosyst Eng. 2015;38:307–13.
92. Huang Y, Ren J, Qu X. Nanozymes: classification, catalytic mechanisms, activity regulation, and applications. Chem Rev. 2019;119:4357–412.
93. Wang YH, Huang KJ, Wu X. Recent advances in transition-metal dichalcogenides based electrochemical biosensors: a review. Biosens Bioelectron. 2017;97:305–16.
94. Luo Y, Alocilja EC. Portable nuclear magnetic resonance biosensor and assay for a highly sensitive and rapid detection of foodborne bacteria in complex matrices. J Biol Eng. 2017;11:1–8.
95. Park YW, Kim SM, Lee JY, Jang W. Application of biosensors in smart packaging. Mol Cell Toxicol. 2015;11:277–85.
96. Wu Y, Belmonte I, Sykes KS, Xiao Y, White RJ. A perspective on the future role of aptamers in analytical chemistry. Anal Chem. 2019;91:15335–44.
97. Xie Y, Wang J, Wu Y, Ren C, Song C, Yang J, Yu H, Giesy JP, Zhang X. Using in situ bacterial communities to monitor contaminants in river sediments. Environ Pollut. 2016;212:348–57.
98. Xu Y, Dai Y, Li C, Zhang H, Guo M, Yang Y. PC software-based portable cyclic voltammetry system with PB-MCNT-GNPs-modified electrodes for E. coli detection. Rev Sci Instrum. 2020;91:014103.
99. Xu Y, Cheng G, He P, Fang Y. A review: electrochemical aptasensors with various detection strategies. Electroanalysis. 2009;21:1251–9. https://doi.org/10.1002/elan.200804561.
100. Zhou Y, Liu B, Yang R, Liu J. Filling in the gaps between nanozymes and enzymes: challenges and opportunities. Bioconjug Chem. 2017;28:2903–9.
101. Sun Z, Wang W, Wen H, Gan C, Lei H, Liu Y. Sensitive electrochemical immunoassay for chlorpyrifos by using flake-like Fe_3O_4 modified carbon nanotubes as the enhanced multienzyme label. Anal Chim Acta. 2015;899:91–9.

Chapter 12
Biosensor-Based Disease Detection System Integrated with Computation Tools

Surbhi Sharma, Shivangi Verma, Prateek Saxena, Agrima Saxena, and Shravan Kumar

Abstract In recent years, smart and sustainable nanomaterial-based biosensing technologies have got significant attention. It has immense potential to revolutionize several fields, including environmental monitoring, food safety, and healthcare. The application of nanomaterials in biosensors embarks unique advantages like sensitivity, selectivity, and rapid response, which make it one of the most prominent technologies for the identification of biomolecules with accurate precision. The creation of a graphene-based biosensor that exhibits exceptional sensitivity and specificity in identifying biomarkers for cancer diagnosis underscores the potential of nanomaterials in medical applications. Furthermore, incorporating intelligent features into biosensors based on nanomaterials has improved their capacity for remote sensing and real-time monitoring. Nanotechnology has the potential to be used in environmental monitoring and management. It demonstrated a smart biosensing platform that uses functionalized nanoparticles for continuous monitoring of environmental pollutants. Including their sensing capabilities, sustainable aspects of nanomaterials-based biosensors have also been explored up to a certain extent. Several sustainable materials like biocompatible polymers and green synthesis methods have also been observed to prevent environmental impact while maintaining sensor performance. One development that adds to the environmentally friendly nature of nanomaterial-based sensors is the sustainable biosensing platform that was created using biodegradable polymers. Intelligent biosensing systems that can make decisions on their own and diagnose themselves have also been made possible by developments in data analytics and signal processing techniques. In a nutshell, there is great potential for addressing important issues in food safety, environmental monitoring, and healthcare through the integration of smart functionalities, sustain-

Surbhi Sharma, Shivangi Verma and Prateek Mishra contributed equally with all other contributors.

S. Sharma · S. Verma · P. Mishra · A. Saxena · S. Kumar (✉)
Department of Biochemical Engineering, Harcourt Butler Technical University, Kanpur, India

S. Mondal et al. (eds.), *Smart and Sustainable Nanomaterials in Digital Healthcare and Theranostic*, https://doi.org/10.1007/978-981-95-9386-6_12

able materials, and intelligent data analytics in nanomaterial-based biosensing technologies. To fully realize the promise of intelligent and sustainable biosensing technologies, more research and innovation in this area are required.

Keywords Biosensors · Nanomaterials · Sustainable · Environmentally friendly · Biosensing

12.1 Introduction

Biosensors are advanced technologies that have a convergence of Biology, Computer Science, and Technology. The invention of biosensors first took place in the year 1962 by Clark and Lyons to estimate the level of glucose present in biological samples utilizing the characteristics and strategy of electrochemical detection of oxygen and hydrogen Peroxide [58, 116]. The difference between biosensors and traditional sensors is that biosensors work specifically on the biological processes and identify the particular toxins in the environment or trace out some specific compounds in the biological systems. Apart from that, they are highly sensitive, cost-effective, and give accurate results most of the time, unlike traditional sensors that measure temperature and pressure. There is a vast role of biosensors in multiple fields. Several foodborne pathogens are present in the food products; in detecting them, biosensors convert several biochemical, biological, and chemical signals into electrical signals. According to World Health Statistics (2023), it has been found that the number of deaths is caused by non-communicable diseases as compared to communicable diseases. The mortality rate is 71% due to non-communicable diseases because in most cases early diagnosis of diseases like cancer can't be detected easily [54]. While communicable diseases can be cured easily by taking certain measures. The researchers are trying to modify the biosensors that can give accurate results in the diagnosis of a disease and be cost-effective at the same time [42]. Microorganism-based biosensors also have wide applications in the field of environmental sciences for tracing out toxins in the soil or detecting the quality of soil for agricultural purposes [10]. Biosensors have also been used in the detection of bioterrorism agents by enabling early signs and response [78]. The combination of biology and technology has brought unprecedented innovation in the health sector. At the forefront of this revolution lies the combination of biosensors with computational tools for tracking diseases. This collective approach promised to transform the old methods of diagnosis of diseases by enabling more precise, personalized, and cost-effective healthcare for patients [67]. A biosensor is an analytical device that transmits biological signals into estimated electrical signals. This device has now become a powerful tool in the detection of multiple biological parameters. These sensors are fully equipped with biological recognition elements like enzymes and antibodies, and they target the specific molecules and generate signals that provide information about the physiological state of any individual. For example, the advancement of diabetes mellitus monitoring and its treatment has combined with the introduction of the biological sensors, which have significantly improved polymeric control and stopped the onset of progression associated with diabetes [16, 83]. Despite these, the full potential of the biosensors can be only utilized when they are coupled with computational tools. The integration of biosensors with sophisticated algorithms and data analysis techniques [33]. We filter the important information from the raw sensor data. This combination of biosensors not only helps in the monitoring of diseases but also helps in the prediction of disease and progression, monitoring treatment and efficiency even providing preventative measures. While the potential of biosensors and computer tools is vast, some of the challenges remain. Developing biosensors with advanced computational tools that can give precise and accurate results is a big challenge. In addition to this, data privacy and security are of utmost importance to protect patient information. If we overcome these challenges, then the future of disease diagnosis lies in the combination of biosensors and computational tools. By harnessing the power of these devices, we can transform the healthcare sector to improve patient outcomes and save their lives [125]. Biosensors generally portray the cutting edge between biology and technology that has the potential to recognize certain patterns in the target element.

The sample generates some specific signals. This chapter delves into the world of biosensors, exploring their evolution, applications, and the transformative potential they hold for various fields. While biosensors have been instrumental in detecting foodborne pathogens, monitoring environmental pollutants, and even aiding in bioterrorism detection, their true power lies in their ability to revolutionize healthcare. By combining biosensors with computational tools, we can usher in a new era of disease diagnosis, prognosis, and prevention. The main attention in this chapter is given to the relationship between biosensors and computational tools technologies. The old diagnostic methods often involve invasive and time-consuming laboratory analysis by the modernization of diagnostic methods, all these processes have become non-invasive, efficient, consume less time, and give accurate results that health professionals might miss by using old diagnostic methods [71]. By the use of such biosensors, we can get deep insights into the health of the person and can give the proper treatment to the patients based on their medical history and disease. This work differentiates itself from the previous studies by giving the main focus on the modernization of healthcare through the integration of computational tools and techniques. Most of the research work done up till now has focused on the application of biosensors in specific areas. This chapter provides a comprehensive overview of the technology and highlights its principles and potential for human health. Furthermore, it addresses the challenges assigned to the computational tools and their future directions in this field. Overall, by overcoming certain challenges, we can save countless lives and create a society free from previously incurable diseases.

12.2 Overview of Computation Tools in Healthcare

The healthcare industry is undergoing modernization by converting traditional treatment methods to digital processes and technology. Current advancements and suggestions from academic institutions, the biotechnology sector, nonprofit foundations, regulators, and technology companies for incorporating relevant computational evidence into clinical development and healthcare [96]. The computational tools in the healthcare sector that can play a major role in the diagnosis and treatment of the patient are Artificial Intelligence, Big Data, the Internet of Things, and Machine Learning [69, 70], which are represented in Fig. 12.1.

Computational tools are referred to as the software tools and programs that are specifically designed to process and analyze the medical data of patients. These tools can range from simple data management to complex artificial intelligence (AI) tenets [36]. The main aim of these computational tools is to extract only information from the healthcare data that can improve the patients' lives and decrease the mortality rate of the population [26]. A detailed explanation of the key areas of application of computational tools in the healthcare sectors is given in Table 12.1.

The combination of two diverse fields, biology and computational tools, has provided immense potential in the healthcare sectors [47]. That has resulted in the improvement of patient outcomes and has enhanced its efficiency. From EHR (electric health records) simplifying data management to [114] artificial intelligence in the diagnosis and treatment [60]. The impact of this technology is overpowering. Wearable health has empowered patients to take control of their health and take all the preventive measures to improve their health [41, 117] (Stan 2013). Telemedicine has expanded its access to care for underserved populations. Telemedicine is the term for the utilization of technology to provide Remote clinical care is still a potential but underutilized approach for patients [123]. However, the instant evolution of healthcare technology portrays some of the challenges as well. There is a need for powerful data privacy and security and a platform to address the ethical implications of filling the gaps between the digital divide which are critical considerations [37]. In addition to these, the successful implications of these advanced tools require a

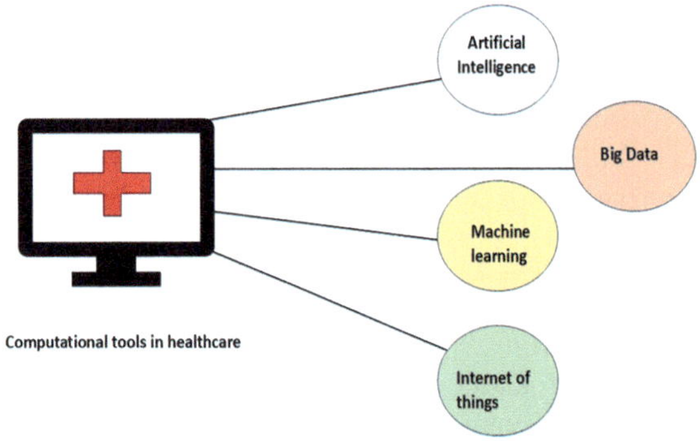

Fig. 12.1 Representing computational tools that are used in the healthcare sector

Table 12.1 The key application of computational tools in healthcare

Healthcare areas	Applications	References
Patient Management	Electronic Health Records (EHRs): Digital archives of medical records for patients that facilitate effective data exchange and access.	[45, 57]
	Patient portals: Online tools that let Patients make and access appointments, view their medical records, and get in touch with doctors.	[107, 112]
	Patient-controlled records that are accessible to healthcare practitioners are called personal health records, or PHRs.	[1]
Clinical Decision Support Systems (CDSS)	Tools include medication interaction checks, diagnosis help, and treatment plans that offer up-to-date data and suggestions to aid in clinical decision-making.	[73, 76]
Medical Imaging	Algorithms for image processing and analysis, such as those used in computer-aided diagnosis (CAD), segmentation, and picture enhancement. Examples include looking for malignancies on mammograms or looking for abnormalities in the brain on MRI scans.	[15]
Drug Discovery and Development	Computational methods for developing compounds, determining medicinal targets, forecasting toxicity and efficacy, and quickening clinical trials	[40, 109]
Population Health Management	Instruments for examining big groups to find patterns, risk factors, and chances for prophylactic treatment. Predicting disease outbreaks or identifying patient populations at high risk are two examples.	[74]
Genomics and Precision Medicine	Computational methods for analyzing genetic data to understand disease mechanisms and develop personalized treatment plans.	[30, 120]

skilled workplace capable of harnessing their potential. As the new versions of these technologies are going to be launched the healthcare sector will undergo more advanced transformations. The collaborative efforts of both the fields of biology and technology will maximize their potential in the future while mitigating the risks.

These advancements highlight the challenges we can face in healthcare systems that are more patient-centric, efficient, and equitable. By embracing innovation and addressing the associated challenges, we can create a healthcare system that is more patient-centric, efficient, and equitable [28]. The future of healthcare is linked with the future of technology where machine learning, big data, artificial intelligence, and the Internet of Things will play a crucial role. As we move ahead it is of utmost importance to protect human-centered design, ethical considerations, and safety of the patients to ensure that computational tools truly serve the best interests of patients and healthcare professionals.

12.2.1 Role of Computation Tools in Disease Detection

Computational tools are one of the advanced fields in the healthcare sector, most specifically in the diagnosis of several diseases [51]. They provide us with an unprecedented capability to identify vast amounts of data, trace out certain kinds of patterns, and make predictions that ultimately lead to more accurate diagnoses [10]. Some of the key roles of the computational tools related to healthcare are discussed below:

(a) *Analysis of the Data and Recognition of the Patterns*

   (i) A large amount of data is produced in the electrical health record by the use of which one can diagnose health problems in the body [86].
   (ii) To detect certain abnormalities in the body medical images are been processed like CT scans, X-rays, and MRIs [82].
   (iii) Analysis of the genomic data to find some genetic markers that are related to diseases [113].
   (iv) Studying many electrical health records to trace risks and early warning signs of the body to prevent it before worsening and becoming difficult to treat [39].

(b) *Predictive Modeling*

   (i) To predict the outbreaks of diseases based on epidemiological data (Jia et al. 2019).
   (ii) Forecasting the progression of the diseases and generating treatment responses according to the disease [52].
   (iii) Based on data from the patient, personalized treatment plans are developed [21].

(c) *Drug Discovery*

   (i) Identifying potential drug targets by analyzing protein structures and interactions [126].
   (ii) Simulating drug interactions to accelerate drug development [66].

(d) *Remote Sensing and Telemedicine*

   (i) The application of wearable devices and sensors can enable remote patient monitoring [95, 99].
   (ii) Patients who are at a far distance from the hospital can also get virtual consultations from the doctors with this computerized device [98].

These are some roles that are discussed in the above points that not only advanced treatments and diagnosis with the help of these tools, but also allow other health professionals to treat the diseases of their patients living far from the hospital by the application of remote sensing technologies [8]. Altogether after overcoming certain challenges of computational integration of these tools with healthcare will provide effective and low-cost treatments to patients [3, 6].

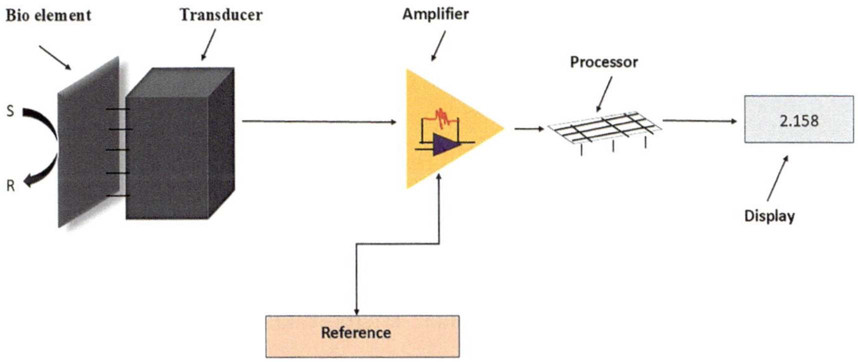

Fig. 12.2 Working of biosensors

12.3 Biosensor Fundamentals

Biosensors are modern and advanced devices composed of a combination of advanced computational tools and biological components. With the help of the physical transducer, it is easy to quantify the target product in the sample. It operates by converting biological signals into measurable electrical signals as shown in Fig. 12.2. This technology has changed and brought many breakthroughs in several areas like food, healthcare, environment, and biodefense systems.

12.3.1 Parts in Biosensors

A typical biosensor consists of three primary parts:

(a) *Bioreceptor:* A bioreceptor is a biological component of a biosensor that specifically interacts with some specific target molecule or an analyte [121]. They specifically interact with the analyte and form a complex.

(b) *Transducer:* These components are used to convert biological signals into measurable electrical signals [108]. Transducers can be electrochemical, optical piezoelectric, or thermal, depending on the nature of the analysis and desired output signal.

(c) *Detector:* The electronic component processes electrical signals from the transducer and provides a quantitative output, such as a numerical display or a digital reading [43].

12.3.2 Types of Biosensors

Biosensors are classified into two parts:

12.3.2.1 Based on the Biological Component

(a) *Enzyme-based biosensors*: these utilize enzymes as receptors to catalyze specific reactions [22].

(b) *Microbial biosensors*: employs whole microorganisms to trace specific compounds [14].

(c) *Immunosensors:* they work for antibodies or antigens as receptors for specific analyte detection [65].

(d) *Nucleic acid-based biosensors*: utilize DNA or RNA probes for detecting specific types of genetic sequences [46].

12.3.2.2 Based on the Transducer

(a) *Electrochemical biosensor*: An electrochemical transducer and a biological recognition element are combined in an electrochemical biosensor to identify particular analytes [124]. For these biosensors to function, a biological response must be transformed into an electrical signal that can be measured and examined. The biological component—such as an enzyme, antibody, or nucleic acid—usually interacts with the target molecule to alter the system's electrochemical characteristics. Following this alteration, a quantifiable electrical response is produced, yielding either quantitative or qualitative data. Because of their great sensitivity and specificity, electrochemical biosensors are widely employed in environmental monitoring, medical diagnostics, and food safety [55].

(b) *Optical biosensor*: A device that employs light to identify biological substances is called an optical biosensor. It combines an optical transducer with a biorecognition component, like an enzyme, antibody, or nucleic acid [104]. The biorecognition element and the target analyte interact to modify optical characteristics such as absorbance, refractive index, and fluorescence. To find out if the analyte is present or at what concentration, this change is monitored and examined. Because optical biosensors have great sensitivity, specificity, and real-time results, they are frequently employed in environmental monitoring, medical diagnostics, and food safety.

(c) *Piezoelectric biosensor:* A device that uses piezoelectric materials to identify biological interactions is called a piezoelectric biosensor. The piezoelectric effect, which occurs when mechanical stress on a material produces an electrical charge, is used by these sensors. Usually, an enzyme, antibody, or nucleic acid biorecognition element is affixed to the piezoelectric material of the biosensor [44]. The binding of the target analyte to the biorecognition element results in a displacement of mass on the sensor surface, which in turn induces a shift in the frequency of vibrations of the piezoelectric material. The existence or concentration of the analyte is ascertained by measuring and analyzing this shift. Piezoelectric biosensors are highly appreciated for their quick response times and great sensitivity.

12.4 Public Health Surveillance Using Biosensors

A vital component of contemporary healthcare systems [77], public health surveillance acts as an early warning system for potential health risks. Since biosensors can provide precise, real-time data on a range of health variables [20], their integration into public health surveillance systems has the potential to completely transform this area of study. This paper investigates the use of biosensors in public health surveillance, looking at their benefits, uses, difficulties, and potential future developments. Analytical tools known as biosensors translate a biological reaction into an electrical signal [103]. A bioreceptor, transducer, and electronic system are usually included. The transducer transforms the interaction between the bioreceptor and the target analyte (such as viruses, biomarkers, or chemicals) into a signal that can be measured. This signal is processed by the electronic system so that analysis and decision-making may be done with it.

12.4.1 The Role of Biosensors in Public Health Surveillance

The real-time data that biosensors can deliver is one of their biggest advantages [59]. The discovery of epidemics may be delayed by the reliance on traditional public health surveillance approaches on laboratory testing and periodic reporting. On the other hand, biosensors can instantly provide data to health authorities while continuously monitoring biological or environmental samples. This capacity makes it possible to respond to new health risks more quickly, potentially lessening their effects. Biosensors can be made with great sensitivity and specificity to identify particular infections or biomarkers [64]. This accuracy guarantees that public health responses are founded on correct information by lowering the possibility of false positives and negatives. Biosensors, for instance, can distinguish between different influenza strains, enabling more specialized vaccination and treatment plans. Biosensors can be applied in a variety of contexts, including households, public areas, and medical facilities [32]. A vast array of health indicators, such as chronic disorders, environmental pollutants, and infectious infections, can be tracked by them. Because of their adaptability, biosensors are useful instruments in a wide range of public health programs, from monitoring the spread of disease to evaluating urban air quality. Infectious illness surveillance is one area where biosensors are especially helpful. They can identify pathogens in surfaces, water, air, and bodily fluids, giving important information on the dynamics of disease transmission and prevalence. For example, biosensors were created to identify SARS-CoV-2 in wastewater during the COVID-19 pandemic providing an early warning system for community outbreaks [17]. Public health is greatly impacted by environmental conditions, which biosensors can assist in monitoring.

Toxins, pollutants, and allergies in the soil, water, and air can all be found using sensors. For instance, biosensors can track the amount of volatile organic compounds and particulate matter in the air, which can be used to determine the efficacy of environmental restrictions and pinpoint areas of pollution. The treatment of chronic illnesses is another area in which biosensors can be used. For example, glucose monitoring devices for diabetics allow for continuous monitoring of blood sugar levels, improving disease management and lowering complications. In a similar vein, biosensors that identify cardiovascular disease biomarkers can facilitate prompt diagnosis and treatment. Biosensors have a lot of potential to improve surveillance of public health. Their capacity to deliver precise, up-to-date information on an extensive array of health metrics can greatly enhance illness identification, environmental tracking, and the management of chronic conditions. The broad use of biosensors in public health is probably going to be fueled by continued technological improvements and international cooperation, notwithstanding obstacles about financial constraints, data administration, and technical constraints. We can build a more adaptable and efficient public health infrastructure by incorporating biosensors into monitoring systems, which will eventually improve health outcomes for populations all around the world.

12.4.2 Technological Developments

Continuous developments in materials science, data analytics, and nanotechnology are probably going to improve and lower the cost of biosensors. For example, machine learning advancements can enhance data interpretation and predictive capacities, while nanomaterials can boost sensor sensitivity and specificity. There is a lot of potential for integrating biosensors with mobile apps and digital health platforms. Personalized health interventions and real-time data sharing can be facilitated by this kind of integration [53]. Using biometric data, a smartphone app that is linked to a biosensor, for instance, might notify users when pollution levels are high or remind them to take their prescription. Global health endeavors could be transformed by biosensor technology. Biosensors can help in efforts to alleviate health disparities and respond to pandemics by providing real-time data on disease prevalence and environmental variables [122]. International financing and cooperation are necessary to guarantee that biosensor technology benefits people all over the world.

12.5 System Integration and Validation

In the lifespan of complex system development, system integration and validation are essential procedures, especially in sectors like software development, telecommunications, automotive, and aerospace [115]. These procedures make sure that different parts and subsystems act together harmoniously to provide the required functionality and performance. This essay explores the significance of system integration and validation, as well as the methods used, difficulties encountered, and successful strategies.

12.5.1 System Integration and Validation's Significance

12.5.1.1 Providing Coherent Functions

Any complex system must have faultless interactions between its many subsystems and components to accomplish its overall goals. Integrating these components into a single, functional entity is known as system integration [118].

Validation ensures that the integrated system satisfies user requirements and necessary specifications. If components are not rigorously integrated and validated, they may function flawlessly separately but malfunction when combined, resulting in expensive failures and sometimes hazardous circumstances.

12.5.1.2 Mitigation of Risk

Early system integration and validation throughout the development lifecycle help detect and reduce risks before they become serious problems [72]. Early identification of integration issues or validation failures enables prompt fixes, lowering the risk of expensive rework or development delays later on.

12.5.1.3 Observance of Standards

Strict regulatory standards that specify certain requirements for performance, safety, and dependability apply to many businesses. Procedures for system integration and validation guarantee that the finished product conforms with these criteria, protecting users' safety and averting financial and legal consequences [5].

12.6 Applications of Integrated Systems in Disease Detection

Disease detection has undergone revolutionary modifications as a result of the incorporation of biosensors with computational technologies. By combining the advantages of both technologies, this union improves the precision, effectiveness, and range of diagnostic procedures. Key applications of these integrated systems in various disease detection domains are highlighted in the following sections.

(a) *Early Identification of Cancer*

The results of cancer treatments and survival rates are greatly enhanced by early identification. The identification of cancer biomarkers in their early stages is greatly aided by integrated systems that include biosensors and computational techniques [2]. Initial data can be obtained by using biosensors that are engineered to identify particular proteins, DNA alterations, or circulating tumor cells. After that, computational techniques evaluate this data to identify benign and malignant disorders [50]. Large datasets can be used to train machine learning algorithms to identify patterns that point to early cancer, allowing for faster detection and treatment.

(b) *Monitoring of Infectious Diseases*

Effective containment and treatment of infectious diseases depend heavily on the prompt and precise diagnosis of these illnesses. In this situation, integrated systems are especially beneficial. Biosensors can identify pathogens in bodily fluids, including bacteria, viruses, and fungi [25]. Real-time sensor data analysis is made possible by computational techniques, which also allow for fast infectious agent identification. This method is particularly helpful during illness outbreaks, such as those caused by the influenza virus, COVID-19, or Ebola, when prompt detection can stop the disease's spread and guide public health measures [63]. These systems can also track pathogen mutations, which aids in the creation of potent vaccinations and therapies.

(c) *Management of Chronic Diseases*

To properly manage chronic diseases like diabetes, cardiovascular disease, and chronic respiratory disorders, continuous monitoring is necessary. Relevant biomarkers can be continuously tracked thanks to integrated systems [24]. For example, glucose sensors allow diabetics to monitor their blood sugar levels in real time. This data is analyzed by computational techniques to forecast patterns, spot possible issues, and suggest changes to medication or lifestyle. This ongoing feedback loop lowers the risk of serious consequences and hospital stays by assisting individuals and healthcare professionals in managing chronic illnesses more proactively [110].

(d) *Diagnosis of Neurological Disease*

Because neurological disorders including Parkinson's, Alzheimer's, and multiple sclerosis are complicated, diagnosing them can be difficult. Integrated technologies that analyze biomarkers in blood or cerebrospinal fluid can help in early and accurate detection [51]. These biomarkers are detected by biosensors, and patterns linked to certain neurological diseases are found by computer methods interpreting the data. To offer a thorough evaluation of brain health, sophisticated algorithms can also examine imaging data from PET or MRI scans. The management and treatment of neurological illnesses can be greatly enhanced by the early diagnosis made possible by these integrated systems.

(e) *Screening for Cardiovascular Disease*

In the world, cardiovascular illnesses rank among the top causes of death. Heart attacks and strokes are examples of serious events that can be avoided by early detection and surveillance. Biosensors are employed by integrated systems to identify heart health biomarkers, including troponin, cholesterol, and C-reactive protein [100]. To evaluate cardiovascular risk, computational methods evaluate these biomarker levels in combination with additional patient data, such as blood pressure and electrocardiogram (ECG) values. By identifying high-risk patients and suggesting preventive steps, predictive analytics can lower the frequency of acute cardiovascular events.

(f) *Detection of Respiratory Diseases*

The early diagnosis and management of respiratory disorders, such as tuberculosis, asthma, and chronic obstructive pulmonary disease (COPD) [101], are enhanced by the integration of biosensors and computational techniques. Biosensors can identify certain infections in respiratory secretions, assess parameters related to lung function, and find inflammatory indicators. This data is analyzed by computational tools to diagnose the condition, track its course, and assess the effectiveness of treatment. For example, people with asthma can better manage their condition and prevent severe exacerbations by having real-time lung function monitored.

(g) *Diagnostics at the Point of Care*

Point-of-care diagnostics is one of the most important uses of integrated systems. Rapid on-site testing is made possible by these methods, which do not require elaborate laboratory equipment. To swiftly identify illnesses, portable biosensors can be utilized at homes, in clinics, or even in emergency rooms [33]. The instantaneous data analysis made possible by computational tools enables healthcare professionals to act quickly and intelligently. This capacity is especially helpful in underserved or isolated locations where access to cutting-edge medical facilities may be restricted.

(h) *Individualized Medical Care*

The goal of personalized medicine is to adjust medical care to each patient's unique needs. This method relies heavily on integrated systems, which offer comprehensive insights into each patient's biological profile. Multiple indicators can be monitored by biosensors at once, giving a complete picture of the patient's health [18]. This data is analyzed by computational algorithms to determine the best courses of action and forecast the patient's reaction to particular treatments. Better patient results result from this tailored strategy, which maximizes benefits and increases therapeutic efficacy.

(i) *Pandemic Response and Preparation*

The necessity for reliable mechanisms to identify and track infectious diseases globally was highlighted by the COVID-19 pandemic [61]. For pandemic preparedness and response, integrated systems incorporating biosensors and computational tools are crucial. Pathogens can be quickly detected by biosensors, and data can be analyzed by computational tools to follow the disease's spread and pinpoint new hotspots. Public health authorities can lessen the effects of the epidemic by implementing targeted measures and allocating resources effectively thanks to this real-time surveillance.

The field of disease detection has expanded its possibilities with the combination of biosensors and computational techniques. Many applications that improve the precision, effectiveness, and scope of diagnostic procedures are provided by these integrated systems, ranging from customized care and pandemic preparedness to early cancer detection and infectious disease surveillance [119]. The ability of these systems to revolutionize healthcare is becoming more and more clear as technology advances, offering a future in which illnesses are identified early, treated more successfully, and managed more effectively.

12.7 Case Studies and Examples

Healthcare delivery is changing as a result of the convergence of biosensors, data science, and artificial intelligence. This section explores real-world case studies and examples that show how computational tools are used in diverse healthcare sectors. The case studies related to the integration of computational tools in healthcare are listed in Table 12.2.

12.8 Challenges and Future Directions

Computational tools have made very significant changes in the healthcare sectors from diagnosis and treatment to patient management and research [9]. But several challenges persist in this advanced technology, which need to be highlighted in this particular subheading. Artificial intelligence can process and analyze large sets of data without consuming much time and the chances of errors are minimal compared to humans [56]. Computer vision tools can now obtain medical images like CT scans, MRIs, and X-rays often revealing issues that humans might miss. Machine learning (ML) algorithms have been employed in the healthcare system to assess a range of medical data, including data from electronic health records (EHRs) and genetic and physiological imaging data [105]. Cloud IoT is a multitasking computational tool that is integrated with the system and can perform several functions and costs low as compared to the traditional diagnosis methods [4]. These techniques excel at identifying connections and patterns in huge, complex datasets that are too complex for people to examine [31].

Table 12.2 Case studies and examples

Area	Case studies	Explanation	Examples	References
Precision medicine and genomics	Personalized Cancer Treatment	With its varied genetic and molecular characteristics, cancer is a complicated disease. Conventional one-size-fits-all therapies frequently don't work very well. Large-scale genomic data is analyzed using computational technologies in order to pinpoint certain genetic alterations linked to cancer. Plans for individualized treatment are created using this data.	Platforms for genome sequencing is provided by businesses like Illumina, and platforms for genomic data analysis that support treatment choices are provided by Foundation Medicine	[34, 75]
Remote patient monitoring and wearable devices	Chronic disease management	Chronic conditions like diabetes, heart disease, and high blood pressure necessitate ongoing care and lifestyle adjustments. Biosensor-equipped wearables gather data in real-time on blood glucose levels, vital signs, and other characteristics. This data is analyzed by computational techniques to find patterns, abnormalities, and possible health hazards.	Apple Watch offers useful data for users and healthcare providers with its heart rate tracking and ECG features combined with health apps.	[49, 80]
Drug discovery and development	Accelerating drug development	Conventional drug discovery is a costly and time-consuming procedure. To find possible drug candidates, forecast drug interactions, and improve drug formulations, computational approaches such as molecular modeling, simulations, and machine learning are employed.	Computational drug discovery platforms are used by companies such as Schrödinger and atomwise to expedite the creation of novel treatments.	[38, 89]

(continued)

Table 12.2 (continued)

Area	Case studies	Explanation	Examples	References
Medical imaging and image analysis	Early disease detection	It is essential to diagnose illnesses including cancer, cardiovascular disease, and neurological disorders accurately and promptly. To identify anomalies and aid in diagnosis, computational technologies like image recognition and deep learning examine medical pictures (X-rays, CT scans, and MRIs).	By analyzing mammograms, AI-powered systems can identify breast cancer early on and improve patient outcomes.	[62, 102]
Electronic health records (EHR) and data analytics	Population health management	It is difficult to maximize healthcare service while also comprehending the health demands of a population. Analysis of population health trends, disease outbreaks, and resource allocation are made possible by the combination of EHR data and computational tools.	Healthcare institutions can recognize patient groups at high risk, forecast illness outbreaks, and carry out focused interventions.	[11, 88]

12.8.1 Problem Statement of Computational Tools

The advancements of computational technologies such as AI and ML have been some of the obstacles that prevent their complete merger into the medical field [7]. Such kind of difficulties include problems related to algorithm transparency, data security, and the existence of some biases in the AI models [27, 35]. The challenges in integrating with the current healthcare platform are hampering their broad application. Even cloud IOT is most frequently used in healthcare; nowadays, it is a multitasking tool that can store all data and also monitor health as well. Besides these functions, it has some major drawbacks as there are high chances that cloud IoT can be easily hacked by any hacker and they can fetch all the information and can create huge damage to the healthcare system [97]. There are clear gaps observed in some of the biased Artificial Intelligence, ML and Cloud IoT applications that are unethical which can put the safety of the patients in danger [85]. To overcome these challenges, it is essential to improve the focus on the overall healthcare system consequences.

12.8.2 Challenges and Limitations in the Prior Systematic Review

Table 12.3 (Nadella et al. 2023) provides a structured overview of the challenges and limitations that are observed in the prior systemic review on artificial intelligence and machines.

Learning, and cloud IoT learning in healthcare details the names of the "authors", "the years of publication", "the titles of the papers", the techniques used, the methodology used, and any particular restrictions found.

12.8.3 Areas for Improvement

The addition of computational technologies in the healthcare area has shown immense improvement in the detection of diseases and has maximized its impact over the period [60]. Figure 12.3 is a depiction of the areas of improvement in the field of computational tools in healthcare sectors.

Several critical aspects need to be improved before computational technologies can be effectively integrated into healthcare [106]. Improving data accessibility and quality is the most important thing to do. Even with the improvements made to EHRs, data is still frequently missing, inconsistent, and fragmented [92]. To overcome these obstacles, standards, interoperability, and safe data sharing are necessary. Second, trust and adoption are hampered by complicated algorithms' black-box character [12]. It's critical to create interpretable models that offer concise justifications for choices, especially in high-stakes healthcare applications. Thirdly, to guarantee justice and equity in the healthcare system, algorithmic bias must be addressed. Prioritizing methods for locating and reducing biases in data and models is necessary. Furthermore, the end-user should be considered in the design of computational tools. Designing with the needs of the user in mind is essential to producing supportive, effective, and user-friendly technologies. Lastly, it is critical to preserve patient data. Strong security protocols and adherence to privacy laws are crucial. A thoughtful approach and creative solutions are needed to strike a balance between data sharing and privacy concerns (Tyagi et al. 2020). The healthcare sector may fully utilize computational technologies to improve patient outcomes, increase efficiency, and spur innovation by tackling this area (Hussain et al. 2022).

12.8.4 Future Directions

In the area of healthcare, AI and ML present a trajectory marked by the interaction of technologies [13]. They are completely interdisciplinary, they are collaborative at the same time. AI continues to place an emerging focus on its innovative method of

Table 12.3 Prior studies on the systemic review

Name of the paper	Author	Published Year	Procedure	Methods	Drawbacks
"Challenges in Implementing AI in Healthcare"	Smith et al.	2018	A systematic review of the literature	Qualitative analyses	Insufficient access to high-quality data and the absence of defined procedures for implementing AI
"A Review of ML Applications in Healthcare"	Johnson and Khoshgoftaar	2019	Meta-analysis of previous research	Quantitative analysis	Variability in research methodologies, variability in results as reported, restricted generalizability
"Future Directions in AI-driven Clinical Decision Support"	Rajkumar et al.	2021	Thorough analysis of new developments and areas in need of research	Qualitative synthesis	Insufficient data on long-term effects and difficulties incorporating AI into therapeutic processes
"Addressing Bias in AI Algorithms for Healthcare"	Wang and Summers	2018	An organized analysis of prejudice reduction methods	Comparative analysis	Strategies for mitigating bias has limited effectiveness and may have unforeseen consequences
"Challenges and opportunities in IoT healthcare systems: a systematic review"	Selvaraj and Sundaravaradhan [93]	2020	A systematic review of the literature	Qualitative analyses	The main drawbacks of the current systems are their high power consumption, lack of resources, and security problems brought on by the use of several devices

federated learning and decentralization architecture. Blockchain technology and the Internet of Medical Things (IoMT) are two more disruptive technologies that AI is combining with the potential to revolutionize data management systems for security requirements in patient-centric care delivery [91]. To effectively navigate the ethical, legal, and societal ramifications of artificial intelligence in healthcare, interdisciplinary collaboration between physicians, data scientists, ethicists, experts, and

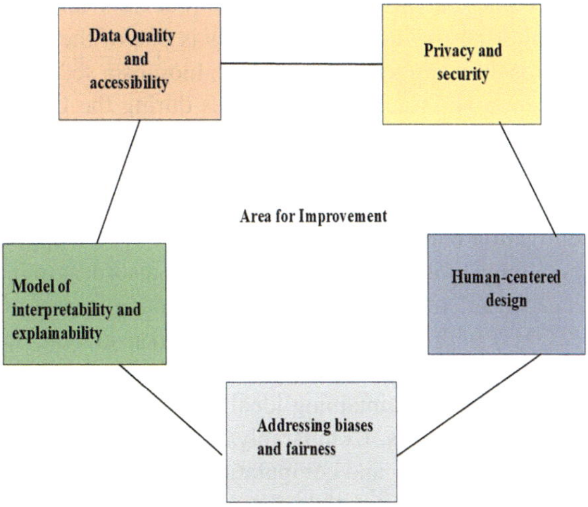

Fig. 12.3 The area of improvement in the computation tools for healthcare advancements

policymakers will be essential [19]. Our future research projects must plan for the development of AI-driven solutions that enable people to enhance health outcomes and advance fair access to high-quality care by adopting a patient-centered approach. A future of clinical decision support that is ready to break through current barriers and usher in a new era of precision medicine and individualized healthcare delivery is made possible by the synergistic potential of AI and human expertise. Healthcare could be drastically changed by AI and ML by enhancing diagnosis, tailoring therapies, and maximizing results (Mannan et al. 2024). Even though these technologies have a lot to offer, issues like bias, data privacy, and regulatory barriers need to be resolved. To create moral and practical AI solutions that put patient care, efficiency, and fair access to healthcare first, expert collaboration is essential.

12.9 Conclusion

Biosensor-based illness detection systems combined with computational tools represent a breakthrough in public health management and medical diagnosis. Biosensors provide accurate, real-time monitoring of several biomarkers linked to diseases by converting biological responses into measurable signals. These systems offer a strong foundation for early illness identification, ongoing health monitoring, and tailored medication when combined with cutting-edge computational technologies. Enhancing data processing and interpretation capabilities is the main benefit of combining biosensors with computational tools. Large volumes of data are produced by biosensors, which can make manual analysis difficult. These data can be processed effectively by computational tools, such as machine learning algorithms and data analytics software, which can then spot trends and anomalies that can point to the existence of a disease. This combination not only expedites the diagnostic procedure but also enhances the precision and dependability of the outcomes. Monitoring for infectious diseases is one of the key areas in which this integrated approach is applied. For example, biosensor technology was essential to the quick detection and tracking of the virus during the COVID-19 epidemic. These efforts were further strengthened by computational tools, which made it possible to track infection rates in real-time and forecast outbreak situations. This combination gave health authorities important information that helped them create containment and mitigation plans that worked. Furthermore, the application of biosensors and computational tools goes beyond infectious disorders to include chronic ailments including cancer, diabetes, and cardiovascular diseases. Continuous glucose monitors (CGMs) with biosensors can track blood glucose levels in real-time for diabetes treatment. Through the analysis of these data by computational techniques, patients are assisted in maintaining ideal glucose levels through individualized recommendations and alerts. Comparably, in oncology, biosensors can identify cancer biomarkers early on, and computational tools make it easier to analyze these markers to forecast the course of the disease and customize treatment regimens. The promise of this integrated approach is further demonstrated by the development of wearable biosensors. Biosensors are integrated into wearable technology, including fitness trackers and smartwatches, to continuously monitor vital signs, physical activity, and other health indicators. These gadgets are connected to computer systems that examine the gathered information to give users useful health-related insights. Continuous monitoring facilitates the early identification of possible health problems, thereby advancing preventative healthcare and enhancing general well-being. The combination of biosensor-based systems with computational tools presents several difficulties despite the clear advantages. One of the main issues is privacy and data security. As these systems gather and handle private health data, it is critical to guarantee data security and regulatory compliance. Additionally, to preserve confidence in biosensors' diagnostic skills, their accuracy and dependability must be regularly verified. The pricing and availability of these sophisticated diagnostic tools provide another difficulty. Even if the technology has a lot of potential, it is crucial to make sure that a variety of people, especially those living in low-resource environments, can use it. To create affordable solutions and encourage fair access to new technologies, researchers, healthcare professionals, and legislators must work together. To sum up, the amalgamation of computational tools and biosensor-based illness detection systems signifies a revolutionary advancement in healthcare diagnostics. This synergy offers significant advantages in the contexts of infectious and chronic diseases by improving the precision, speed, and personalization of disease identification and management. To fully exploit the promise of these interconnected systems, it will be imperative to solve issues with data security, accuracy, and accessibility as technology continues to advance. In the end, this strategy has the potential to improve health outcomes worldwide, facilitate prompt interventions, and open the door for a period when proactive and individualized healthcare is the standard.

References

1. Abaid Z, Shaghaghi A, Gunawardena R, Seneviratne S, Seneviratne A, Jha S. Health access broker: secure, patient-controlled management of personal health records in the cloud. Adv Intell Syst Comput. 2021;1267:111–21. https://doi.org/10.1007/978-3-030-57805-3_11.
2. Abouali H, Hosseini SA, Purcell E, Nagrath S, Poudineh M. Recent advances in device engineering and computational analysis for characterization of cell-released cancer biomarkers. Cancer. 2022;14(2):288. https://doi.org/10.3390/cancers14020288.
3. Aceto G, Persico V, Pescapé A. Industry 4.0 and health: internet of things, big data, and cloud computing for healthcare 4.0. J Ind Inf Integr. 2020;18:1–14. https://doi.org/10.1016/j.jii.2020.100129.
4. Adewole KS, Akintola AG, Jimoh RG, Mabayoje MA, Jimoh MK, Usman- Hamza FE, Balogun AO, Sangaiah AK, Ameen AO. Cloud-based IoMT framework for cardiovascular disease prediction and diagnosis in personalized E- health care. In: Intelligent IoT Systems in Personalized Health Care (Issue July); 2020. https://doi.org/10.1016/B978-0-12-821187-8.00005-8.
5. Agirre JA, Etxeberria L, Barbosa R, Basagiannis S, Giantamidis G, Bauer T, Ferrari E, Labayen Esnaola M, Orani V, Öberg J, Pereira D, Proença J, Schlick R, Smrčka A, Tiberti W, Tonetta S, Bozzano M, Yazici A, Sangchoolie B. The VALU3S ECSEL project: verification and validation of automated systems safety and security. Microprocess Microsyst. 2021;87:104349. https://doi.org/10.1016/J.MICPRO.2021.104349.
6. Ahmad F, Muhmood T. Clinical translation of nanomedicine with integrated digital medicine and machine learning interventions. Colloids Surf B: Biointerfaces. 2024;241(June). https://doi.org/10.1016/j.colsurfb.2024.114041.
7. Ahmad Z, Rahim S, Zubair M, Abdul-Ghafar J. Artificial intelligence (AI) in medicine, current applications and future role with special emphasis on its potential and promise in pathology: present and future impact, obstacles including costs and acceptance among pathologists, practical and philosoph. Diagn Pathol. 2021;16(1):1–16. https://doi.org/10.1186/s13000-021-01085-4.
8. Ahmad I, Asghar Z, Kumar T, Li G, Manzoor A, Mikhaylov K, Shah SA, Hoyhtya M, Reponen J, Huusko J, Harjula E. Emerging technologies for next generation remote health care and assisted living. IEEE Access. 2022;10:56094–132. https://doi.org/10.1109/ACCESS.2022.3177278.
9. Ahmad A, Tariq A, Hussain HK, Yousaf Gill A. Revolutionizing healthcare: how deep learning is poised to change the landscape of medical diagnosis and treatment. J Comput Netw Archit High Perform Comput. 2023;5(2):458–71. https://doi.org/10.47709/cnahpc.v5i2.2350.
10. Ahmed Z, Mohamed K, Zeeshan S, Dong XQ. Artificial intelligence with multi-functional machine learning platform development for better healthcare and precision medicine. Database. 2020;2020:1–35. https://doi.org/10.1093/database/baaa010.
11. Alahmadi A, Belet S, Black A, Cromer D, Flegg JA, House T, Jayasundara P, Keith JM, McCaw JM, Moss R, Ross JV, Shearer FM, Tun STT, Walker J, White L, Whyte JM, Yan AWC, Zarebski AE. Influencing public health policy with data-informed mathematical models of infectious diseases: recent developments and new challenges. Epidemics. 2020;32:100393. https://doi.org/10.1016/J.EPIDEM.2020.100393.
12. Albahri AS, Duhaim AM, Fadhel MA, Alnoor A, Baqer NS, Alzubaidi L, Albahri OS, Alamoodi AH, Bai J, Salhi A, Santamaría J, Ouyang C, Gupta A, Gu Y, Deveci M. A systematic review of trustworthy and explainable artificial intelligence in healthcare: assessment of quality, bias risk, and data fusion. Inf Fusion. 2023;96:156–91. https://doi.org/10.1016/j.inffus.2023.03.008.
13. Allam A, Feuerriegel S, Rebhan M, Krauthammer M. Analyzing patient trajectories with artificial intelligence. J Med Internet Res. 2021;23(12):1–14. https://doi.org/10.2196/29812.

14. Arlyapov VA, Plekhanova YV, Kamanina OA, Nakamura H, Reshetilov AN. Microbial biosensors for rapid determination of biochemical oxygen demand: approaches, tendencies and development prospects. Biosensors. 2022;12(10). https://doi.org/10.3390/bios12100842.
15. Bagchi S, Tay KG, Huong A, Debnath SK. Image processing and machine learning techniques used in computer-aided detection system for mammogram screening-A review. Int J Electr Comput Eng. 2020;10(3):2336–48. https://doi.org/10.11591/ijece.v10i3.pp2336-2348.
16. Bailey TS. Clinical implications of accuracy measurements of continuous glucose sensors. Diabetes Technol Ther. 2017;19(S2):S51–4. https://doi.org/10.1089/dia.2017.0050.
17. Barceló D. Wastewater-based epidemiology to monitor COVID-19 outbreak: present and future diagnostic methods to be in your radar. Case Stud Chem Environ Eng. 2020;2:100042. https://doi.org/10.1016/J.CSCEE.2020.100042.
18. Beduk T, Beduk D, Hasan MR, Guler Celik E, Kosel J, Narang J, Salama KN, Timur S. Smartphone-based multiplexed biosensing tools for health monitoring. Biosensors. 2022;12(8):583. https://doi.org/10.3390/bios12080583.
19. Bekbolatova M, Mayer J, Ong CW, Toma M. Transformative potential of AI in healthcare: definitions, applications, and navigating the ethical landscape and public perspectives. Healthcare (Switzerland). 2024;12(2):125. https://doi.org/10.3390/healthcare12020125.
20. Bhatia D, Paul S, Acharjee T, Ramachairy SS. Biosensors and their widespread impact on human health. Sensors Int. 2024;5:100257. https://doi.org/10.1016/J.SINTL.2023.100257.
21. Bica I, Alaa AM, Lambert C, van der Schaar M. From real-world patient data to individualized treatment effects using machine learning: current and future methods to address underlying challenges. Clin Pharmacol Ther. 2021;109(1):87–100. https://doi.org/10.1002/cpt.1907.
22. Bollella P, Katz E. Enzyme-based biosensors: tackling electron transfer issues. Sensors (Switzerland). 2020;20(12):1–32. https://doi.org/10.3390/s20123517.
23. Bustin SA, Jellinger KA. Advances in molecular medicine: unravelling disease complexity and pioneering precision healthcare. Int J Mol Sci. 2023;24(18):14168. https://doi.org/10.3390/ijms241814168.
24. Castelli FA, Rosati G, Moguet C, Fuentes C, Marrugo-Ramírez J, Lefebvre T, Volland H, Merkoçi A, Simon S, Fenaille F, Junot C. Metabolomics for personalized medicine: the input of analytical chemistry from biomarker discovery to point-of-care tests. Anal Bioanal Chem. 2022;414(2):759. https://doi.org/10.1007/s00216-021-03586-z.
25. Castillo-Henríquez L, Brenes-Acuña M, Castro-Rojas A, Cordero-Salmerón R, Lopretti-Correa M, Vega-Baudrit JR. Biosensors for the detection of bacterial and viral clinical pathogens. Sensors (Switzerland). 2020;20(23):1–26. https://doi.org/10.3390/s20236926.
26. Chawla NV, Davis DA. Bringing big data to personalized healthcare: a patient-centered framework. J Gen Intern Med. 2013;28(SUPPL.3):660–5. https://doi.org/10.1007/s11606-013-2455-8.
27. Cheng L, Varshney KR, Liu H. Socially responsible AI algorithms: issues, purposes, and challenges. J Artif Intell Res. 2021;71:1137–81. https://doi.org/10.1613/JAIR.1.12814.
28. Chibuike MC, Grobbelaar SS, Botha A. Overcoming challenges for improved patient-centric care: a scoping review of platform ecosystems in healthcare. IEEE Access. 2024;12(November 2023):14298–313. https://doi.org/10.1109/ACCESS.2024.3356860.
29. Chu SS, Nguyen HA, Zhang J, Tabassum S, Cao H. Towards multiplexed and multimodal biosensor platforms in real-time monitoring of metabolic disorders. Sensors. 2022;22(14):5200. https://doi.org/10.3390/s22145200.
30. Collin CB, Gebhardt T, Golebiewski M, Karaderi T, Hillemanns M, Khan FM, Salehzadeh-Yazdi A, Kirschner M, Krobitsch S, Kuepfer L. Computational models for clinical applications in personalized medicine—guidelines and recommendations for data integration and model validation. J Pers Med. 2022;12(2):166. https://doi.org/10.3390/jpm12020166.
31. Collins C, Dennehy D, Conboy K, Mikalef P. Artificial intelligence in information systems research: a systematic literature review and research agenda. Int J Inf Manag. 2021;60:102383. https://doi.org/10.1016/J.IJINFOMGT.2021.102383.

32. Cui F, Zhou HS. Diagnostic methods and potential portable biosensors for coronavirus disease 2019. Biosens Bioelectron. 2020;165:112349. https://doi.org/10.1016/J.BIOS.2020.112349.
33. Cui F, Yue Y, Zhang Y, Zhang Z, Zhou HS. Advancing biosensors with machine learning. ACS Sens. 2020;5(11):3346–64. https://doi.org/10.1021/acssensors.0c01424.
34. Cuppen E, Elemento O, Rosenquist R, Nikic S, IJzerman M, Zaleski ID, Frederix G, Levin L-Å, Mullighan CG, Buettner R, Pugh TJ, Grimmond S, Caldas C, Andre F, Custers I, Campo E, van Snellenberg H, Schuh A, Nakagawa H, et al. Implementation of whole-genome and transcriptome sequencing into clinical cancer care. JCO Precis Oncol. 2022;6:1–11. https://doi.org/10.1200/po.22.00245.
35. Daneshjou R, Smith MP, Sun MD, Rotemberg V, Zou J. Lack of transparency and potential bias in artificial intelligence data sets and algorithms: a scoping review. JAMA Dermatol. 2021;157(11):1362–9. https://doi.org/10.1001/jamadermatol.2021.3129.
36. Diaz O, Kushibar K, Osuala R, Linardos A, Garrucho L, Igual L, Radeva P, Prior F, Gkontra P, Lekadir K. Data preparation for artificial intelligence in medical imaging: a comprehensive guide to open-access platforms and tools. Phys Med. 2021;83:25–37. https://doi.org/10.1016/J.EJMP.2021.02.007.
37. Galetsi P, Katsaliaki K, Kumar S. Exploring benefits and ethical challenges in the rise of mHealth (mobile healthcare) technology for the common good: an analysis of mobile applications for health specialists. Technovation. 2023;121:102598. https://doi.org/10.1016/J.TECHNOVATION.2022.102598.
38. Gangwal A, Lavecchia A. Unleashing the power of generative AI in drug discovery. Drug Discov Today. 2024;29(6):103992. https://doi.org/10.1016/J.DRUDIS.2024.103992.
39. Garcelon N, Burgun A, Salomon R, Neuraz A. Electronic health records for the diagnosis of rare diseases. Kidney Int. 2020;97(4):676–86. https://doi.org/10.1016/J.KINT.2019.11.037.
40. Gaurav D, Rodriguez FO, Tiwari S, Jabbar MA. Review of machine learning approach for drug development process. In: Deep learning in biomedical and health informatics, August; 2021. p. 53–77. https://doi.org/10.1201/9781003161233-3.
41. Greiwe J, Nyenhuis SM. Wearable technology and how this can be implemented into clinical practice. Curr Allergy Asthma Rep. 2020;20(8):36. https://doi.org/10.1007/s11882-020-00927-3.
42. Haleem A, Javaid M, Singh RP, Suman R, Rab S. Biosensors applications in medical field: a brief review. Sensors Int. 2021;2:100100. https://doi.org/10.1016/J.SINTL.2021.100100.
43. He Y, Li M, Meng Z, Chen S, Huang S, Hu Y, Zou X. An overview of acoustic emission inspection and monitoring technology in the key components of renewable energy systems. Mech Syst Signal Process. 2021;148:107146. https://doi.org/10.1016/J.YMSSP.2020.107146.
44. He JH, He CH, Qian MY, Alsolami AA. Piezoelectric biosensor based on ultrasensitive MEMS system. Sensors Actuators A Phys. 2024;376:115664. https://doi.org/10.1016/J.SNA.2024.115664.
45. Holmes JH, Beinlich J, Boland MR, Bowles KH, Chen Y, Cook TS, Demiris G, Draugelis M, Fluharty L, Gabriel PE, Grundmeier R, Hanson CW, Herman DS, Himes BE, Hubbard RA, Kahn CE, Kim D, Koppel R, Long Q, et al. Why is the electronic health record so challenging for research and clinical care? Methods Inf Med. 2021;60(1–2):32–48. https://doi.org/10.1055/s-0041-1731784.
46. Huo B, Hu Y, Gao Z, Li G. Recent advances on functional nucleic acid-based biosensors for detection of food contaminants. Talanta. 2021:222. https://doi.org/10.1016/j.talanta.2020.121565.
47. Iqbal N, Kumar P. From data science to bioscience: emerging era of bioinformatics applications, tools and challenges. Proc Comput Sci. 2022;218(2022):1516–28. https://doi.org/10.1016/j.procs.2023.01.130.
48. Iqbal MJ, Javed Z, Sadia H, Qureshi IA, Irshad A, Ahmed R, Malik K, Raza S, Abbas A, Pezzani R, Sharifi-Rad J. Clinical applications of artificial intelligence and machine learning

in cancer diagnosis: looking into the future. Cancer Cell Int. 2021;21(1):1–11. https://doi.org/10.1186/s12935-021-01981-1.
49. Isakadze N, Martin SS. How useful is the smartwatch ECG? Trends Cardiovasc Med. 2020;30(7):442–8. https://doi.org/10.1016/J.TCM.2019.10.010.
50. Jasti VDP, Zamani AS, Arumugam K, Naved M, Pallathadka H, Sammy F, Raghuvanshi A, Kaliyaperumal K. Computational technique based on machine learning and image processing for medical image analysis of breast cancer diagnosis. Security Commun Netw. 2022;2022:1. https://doi.org/10.1155/2022/1918379.
51. Jayatilake SMDAC, Ganegoda GU. Involvement of machine learning tools in healthcare decision making. J Healthc Eng. 2021;2021:6679512. https://doi.org/10.1155/2021/6679512.
52. Jin C, Yu H, Ke J, Ding P, Yi Y, Jiang X, Duan X, Tang J, Chang DT, Wu X, Gao F, Li R. Predicting treatment response from longitudinal images using multi-task deep learning. Nat Commun. 2021;12(1):1–11. https://doi.org/10.1038/s41467-021-22188-y.
53. Kamel Boulos MN, Zhang P. Digital twins: from personalised medicine to precision public health. J Pers Med. 2021;11(8):745. https://doi.org/10.3390/jpm11080745.
54. Kaur A, Rohilla R, Rana S, Rani S, Prabhakar N. Recent advances in protein biomarkers based enzymatic biosensors for non-communicable diseases. TrAC Trends Anal Chem. 2024;174:117683. https://doi.org/10.1016/J.TRAC.2024.117683.
55. Khanmohammadi A, Jalili Ghazizadeh A, Hashemi P, Afkhami A, Arduini F, Bagheri H. An overview to electrochemical biosensors and sensors for the detection of environmental contaminants. J Iran Chem Soc. 2020;17(10):2429–47. https://doi.org/10.1007/s13738-020-01940-z.
56. Korteling JE, van de Boer-Visschedijk GC, Blankendaal RAM, Boonekamp RC, Eikelboom AR. Human- versus artificial intelligence. Front Artif Intell. 2021;4(March):1–13. https://doi.org/10.3389/frai.2021.622364.
57. Kotecha D, Asselbergs FW, Achenbach S, Anker SD, Atar D, Baigent C, Banerjee A, Beger B, Brobert G, Casadei B, Ceccarelli C, Cowie MR, Crea F, Cronin M, Denaxas S, Derix A, Fitzsimons D, Fredriksson M, Gale CP, et al. CODE-EHR best-practice framework for the use of structured electronic health-care records in clinical research. Lancet Digit Health. 2022;4(10):e757–64. https://doi.org/10.1016/S2589-7500(22)00151-0.
58. Kula MR. Advances in biochemical engineering. Bioelectrochem Bioenerg. 1980;7(2). https://doi.org/10.1016/0302-4598(80)87020-6.
59. Kulkarni MB, Ayachit NH, Aminabhavi TM. Biosensors and microfluidic biosensors: from fabrication to application. Biosensors. 2022;12(7). https://doi.org/10.3390/bios12070543.
60. Kumar Y, Koul A, Singla R, Ijaz MF. Artificial intelligence in disease diagnosis: a systematic literature review, synthesizing framework and future research agenda. J Ambient Intell Humaniz Comput. 2023;14(7):8459–86. https://doi.org/10.1007/s12652-021-03612-z.
61. Lee HA, Kung HH, Lee YJ, Chao JCJ, Udayasankaran JG, Fan HC, Ng KK, Chang YK, Kijsanayotin B, Marcelo AB, Hsu CY. Global infectious disease surveillance and case tracking system for COVID-19: development study. JMIR Med Inform. 2020;8(12):1–18. https://doi.org/10.2196/20567.
62. Leibig C, Brehmer M, Bunk S, Byng D, Pinker K, Umutlu L. Combining the strengths of radiologists and AI for breast cancer screening: a retrospective analysis. Lancet Digit Health. 2022;4(7):e507–19. https://doi.org/10.1016/S2589-7500(22)00070-X.
63. Leite GS, Albuquerque AB, Pinheiro PR. Applications of technological solutions in primary ways of preventing transmission of respiratory infectious diseases—a systematic literature review. Int J Environ Res Public Health. 2021;18(20):10765. https://doi.org/10.3390/ijerph182010765.
64. Leva-Bueno J, Peyman SA, Millner PA. A review on impedimetric immunosensors for pathogen and biomarker detection. Med Microbiol Immunol. 2020;209(3):343–62. https://doi.org/10.1007/s00430-020-00668-0.

65. Li Z, Zhang J, Huang Y, Zhai J, Liao G, Wang Z, Ning C. Development of electroactive materials-based immunosensor towards early-stage cancer detection. Coord Chem Rev. 2022;471:214723. https://doi.org/10.1016/J.CCR.2022.214723.
66. Lin X, Li X, Lin X. A review on applications of computational methods in drug screening and design. Molecules. 2020;25(6):1–17. https://doi.org/10.3390/molecules25061375.
67. Lin Y, Bariya M, Javey A. Wearable biosensors for body computing. Adv Funct Mater. 2021;31(39):1–21. https://doi.org/10.1002/adfm.202008087.
68. Lu L, Zhang J, Xie Y, Gao F, Xu S, Wu X, Ye Z. Wearable health devices in health care: narrative systematic review. JMIR Mhealth Uhealth. 2020;8(11):e18907. https://doi.org/10.2196/18907.
69. Manickam P, Mariappan SA, Murugesan SM, Hansda S, Kaushik A, Shinde R, Thipperudraswamy SP. Artificial Intelligence (AI) and Internet of Medical Things (IoMT) assisted biomedical systems for intelligent healthcare. Biosensors. 2022;12(8):562. https://doi.org/10.3390/bios12080562.
70. Mansour RF, El Amraoui A, Nouaouri I, DIaz VG, Gupta D, Kumar S. Artificial intelligence and internet of things enabled disease diagnosis model for smart healthcare systems. IEEE Access. 2021;9:45137–46. https://doi.org/10.1109/ACCESS.2021.3066365.
71. Marziyeh Ghoreshi Beyrami S, Ghaderyan P. A robust, cost-effective and non- invasive computer-aided method for diagnosis three types of neurodegenerative diseases with gait signal analysis. Measurement. 2020;156:107579. https://doi.org/10.1016/J.MEASUREMENT.2020.107579.
72. Masso J, Pino FJ, Pardo C, García F, Piattini M. Risk management in the software life cycle: a systematic literature review. Comput Stand Interfaces. 2020;71(March 2019):103431. https://doi.org/10.1016/j.csi.2020.103431.
73. Mebrahtu TF, Skyrme S, Randell R, Keenan AM, Bloor K, Yang H, Andre D, Ledward A, King H, Thompson C. Effects of computerised clinical decision support systems (CDSS) on nursing and allied health professional performance and patient outcomes: a systematic review of experimental and observational studies. BMJ Open. 2021;11(12). https://doi.org/10.1136/bmjopen-2021-053886.
74. Mhasawade V, Zhao Y, Chunara R. Machine learning and algorithmic fairness in public and population health. Nat Machine Intell. 2021;3(8):659–66. https://doi.org/10.1038/s42256-021-00373-4.
75. Mottini C, Napolitano F, Li Z, Gao X, Cardone L. Computer-aided drug repurposing for cancer therapy: approaches and opportunities to challenge anticancer targets. Semin Cancer Biol. 2021;68:59–74. https://doi.org/10.1016/J.SEMCANCER.2019.09.023.
76. Muhiyaddin R, Abd-Alrazaq AA, Househ M, Alam T, Shah Z. The impact of Clinical Decision Support Systems (CDSS) on physicians: a scoping review. Stud Health Technol Inform. 2020;272:470–3. https://doi.org/10.3233/SHTI200597.
77. Newaz AI, Sikder AK, Rahman MA, Uluagac AS. A survey on security and privacy issues in modern healthcare systems. ACM Trans Comput Healthc. 2021;2(3):1–44. https://doi.org/10.1145/3453176.
78. O'Brien C, Varty K, Ignaszak A. The electrochemical detection of bioterrorism agents: a review of the detection, diagnostics, and implementation of sensors in biosafety programs for Class A bioweapons. Microsyst Nanoeng. 2021;7(1):16. https://doi.org/10.1038/s41378-021-00242-5.
79. Özdemir V, Arga KY, Aziz RK, Bayram M, Conley SN, Dandara C, Endrenyi L, Fisher E, Garvey CK, Hekim N, Kunej T, Şardaş S, Von Schomberg R, Yassin AS, YIlmaz G, Wang W. Digging deeper into precision/personalized medicine: cracking the sugar code, the third alphabet of life, and sociomateriality of the cell. OMICS. 2020;24(2):62–80. https://doi.org/10.1089/omi.2019.0220.
80. Park M, Heo YJ. Biosensing technologies for chronic diseases. Biochip J. 2021;15(1):1–13. https://doi.org/10.1007/s13206-021-00014-3.

81. Pearson JE, Gill A, Vadgama P. Analytical aspects of biosensors. Ann Clin Biochem. 2000;37(2):119–45. https://doi.org/10.1258/0004563001899131.
82. Prabhu Kavin B, Ganapathy S, Suthanthiramani P, Kannan A. A modified digital signature algorithm to improve the biomedical image integrity in cloud environment. In: Advances in computational techniques for biomedical image analysis: methods and applications (Issue January); 2020. https://doi.org/10.1016/B978-0-12-820024-7.00013-X.
83. Pullano SA, Greco M, Bianco MG, Foti D, Brunetti A, Fiorillo AS. Glucose biosensors in clinical practice: principles, limits and perspectives of currently used devices. Theranostics. 2022;12(2):493–511. https://doi.org/10.7150/thno.64035.
84. Purohit B, Vernekar PR, Shetti NP, Chandra P. Biosensor nanoengineering: design, operation, and implementation for biomolecular analysis. Sensors Int. 2020;1(September):100040. https://doi.org/10.1016/j.sintl.2020.100040.
85. Rasheed K, Qayyum A, Ghaly M, Al-Fuqaha A, Razi A, Qadir J. Explainable, trustworthy, and ethical machine learning for healthcare: a survey. Comput Biol Med. 2022;149:106043. https://doi.org/10.1016/J.COMPBIOMED.2022.106043.
86. Rayan RA, Tsagkaris C, Zafar I, Moysidis DV, Papazoglou AS. Big data analytics for health. In: Big data analytics for healthcare: datasets, techniques, life cycles, management, and applications; 2022. p. 83–92. https://doi.org/10.1016/B978-0-323-91907-4.00002-9.
87. Rodrigues JF, Florea L, de Oliveira MCF, Diamond D, Oliveira ON. Big data and machine learning for materials science. Discov Mater. 2021;1(1):12. https://doi.org/10.1007/s43939-021-00012-0.
88. Rosenfeld R, Tibshirani RJ. Epidemic tracking and forecasting: lessons learned from a tumultuous year. Proc Natl Acad Sci USA. 2021;118(51):1–6. https://doi.org/10.1073/pnas.2111456118.
89. Sadybekov AV, Katritch V. Computational approaches streamlining drug discovery. Nature. 2023;616(7958):673–85. https://doi.org/10.1038/s41586-023-05905-z.
90. Sargazi S, Fatima I, Hassan Kiani M, Mohammadzadeh V, Arshad R, Bilal M, Rahdar A, Díez-Pascual AM, Behzadmehr R. Fluorescent-based nanosensors for selective detection of a wide range of biological macromolecules: a comprehensive review. Int J Biol Macromol. 2022;206:115–47. https://doi.org/10.1016/J.IJBIOMAC.2022.02.137.
91. Sarker B, Bin Sharif N, Atikur Rahman M, Shahariar Parvez AHM. AI, IoMT and Blockchain in healthcare. J Trends Comput Sci Smart Technol. 2023;5(1):30–50. https://doi.org/10.36548/jtcsst.2023.1.003.
92. Sarwar T, Seifollahi S, Chan J, Zhang X, Aksakalli V, Hudson I, Verspoor K, Cavedon L. The secondary use of electronic health records for data mining: data characteristics and challenges. ACM Comput Surv. 2023;55(2):1. https://doi.org/10.1145/3490234.
93. Selvaraj S, Sundaravaradhan S. Challenges and opportunities in IoT healthcare systems: a systematic review. SN Appl Sci. 2020;2(1):1–8. https://doi.org/10.1007/s42452-019-1925-y.
94. Sempionatto JR, Lasalde-Ramírez JA, Mahato K, Wang J, Gao W. Wearable chemical sensors for biomarker discovery in the omics era. Nat Rev Chem. 2022;6(12):899–915. https://doi.org/10.1038/s41570-022-00439-w.
95. Seshadri DR, Davies EV, Harlow ER, Hsu JJ, Knighton SC, Walker TA, Voos JE, Drummond CK. Wearable sensors for COVID-19: a call to action to harness our digital infrastructure for remote patient monitoring and virtual assessments. Front Digital Health. 2020;2(June):1–11. https://doi.org/10.3389/fdgth.2020.00008.
96. Shah P, Kendall F, Khozin S, Goosen R, Hu J, Laramie J, Ringel M, Schork N. Artificial intelligence and machine learning in clinical development: a translational perspective. Npj Digit Med. 2019;2(1):69. https://doi.org/10.1038/s41746-019-0148-3.
97. Shah JL, Bhat HF, Khan AI. Integration of cloud and IoT for smart e- healthcare. In: Healthcare paradigms in the internet of things ecosystem (Issue January 2021); 2020. https://doi.org/10.1016/B978-0-12-819664-9.00006-5.

98. Shaik T, Tao X, Higgins N, Li L, Gururajan R, Zhou X, Acharya UR. Remote patient monitoring using artificial intelligence: current state, applications, and challenges. Wiley Interdiscip Rev: Data Min Knowl Discov. 2023;13(2):1–31. https://doi.org/10.1002/widm.1485.
99. Sharma N, Mangla M, Mohanty SN, Gupta D, Tiwari P, Shorfuzzaman M, Rawashdeh M. A smart ontology-based IoT framework for remote patient monitoring. Biomed Signal Process Control. 2021;68:102717. https://doi.org/10.1016/J.BSPC.2021.102717.
100. Shinde R, Juwarwala I, Modi V, Chandarana V. Utility of cardiac biomarkers and biosensors for diagnosis of acute myocardial infarction. Glob Transl Med. 2023;2(2):0403. https://doi.org/10.36922/gtm.0403.
101. Shukla SD, Vanka KS, Chavelier A, Shastri MD, Tambuwala MM, Bakshi HA, Pabreja K, Mahmood MQ, O'Toole RF. Chronic respiratory diseases: an introduction and need for novel drug delivery approaches. In: Targeting chronic inflammatory lung diseases using advanced drug delivery systems. Elsevier Inc.; 2020. https://doi.org/10.1016/B978-0-12-820658-4.00001-7.
102. Siddiq M. ML-based medical image analysis for anomaly detection in CT scans, X-rays, and MRIs. Devotion J Res Community Service. 2020;2(1):53–64. https://doi.org/10.59188/devotion.v3i13.469.
103. Singh S, Kumar V, Dhanjal DS, Datta S, Prasad R, Singh J. Biological biosensors for monitoring and diagnosis; 2020. p. 317–35. https://doi.org/10.1007/978-981-15-2817-0_14.
104. Singh AK, Mittal S, Das M, Saharia A, Tiwari M. Optical biosensors: a decade in review. Alex Eng J. 2023;67:673–91. https://doi.org/10.1016/J.AEJ.2022.12.040.
105. Singha A, Thakur RS, Patel T. Deep learning applications in medical image analysis. In: Biomedical Data Mining for Information Retrieval (Issue August); 2021. https://doi.org/10.1002/9781119711278.ch11.
106. Stead WW, Lin HS. Computational technology for effective health care: immediate steps and strategic directions; 2009. p. 1–120. https://doi.org/10.17226/12572.
107. Stewart MT, Hogan TP, Nicklas J, Robinson SA, Purington CM, Miller CJ, Vimalananda VG, Connolly SL, Wolfe HL, Nazi KM, Netherton D, Shimada SL. The promise of patient portals for individuals living with chronic illness: qualitative study identifying pathways of patient engagement. J Med Internet Res. 2020;22(7):1–10. https://doi.org/10.2196/17744.
108. Suresh Kumar V, Krishnamoorthi C. Development of electrical transduction based wearable tactile sensors for human vital signs monitor: fundamentals, methodologies and applications. Sensors Actuators A Phys. 2021;321:112582. https://doi.org/10.1016/J.SNA.2021.112582.
109. Swamy MK. Plant-derived bioactives: chemistry and mode of action. In: Plant-derived bioactives: chemistry and mode of action, June; 2020. p. 1–589. https://doi.org/10.1007/978-981-15-2361-8.
110. Tenison E, Smink A, Redwood S, Darweesh S, Cottle H, Van Halteren A, Van Den Haak P, Hamlin R, Ypinga J, Bloem BR, Ben-Shlomo Y, Munneke M, Henderson E, Portillo MC. Proactive and integrated management and empowerment in Parkinson's disease: designing a new model of care. Parkinson's Dis. 2020:2020. https://doi.org/10.1155/2020/8673087.
111. Tu J, Torrente-Rodríguez RM, Wang M, Gao W. The era of digital health: a review of portable and wearable affinity biosensors. Adv Funct Mater. 2020;30(29):1–30. https://doi.org/10.1002/adfm.201906713.
112. Turvey CL, Fuhrmeister LA, Klein DM, Howren MB, Chasco EE. Patient and provider experience of electronic patient portals and secure messaging in mental health treatment. Telemed e-Health. 2023;28(2):189–98. https://doi.org/10.1089/tmj.2020.0395.Patient.
113. Umlai UKI, Bangarusamy DK, Estivill X, Jithesh PV. Genome sequencing data analysis for rare disease gene discovery. Brief Bioinform. 2022;23(1):1–28. https://doi.org/10.1093/bib/bbab363.
114. Upadhyay S, Hu HF. A qualitative analysis of the impact of electronic health records (EHR) on healthcare quality and safety: clinicians' lived experiences. Health Services Insights. 2022;15. https://doi.org/10.1177/11786329211070722.

115. Valerdi R, Sullivan BP. Engineering systems integration, testing, and validation. In: Handbook of engineering systems design: with 178 figures and 54 tables; 2022. p. 679–708. https://doi.org/10.1007/978-3-030-81159-4_20.
116. Vigneshvar S, Sudhakumari CC, Senthilkumaran B, Prakash H. Recent advances in biosensor technology for potential applications - an overview. Front Bioeng Biotechnol. 2016;4(FEB):1–9. https://doi.org/10.3389/fbioe.2016.00011.
117. Volpato L, del Río Carral M, Senn N, Delefosse MS. General practitioners' perceptions of the use of wearable electronic health monitoring devices: qualitative analysis of risks and benefits. JMIR Mhealth Uhealth. 2021;9(8):e23896. https://doi.org/10.2196/23896.
118. Walonoski J, Hall D, Bates KM, Farris MH, Dagher J, Downs ME, Sivek RT, Wellner B, Gregorowicz A, Hadley M, Campion FX, Levine L, Wacome K, Emmer G, Kemmer A, Malik M, Hughes J, Granger E, Russell S. The "coherent data set": combining patient data and imaging in a comprehensive, synthetic health record. Electronics (Switzerland). 2022;11(8):1199. https://doi.org/10.3390/electronics11081199.
119. Wang Q, Su M, Zhang M, Li R. Integrating digital technologies and public health to fight covid-19 pandemic: key technologies, applications, challenges and outlook of digital healthcare. Int J Environ Res Public Health. 2021;18(11):6053. https://doi.org/10.3390/ijerph18116053.
120. Wang YC, Wu Y, Choi J, Allington G, Zhao S, Khanfar M, Yang K, Fu PY, Wrubel M, Yu X, Mekbib KY, Ocken J, Smith H, Shohfi J, Kahle KT, Lu Q, Jin SC. Computational genomics in the era of precision medicine: applications to variant analysis and gene therapy. J Personal Med. 2022;12(2):175. https://doi.org/10.3390/jpm12020175.
121. Wang X, Zhou J, Wang H. Bioreceptors as the key components for electrochemical biosensing in medicine. Cell Rep Phys Sci. 2024;5(2):101801. https://doi.org/10.1016/j.xcrp.2024.101801.
122. Williams A, Aguilar MR, Pattiya Arachchillage KGG, Chandra S, Rangan S, Ghosal Gupta S, Artes Vivancos JM. Biosensors for public health and environmental monitoring: the case for sustainable biosensing. ACS Sustain Chem Eng. 2024;12(28):10296–312. https://doi.org/10.1021/acssuschemeng.3c06112.
123. Woodall T, Ramage M, LaBruyere JT, McLean W, Tak CR. Telemedicine services during COVID-19: considerations for medically underserved populations. J Rural Health. 2021;37(1):231–4. https://doi.org/10.1111/jrh.12466.
124. Wu J, Liu H, Chen W, Ma B, Ju H. Device integration of electrochemical biosensors. Nat Rev Bioeng. 2023;1(5):346–60. https://doi.org/10.1038/s44222-023-00032-w.
125. Zeadally S, Bello O. Harnessing the power of internet of things based connectivity to improve healthcare. Internet of Things. 2021;14:100074. https://doi.org/10.1016/J.IOT.2019.100074.
126. Zhao T, Hu Y, Valsdottir LR, Zang T, Peng J. Identifying drug-target interactions based on graph convolutional network and deep neural network. Brief Bioinform. 2021;22(2):2141–50. https://doi.org/10.1093/bib/bbaa044.

Chapter 13
Nanocomposites for Implants

Khushi Dedhia, Akhilesh Airun, and Mrinmoy Misra

Abstract This chapter explores the transformative impact of nanocomposites on biomedical implants, emphasizing their enhanced properties and diverse applications across various medical fields. Nanocomposites, which feature nanoscale phases integrated into solid materials, offer significant improvements in mechanical strength, biocompatibility, and bioactivity for implants. The chapter covers advancements in ceramic, polymer, and metallic matrix nanocomposites, highlighting their roles in orthopedic, dental, and surgical implants, with particular focus on antimicrobial coatings to combat infection and enhance implant longevity. It also examines specialized nanoimplants for neurological, cardiovascular, and drug delivery applications, showcasing how nanocomposites enable precise targeting, controlled drug release, and improved integration with biological tissues. Overall, the chapter illustrates how nanocomposite technology is revolutionizing implant design and functionality, leading to more effective and safer medical treatment.

Keywords Nanocomposite · Nanoimplants · Medical Fields · Biocompatibility · Coating

13.1 Introduction to Nanocomposites for Implants

A nanocomposite is a solid material with multiple phases, where one of the phases has dimensions of less than 100 nanometers. There are many types of nanocomposite implants such as ceramic, polymer, and metallic matrix nanocomposites, which offer a wide range of properties with different chemical and mechanical features [9, 24, 25]. They also exhibit indispensable bioactivity. These biomedical implants can

K. Dedhia · A. Airun · M. Misra (✉)
Mechatronics Engineering Department, School of Engineering, Manipal University Jaipur, Jaipur, India
e-mail: mrinmoy.mishra@jaipur.manipal.edu

S. Mondal et al. (eds.), *Smart and Sustainable Nanomaterials in Digital Healthcare and Theranostic*, https://doi.org/10.1007/978-981-95-9386-6_13

be implanted in orthopedic, dental, and surgical applications. Orthopedic implants are extensively employed across various clinical applications, including soft tissue reconstruction, joint replacement, bone repair and regeneration, artificial bone substitutes, and dental implants. For these implants, this material should possess various features and capabilities such as antibacterial, anti-corrosive, and illness-free. These capabilities of nanocomposites will be developed by mixing some types of materials in nanocomposites. Such properties can be tailored in nanocomposites by incorporating functional constituents such as Zn, Ag, polymers, oxides, and engineered alloys, alongside traditional biomedical metals like cobalt–chromium, stainless steel, and titanium-based alloys [32].

Medical alloys based on zinc (Zn) are thought to be biodegradable substances with a lot of promise. Zinc alloy systems that have osteogenic qualities can be enhanced by hydroxyapatite (HA). Zinc is necessary for gene expression, signal transduction, and the synthesis and mineralization of new bone in the human body. On the other hand, excessive concentrations of zinc ions on the surface of zinc alloy implants may obstruct cell adherence and proliferation, delaying osseointegration. By altering the surface of Zn alloy implants to create a coating with superior biocompatibility [14, 28, 30]. Due to its low modulus of elasticity equivalent to human bone and superior biodegradability in physiological conditions, magnesium alloy implants have drawn a lot of attention. However, Mg-based implants break down more quickly than is usually necessary for bone repair. This could lead to an increase in humoral pH and an early loss of mechanical integrity before bone mending and regeneration occur.

As we know, the implants are medical devices that replace or support damaged tissues and organs. They have a range of advantages and disadvantages. Orthopedic implants, like bone plates and joint replacements, aid in pain relief and mobility restoration, but they may eventually develop problems like infection or implant failure. While neurological implants, such as cochlear implants or deep brain stimulators, enhance abilities like hearing, movement, and cognition, they also come with risks like high costs, malfunctioning devices, and surgical complications. Dental implants offer a long-term solution for missing teeth, improving both function and appearance. However, if not properly maintained, they may be vulnerable to infection and bone loss. Although they guarantee healthy heart function, cardiovascular implants like pacemakers and stents can have problems like blood clots or battery drain. Implants greatly enhance patients' quality of life, but they can also present problems, such as rejection risk, device malfunction, and ongoing maintenance needs. The benefits, limitation and examples of different type implants are mentioned in Table 13.1.

Table 13.1 Different type benefits, limitation and examples of implants

Application	Benefits	Limitations	Examples
Bone implants	(a) Enhanced biocompatibility and osseointegration (b) Increased mechanical strength (c) Improved wear and corrosion resistance	(a) Potential toxicity of nanoparticles (b) Challenges in achieving uniform dispersion	(a) Hydroxyapatite (HA)/carbon nanotube (CNT) nanocomposites for bone regeneration (b) Nanotitanium coatings
Dental implants	(a) Reduced risk of bacterial infection (b) Improved integration with jawbone Longer implant lifespan	(a) Risk of nanoparticle leaching (b) Expensive manufacturing	Titanium dioxide (TiO_2) nanocomposites for antibacterial surfaces
Joint replacement implants	(a) High wear resistance (b) Reduced risk of implant loosening (c) Improved load-bearing capacity	(a) Risk of mechanical failure if nanoparticles agglomerate (b) Long-term biostability concerns	Ultra-high-molecular-weight polyethylene (UHMWPE) reinforced with carbon nanotubes
Craniofacial implants	(a) Enhanced aesthetic and mechanical properties (b) Lightweight materials (c) Faster tissue integration	(a) Limited clinical trials (b) Complex fabrication methods	(a) Bioactive glass-ceramic nanocomposites (b) Polymeric nanocomposites reinforced with HA
Cardiovascular stents	(a) Controlled drug release to prevent restenosis Reduced thrombosis risk Enhanced flexibility	(a) Complex manufacturing of nano-coatings (b) Limited long-term performance data	(a) Polymer nanocomposites with drug-eluting properties (b) TiO_2 nanocomposites for biocompatible coatings
Spinal implants	(a) Improved strength-to-weight ratio (b) Reduced implant failure rates (c) Accelerated bone fusion	(a) High cost of materials (b) Regulatory hurdles for clinical use	(a) HA-reinforced polymer composites for spinal cages (b) Graphene oxide coatings for spinal fixation devices
Cochlear implants	(a) Improved biocompatibility for long-term use (b) Lightweight design (c) Enhanced conductivity for signal transfer	(a) Complexity in nano-coating application (b) Expensive production techniques	Conductive polymer nanocomposites with carbon nanotubes

(continued)

Table 13.1 (continued)

Application	Benefits	Limitations	Examples
Vascular grafts	(a) Improved flexibility and mechanical stability (b) Enhanced hemocompatibility (c) Resistance to clot formation	(a) Durability under high-pressure blood flow (b) Manufacturing and sterilization challenges	Electrospun polymer nanocomposites with silver nanoparticles
Neurological implants	(a) Restore lost functions (b) Provide effective pain management through neural stimulation (c) Improve quality of life and daily independence (d) Minimally invasive with reduced recovery time (e) Offer targeted, precise therapy with fewer side effects. (f) Provide long-term symptom management	(a) Surgical risks like infection and nerve damage (b) Potential device malfunctions or failure. (c) Limited lifespan, requiring replacement (d) Invasive nature causing discomfort (e) Risk of tissue rejection	(a) Gold nanoparticles for improving the biocompatibility (b) Graphene-based materials used in neural implants for enhanced signal transmission (c) Silicon nanowires for high-performance neural probes in brain-machine interfaces

13.2 Preparation of Coatings for Implants

These coatings need to be done in lab and then after getting ready they will be ready for implants. Coating implants involves lab-based techniques like Micro Arc Oxidation (MAO), also known as Plasma Electrolytic Oxidation (PEO) [6, 12]. MAO creates oxide coatings on metals such as titanium (Ti) by applying high voltage (up to 600 V) in an alkaline electrolyte, such as diluted KOH. The process consists of three main stages: first, electrochemical oxidation occurs as the metal acts as the anode in the electrolyte, leading to the formation of an oxide layer; second, plasma chemistry is involved, where increasing voltage generates spark discharges that produce a high-temperature plasma, affecting the coating's chemical properties; and third, thermal diffusion happens as the high temperatures from the sparks enhance diffusion within the electrolyte, altering the coating's composition and structure. The MAO process typically uses stainless steel cathodes, with treatment times ranging from 5 to 180 minutes, current densities between 500 and 2000 A/m^2, and voltages up to 1000 V.

13.2.1 PLA-nHA Coatings for Implants

Poly(lactic acid) (PLA) is a widely used biodegradable polymer in medical implants, but its hydrophobic nature and limited bioactivity can impact its performance [3, 4]. To enhance PLA's suitability for implants, researchers incorporate nanohydroxy-apatite (nHA)—a bioceramic similar to natural bone mineral-into the PLA matrix, creating PLA-nHA coatings. These coatings offer several advantages:

- *Enhanced Biocompatibility*: nHA significantly improves the biocompatibility of PLA, facilitating better integration with surrounding bone tissue.
- *Increased Osseoconductivity*: By promoting bone growth on the surface, nHA enhances the material's ability to support and encourage new bone formation.
- *Controlled Degradation*: The inclusion of nHA allows for a more controlled degradation of PLA, aligning the breakdown rate of the implant with the rate of bone tissue regeneration.

13.2.2 Methods for Preparing PLA-nHA Coatings

PLA-nHA coatings can be prepared using three main methods: solvent casting, where PLA and nHA are dissolved in a solvent, applied to the implant, and left to dry, forming a thin film; electrospinning, which uses an electric field to create fine PLA-nHA nanofibers that form a porous coating on the implant surface; and dip coating, where the implant is dipped in a PLA-nHA solution, and a thin layer of the coating forms as the solvent evaporates [4].

13.3 Antibiotic Coatings

Researchers have developed an Ag nanoparticle (ANPs)/TaC coating for titanium alloy implants using a double cathode glow discharge technique [3]. This coating, with an outer layer rich in Ag and an inner layer containing Ag nanoparticles embedded in a nanoscale TaC matrix, aims to improve the antibacterial properties of implants. The coating showed high hardness and elasticity. Tests against bacteria like Salmonella, E. coli, and S. aureus were conducted after sterilizing samples and incubating the bacteria. In a separate study, gelatin-curcumin nanocomposites were explored as coatings for dental implant healing abutments. Gelatin serves as a biocompatible base, while curcumin provides anti-inflammatory and healing benefits. The combination aims to enhance bone integration, reduce inflammation, and speed up healing. Initial tests showed that the coating is biocompatible and releases curcumin effectively, but more research and clinical trials are needed to confirm its long-term effectiveness and safety.

Additionally, the antibiotic coating methods offer significant benefits in medical applications, particularly in implants and medical devices, by preventing infections. By applying a layer of antibiotics to the surface of implants, such as orthopedic devices or catheters, it helps in the controlled release of the drug and the risk of postoperative infections. This method promotes faster healing, reduces the need for systemic antibiotic treatments, and minimizes the development of antibiotic-resistant bacteria, making it a highly effective strategy for improving patient outcomes and ensuring the longevity of medical implants.

The need for enhanced implants:

I. *Infection Risk:* Bacterial colonization on implant surfaces can lead to infections, a significant complication that can lead to implant failure and additional surgeries.
II. *Biocompatibility Issues:* Some implant materials, while generally safe, may not perfectly integrate with surrounding bone tissue, potentially hindering long-term stability.

Silver-doped MgO nanocomposite coatings: Silver-doped MgO nanocomposite coatings combine silver and magnesium oxide to tackle challenges in implant technology [26]. Silver nanoparticles provide strong antimicrobial properties, reducing the risk of infections, while magnesium oxide (MgO) offers good biocompatibility, promoting better bone integration and potentially degrading at a rate that matches bone regeneration. This dual approach leads to reduced infection rates, improved osseointegration, and biodegradability, which can align with natural bone healing processes. While stainless steel 316 L is widely used in orthopedic implants for its strength and cost-effectiveness, its susceptibility to infections and poor integration with surrounding tissues remain significant issues. Advanced coatings that enhance corrosion resistance, wear resistance, and biological compatibility are crucial for overcoming these limitations and improving implant longevity and performance.

13.4 Antibacterial Coating of Implants

Antimicrobial coatings are a rapidly evolving field with the potential to revolutionize implant success [8, 15, 23]. By continuously refining existing technologies and exploring novel strategies, researchers are paving the way for a future where implants offer long-term functionality with minimal infection risk. Antimicrobial coatings are a rapidly evolving field with the potential to revolutionize implant success. By continuously refining existing technologies and exploring novel strategies, researchers are paving the way for a future where implants offer long-term functionality with minimal infection risk. Furthermore, antibacterial coatings, typically made from materials like silver, copper, or antibiotic-loaded polymers, release antimicrobial agents gradually, inhibiting bacterial growth and biofilm formation on the implant surface. Overall, antibacterial coatings enhance the safety, longevity, and success of medical implants, improving patient outcomes. For example, the antimicrobial properties of silver nanoparticles (Ag NPs) in conjunction with antibiotics have been the subject of numerous investigations [2]. The use of Ag nanoparticles (Ag NPs) in combination with antibiotics such as ampicillin, kanamycin, and chloramphenicol has been reported. Notably, the combination of Ag NPs and chloramphenicol together were found to reduce the growth of S. aureus, S. typhimurium, and E. coli by about 50%. By contrast, the Ag NPs and kanamycin combination inhibited these same bacterial strains by almost 95%. The study came to the conclusion that Ag NPs' disruption of the bacterial membrane's integrity and potential, which raises membrane permeability and facilitates antibiotic penetration, is what gives the combined treatment its increased efficacy. Sublethal concentrations of AgNPs and half the antibiotics' minimum inhibitory concentration were used in these tests.

13.5 Antimicrobial Coatings

Antimicrobial coatings provide crucial protection against infections on implants by preventing bacterial adhesion and growth [1]. They work through several mechanisms: directly killing bacteria with antimicrobial agents like silver nanoparticles, altering the surface chemistry to discourage bacterial colonization, and slowly releasing antimicrobial agents over time. For example, silver nanoparticles can disrupt bacterial cell membranes, bind to proteins, and generate reactive oxygen species, all of which inhibit bacterial growth. In testing, coatings with hierarchical etched surfaces and chitosan, combined with silver oxide nanoparticles, showed significant improvements in antibacterial performance, reducing bacterial colonies by over 86% compared to untreated surfaces. These coatings also foster better calcium phosphate formation, essential for bone integration, mimicking the natural bone structure and potentially enhancing bone healing and stability. Antimicrobial coatings significantly reduce the risk of post-surgical infections, promote faster healing, and minimize the need for systemic antibiotics, ultimately improving the success rate, longevity, and safety of medical implants.

13.6 Types of Nanoimplants

Nanoimplants represent a cutting-edge innovation in the field of medical technology, leveraging the unique properties of nanomaterials to create highly specialized implants that can perform a wide range of functions within the human body. Due to their nanoscale size and remarkable versatility, nanoimplants are increasingly being applied across various medical disciplines, offering new solutions for diagnosis, treatment, and tissue repair. These tiny, yet powerful devices are designed to interact with biological systems at the cellular and molecular levels, enabling precision-targeted therapies, real-time monitoring, and enhanced integration with bodily tissues. Nanoimplants are being developed for a wide range of medical uses, each tailored to address specific challenges. The nanoimplants are categorized as neurological implants, cardiovascular implants, ophthalmic implants, dermal implants, respiratory implants, reproductive implants, ENT (Ear, Nose, and Throat) implants, maxillofacial implants, orthopedic implants, and tissue implants.

13.6.1 Neurological Implants

Neurological implants are highly advanced devices designed to interact directly with the nervous system for diagnostic, therapeutic, or research purposes [22]. They have a wide range of applications, such as recording or stimulating neural activity, delivering drugs or other substances to specific areas of the nervous system, or interfacing with prosthetic devices to restore lost sensory or motor functions. The nanocomposite for neurological implants includes:

13.6.1.1 Deep Brain Stimulation (DBS) Implants

DBS involves implantable electrical stimulation devices that target specific brain regions and mitigate neurological symptoms [5]. It is effective for involuntary movement disorders and is being investigated for use in treating epilepsy, psychiatric conditions, and other ailments. The DBS implants are sophisticated devices used to manage neurological conditions like Parkinson's disease, essential tremor, and dystonia. By sending electrical signals to targeted areas of the brain, these implants help regulate abnormal neural activity, thereby reducing symptoms. Technological advancements have improved the accuracy and functionality of DBS systems, with innovations in electrode design and programming. DBS implants offer a flexible, adjustable treatment option that can provide significant symptom relief for patients with movement disorders and hold potential for treating other neurological issues as well. Nanocomposite materials are revolutionizing deep brain stimulation (DBS) implants by integrating nanoscale elements to enhance their performance across several key areas. These materials, such as graphene or carbon nanotube composites, improve electrical conductivity, allowing for more precise and effective neural stimulation. They also enhance biocompatibility by reducing inflammatory responses and integrate better with brain tissue. Additionally, nanocomposites strengthen mechanical properties and flexibility, ensuring durability and adaptability within the brain. By customizing the properties of these materials, researchers can tailor DBS implants to meet specific patient needs, potentially transforming the field of neurostimulation and improving treatment outcomes for neurological conditions.

13.6.1.2 Neural Prosthetics and Neural Recording Implants

Neural prosthetics represent an advanced field in biomedical technology aimed at restoring lost sensory and motor functions due to injury or disease by directly interfacing with the nervous system. These implants are engineered to bypass or repair damaged neural pathways, helping individuals regain vital abilities such as hearing, vision, and movement. By translating neural signals into actionable outputs, neural prosthetics have the potential to greatly enhance the quality of life for those with disabilities. This area integrates electronics, neuroscience, and rehabilitation to develop devices that seamlessly work with the nervous system. Additionally, neural recording implants play a crucial role in neuroscience research by capturing, amplifying, digitizing, and transmitting brain signals. These implants enable scientists to study neural dynamics, map brain activity, and explore new treatments for neurological disorders [16, 19]. The nanocomposite materials are transforming neural prosthetics and neural recording implants by enhancing their electrical properties, biocompatibility, mechanical strength, and signal resolution. This integration of nanotechnology not only improves the performance and longevity of these implants but also paves the way for more personalized and effective treatments for neurological conditions [31].

13.6.1.3 Drug Delivery Implants

Localized and site-specific drug delivery is a highly effective method for treating brain diseases compared to traditional systemic drug administration [18]. This approach focuses on administering medication directly to the targeted area within the brain, which reduces the risk of widespread side effects and enhances treatment efficacy. Achieving this precision requires advanced technology and miniaturized implants or devices that allow for controlled drug delivery with minimal invasiveness. These sophisticated systems, often incorporating microelectromechanical systems (MEMS) and advanced materials, enable drugs to be delivered precisely where needed through minimally invasive procedures. The success of this technique hinges on the development of innovative drug delivery technologies that address the specific challenges of targeting precise brain regions while ensuring patient safety and comfort. Nanocomposite materials are revolutionizing drug delivery implants by enhancing their functionality, precision, and overall effectiveness. These materials blend nanoscale components with traditional substrates to develop advanced systems with several benefits.

I. *Enhanced Drug Loading and Release Control:*

Nanocomposites improve drug delivery by allowing precise control over how drugs are loaded and released. Materials like mesoporous silica nanoparticles or polymer-based composites can be engineered with large surface areas and adjustable pore sizes, enabling significant drug loading and controlled, sustained release.

This customization ensures drugs are delivered at consistent and optimal rates over time.

II. *Targeted Delivery and Specificity:*

A major advantage of nanocomposites is their ability to enhance targeting accuracy. By attaching specific ligands or antibodies to nanocomposites, drug delivery systems can precisely target particular cells or tissues. This targeted approach reduces off-target effects and improves therapeutic efficacy, as seen with drugs directed to cancerous cells or inflamed areas, thereby improving treatment outcomes and minimizing side effects.

III. *Biocompatibility and Reduced Toxicity:*

Nanocomposites can be designed to improve the biocompatibility of drug delivery implants, mitigating potential toxicity and adverse reactions. Integrating biocompatible materials, such as biodegradable polymers or metals, helps ensure that the implants are well-tolerated by the body. These materials can also be crafted to degrade over time, reducing long-term toxicity and easing removal if necessary.

IV. *Versatile Delivery Mechanisms:*

Nanocomposites support various drug delivery methods, including oral, injectable, and implantable systems. They can enhance drug solubility and stability for oral and injectable routes, leading to better absorption and bioavailability. For implantable systems, nanocomposites enable localized drug release at the target site, providing effective therapy while minimizing systemic exposure.

V. *Stability and Extended Shelf Life:*

Nanocomposites also improve the stability and shelf life of drug formulations. Encapsulating drugs within nanocomposite materials can protect them from environmental degradation due to factors like light or moisture, thus extending their effectiveness over longer periods.

VI. *Customizable Features:*

The flexibility of nanocomposites allows for customization to meet specific drug and delivery needs. Researchers can modify the size, surface properties, and composition of these materials to create specialized drug delivery systems that cater to particular therapeutic requirements.

Research into nanocomposites for drug delivery continues to explore new methods for increasing delivery efficiency, targeting precision, and ensuring patient safety. Innovations like stimuli-responsive nanocomposites that release drugs in response to environmental changes and hybrid systems combining multiple delivery strategies are being developed, promising further advancements in personalized medicine and targeted therapies. The nanocomposite materials are advancing drug delivery implants by improving control over drug release, enhancing targeting, and boosting biocompatibility. These materials offer versatile and customizable solutions that enhance therapeutic effectiveness and patient safety, leading to more tailored and efficient drug delivery systems.

13.6.2 Cardiovascular Implants

Cardiovascular implants are medical devices designed to treat or manage conditions affecting the heart and blood vessels. These implants play a crucial role in various cardiovascular procedures and treatments. Nanocomposites are significantly advancing cardiovascular implants by improving their functionality, durability, and interaction with biological tissues [29]. These advanced materials combine nanoscale elements with traditional substrates to enhance various aspects of cardiovascular devices such as stents, valves, and vascular grafts. The use of nanocomposite for cardiovascular implants has several benefits as mentioned below.

I. *Enhanced Biocompatibility:*

Nanocomposites can be tailored to enhance the biocompatibility of cardiovascular implants. By integrating nanoscale fillers like carbon nanotubes or nanoparticles with biocompatible polymers, these implants are better able to integrate with surrounding tissues and minimize adverse reactions. This improved compatibility is vital for reducing complications and ensuring the long-term success of the implants.

II. *Improved Mechanical Properties*

The mechanical performance of cardiovascular implants is critical for their functionality. Nanocomposites strengthen and increase the flexibility of traditional materials. For example, composites reinforced with carbon nanotubes or nanoclays offer superior mechanical properties, making the implants more robust and adaptable to the stresses of the cardiovascular system.

III. *Advanced Drug Delivery and Coatings*

Nanocomposites enable the development of sophisticated drug-eluting coatings for cardiovascular implants. These coatings can release medications like anticoagulants or anti-inflammatory drugs in a controlled manner directly at the site of the implant. This targeted drug delivery can help prevent issues such as restenosis and support more effective healing.

IV. *Enhanced Imaging and Diagnostics*

Nanocomposites can also improve imaging and diagnostic capabilities for cardiovascular implants. Incorporating nanoparticles with contrast-enhancing properties into implant materials can provide clearer, more detailed images during diagnostic procedures. This improvement facilitates better monitoring of the implant's condition and the patient's health.

V. *Reduced Thrombogenicity:*

Minimizing the risk of blood clot formation is crucial for cardiovascular implants. Nanocomposites can be designed with properties that reduce thrombogenicity. By incorporating anticoagulant agents or modifying surface coatings at the nanoscale, these materials help prevent blood clots and maintain the implant's functionality over time.

VI. *Customization and Versatility:*

The flexibility of nanocomposites allows for precise customization of cardiovascular implants. Researchers can adjust the size, composition, and surface features of these materials to meet specific therapeutic needs or patient conditions. This adaptability results in more personalized and effective cardiovascular devices.

13.6.3 Ophthalmic Implants

Nanocomposites are increasingly influencing the field of ophthalmic implants by offering substantial improvements in performance, biocompatibility, and functionality [20]. These advanced materials blend nanoscale components with traditional substrates to address various challenges in ophthalmology, providing innovative solutions for drug delivery, mechanical reinforcement, and optical enhancement. Biocompatibility is critical for ophthalmic implants due to the sensitive nature of eye tissues. Nanocomposites enhance biocompatibility by incorporating biocompatible nanoscale materials such as titanium dioxide, silica nanoparticles, or graphene into implant matrices. These materials help to minimize inflammatory responses and irritation, ensuring that the implants integrate seamlessly with the eye's delicate structures. By improving tissue compatibility, nanocomposites reduce the risk of complications and improve patient comfort. Nanocomposites revolutionize drug delivery in ophthalmic implants by enabling controlled and sustained release of therapeutic agents. Drug-eluting contact lenses or intraocular lenses can be coated with nanocomposites designed to gradually release medications such as anti-inflammatory drugs, antibiotics, or growth factors. This controlled delivery system enhances the therapeutic efficacy of the implants, reduces the need for frequent drug administration, and supports more effective management of chronic eye conditions or postoperative care. The mechanical integrity of ophthalmic implants is vital for their performance and longevity. Nanocomposites can significantly enhance the mechanical properties of these implants. By reinforcing traditional materials with nanoscale fillers like carbon nanotubes, graphene, or nanoclays, researchers can develop implants with improved strength, durability, and flexibility. This enhancement is crucial for devices such as corneal implants or lens replacements, which must withstand the dynamic conditions of the eye while maintaining their functionality. Nanocomposites can also be engineered to optimize the optical properties of ophthalmic implants. Nanoscale materials such as gold or silver nanoparticles can be integrated to enhance light transmission and minimize optical distortions. This optimization is essential for intraocular lenses, artificial corneas, and other optical implants, ensuring they provide clear and accurate visual acuity without interfering with natural vision. Incorporating nanocomposites into ophthalmic implants can enhance imaging and diagnostic capabilities. Nanoparticles with contrast-enhancing properties can be integrated into implants to improve the quality of images obtained during diagnostic procedures. Enhanced imaging allows for more precise monitoring of implant performance and better assessment of the patient's condition, facilitating accurate diagnoses and effective treatment planning. Further, nanocomposites contribute to reducing the risk of complications associated with ophthalmic implants. Materials with inherent antimicrobial properties, such as those incorporating silver nanoparticles, can help prevent infections around the implant site. Additionally, nanocomposites with anti-fogging properties can be used in lenses to prevent cloudiness, improving the implant's longevity and performance. Furthermore, the versatility of nanocomposites allows for the customization of ophthalmic implants to meet specific patient needs. By adjusting the size, surface properties, and composition of nanocomposites, researchers can develop implants that address individual conditions or preferences. This adaptability enables the creation of highly specialized and effective ophthalmic solutions tailored to the unique requirements of each patient. Future research into nanocomposites for ophthalmic implants is poised to explore new frontiers in the field. Innovations such as stimuli-responsive materials, which release drugs or change properties in response to environmental cues, and multi-functional implants that integrate therapeutic and diagnostic capabilities are on the horizon. These advancements promise to further enhance the performance, safety, and effectiveness of ophthalmic implants, paving the way for more sophisticated and personalized eye care solutions. Nanocomposites are significantly advancing ophthalmic implants by improving biocompatibility, drug delivery, mechanical strength, and optical performance. Their ability to be customized and their potential for future innovations make them a pivotal area of research for developing cutting-edge solutions in ophthalmology. As the field progresses, nanocomposites are expected to play an increasingly vital role in enhancing the functionality and effectiveness of ophthalmic implants, offering new opportunities for improved patient outcomes and advanced eye care technologies.

13.6.4 Dermal Implants

Dermal implants encompass a wide array of medical devices designed to address various needs, ranging from aesthetic improvements to therapeutic interventions. Dermal fillers are injectable substances, such as hyaluronic acid or collagen, used to add volume, smooth wrinkles, and enhance facial contours, primarily for cosmetic purposes. Implantable drug delivery systems are devices placed beneath the skin to administer medication over an extended period, offering controlled treatment for chronic conditions like pain or hormone deficiencies, with advanced nanoimplants enhancing delivery accuracy. Skin grafts and substitutes are utilized to replace or repair damaged skin from burns or injuries, using natural materials (autografts or allografts) or synthetic biocompatible polymers, with modern versions incorporating nanostructured scaffolds to improve tissue regeneration. Electrodes and sensors are implanted to monitor physiological parameters such as glucose levels in diabetics or enable myoelectric control for prosthetics, providing real-time data essential for health management. Cosmetic implants, including silicone implants for breast augmentation and bioabsorbable implants for facial enhancements, modify physical appearance, offering both cosmetic and reconstructive benefits. These implants play a significant role in both improving aesthetics and addressing critical medical conditions, reflecting their broad applicability and importance in modern medicine. Nanocomposites are significantly advancing dermal implants by enhancing their performance, biocompatibility, and preventing infection [17]. These materials integrate nanoscale components, such as carbon nanotubes, graphene, or nanoparticles, into traditional implant substrates to improve various aspects of dermal implants. Nanocomposites enhance mechanical properties, such as strength and flexibility, which are crucial for ensuring durability and comfort in implants like dermal fillers or prosthetic devices. They also offer superior biocompatibility, reducing the risk of inflammation and promoting better integration with skin tissues. Additionally, nanocomposites can be designed to support controlled drug delivery, releasing medications such as anti-inflammatory agents or growth factors to aid in wound healing and tissue regeneration. This combination of enhanced mechanical performance, biocompatibility, and therapeutic capabilities makes nanocomposites a promising technology for improving the efficacy and safety of dermal implants.

13.6.5 Respiratory Implants

Respiratory implants are a specialized group of medical devices and systems developed to support, monitor, or treat various respiratory conditions. Unlike traditional methods like ventilators and oxygen therapy, which mainly provide external assistance, respiratory implants are more invasive and are typically used when standard treatments are no longer effective. These implants function directly within the body to improve or restore respiratory function, offering solutions for complex and severe conditions. Examples include artificial lungs, which are used when the natural lungs cannot function properly, providing essential support during lung transplants or as a long-term solution for chronic respiratory failure. Bronchial stents are another type, designed to keep airways open, ensuring adequate airflow in patients with obstructions caused by tumors or chronic diseases. Devices like diaphragm pacing systems and phrenic nerve stimulators are used to stimulate the diaphragm or phrenic nerve, helping to maintain or restore breathing in patients with conditions such as spinal cord injuries or central sleep apnea. These implants offer an alternative to mechanical ventilation by directly engaging the body's natural respiratory muscles. In cases of severe lung disease, such as emphysema, lung volume reduction coils compress and reduce damaged lung tissue, enhancing lung function by allowing healthier tissue to expand more effectively. Additionally, implantable pulmonary drug delivery systems are designed to administer medications directly to the lungs, ensuring targeted treatment with minimized systemic side effects. Nanocomposites are revolutionizing respiratory implants by enhancing their functionality, durability, and biocompatibility. These advanced materials, which blend nanoscale components with traditional substrates, offer several key benefits. They improve the mechanical properties of implants, such as strength and flexibility, which are essential for devices like tracheal stents or artificial lungs. Nanocomposites also enhance biocompatibility, reducing the risk of adverse reactions and promoting better integration with the respiratory tissues. Additionally, they can be engineered to provide controlled drug delivery, releasing medications like anti-inflammatory agents or antibiotics directly to the respiratory system, thus aiding in the management of chronic conditions and promoting healing. Furthermore, nanocomposites offer potential advancements in antimicrobial properties, helping to prevent infections associated with respiratory implants. Overall, the integration of nanocomposites in respiratory implants enhances their performance and patient outcomes by improving their mechanical, biological, and therapeutic attributes.

The respiratory implants and their uses are mentioned below.

13.6.5.1 Artificial Lungs

Artificial lungs are advanced medical devices designed to take over the critical function of gas exchange when the natural lungs are unable to do so effectively. These devices are vital for patients experiencing severe respiratory failure, where the lungs can no longer provide adequate oxygen to the bloodstream or remove carbon dioxide efficiently. Artificial lungs can be used both temporarily and for long-term support, depending on the specific needs of the patient. In a temporary role, artificial lungs are often employed during lung transplant procedures. For patients awaiting a transplant or those undergoing surgery, these devices ensure continuous oxygenation and carbon dioxide removal, crucial for maintaining life when the natural lungs are failing or have been removed, and the new lungs are not yet fully operational. For chronic conditions like advanced chronic obstructive pulmonary disease (COPD), pulmonary fibrosis, or acute respiratory distress syndrome (ARDS), artificial lungs can serve as long-term support. They may be used as a bridge to lung transplantation or as a permanent solution when transplantation is not feasible. These devices typically work through systems like extracorporeal membrane oxygenation (ECMO), where blood is circulated outside the body, oxygenated, and then returned. Ongoing advancements in artificial lung technology aim to enhance their efficiency, portability, and compatibility with the body, providing critical respiratory support for patients with life-threatening lung conditions. Nanocomposites are significantly advancing the development of artificial lungs by enhancing their performance, biocompatibility, and overall effectiveness. By incorporating nanoscale materials such as carbon nanotubes, graphene, or silica nanoparticles into traditional materials, nanocomposites improve the mechanical strength and flexibility of artificial lungs, making them more resilient and adaptable to the dynamic conditions of the respiratory system. These materials also enhance gas permeability and exchange efficiency, which is crucial for the effective oxygenation of blood. Additionally, nanocomposites can be engineered to optimize biocompatibility, reducing the risk of immune response and improving integration with lung tissues. Furthermore, they can support controlled drug delivery, enabling the release of medications that can help manage complications or support lung function. Collectively, these improvements make nanocomposites a promising technology for developing more effective and reliable artificial lungs, contributing to better patient outcomes and quality of life for those with severe respiratory conditions.

13.6.6 ENT (Ear, Nose, Throat) Implants

ENT (Ear, Nose, and Throat) implants are specialized medical devices designed to treat conditions affecting the ear, nose, and throat regions. Key types include cochlear implants, which provide sound to those with severe hearing loss by stimulating the auditory nerve; bone-anchored hearing aids (BAHA), which transmit sound through the skull bone for individuals with conductive hearing loss; and sinus implants, which help maintain sinus drainage and reduce symptoms of chronic sinusitis. Other implants include septal implants for correcting nasal septum deviations, tympanostomy tubes for treating ear infections and fluid accumulation, and voice prostheses for restoring speech in patients who have undergone laryngectomy. These devices aim to improve auditory function, nasal airflow, sinus health, and overall quality of life.

Nanocomposites are significantly advancing the field of ENT (Ear, Nose, Throat) implants by improving their biocompatibility, mechanical strength, and overall functionality [13, 27]. These innovative materials blend nanoscale components with traditional implant substrates, offering numerous enhancements across various types of ENT devices, such as hearing aids, nasal implants, and throat prosthetics. Nanocomposites greatly improve the biocompatibility of ENT implants, which is essential for minimizing adverse reactions and ensuring smooth integration with sensitive tissues. By integrating biocompatible nanoscale materials like titanium dioxide or silica into implants, the risk of inflammation and irritation is reduced, allowing for better acceptance by the ear, nose, and throat tissues. The mechanical attributes of ENT implants are crucial for their effectiveness and durability. Nanocomposites reinforce traditional implant materials, such as polymers or metals, with nanoscale fillers like carbon nanotubes or graphene. This reinforcement enhances the strength, flexibility, and longevity of the implants, making them more resistant to wear and tear, which is particularly important for devices such as hearing aids and nasal splints. Nanocomposites enhance the functionality of ENT implants in various ways. For hearing aids, they improve acoustic performance and device efficiency. In nasal implants, they offer better structural support and flexibility, facilitating improved airflow and comfort. For throat prosthetics, nanocomposites increase durability and resistance to infection, ensuring reliable and long-lasting performance. The use of nanocomposites in ENT implants allows for sophisticated drug delivery systems. Drug-eluting nasal implants, for example, can be designed with nanocomposite coatings that provide controlled release of medications like anti-inflammatory agents or antibiotics. This targeted delivery helps manage conditions such as inflammation and infection more effectively and reduces the frequency of medication administration. Nanocomposites can be engineered with inherent antimicrobial properties, which is beneficial for preventing infections in ENT implants. Incorporating nanoparticles like silver or copper helps inhibit microbial growth, reducing the risk of infections and contributing to the long-term success and safety of the implants. Nanocomposites improve imaging and diagnostic capabilities for ENT implants. By integrating nanoparticles that enhance contrast, these materials facilitate clearer and more detailed imaging during diagnostic procedures. This enhancement allows for better monitoring of implant performance and a more accurate assessment of the patient's condition. The adaptability of nanocomposites allows for precise customization of ENT implants to meet individual patient needs. Adjusting the size, composition, and surface characteristics of these materials enables the creation of specialized implants tailored to specific conditions, resulting in more effective and personalized treatment solutions. Ongoing research into nanocomposites for ENT implants is exploring exciting innovations such as self-repairing materials that can mend themselves and smart implants that respond to environmental changes. These advancements hold the promise of further improving the performance and outcomes of ENT devices.

13.6.7 Cochlear Implants

Cochlear implants are advanced electronic devices designed to provide a sense of sound to individuals with severe to profound hearing loss who do not benefit from conventional hearing aids. These implants are surgically placed in the inner ear and work by bypassing damaged or non-functional components of the auditory system. The device consists of a microphone, a speech processor, and an electrode array. The microphone captures sound from the environment, which is then processed into electrical signals by the speech processor. These signals are transmitted to the electrode array implanted in the cochlea, a spiral-shaped structure in the inner ear. The electrodes directly stimulate the auditory nerve fibers, allowing the brain to interpret these signals as sound. This process effectively restores auditory perception and helps users to detect, recognize, and understand sounds, thereby significantly improving their ability to communicate and interact with their surroundings. Nanocomposites are transforming cochlear implants by offering enhanced functionality and performance. By integrating nanoscale materials such as graphene or carbon nanotubes, these advanced composites improve the efficiency of electrical signal transmission, crucial for stimulating auditory nerves accurately.

13.6.7.1 Middle Ear Implants

Middle ear implants are advanced hearing devices implanted surgically to treat hearing loss by directly stimulating the middle ear's structures. Unlike traditional hearing aids that amplify sound to assist hearing, middle ear implants work by transforming sound waves into mechanical vibrations. These devices are designed to interact with the middle ear's natural components, such as the ossicles (the tiny bones in the ear). The implant typically includes a small sensor or microphone that captures sound, a processor that converts this sound into vibrations, and a transducer that transmits these vibrations directly to the ossicles. By bypassing damaged parts of the ear and directly stimulating the middle ear, these implants can improve sound transmission to the inner ear, enhancing auditory perception for individuals with certain types of hearing impairment. This approach can offer a more natural hearing experience compared to the amplified sound produced by conventional hearing aids.

13.6.7.2 Bone-Anchored Hearing Aids (BAHA)

The BAHA are a specialized hearing solution designed to assist individuals with conductive or mixed hearing loss. Unlike traditional hearing aids, which amplify sound, BAHA devices use a different approach to address hearing impairment. The system involves surgically implanting a titanium fixture, often referred to as a fixture or implant, into the bone behind the ear. This titanium post is integrated into the skull bone, creating a stable anchor. The device works by converting sound vibrations into mechanical vibrations, which are transmitted directly through the bone to the inner ear. This method bypasses damaged parts of the ear canal or middle ear and directly stimulates the cochlea, allowing individuals with certain types of hearing loss to perceive sound more effectively. BAHA devices are particularly beneficial for individuals who have conductive hearing loss, where sound transmission through the outer or middle ear is impaired, or mixed hearing loss, which involves both conductive and sensorineural components. For these individuals, who might not gain adequate benefit from conventional air-conduction hearing aids, BAHA offers a viable alternative by providing a clear and direct pathway for sound to reach the inner ear. This can significantly improve auditory experiences and overall communication abilities for those affected by specific hearing impairments. Nanocomposite coatings are revolutionizing Bone-Anchored Hearing Aids (BAHA) by integrating nanoscale materials to address critical challenges. These coatings enhance osseointegration by improving the bond between the implant and bone, ensuring a stable and long-lasting attachment. They also provide increased resistance to environmental factors like moisture and wear, thereby extending the lifespan of the implant. Additionally, nanocomposite coatings can incorporate antimicrobial agents, reducing the risk of infections around the implant site. Their customizable nature allows for tailored surface properties, optimizing the device for individual patient needs and improving overall comfort and functionality.

13.6.7.3 Nasal Stents

Nasal stents are specialized medical devices designed to maintain open nasal passages and improve airflow for patients suffering from nasal obstruction or related conditions. These implants are generally made from biocompatible materials such as silicone, which is chosen for its durability and compatibility with human tissue. The primary function of nasal stents is to keep the nasal passages unobstructed, allowing for improved breathing and reduced symptoms associated with nasal congestion or sleep apnea. The insertion of these stents is typically performed through a minor surgical procedure. Once in place, nasal stents work by physically supporting the nasal passages to prevent them from collapsing or becoming blocked, which can help alleviate symptoms and enhance overall respiratory function. Nasal stents are especially beneficial for individuals who have structural abnormalities, chronic nasal congestion, or conditions that affect airflow through the nasal passages. By ensuring that the nasal passages remain open, these implants can contribute significantly to better breathing, improved sleep quality, and overall comfort for patients dealing with nasal obstructions. Nanocomposites are enhancing nasal stents by improving their functionality and patient comfort. Incorporating nanoscale materials into the stent coatings boosts their mechanical strength and flexibility, ensuring a better fit and durability. These advanced materials also improve biocompatibility, reducing the risk of irritation and promoting seamless integration with nasal tissues. Additionally, nanocomposites can be designed for controlled drug release, providing localized treatment to reduce inflammation and support healing. The incorporation of antimicrobial nanoparticles helps prevent infections, further contributing to the stent's effectiveness and safety.

13.6.7.4 Nasal Valve Implants

Nasal valve implants are advanced medical devices designed to support and stabilize the nasal valve area, which is a critical region within the nasal passages responsible for regulating airflow. The nasal valve is a narrow segment of the nasal airway, and its proper function is essential for maintaining effective breathing. When this area becomes weakened or collapses, it can lead to issues such as nasal congestion and obstructed airflow, which can significantly impact a person's ability to breathe comfortably. These implants are surgically placed within the nasal passages to reinforce the nasal valve, thereby preventing its collapse and improving the flow of air through the nose. By providing structural support to this key area, nasal valve implants help to alleviate symptoms associated with nasal valve dysfunction, such as difficulty breathing, reduced airflow, and chronic nasal congestion. The use of nasal valve implants is particularly beneficial for individuals with structural abnormalities or functional impairments in the nasal valve area, offering a solution for those who do not respond well to non-surgical treatments. These implants work by enhancing the stability of the nasal valve, allowing for more efficient and unobstructed breathing, and thus improving overall respiratory health and quality of life.

Nanocomposites enhance nasal valve implants by improving their mechanical properties, biocompatibility, and performance. The incorporation of nanoscale materials like graphene or titanium dioxide strengthens the implants, ensuring better durability and flexibility. These materials also promote better integration with nasal tissues, reducing irritation and improving comfort. Additionally, nanocomposites can feature controlled drug release for localized treatment and antimicrobial properties to prevent infections, enhancing the overall effectiveness and safety of nasal valve implants.

13.6.7.5 Sinus Implants

Sinus implants are specialized medical devices used to address and manage chronic sinus conditions, such as sinusitis. These implants are designed to be placed within the sinus cavities, where they serve several important functions to aid in the treatment and management of sinus issues. Made from biocompatible materials either absorbable or non-absorbable polymers sinus implants are engineered to integrate seamlessly with the surrounding tissues. Their primary purpose is to provide structural support to the sinus walls, which helps in maintaining proper sinus drainage and reducing the likelihood of blockages. By keeping the sinus passages open, these implants facilitate better airflow and drainage, which can alleviate symptoms and improve overall sinus function. Additionally, sinus implants often play a role in delivering medications directly to the affected areas. This targeted delivery method ensures that the medication is applied precisely where it is needed, potentially increasing its effectiveness while minimizing systemic side effects. For example, some sinus implants are designed to release anti-inflammatory or antimicrobial agents gradually over time, helping to reduce inflammation and combat infection more effectively. Overall, sinus implants are valuable tools in the management of chronic sinus conditions. They help support tissue healing, maintain sinus openness, and enable localized treatment, contributing to improved patient outcomes and quality of life. Nanocomposites are advancing sinus implants by enhancing their biocompatibility, strength, and functionality. These materials integrate nanoscale components to improve the mechanical properties of the implants, ensuring durability and flexibility within the sinus cavity. They also promote better tissue integration, reducing irritation and the risk of adverse reactions. Additionally, nanocomposites can be engineered for controlled drug release, providing targeted treatment to reduce inflammation and support healing, while antimicrobial properties help prevent infections, thereby improving the overall effectiveness and safety of sinus implants.

13.6.7.6 Tracheal and Laryngeal Implants

These implants are designed to support the trachea or larynx, providing crucial assistance when these structures are weakened or damaged. Their primary function is to maintain the integrity of the airway and help preserve vocal function, which is essential for individuals with conditions like tracheomalacia or vocal cord paralysis. Tracheomalacia involves the softening of the trachea's cartilage, which can lead to airway collapse and breathing difficulties. Implants used in such cases work by reinforcing the tracheal walls to prevent collapse, thereby ensuring that the airway remains open and unobstructed. Similarly, for patients with vocal cord paralysis, these implants can stabilize the larynx, which helps in sustaining normal vocalization and preventing voice loss. By providing structural reinforcement, these implants help restore normal airflow and support effective communication. They are particularly valuable in cases where conventional treatments might not be sufficient, offering an enhanced quality of life through improved respiratory and vocal capabilities. Nanocomposites are advancing tracheal and laryngeal implants by integrating nanoscale materials to enhance various aspects of these devices. These advanced coatings improve the structural integrity and flexibility of implants, allowing them to withstand the stresses of breathing and vocalization [33]. They also facilitate superior integration with the surrounding tissues, minimizing irritation and promoting natural healing. Additionally, nanocomposites can incorporate specific functional features, such as drug-eluting properties for targeted therapeutic delivery or antimicrobial agents to reduce infection risks, thereby optimizing the performance and safety of tracheal and laryngeal implants.

13.6.8 Dental Implants

Dental implants are a prominent type of maxillofacial implant specifically designed to replace missing teeth by surgically embedding artificial tooth roots into the jawbone [7]. This procedure begins with the placement of a small titanium post or screw into the bone, which acts as a stable foundation for attaching dental prosthetics. Over time, the implant integrates with the bone through a process called osseointegration, creating a strong and durable base. Once the implant has securely fused with the bone, it can support various types of dental restorations such as crowns, bridges, or dentures. Crowns are individual replacement teeth that are placed on top of the implant, while bridges consist of multiple crowns connected together to replace several adjacent missing teeth. Dentures, which can be either partial or complete, are removable appliances designed to replace multiple teeth. The use of dental implants offers several advantages over traditional tooth replacement options. They provide a more natural appearance and function by mimicking the look and feel of natural teeth. Additionally, dental implants help preserve the integrity of the jawbone by stimulating bone growth, which can prevent the bone loss that often occurs after tooth loss. This preservation of bone structure also helps maintain facial aesthetics and overall oral health. Nanocomposite coatings are revolutionizing dental implants by offering several key advancements in their performance and patient outcomes. These coatings, which incorporate nanoscale materials such as titanium dioxide, hydroxyapatite, or graphene, are engineered to enhance specific aspects of dental implants. Nanocomposite coatings improve the surface properties of dental implants, facilitating better osseointegration with the surrounding bone. The nanoscale texture of these coatings promotes stronger and faster bone growth around the implant, leading to a more secure and stable placement. By integrating nanoscale fillers, these coatings enhance the mechanical strength and wear resistance of dental implants. This reinforcement helps the implants withstand the forces of chewing and biting, extending their lifespan and reducing the likelihood of mechanical failure. Some nanocomposite coatings are designed with antimicrobial agents, such as silver or copper nanoparticles, which inhibit bacterial growth on the implant surface. This reduces the risk of peri-implant infections and supports better oral health around the implant site. Nanocomposite coatings can be engineered to release therapeutic agents gradually. For instance, coatings can include medications such as antibiotics or anti-inflammatory drugs, which are slowly released to prevent infection and manage inflammation at the implant site. These coatings can be tailored to match the natural appearance of teeth more closely. Nanocomposites can be designed to mimic the color and translucency of natural teeth, improving the aesthetic outcome and blending seamlessly with the surrounding dental structures. The advanced surface characteristics of nanocomposite coatings make it harder for bacterial biofilms to adhere. This helps in maintaining oral hygiene and reduces the need for frequent cleaning or adjustments. The coatings offer the ability to precisely control surface roughness and porosity. This customization allows for the optimization of implant surface characteristics to meet individual patient needs and specific clinical requirements. Further, the durability of nanocomposite coatings ensures that dental implants remain effective and visually appealing over time. The coatings resist degradation from oral fluids and mechanical stress, contributing to the long-term success of the implant. By enhancing the biocompatibility and reducing irritation, nanocomposite coatings can contribute to a more comfortable experience for patients. This improved compatibility minimizes discomfort and enhances the overall satisfaction with the dental implant.

13.6.8.1 Mandibular Reconstruction Plates

Mandibular reconstruction plates are specialized implants used to restore and stabilize the mandible, or lower jaw, following various medical challenges such as trauma, surgical removal of tumors, or congenital deformities. These implants are essential in reconstructive surgery to reestablish the structural integrity and functionality of the jawbone. Typically made from biocompatible metals like titanium, these plates are designed to match the contour of the mandible precisely. Titanium is favored due to its strength, lightweight properties, and compatibility with human tissue, which minimizes the risk of rejection or complications. The plates are custom-shaped and sized to fit the unique anatomy of each patient's jaw, ensuring a secure and effective reconstruction. The implantation process involves surgically positioning the plates against the jawbone. Once in place, the plates are secured with screws or other fixation devices to hold the bone fragments or reconstructed sections in the correct position. This stabilization is crucial for proper healing and function, allowing the mandible to regain its strength and support for chewing, speaking, and other essential functions. Mandibular reconstruction plates play a vital role in both functional and aesthetic recovery. They help to restore the jaw's alignment and support facial structure, improving the overall appearance and enabling normal jaw movement. Their use is a key component in comprehensive care for patients undergoing significant jaw reconstruction. Nanocomposites are improving mandibular reconstruction plates by integrating nanoscale materials to enhance their mechanical strength, biocompatibility, and functionality. For example, titanium dioxide or graphene nanoparticles are used to increase the plates' durability and resistance to stress, while antimicrobial agents like silver nanoparticles help prevent post-surgical infections. These coatings also support better bone integration and can deliver growth factors or antibiotics to the implant site, aiding in faster recovery and improved outcomes. Real-world applications include custom mandibular plates used in surgeries for trauma or congenital defects, where these advanced materials ensure better performance and patient safety.

13.6.8.2 Maxillary Reconstruction Plates

Maxillary reconstruction plates are specialized implants designed to stabilize and reconstruct the maxilla, or upper jaw, particularly following trauma, tumor removal, or congenital abnormalities. These implants are crucial in restoring both the structural integrity and functional aspects of the upper jaw, which plays a key role in facial aesthetics, chewing, and speech. Typically made from durable, biocompatible materials such as titanium, these plates are engineered to fit the specific contours of the maxilla. Titanium is chosen for its strength, light weight, and compatibility with bone, which helps reduce the risk of adverse reactions and ensures long-term stability. The plates are custom fabricated to match the unique anatomical features of each patient's maxilla, ensuring precise alignment and support. During the surgical procedure, the reconstruction plates are carefully positioned and secured to the maxilla using screws or other fixation devices. This placement helps to stabilize the bone segments, facilitating proper healing and alignment. The goal is to restore the natural shape and function of the upper jaw, which is essential for effective mastication (chewing), articulation (speaking), and overall facial symmetry. In addition to their functional benefits, maxillary reconstruction plates also play a significant role in aesthetic restoration. By re-establishing the correct contour and position of the upper jaw, these implants help to improve facial appearance and symmetry, which can be particularly important for patients recovering from traumatic injuries or surgical interventions. Nanocomposites are enhancing maxillary reconstruction plates by improving their strength, biocompatibility, and functionality. For instance, adding graphene or titanium dioxide nanoparticles increases the durability and mechanical resilience of the plates, ensuring they endure the stresses of daily use. Antimicrobial nanoparticles, such as silver, help reduce infection risks. These advanced plates also promote better bone integration and can deliver growth factors or antibiotics to support healing. In practice, nanocomposite-coated maxillary plates are used in surgeries for trauma or congenital defects, offering improved performance and faster recovery for patients.

13.6.8.3 Temporomandibular Joint (TMJ) Implants

TMJ implants are specialized devices designed to treat disorders of the temporomandibular joint (TMJ), which connects the lower jaw to the skull. These implants address various issues, including pain, limited movement, and joint dysfunction. They include prosthetic discs that replace damaged natural discs to restore smooth jaw movement, screws and plates that stabilize and support the joint and surrounding structures, and complete joint replacement systems for severe cases where the entire joint needs to be replaced. By mimicking the function of natural TMJ components, these implants aim to alleviate symptoms, restore normal jaw function, and improve overall quality of life for individuals with TMJ disorders. Nanocomposites enhance temporomandibular joint (TMJ) implants by boosting their strength, biocompatibility, and osseointegration. They incorporate materials like graphene for durability and antimicrobial agents to reduce infection risks. These advanced implants improve overall performance and patient outcomes in surgeries for joint repair or replacement.

13.6.9 Orbital Implants

Orbital implants are essential devices used in the management of eye loss following procedures such as enucleation, which involves the surgical removal of the eye due to trauma, disease, or other conditions [21]. These implants are placed in the orbital socket, where they provide critical support and a stable foundation for the placement of an ocular prosthesis, or artificial eye. The primary role of these implants is to maintain the structural integrity of the eye socket and ensure proper alignment and function of the prosthesis. By filling the void left by the removed eye, orbital implants help to preserve the cosmetic appearance of the eye area and support the prosthetic eye's movement, contributing to a more natural look and improving the overall aesthetic outcome for the patient. Nanocomposites enhance orbital implants by improving their strength, biocompatibility, and integration with surrounding tissues. They use materials like titanium dioxide for better durability and graphene for strength, while antimicrobial nanoparticles help prevent infections. These advancements ensure more effective, comfortable, and long-lasting outcomes in surgeries to replace or reconstruct the orbital area.

13.6.9.1 Facial Fracture Fixation Devices

Maxillofacial implants are specialized devices used to stabilize and repair fractures in the facial region resulting from trauma or injury. These implants include various fixation devices such as screws, plates, and wires, each designed to address specific needs in facial reconstruction. Screws and plates are often employed to secure broken or displaced bones, ensuring they are properly aligned and held in place during the healing process. Wires may be used to provide additional support or to stabilize smaller bone fragments. By meticulously realigning fractured bones and maintaining their position, maxillofacial implants play a vital role in facilitating effective healing and restoring normal facial structure and function. These implants are crucial for both the aesthetic and functional recovery of individuals who have suffered facial injuries or undergone reconstructive surgeries. Nanocomposite coatings for facial fracture fixation devices significantly enhance their functionality by offering targeted improvements [10]. They can provide a smoother surface to minimize irritation and discomfort, and tailored surface properties to promote optimal tissue healing. The incorporation of specific nanomaterials allows for adjustable porosity, aiding in better bone regeneration and integration. Additionally, these coatings can be designed to include smart features, such as self-healing properties or responsive drug delivery systems, which adapt to the healing process and improve patient outcomes.

13.6.10 Orthopedic Implants

Orthopedic implants are essential medical devices designed to support, replace, or repair damaged or missing bones and joints within the musculoskeletal system. These implants are integral to a range of orthopedic procedures, helping to restore functionality, stability, and movement in patients with bone fractures, joint disorders, or degenerative conditions. By providing a structural foundation for healing and rehabilitation, orthopedic implants enable improved mobility and quality of life for individuals undergoing surgery or recovering from injuries. Their application spans various types of implants, including plates, screws, prosthetic joints, and more, each tailored to address specific needs and promote effective recovery. Among different materials, the nanocomposites for orthopedic implants introduce advanced capabilities that extend beyond traditional material improvements [11]. These innovative materials can be engineered to exhibit unique properties, such as enhanced bone growth stimulation through bioactive surface modifications. This promotes faster and more effective bone integration. Additionally, nanocomposites can be designed to adapt to mechanical stresses dynamically, reducing the likelihood of implant failure and discomfort. They also enable the development of implants with tailored thermal conductivity to better match the surrounding tissue environment, thereby reducing post-surgical complications. In practical applications, these features are crucial in improving the long-term success and functionality of implants used in joint replacements, fracture repairs, and spinal surgeries.

13.6.10.1 Joint Implants

Joint implants are prosthetic devices designed to replace joints that have been damaged or diseased, such as those in the hip, knee, shoulder, elbow, or ankle. These implants are carefully crafted from materials like metal, ceramic, or plastic to closely mimic the natural movement and function of the original joint. The design and materials of joint implants are selected to provide durability and compatibility with the human body, allowing for improved mobility and pain relief. They are used in a variety of surgical procedures to restore joint function and enhance the overall quality of life for patients suffering from conditions such as arthritis, severe joint injuries, or degenerative diseases. Nanocomposites in joint implants offer innovative enhancements by incorporating nanoscale materials to achieve specific improvements. For instance, these composites can be tailored to feature surfaces that enhance lubrication, reducing friction and wear at the implant interface. They can also be designed to adapt to dynamic loading conditions, providing improved shock absorption and comfort. Advanced nanocomposites might include properties that promote cellular growth or tissue regeneration, accelerating healing around the joint. These features contribute to more effective joint function and a reduced risk of complications in joint replacement and repair surgeries.

13.6.10.2 Bone Plates and Screws

Bone plates and screws are essential implants used in orthopedic surgery to stabilize fractured bones during the healing process. Constructed primarily from metal, these implants are designed to provide structural support and ensure proper alignment of fractured bone segments. The bone plates are securely attached to the surface of the bone, and screws are used to fasten the plate in place, effectively holding the bone fragments together. This fixation technique aids in maintaining the correct alignment and positioning of the fractured bones, facilitating optimal healing and recovery. The use of bone plates and screws is critical in managing complex fractures, promoting bone regeneration, and restoring function to the affected area. Nanocomposites in bone plates and screws offer advanced benefits such as enhanced fatigue resistance and optimized bone healing. These materials can be engineered to include nanostructured surfaces that improve the mechanical interlock between the implant and bone, facilitating quicker and more secure fixation. Additionally, they may incorporate responsive elements that release growth factors or therapeutic agents to promote bone regeneration at the fracture site. Nanocomposites also enable the creation of implants with tailored thermal and electrical properties, which can improve the overall functionality and integration of the fixation devices in various orthopedic applications.

13.6.10.3 Intramedullary Nails

Intramedullary nails are specialized implants designed to stabilize and support fractures in long bones like the femur and tibia. Inserted into the medullary canal—the central cavity within the bone shaft-these nails provide internal support to maintain the alignment of fractured bone segments. This technique is particularly valuable in cases where traditional external fixation methods, such as plates and screws, may not be suitable due to the fracture's location, complexity, or the patient's overall condition. By aligning and immobilizing the bone from within, intramedullary nails facilitate proper healing and enable patients to regain function more effectively. They are often chosen for their ability to promote quicker recovery and reduce the risk of complications associated with other fixation methods. Nanocomposites for intramedullary nails enhance their performance through several advanced features. These materials can be engineered to include nanoscale reinforcements that improve their impact resistance and flexibility, accommodating the dynamic forces experienced during movement and healing. They also enable the development of bioactive coatings that encourage bone cell adhesion and growth directly on the nail surface, promoting faster and more effective bone union. Additionally, nanocomposites can incorporate temperature-sensitive elements that respond to changes in the body's thermal environment, optimizing healing conditions. These innovations result in more robust, adaptable, and biologically compatible intramedullary nails.

13.6.11 Spinal Implants

Spinal implants are essential devices used to manage a range of spinal disorders, including degenerative disc disease, spinal fractures, and structural abnormalities such as scoliosis. These implants come in several forms, each serving a specific function to support and restore spinal health. Spinal fusion implants are designed to promote the union of adjacent vertebrae to provide long-term stability. Artificial discs replace damaged natural discs to maintain spinal mobility and alleviate pain. Rods and screws are used to stabilize the spine and correct deformities by securing vertebrae in the correct position. Cages are inserted between vertebrae to support spinal fusion and enhance structural integrity. Together, these implants help in realigning the spine, reducing pain, and improving overall function, offering significant benefits for individuals suffering from complex spinal conditions. Nanocomposites for spinal implants offer sophisticated advancements by integrating nanoscale materials to achieve specific functional improvements. These composites can be designed with self-healing properties that repair micro-damage over time, enhancing the implant's longevity and reliability. They may also include nanostructured surfaces that improve the interface between the implant and vertebrae, promoting more effective spinal fusion and stability. Additionally, these materials can be tailored to possess adaptive mechanical properties that adjust to the stresses placed on the spine, ensuring better support and comfort. The incorporation of drug-eluting nanocomposites can facilitate localized therapy to manage inflammation and infection, further supporting successful spinal recovery.

13.6.11.1 External Fixators

External fixators are temporary orthopedic devices used to stabilize fractures or correct deformities by providing external support. They consist of metal pins or screws that are surgically inserted into the affected bone through the skin. These pins are then connected to an external frame that extends outside the body. The frame holds the pins in place, thereby stabilizing the bone and maintaining proper alignment during the healing process. This method is particularly useful in managing complex fractures, correcting bone deformities, or when internal fixation methods are not feasible. External fixators allow for adjustments to be made to the alignment of the bones throughout the healing period and facilitate access for ongoing medical care or infection control, making them a versatile tool in orthopedic treatments. Nanocomposites in external fixators enhance their functionality through several advanced features. They can be engineered to incorporate nanoscale reinforcements that provide superior rigidity and resistance to mechanical stresses, crucial for stabilizing fractures effectively. Additionally, these composites can be designed with anti-corrosive properties to prolong the lifespan of the fixator in various environmental conditions. Nanocomposite coatings may include smart materials that adapt to changes in the mechanical load, improving overall stability. Furthermore, they can feature bioactive surfaces that encourage tissue regeneration around the fixation site, promoting faster and more effective healing.

13.6.12 Tissue Implants

Tissue implants, also known as tissue grafts or transplants, are crucial medical devices used to replace or repair damaged or diseased tissues within the body. These implants can be sourced from the patient's own body (autografts), from donors (allografts), from animals (xenografts), or be synthetic materials (alloplasts). Autografts are preferred for their low risk of rejection, while allografts and xenografts are utilized in various surgical procedures with careful matching to minimize immune response. Alloplasts, made from biocompatible materials, are employed in diverse fields such as orthopedics, reconstructive surgery, cardiovascular surgery, and dentistry. They play a vital role in restoring function, repairing tissues, and improving patient outcomes by integrating with the surrounding tissues and promoting effective healing. Nanocomposites for tissue implants offer advanced capabilities by integrating nanoscale materials to enhance implant functionality. These materials can be engineered to create highly porous structures that mimic natural tissue architecture, facilitating better cell infiltration and tissue integration. Additionally, nanocomposites can be designed with stimuli-responsive elements that trigger specific biological responses, such as promoting cellular differentiation or accelerating tissue repair in response to environmental changes. They also enable the incorporation of growth factors or anti-inflammatory agents directly into the implant matrix, providing localized therapeutic effects to support healing. This customization leads to more effective and adaptable tissue implants, tailored to individual patient needs and specific clinical applications.

13.6.12.1 Bone Grafts

Bone grafts are essential for repairing bone defects and promoting healing across various surgical disciplines, including orthopedics, dental implants, and maxillofacial surgery. These grafts can be derived from several sources: autografts, which are taken from the patient's own body, offer high compatibility and minimal risk of rejection; allografts, sourced from donors of the same species, are processed to reduce immune response and disease risk; xenografts, obtained from animals, are specially treated to minimize immune reactions; and alloplasts, synthetic materials designed to replicate natural bone properties, provide an alternative when biological grafts are not suitable. Each type of graft is selected based on the specific needs of the patient and the nature of the surgical procedure, aiming to restore bone function, support healing, and enhance overall outcomes. Nanocomposites for bone grafts advance their functionality through several innovative approaches. These materials can be engineered to feature enhanced bioactivity, promoting superior bone cell adhesion and proliferation directly at the graft site. They can also incorporate biodegradable components that gradually dissolve as natural bone regenerates, seamlessly integrating with the surrounding tissue. Additionally, nanocomposites may include controlled-release systems for delivering osteogenic factors or antibiotics, optimizing the healing process and preventing infections. The incorporation of nanoscale reinforcements improves the mechanical properties of the graft, providing the necessary support during the bone healing phase.

13.6.12.2 Skin Grafts

Skin grafts are essential for repairing damaged or lost skin due to conditions such as burns, wounds, or surgical procedures. These grafts can be categorized based on their source: autografts, which are taken from the patient's own skin, provide the best compatibility and reduce the risk of rejection; allografts, which come from donors of the same species, are often used temporarily while the patient's skin heals but may carry a risk of immune rejection; xenografts, sourced from animals, serve as temporary coverings to protect the wound and aid in healing; and alloplasts, which are synthetic materials that replicate the properties of natural skin, offer an alternative when biological grafts are unsuitable or unavailable. The choice of graft depends on factors such as the wound's characteristics, the patient's health, and the desired healing outcome. Nanocomposites for skin grafts improve their effectiveness by integrating advanced materials that support enhanced healing and functionality. They can be engineered to include nanoscale fibers or particles that mimic the extracellular matrix, promoting better cellular attachment and growth. These composites often incorporate hydrogels or bioactive coatings that provide moisture control and facilitate nutrient exchange, creating an optimal environment for skin regeneration. Additionally, they may feature antimicrobial properties to reduce infection risks and include smart materials that respond to changes in the graft site, such as adjusting moisture levels or releasing growth factors as needed.

13.6.12.3 Tendon and Ligament Grafts

Tendon and ligament grafts are critical in addressing injuries or tears in tendons and ligaments, often seen in sports medicine and orthopedic surgeries. These grafts are employed to restore functionality and stability to affected joints and muscles. Autografts involve using tendons or ligaments harvested from the patient's own body, such as from the hamstring or patellar tendon, which offers a high degree of compatibility and reduces the risk of rejection or disease transmission. Allografts, on the other hand, are sourced from donors of the same species, providing an alternative when autografts are not feasible due to various reasons like the need for a larger graft or multiple surgeries. Both types of grafts are carefully matched to ensure proper integration and healing, with their choice influenced by factors such as the specific injury, patient health, and surgical objectives. Nanocomposites for tendon and ligament grafts enhance their performance through specialized features. They can be engineered with nanoscale fibers or structures that replicate the mechanical properties of natural tendons and ligaments, improving strength and elasticity. These materials often include bioactive components that support tendon and ligament cell growth, ensuring better integration with host tissues. Additionally, they can incorporate nanostructured surfaces that facilitate improved collagen alignment and healing, while some designs offer controlled release of anti-inflammatory agents or growth factors to accelerate recovery and reduce complications.

13.6.12.4 Corneal Grafts

Corneal grafts, also known as corneal transplants, are surgical procedures used to replace damaged or diseased corneal tissue to restore vision and improve eye health. These grafts are essential in treating various corneal conditions, such as scarring, thinning, or degenerative diseases that impair vision. These implants are often used when donor tissue is not available or suitable. Corneal grafts aim to restore clear vision by replacing the damaged cornea with healthy tissue or a biocompatible synthetic alternative, ultimately improving the quality of life for individuals with severe corneal issues. Nanocomposites for corneal grafts offer significant advancements by integrating unique materials to address specific challenges. They can feature nanoscale coatings that enhance optical clarity and reduce light scattering, improving visual outcomes. These materials often include nano-engineered hydrogels that provide optimal hydration and match the natural corneal environment. Additionally, nanocomposites may incorporate bioactive molecules that promote corneal epithelial cell growth and integration, facilitating faster and more effective graft healing. They can also be designed to exhibit anti-inflammatory properties to minimize graft rejection and support long-term stability.

13.6.12.5 Heart Valve Grafts

Heart valve grafts are critical components used in cardiovascular surgery to replace damaged or diseased heart valves, which are essential for maintaining proper blood flow through the heart. These grafts help restore normal valve function, which is vital for effective heart operation. There are two main types of heart valve grafts: allografts and xenografts. Allografts are obtained from human donors and are carefully matched to the recipient to reduce the risk of rejection. Xenografts, on the other hand, are derived from animal tissues, such as porcine (pig) or bovine (cow) valves, and are specially treated to minimize the chances of immune response from the recipient. Both types of grafts are used to address a range of valve-related issues, such as stenosis (narrowing of the valve) or regurgitation (leakage of the valve), and are selected based on factors like patient age, overall health, and the specific valve being replaced. The successful integration of these grafts helps in restoring heart function and improving the patient's quality of life. Nanocomposites for heart valve grafts enhance their performance by incorporating advanced material properties. These composites can include nanoscale coatings that improve hemocompatibility, reducing blood clot formation and enhancing the graft's durability. They can be engineered with nano-textured surfaces that support endothelial cell growth, promoting better integration with the native heart tissue. Additionally, these materials may feature responsive elements that adjust to physiological changes, such as altering stiffness to match the natural valve's function. Advanced nanocomposites also enable localized drug delivery systems to provide targeted anti-inflammatory or anticoagulant treatments, optimizing graft function and longevity.

13.6.12.6 Vascular Grafts

Vascular grafts are medical devices employed in cardiovascular procedures to replace or bypass damaged or obstructed blood vessels. These grafts are crucial for restoring normal blood flow and are often used in surgeries such as coronary artery bypass grafting (CABG) and peripheral artery bypass surgery. Vascular grafts can be categorized into alloplasts and xenografts. Allopath are synthetic materials designed to mimic the function of natural blood vessels, often made from materials like polytetrafluoroethylene (PTFE) or expanded polytetrafluoroethylene (ePTFE). These synthetic grafts are favored for their durability and biocompatibility. Xenografts, conversely, are derived from animal tissues, such as bovine or porcine sources, and are processed to minimize the risk of rejection and infection. The choice between alloplasts and xenografts depends on various factors, including the patient's condition, the location of the graft, and the specific requirements of the surgery. Both types of grafts play a vital role in managing vascular diseases by providing a pathway for blood flow and improving overall cardiovascular health. Among different materials, the nanocomposites for vascular grafts provide several cutting-edge improvements by incorporating specialized nanoscale materials. These materials can enhance the graft's mechanical flexibility and strength, allowing it to better withstand the dynamic forces of blood flow. They may feature nanostructured surfaces that improve endothelial cell adhesion and promote rapid vascularization, facilitating seamless integration with the host vessel. Additionally, nanocomposites can be designed with embedded drug delivery systems to release agents that prevent restenosis or reduce inflammation at the graft site.

13.6.12.7 Dermal Matrices

Dermal matrices are advanced biomaterials employed in plastic and reconstructive surgery to manage and repair soft tissue defects resulting from trauma, burns, or surgical procedures. These matrices act as scaffolds that support and guide the regeneration of damaged skin and underlying tissues by providing a structured foundation for cellular growth and tissue integration. Composed of various materials, dermal matrices can include autografts (tissues taken from the patient's own body), allografts (tissues from human donors), xenografts (tissues from animals), and alloplasts (synthetic materials). Each type offers unique advantages in terms of biocompatibility, integration, and functionality, facilitating optimal healing and restoration of both form and function in affected areas. Nanocomposites for dermal matrices enhance their performance by incorporating nanoscale materials that improve strength, flexibility, and biocompatibility. These advanced materials promote better tissue integration and support enhanced healing by mimicking natural skin properties and offering controlled drug release for infection management. The use of nanocomposites in dermal matrices facilitates more effective repair and regeneration of soft tissue defects from trauma, burns, or surgery.

13.6.12.8 Cartilage Grafts

Cartilage grafts are medical implants used to repair or replace damaged cartilage in joints, playing a vital role in orthopedic and reconstructive surgery. These grafts address cartilage loss or damage, which can occur due to injury, arthritis, or degenerative conditions. Cartilage grafts can be classified into three main types: autografts, which are harvested from the patient's own body; allografts, which are obtained from donor tissues; and alloplasts, which are synthetic materials designed to mimic the properties of natural cartilage. Each type of graft offers specific benefits in terms of integration, biocompatibility, and functionality, aimed at restoring joint function, reducing pain, and improving overall joint health. Nanocomposites for cartilage grafts enhance the repair and replacement of damaged cartilage by integrating nanoscale materials that improve mechanical strength and flexibility. These advanced materials mimic the natural cartilage structure, promoting better integration and function. Additionally, nanocomposites can support controlled release of growth factors to stimulate cartilage regeneration and reduce inflammation. This leads to more effective and durable outcomes in orthopedic and reconstructive surgeries involving cartilage grafts.

References

1. Alt V. Antimicrobial coated implants in trauma and orthopaedics–a clinical review and risk-benefit analysis. Injury. 2017;48:599–607. https://doi.org/10.1016/J.INJURY.2016.12.011.
2. Bruna T, Maldonado-Bravo F, Jara P, Caro N. Silver nanoparticles and their antibacterial applications. Int J Mol Sci. 2021;22:7202. https://doi.org/10.3390/IJMS22137202.
3. Chen X, Gao C, Jiang J, et al. 3D printed porous PLA/nHA composite scaffolds with enhanced osteogenesis and osteoconductivity in vivo for bone regeneration. Biomed Mater. 2019;14:065003. https://doi.org/10.1088/1748-605X/AB388D.
4. Chen Q, Zhu X, Jiang Y, et al. Development and characterization of MAO/PLA-nHA nanocomposite coatings on pure zinc for orthopedic applications. Surf Coat Technol. 2024;478:130452. https://doi.org/10.1016/J.SURFCOAT.2024.130452.
5. Coffey RJ. Deep brain stimulation devices: a brief technical history and review. Artif Organs. 2009;33:208–20. https://doi.org/10.1111/J.1525-1594.2008.00620.X.
6. Costa RC, Nagay BE, Dini C, et al. The race for the optimal antimicrobial surface: perspectives and challenges related to plasma electrolytic oxidation coating for titanium-based implants. Adv Colloid Interf Sci. 2023;311:102805. https://doi.org/10.1016/J.CIS.2022.102805.
7. Das R, Bhattacharjee C. Titanium-based nanocomposite materials for dental implant systems. In: Applications of nanocomposite materials in dentistry; 2019. p. 271–84. https://doi.org/10.1016/B978-0-12-813742-0.00016-X.
8. Jadon MS, Bhanjana G, Dilbaghi N, et al. Fabrication and evaluation of silver-doped magnesium oxide nanocomposite coatings for orthopaedics applications. J Alloys Compd. 2024;972:172848. https://doi.org/10.1016/J.JALLCOM.2023.172848.
9. Jing W, Feng L, Wang B, et al. Polymer-ceramic fiber nanocomposite coatings on titanium metal implant devices for diseased bone tissue regeneration. J Sci Adv Mater Devices. 2021;6:399–406. https://doi.org/10.1016/J.JSAMD.2021.04.001.
10. Khandan A, Nassireslami E, Saber-Samandari S, Arabi N. Fabrication and characterization of porous bioceramic-magnetite biocomposite for maxillofacial fractures application. Dent Hypotheses. 2020;11:78–85. https://doi.org/10.4103/DENTHYP.DENTHYP_11_20.
11. Kumaravel V, Nair KM, Mathew S, et al. Antimicrobial TiO2 nanocomposite coatings for surfaces, dental and orthopaedic implants. Chem Eng J. 2021;416:129071. https://doi.org/10.1016/J.CEJ.2021.129071.
12. Lashkarara S, fazlali A, Ghaseminezhad K, et al. Mechanism of plasma electrolytic oxidation in Mg3ZnCa implants: a study of double-layer formation and properties through nanoindentation. Sci Rep. 2024;14:1–9. https://doi.org/10.1038/s41598-024-58008-8.
13. Latif R, Noor MM, Yunas J, Hamzah AA. Mechanical energy sensing and harvesting in micromachined polymer-based piezoelectric transducers for fully implanted hearing systems: a review. Polymers. 2021;13:2276. https://doi.org/10.3390/POLYM13142276.

14. Li P, Dai J, Li Y, et al. Zinc based biodegradable metals for bone repair and regeneration: bioactivity and molecular mechanisms. Mater Today Bio. 2024;25:100932. https://doi.org/10.1016/J.MTBIO.2023.100932.
15. Liu C, Xu J, Xie ZH, et al. Antibacterial and corrosion resistant ANPs-TaC nanocomposite coating for biomedical applications. Surf Coat Technol. 2023;474:130056. https://doi.org/10.1016/J.SURFCOAT.2023.130056.
16. Loeb GE. Neural prosthetics: a review of empirical vs. systems engineering strategies. Appl Bionics Biomech. 2018;2018:1435030. https://doi.org/10.1155/2018/1435030.
17. Mebert AM, Alvarez GS, Peroni R, et al. Collagen-silica nanocomposites as dermal dressings preventing infection in vivo. Mater Sci Eng C. 2018;93:170–7. https://doi.org/10.1016/J.MSEC.2018.07.078.
18. Mishra SK, Teotia AK, Kumar A, Kannan S. Mechanically tuned nanocomposite coating on titanium metal with integrated properties of biofilm inhibition, cell proliferation, and sustained drug delivery. Nanomedicine. 2017;13:23–35. https://doi.org/10.1016/J.NANO.2016.08.010.
19. Noshahr FH, Nabavi M, Sawan M. Multi-channel neural recording implants: a review. Sensors. 2020;20:904. https://doi.org/10.3390/S20030904.
20. Orasugh JT, Dutta S, Das D, et al. Utilization of Cellulose Nanocrystals (CNC) biopolymer nanocomposites in Ophthalmic Drug Delivery System (ODDS). J Nanotechnol Res. 2019;1:75–87.
21. Patel M, Betz MW, Geibel E, et al. Cyclic acetal hydroxyapatite nanocomposites for orbital bone regeneration https://home.liebertpub.com/tea. Tissue Eng A. 2009;16:55–65. https://doi.org/10.1089/TEN.TEA.2009.0027.
22. Ramezani M, Ripin ZM. An overview of enhancing the performance of medical implants with nanocomposites. J Compos Sci. 2023;7:199. https://doi.org/10.3390/JCS7050199.
23. Romanò CL, Tsuchiya H, Morelli I, et al. Antibacterial coating of implants: are we missing something? Bone Joint Res. 2019;8:199–206. https://doi.org/10.1302/2046-3758.85.BJR-2018-0316/LETTERTOEDITOR.
24. Sagadevan S, Schirhagl R, Rahman MZ, et al. Recent advancements in polymer matrix nanocomposites for bone tissue engineering applications. J Drug Deliv Sci Technol. 2023;82:104313. https://doi.org/10.1016/J.JDDST.2023.104313.
25. Samudrala CSK, Radhi PKS, Soppari Murthy B. Metal, ceramics and polymer nanocomposites for various applications: a review. Mater Today Proc. 2022;56:1120–8. https://doi.org/10.1016/J.MATPR.2021.10.316.
26. Sharma R, Mehrotra N, Singh I, Pal K. Bioceramic filled PLA based nanocomposites for biomedical application: an experimental investigation. Ceram Int. 2024;50:28662–81. https://doi.org/10.1016/J.CERAMINT.2024.05.177.
27. Shrivas S, Samaur H, Yadav V, Boda SK. Soft and hard tissue integration around percutaneous bone-anchored titanium prostheses: toward achieving holistic biointegration. ACS Biomater Sci Eng. 2024;10:1966–87. https://doi.org/10.1021/ACSBIOMATERIALS.3C01555/ASSET/IMAGES/MEDIUM/AB3C01555_0006.GIF.
28. Su Y, Fu J, Du S, et al. Biodegradable Zn–Sr alloys with enhanced mechanical and biocompatibility for biomedical applications. Smart Mater Med. 2022;3:117–27. https://doi.org/10.1016/J.SMAIM.2021.12.004.
29. Vellayappan MV, Balaji A, Subramanian AP, et al. Multifaceted prospects of nanocomposites for cardiovascular grafts and stents. Int J Nanomed. 2015;10:2785–803. https://doi.org/10.2147/IJN.S80121.
30. Vishwakarma V, Kaliaraj GS, Kirubaharan AMK. Advanced alloys and coatings for bioimplants. Coatings. 2022;12:1525. https://doi.org/10.3390/COATINGS12101525.
31. Zhang H, Shih J, Zhu J, Kotov NA. Layered nanocomposites from gold nanoparticles for neural prosthetic devices. Nano Lett. 2012;12:3391–8. https://doi.org/10.1021/NL3015632/SUPPL_FILE/NL3015632_SI_001.PDF.

32. Zhang E, Zhao X, Hu J, et al. Antibacterial metals and alloys for potential biomedical implants. Bioact Mater. 2021;6:2569–612. https://doi.org/10.1016/J.BIOACTMAT.2021.01.030.
33. Zhao L, Sundaram S, Le AV, et al. Engineered tissue–stent biocomposites as tracheal replacements. Tissue Eng A. 2016;22:1086–97. https://doi.org/10.1089/TEN.TEA.2016.0132.

Chapter 14
Nanocomposites for Wearable Monitoring

Vishal M. Gavande, Jayesh M. Sonawane, Karen Lienkamp, and Won-Ki Lee

Abstract This chapter explores a comprehensive overview of the recent advancements and applications of nanocomposites and nanosensors in wearable monitoring systems. Nanocomposites, characterized by their nano-sized constituents dispersed within a matrix, have revolutionized the landscape of wearable technology owing to their exceptional mechanical, electrical, and thermal properties. These attributes make nanocomposites ideal for crafting lightweight, flexible, and resilient sensors that seamlessly conform to the body's contours, ensuring user comfort and prolonged wearability. Furthermore, the integration of nanosensors within these composites enables precise, rapid, and selective detection of various physiological and environmental parameters crucial for health monitoring applications. The chapter elucidates the synthesis techniques, material properties, fabrication methodologies, and sensing mechanisms underlying nanocomposites and nanosensors tailored for wearable monitoring. It also delineates the challenges, opportunities, and future prospects in this burgeoning field. By elucidating the transformative potential of nanocomposites and nanosensors, this chapter underscores their significance in advancing wearable monitoring technologies and ushering in a new era of personalized healthcare delivery.

Keywords Wearable · Sensors · Nanotechnology · Thin films · Flexibility

V. M. Gavande
Department of Polymer Engineering, Pukyong National University, Busan, South Korea

Department of Materials Science & Engineering, Saarland University, Saarbrücken, Germany

J. M. Sonawane
Department of Microbiology, 418 Morrill Science Center IVN, University of Massachusetts, Amherst, MA, USA

K. Lienkamp
Department of Materials Science & Engineering, Saarland University, Saarbrücken, Germany

W.-K. Lee (✉)
Department of Polymer Engineering, Pukyong National University, Busan, South Korea
e-mail: wonki@pknu.ac.kr

S. Mondal et al. (eds.), *Smart and Sustainable Nanomaterials in Digital Healthcare and Theranostic*, https://doi.org/10.1007/978-981-95-9386-6_14

14.1 Introduction

Wearable monitoring devices are revolutionizing healthcare and fitness tracking, owing to their commendable responses to mechanical, thermal, biological, or environmental stimuli. They offer continuous, real-time data collection, enabling personalized health insights and early detection of potential issues in real time with high accuracy. However, conventional materials used in wearables often face limitations. Here's where nanocomposites come in, offering exciting possibilities for next-generation wearable monitoring devices. Nanocomposites have emerged as promising materials for wearable monitoring applications due to their unique combination of enhanced sensing capabilities with biocompatibility and mechanical flexibility. The general comparisons of traditional materials with nanocomposites regarding flexibility, conductivity, and biocompatibility are given in Table 14.1. Wearable monitoring devices detect strain-induced deformations in the wearer and convert these into measurable electrical signals. These devices are increasingly valued for their ability to non-invasively and continuously monitor vital physiological signals, potentially indicating serious health concerns. Real-time tracking of parameters like body movements, heart rate, respiration rate, steps, muscle activities, and posture provides a comprehensive understanding of bodily responses to various activities and environments [1]. This monitoring aids in the initial diagnosis of health abnormalities, personalized healthcare, remote patient monitoring, and optimizing athletic performance. Access to personal physiological data empowers individuals to make informed lifestyle decisions and supports large-scale health data collection for research, aiding in studying population health trends and validating medical hypotheses. These materials typically consist of a polymer matrix reinforced with nanoparticles or nanofillers, which impart specific functionalities to the composite. Innovations in composite materials and processing techniques have led to the development of advanced devices for a variety of applications, including health monitoring, soft robotics, motion detection, smart textiles, and sports activity tracking.

Conventional metal- or semiconductor-based strain sensors are becoming outdated due to their limited detection range and complex fabrication. Polymer nanocomposite-based sensors, which are more flexible and stretchable, are a versatile alternative [2–4]. These sensors typically include a functional composite structure, transducing electrodes, and connection wires. The composite structures often use conductive nanofillers within a polymer matrix, offering both electrical conductivity and mechanical strength. Common nanofillers are carbon-based materials and other conductive fillers like metallic nanowires, nanoparticles, and Mxenes. Polymers such as PDMS, PU, TPU, Ecoflex, polyimide, and PET serve as flexible

Table 14.1 The comparison of traditional materials with nanocomposites regarding flexibility, conductivity, and biocompatibility

Properties	Traditional materials	Nanocomposites
Flexibility	Low to moderate flexibility: The inherent rigidity of traditional polymers, such as PVC and PET, frequently limits their ability to provide some flexibility Rigid materials: Because metals and ceramics are so brittle and rigid, they are not appropriate for applications that call for dynamic flexibility Rigid ceramics: Ceramics (such as zirconia and alumina) are brittle and incredibly rigid, making them inappropriate for uses that call for mechanical flexibility Limitations on customization: Processing methods like copolymerization or mixing can only slightly modify mechanical characteristics	High flexibility: Introduction of nanoscale fillers, such as clay nanoparticles, graphene, or carbon nanotubes, greatly increases flexibility without sacrificing strength Tunable properties: By altering the kind, size, and dispersion of nanoparticles, mechanical properties can be precisely controlled Enhanced resilience: Nanocomposites are perfect for dynamic environments like wearable technology and robotics because they retain their flexibility under mechanical stress
Conductivity	Polymers: Conventional polymers are usually insulators and should not be used in applications where electrical conductivity is required Metals: Metals, such as copper and aluminum, are heavy, stiff, and prone to corrosion, despite their high conductivity Ceramics: Excellent thermal insulation but poor electrical conductivity; some ceramics, like ITO, may conduct electricity but are costly and brittle Cost and weight issues: Conventional materials have trouble achieving both conductivity and lightweight qualities	Enhanced electrical conductivity: While maintaining materials' small weight, nanofillers such as metallic nanoparticles, graphene, or carbon nanotubes (CNTs) allow for high electrical conductivity Enhancement of thermal conductivity by the use of nanomaterials such as graphene or boron nitride is crucial for electronics heat control Applications: Nanocomposites' exceptional conductivity is advantageous for flexible electronics, sensors, and energy storage devices

(continued)

Table 14.1 (continued)

Properties	Traditional materials	Nanocomposites
Biocompatibility	Biocompatible polymers: While silicone, PMMA, PDMS, UHMWPE, and PCL are biocompatible, they don't have sophisticated features like antibacterial or bioactive qualities Metals: Although stainless steel and titanium are biocompatible, they may be too heavy and rigid for several biomedical uses Ceramics: Although bioceramics (such as bioactive glass and hydroxyapatite) are great for bone regeneration, they are mechanically limited and brittle Challenges: There aren't many ways to combine biocompatibility and multifunctionality, like tissue engineering or drug delivery	Improved biocompatibility: Adding bioactive nanoparticles, such as chitosan, silver nanoparticles, or hydroxyapatite, enhances communication with biological systems Controlled functions: Antibacterial coatings, tissue scaffolding, and medication delivery are all possible with nanocomposites Versatility: Facilitates uses such as implantable medical devices, wound healing, and bone regeneration For instance, functionalized nanoparticles in polymeric nanocomposites offer a compromise between mechanical strength, biodegradability, and biocompatibility

matrices [5–8]. Conductive polymers like PEDOT and polyaniline help form conductive networks [8, 9].

Strain-responsive composites detect strain by altering electrical properties through mechanisms like interface changes, conduction pathways, crack propagation, and tunneling effects. Sensors are classified as resistive, capacitive, or impedimetric, with performance metrics such as gauge factor (GF), durability, linear range, response speed, and stability. High-quality sensors balance these parameters through optimized nanofillers, polymer matrices, and fabrication techniques [3, 8, 12]. Achieving these properties requires careful selection of nanofillers and polymer matrices, along with various techniques, often involving trade-offs between performance parameters. This chapter presents a comprehensive overview of functional nanocomposites in which elucidates the synthesis techniques, material properties, fabrication methodologies, and sensing mechanisms underlying nanocomposites and nanosensors tailored for wearable devices. All types of nanomaterials and their composites and structures for stretchable strain sensors, including carbon-based composites like nanoparticles (NPs), nanowires (NWs), bio-hybrid composites, and ionic liquids along with their sensing performance and applications in wearable monitoring.

14.2 Fundamentals of Nanocomposites

Nanocomposites are materials that incorporate nanoscale fillers into a matrix to create a composite with superior properties. Matrix is the bulk material that surrounds and embeds the nanofillers. Polymers are commonly used as the matrix due to their lightweight nature, processability, and diverse functionalities. Other materials like ceramics and metals can also be used as matrices. Nanofillers are the nanoscale reinforcements incorporated into the matrix. They can be various forms including nanoparticles, nanotubes, nanofibers, and nanoplatelets. The choice of nanofiller significantly impacts the final properties of the nanocomposite. These materials offer unique properties that combine the characteristics of the matrix (continuous phase) and the nanofillers (dispersed phase). This combination can lead to significant improvements in various properties compared to traditional materials. Nanocomposites offer superior performance over traditional materials due to the high surface area and exceptional properties of nanofillers. A well-defined interface between the matrix and nanofillers ensures effective stress transfer, maximizing their benefits. Wearable sensors typically consist of flexible substrates for adaptability, sensing elements to convert signals into electrical outputs, and electrodes to transmit these signals, making them highly efficient for advanced applications [12].

14.2.1 Flexible Substrates

Flexible substrates are essential for wearable sensors as they support conductive components and circuits, and their flexibility or stretchability determines the sensor's performance. Commonly used substrates include polydimethylsiloxane (PDMS) and Ecoflex for their elasticity [13], as well as polyethylene terephthalate (PET) and polyimide (PI) for their bendability [14, 15]. Emerging materials like silk fibroin, cellulose, and sponge are gaining interest for their biocompatibility and biodegradability, expanding options for sensor substrates [13, 16].

14.2.2 Sensing Elements

The choice of sensing elements in wearable sensors depends on the target being monitored. Key sensing elements include:

Enzymes: Such as glucose oxidase, alcohol oxidase, and lactate oxidase, which detect specific molecules like glucose, alcohol, and lactate through electron transfer reactions. The concentration of these molecules is measured by changes in current [17, 18].

Ion-Selective Electrodes: These measure essential ions like H+, Na+, and K+ in body fluids using the Nernst equation to determine ion concentration based on the potential difference between electrodes [10, 19].

Physical Parameters: For monitoring parameters like body motion and heart function, electrical signals such as resistance, current, capacitance, and voltage are directly measured to reflect changes in physiological conditions [11].

14.2.3 Conductive Materials

Sensing elements are essential in wearable sensors, converting various signals into electrical ones, which requires high conductivity. However, accurately detecting subtle body movements and measuring small targets in body fluids present challenges. To improve the sensitivity, reliability, and stability of wearable sensors, nanomaterials are used. These materials are categorized as 0D, 1D, 2D, or 3D, each offering unique properties like high surface area, excellent electrical and optical responsiveness, and multiple active sites. Such properties make nanomaterials highly effective for wearable sensors. They are typically combined with flexible substrates using methods like printing, spray-coating, drop-casting, layer-by-layer deposition, dip-coating, in situ polymerization, or electrochemical deposition. These techniques enhance both the flexibility and performance of wearable sensors.

14.3 Types of Nanomaterials

Wearable sensors benefit from various nanomaterials due to their exceptional properties, including high optical, mechanical, electrical, and a large surface area, along with chemical stability. Polymers, on the other hand, offer skin compatibility, stretchability, flexibility, and durability. Extensive research has explored a range of nanomaterials (1D, 2D, and 3D shapes) for wearable applications.

These materials are studied for their potential to ameliorate the performance and functionality of wearable sensors [20–23]. Carbon-based nanomaterials are prominent due to their high mechanical robustness, flexibility, high conductivity, and ease of processing. Metal nanoparticles and nanowires, including silver nanoparticles (AgNPs) known for their high conductivity and antibacterial properties, and gold nanoparticles (AuNPs) valued for their chemical stability and biocompatibility, are extensively used. Additionally, metal oxide nanoparticles like ZnO and TiO2 offer semiconducting properties crucial for environmental sensing. Polymer nanocomposites such as conductive polymers (polyaniline, polypyrrole, PEDOT) enhance electrical properties while maintaining flexibility, and nanocomposite hydrogels provide soft, stretchable matrices for wearable applications [24–26]. Furthermore, 2D materials like MXenes and transition metal dichalcogenides (TMDs, e.g., MoS_2) are notable for their metallic conductivity, hydrophilicity, and unique electrical and mechanical properties, making them ideal for flexible electronics [27, 28]. These nanomaterials collectively advance the development of wearable sensors, ensuring high sensitivity, functionality, and seamless integration into various applications. Figure 14.1 illustrates the characteristics and applications of nanomaterials and their respective applications.

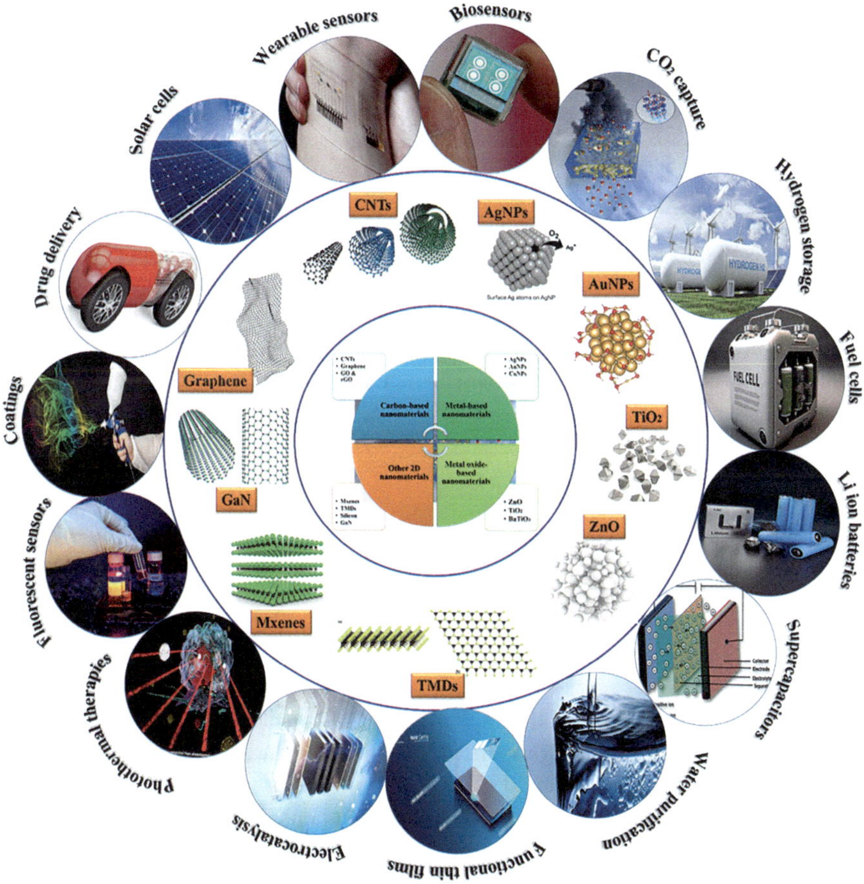

Fig. 14.1 Properties and application of nanomaterials

14.3.1 1D Nanomaterials

14.3.1.1 Carbon Nanotubes (CNTs)

CNTs, with their 1D cylindrical structure, high aspect ratio, and electron mobility, are ideal for wearable electronics. Common fabrication methods include chemical vapor deposition (CVD), arc discharge, and laser ablation, using CH_4, C_2H_4, or C_2H_2 as carbon sources. These techniques allow precise control over the nanotube's length, diameter, and orientation. CNTs can be applied to flexible substrates through vacuum filtration, spin-coating, or spray-coating, forming conductive films that fracture when stretched, thus altering the electric signal [7, 14, 29, 30]. This makes CNTs suitable for strain sensors monitoring joint movement and human-machine interaction.

14.3.1.2 Metal Nanowires

Gold, copper, and silver nanowires are commonly used in wearable monitoring sensors [22, 31]. For example, silver nanowires (AgNWs) are synthesized by reducing a silver precursor (e.g., $AgNO_3$), using molecules like polyol (ethylene glycol), cetyltrimethylammonium bromide, and polyvinyl pyrrolidone as templates, reducing agents, and capping agents, respectively. Gold nanowires can be synthesized similarly. Novel reducing agents, such as WS2 nanosheets, can also be used, where copper ions adsorb to WS2 and reduce to metal nanoparticles, elongating into nanowires. These metal nanowires function similarly to CNTs in sensors, with conductivity changes indicating applied force.

14.3.2 2D Nanomaterials

14.3.2.1 Graphene and Its Derivatives

Discovered by Novoselov et al., graphene is a 2D layer with one-atom thickness, offering excellent mechanical properties, electrical conductivity, Young's modulus, carrier mobility, and surface area [5, 32, 33]. It is widely used in wearable sensors as sensing elements or conductive electrodes. Graphene synthesis methods include chemical vapor deposition (CVD), epitaxial growth, micromechanical exfoliation, and chemical reduction, with laser-assisted technologies emerging recently. Graphene oxide (GO) and reduced graphene oxide (rGO) are derived from graphite oxide and can be synthesized via hydrothermal reduction, chemical, or electrochemical processes.

14.3.2.2 2D Transition Metal Dichalcogenides and Carbide Nanosheets

TMD nanosheets (e.g., MoS_2, WS_2) and MXene nanosheets (e.g., Ti_3C_2, Ti_2C) have high specific areas and electrical conductivity, suitable for electron transfer and high-accuracy detection [24, 27, 28]. TMDs, with a lamellar structure, show diverse properties and can be synthesized by mechanical cleavage, solvent exfoliation, chemical intercalation, and CVD. MXenes, composed of Mn + 1XnTx, are synthesized by etching elements from MAX powders, with variations in etching conditions affecting size and thickness.

14.3.3 3D Nanomaterials

Metal-organic frameworks (MOFs) are 3D nanomaterials with high specific areas and modification potential, used in wearable gas sensors [27, 28, 34]. MOFs are synthesized by hydrothermal or solvothermal methods, with microwave-assisted and ultrasonic methods also employed for size control.

14.3.4 Hybrid Nanomaterials

Hybrid nanomaterials enhance sensing performance by increasing conductivity and addressing biocompatibility or oxidation issues. Core-shell structures, synthesized by replacement reactions or novel methods like laser-assisted technology, are common. For example, AgNWs and $HAuCl_4$ can form Au and Ag nanotubes, and SiO_2@NiO composites can enhance piezoelectric properties [35, 36].

14.3.5 Bio-nanomaterials

Bio-nanomaterials, like cellulose nanofiber and silk fibroin (SF) nanofiber, offer biodegradability and safety for wearable sensors. Cellulose, abundant in nature, can be chemically extracted and processed into nanofibers for health monitoring. SF, obtained from silk fibers, is used for its tensile strength and can also be processed into nanofibers [37, 38]. These advancements in nanomaterials play crucial roles in the development and performance of wearable sensors, enhancing their capabilities and applications in various fields.

14.4 Fabrication Techniques

Fabricating nanocomposite-based wearable strain sensors involves integrating nanomaterials into polymer matrices using various methods. Uniform graphene dispersion within the matrix is crucial for optimizing material properties, which can be achieved through covalent and noncovalent functionalization. Common fabrication techniques include coating, printing, spinning, in-situ polymerization, melt blending, and solution processing, with the choice depending on specific application needs and sensing requirements [39].

14.4.1 Solution Processing

A simple and efficient method for fabricating wearable strain sensors involves dissolving nanomaterials and polymer in a common solvent. External forces like high-speed mechanical stirring and strong ultrasound aid in dispersing the polymer chains into the nanomaterials. Upon solvent evaporation, a polymer nanocomposite forms, which can be applied to create thin films using techniques such as spin coating, drop casting, and dip coating. This approach has been used with various polymer matrices like PU, PDMS, polysilicon, EPDM, and TPU [33, 39].

Hou et al. developed a biodegradable, stretchable sensor using silver nanofibers (AgNFs) and silk fibroin [40]. They created SF films through solution casting, electrospun polyvinyl alcohol (PVA) nanofibers, and coated them with silver via magnetron sputtering to form AgNFs. This AgNF film was then transferred onto the SF film to serve as the sensor's electrode, with Ecoflex used as the dielectric elastomer. The biocompatibility of SF enabled the sensor to be worn on the skin for long-term monitoring with minimal inflammation. Similarly, Lee and his team fabricated solution processed transparent, flexible strain sensor with CNT/PDMS composite and investigated detection of human activities and emotions [41] (Fig. 14.2).

14.4.2 Printing Techniques

Nanocomposites are fabricated using techniques like 3D printing, screen printing, and inkjet printing, each suited to specific needs [7, 23, 39]. Screen printing uses conductive inks applied through a mesh, ideal for low-cost, large-area sensors. Inkjet printing precisely deposits nanocomposite inks onto flexible substrates in fine layers, allowing high customization. 3D printing creates complex 3D structures layer by layer, offering versatility in shaping nanocomposites. Each method plays a vital role in developing functional and adaptable materials.

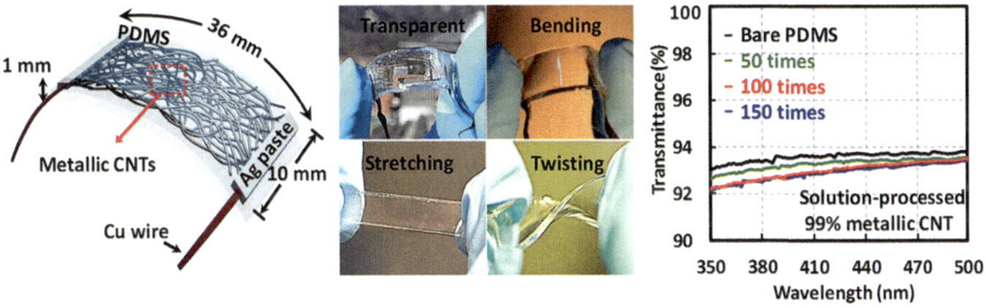

Fig. 14.2 Schematic representation of the transparent CNT–PDMS sandwich composite strain sensor. (Reproduced with permission [41]. Copyright 2017, American Chemical Society)

14.4.3 Coating

This includes spray coating and dip coating. In spray coating, a polymer solution with nanofillers is atomized and sprayed onto a substrate, forming a thin, uniform coating. Dip coating involves dipping nanofibers into a polymer solution, followed by drying. Both methods are effective in creating uniform polymer nanocomposites for various applications [23]. Spray coating has been used to develop PU-GNP nanocomposites [42], while dip coating [32] is employed for fibrous polymer nanocomposite structures.

14.4.4 In-Situ Polymerization

This method involves preparing a uniform dispersion of nanofillers in a solvent with a monomer or prepolymer to establish a stable chemical bond. A suitable initiator is then added to polymerize the monomer or prepolymer, enhancing interaction between the polymer and nanofillers and improving the performance of the polymer nanocomposites. Challenges include controlling the process due to graphene's impact on polymerization rates. Examples include polymers like PU, TPU, NR, PANI, and PVA with different types of conductive nanomaterials [42, 43].

14.4.5 Spinning

To fabricate fibrous polymer nanocomposites, spinning methods such as wet spinning and electrospinning are used. The wet spinning process involves creating a homogeneous composite solution, which is extruded through a spinneret into long fibers that solidify in a coagulation bath (see Fig. 14.3a). Electrospinning is a voltage-driven method that produces fine fibers from a

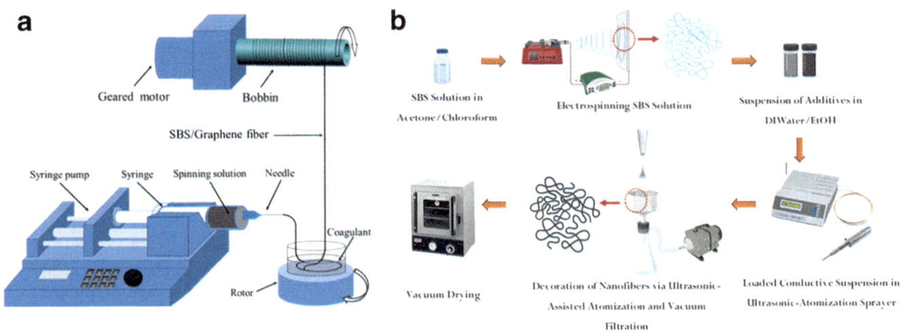

Fig. 14.3 Preparation of fiber-based strain sensors by (**a**) fabrication of poly(styrene-butadiene-styrene)/few layer graphene (SBS/FLG) composite fibers by wet-spinning: Reproduced with permission [46]. Copyright 2017, Elsevier Ltd. (**b**) Electrospinning Poly(styrene-butadiene-styrene) (SBS) fibers modified with graphene and MXene for strain sensing. (Reproduced with permission [47]. Copyright 2022, Elsevier)

polymer solution for fabricating nanofibers. A high voltage applied to the solution ejects a thin jet of polymer, which solidifies into fibers as the solvent evaporates (see Fig. 14.3b) [44, 45].

14.4.6 Melt Blending

This approach efficiently fabricates polymer nanocomposites by enhancing nanofiller dispersion within the polymer matrix. It involves dissolving nanofillers and the polymer in a common solvent, with polymer chain intercalation into the nanomaterials aided by external forces like mechanical stirring and strong ultrasound. Once the solvent evaporates, a nanocomposite is formed. Examples include polymers like PU, TPU, NR, polysilicone, EPDM, EVA, PANI, and PVA with different types of conductive nanomaterials [48].

14.5 Applications in Wearable Monitoring

14.5.1 Health Monitoring

Wearable sensors integrated into clothing or mounted on the skin enable real-time monitoring of physiological and environmental conditions, advancing healthcare from expensive hospital settings to personalized home care. These sensors go beyond traditional biomedical functions, incorporating mechanical sensors for detecting physiological changes such as strain and pressure. They can monitor subtle deformations from activities like blood flow and respiration, as well as larger movements such as joint bending. Continuous ECG monitoring is crucial for managing heart conditions. Nanomaterial-based dry electrodes are effective for long-term ECG sensing without skin irritation [49]. Apexcardiogram (ACG) complements ECG by providing insights into heart volume and pressure changes, with AuNP-based strain sensors detecting temporal cardiac variations. Heart rate can be calculated from ECG's R–R interval or by detecting strain or pressure at various body sites, including the wrist, neck, or foot.

Accurate respiration rate measurement is essential for diagnosing conditions like sleep disorders and asthma [31]. This can be achieved using strain or pressure sensors to measure chest deformation or airflow, such as a graphene-based strain sensor monitoring respiration rate. Temperature changes from mouth or nose breathing can also indicate respiration rate. Continuous body temperature monitoring is crucial for detecting conditions like hypothermia. Sensors like Al_2O_3-doped ZnO/AgNPs attached to the skin can track temperature variations during different activities [50]. Sensors also evaluate body motions to detect diseases such as Parkinson's and epilepsy. For example, AgNW-based strain sensors attached to the knee can record motion amplitude and duration, aiding early diagnosis of nervous system disorders [51].

Modern wearable systems combine sensing with therapeutic capabilities. These systems use multimodal sensors to monitor health parameters and body motions, providing real-time data to users, caregivers, or emergency centers. For example, a graphene-based wearable system includes a strain sensor, LED for alerts, a heater for thermal therapy, and iontophoresis electrodes for drug delivery [23]. This patch can measure tremor signals during hypoglycemic conditions, collect sweat for glucose sensing, and wirelessly monitor glucose levels via Bluetooth [52]. Temperature-controlled drug release can then be triggered by heating the microneedle array, successfully regulating blood glucose levels in diabetic mice [53]. These innovative wearable systems demonstrate significant potential in healthcare, offering real-time monitoring and immediate therapeutic responses to various health conditions. Figure 14.4 depicts nanocomposite-based wearable sensors for healthcare monitoring.

14.5.2 Physical Activity Tracking

Analyzing daily activities and sports performance yields essential insights into overall health, fitness levels, and rehabilitation progress. It also offers valuable quantitative data for assessing athletic performance and developing innovative human-machine interfaces.

14.5.2.1 Strain and Pressure Sensors

Wearable strain sensors, known for their ability to detect extensive strain ranges, are extensively used to monitor various body movements such as bending of finger, forearm muscle activities, and knee motions. For example, a strain sensor made

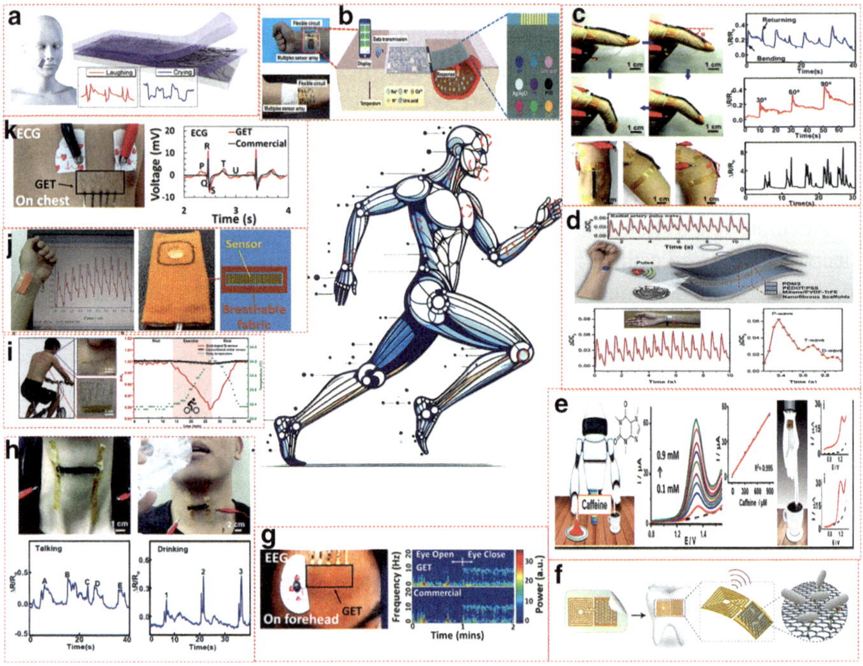

Fig. 14.4 The detailed scenario of nanocomposite-based wearable sensors for healthcare monitoring: (**a**) Emotion detection by CNT-based wearable strain sensor. Reproduced with permission [54] Copyright 2015, American Chemical Society. (**b**) Integrated multiple sensing bandage for monitoring of wounds. Reproduced with permission [55] Copyright 2021, American Chemical Society. (**c**) Monitoring minor human motions by the CNT reinforced PDMS sponge strain sensor [56] Copyright 2017, Royal Society of Chemistry. (**d**) Monitoring heartbeat or pulse by the MXene-based Nanofibrous Scaffolds composite [57] Copyright 2020, American Chemical Society. (**e**) Caffeine monitoring by wearable sensor. Reproduced with permission [58] Copyright 2018, American Chemical Society. (**f**) Pathogenic bacteria detection by graphene-reinforced wearable sensor. Reproduced with permission [59] Copyright 2012, Springer Nature. (**g**) Graphene-based wearable electroencephalogram (EEG), skin hydration, and skin temperature sensor. Reproduced with permission [60] Copyright 2017, American Chemical Society. (**h**) CNT/PDMS sponge strain sensor for monitoring small-strain human motions [56] Copyright 2017, Royal Society of Chemistry. (**i**) Real-time monitoring Au-doped SiNM temperature sensor for respiration monitoring and continuous body temperature [31]. Copyright 2021, WILEY-VCH Verlag GmbH & Co. KGaA, Weinheim. (**j**) Graphene-based pressure sensor for real-time high accuracy pulse wave monitoring under body motion interference [61]. Copyright 2019, Elsevier Ltd. K) ECG wearable sensor based on graphene. (Reproduced with permission [60] Copyright 2017, American Chemical Society)

from carbon nanotubes (CNTs) can distinguish different knee movements, including extending, flexing, marching, squatting, and jumping. Pressure sensors, when attached to the hand, can track the pressure distribution while gripping an object [2]. Additionally, data such as respiration rate, heart rate, and movements of body collected from wearable sensors are crucial for assessing and enhancing performance during rehabilitation and sports activities. Figure 14.5 illustrates the application of pressure sensors in sport monitoring.

Pressure sensors are widely used in sports to monitor plantar pressure by integrating them into shoe insoles. This monitoring is essential for evaluating the gait of athletes. Various gait variables, such as peak/mean pressure and reaction force, are measured. Zhao et al. used a flexible sensor matrix with 16 piezoresistive cells to analyze plantar pressure, showing similar static pressure forces for both feet during standing and dynamic gait cycles (Fig. 14.5a, b) [62]. Barratt et al. assessed commercial insoles' reliability during rowing, noting that the Motion insole overestimated pressure and force variables as shown in Fig. 14.5c [63]. Jeong et al. developed a durable, ultra-wide range pressure sensor suitable for powerlifting, identifying imbalances and incorrect poses (Fig. 14.5d–f) [30]. Similarly, a textile-based wireless pressure sensor was used to monitor pressure during yoga (Fig. 14.5g) [64]. These sensors can also be used as artificial electronic skin, mimicking human tactile sensitivity, as demonstrated by Cho et al. in a prosthetic hand [65]. Additionally, Yang et al. utilized a flexible triboelectric nanogenerator for monitoring pressure in skiing, applicable to insoles or ski pole sleeves [66].

14.5.2.2 Wearable Electrochemical Sensors

Wearable electrochemical sensors facilitate the real-time and continuous monitoring of sweat composition during physical activities [18, 52]. These sensors, integrated into devices such as wristbands or headbands, utilize a multiplexed sensor array combined with a flexible printed circuit board. This setup enables wireless tracking of variations in skin temperature, electrolytes, and sweat metabolites through a dedicated smartphone application, as depicted in Fig. 14.5i. Such real-time sweat analysis provides crucial insights into physiological and metabolic states, aiding in both disease diagnosis and the evaluation of athletic performance (Fig. 14.5h) [68]. Incorporating nanomaterials with high thermal conductivity improves response time and sensitivity.

14.5.3 Electronic Skin for Prosthetics and Intelligent Robotics

A network of wearable sensors can be integrated into prosthetics or robotic systems to replicate the sensory and transduction functions of human skin [14, 15]. This sensor-laden electronic skin, which is mechanically compliant, allows the detection of changes in the surrounding environment, enhancing interactions with it. This capability is particularly crucial for robotic systems operating in challenging or hazardous conditions. To effectively mimic human skin, the electronic skin must exhibit high mechanical compliance, sensitivity, spatiotemporal resolution, and the ability to sense multiple modalities [15]. Pressure sensing arrays can capture spatial pressure distributions from various sources, including static objects, gas flow, water

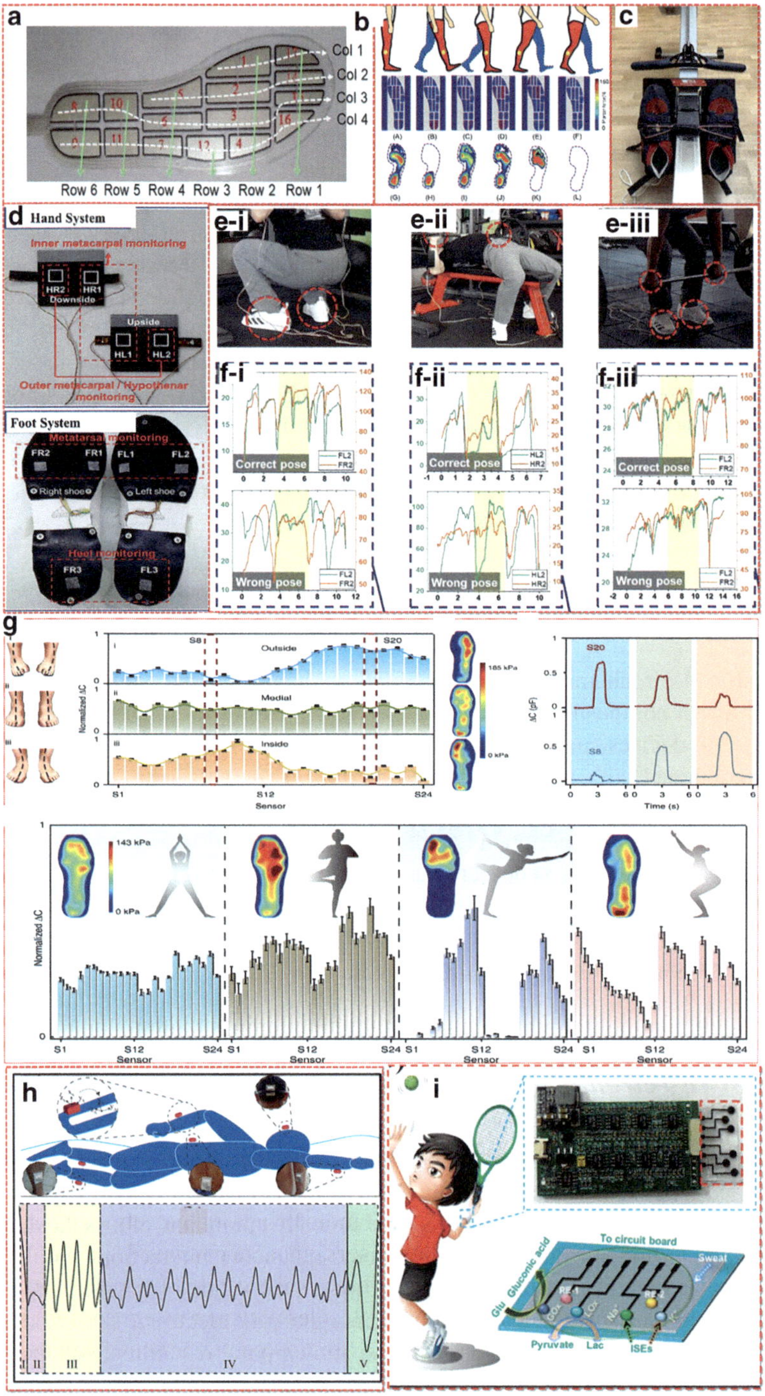

a
Col 1
Col 2
Col 3
Col 4
Row 6 Row 5 Row 4 Row 3 Row 2 Row 1
b
c
d Hand System
Inner metacarpal monitoring
HR2 HR1
Downside
Upside
HL1 HL2
Outer metacarpal / Hypothenar monitoring
Foot System
Metatarsal monitoring
FR2 FR1 FL1 FL2
Right shoe
Left shoe
Heel monitoring
FR3 FL3
e-i
e-ii
e-iii
f-i
f-ii
f-iii
Correct pose
Wrong pose
g
Outside
Medial
Inside
Normalized ΔC
Sensor
185 kPa
0 kPa
S20
S8
ΔC (pF)
Time (s)
143 kPa
h
I II III IV V
i
To circuit board
Sweat
Glu Gluconic acid
Pyruvate
Lac
ISEs

Fig. 14.5 Utilization of pressure-based sensors for monitoring of sport activities, including (**a**) Detection and analysis of plantar pressure during walking and (**b**) captured results of plantar pressure analysis [62]. (**c**) Measurement of plantar pressure using an ergometer [63]. (**d** and **e**) Monitoring hand and foot pressures during powerlifting (i–iii) and (**f**) pressure results for correct and incorrect poses corresponding to the methods (i–iii) [30]. (**g**) Monitoring pressure distribution in four different yoga postures based on the insole system [67]. (**h**) Applications of IMUs in sports monitoring, specifically for analyzing swimming activities [68]. (**i**) Wearable sweat metabolite sensors and their applications in sports monitoring [69]

droplet impacts, finger touches, and acoustic vibrations. For instance, Roh et al. developed a stretchable, ultrasensitive strain sensor using carbon nanotubes (CNTs) combined with a conductive elastomer (PU/PEDOT) [54]. A PDMS layer was treated with O_2 plasma to become hydrophilic, then coated with layers of PU/PEDOT, SWCNT solution, and another PU/PEDOT layer, forming a wearable sensor (Fig. 14.4a). This sensor, featuring high transparency, stretchability, and sensitivity, can be attached to the face to monitor muscle movements and distinguish between laughing and crying.

Integrating sensors with transistors enables active matrix addressing, minimizing signal interference. Advanced electronic skins combine temperature, tactile, humidity, and pressure sensors into single pixels, allowing for multi-stimuli detection and mapping. For example, graphene-based skins can detect changes from hot wind, touch, and breathing [70].

14.5.4 Multifunctional Sensors for Environmental Monitoring

Advanced wearable sensors must distinguish between multiple stimuli like strain, twist, temperature, light, humidity, and gases. Researchers are developing multifunctional sensors that provide real-time tracking of human motion and environmental conditions, streamlining integration and miniaturization. For example, piezoresistive and thermoresistive sensors which are ultrasensitive sensors have been created using PANI hollow nanospheres and a CNT composite, which detects both pressure and temperature through resistance changes [71]. In another example, self-powered multifunctional sensors made from rGO/PVDF nanofibers integrate pressure, gas, and light detection with energy storage capabilities [72]. These multifunctional sensors simplify integration by combining various sensing functions into a single device. The design of these sensors addresses challenges by incorporating features like self-healing, self-powering, self-cleaning, and biocompatibility, enhancing their versatility and functionality.

14.5.4.1 Light Sensors

Light is essential for life, aiding in photosynthesis in plants and supporting ocean plankton. However, excessive light can harm human health and affect plant photosynthesis. Artificial night light pollution also disrupts wildlife. Light sensors, or photodetectors (PDs), convert light into electrical signals. They detect light in the UV, visible, and infrared ranges. These sensors use semiconductor materials like silicon and germanium, which are incorporated into stretchable devices using innovative designs. For example, PDs made from ZnO nanowires or graphene show great potential for stretchability and sensitivity [73, 74]. Researchers have developed multifunctional sensors that combine various functions, like pressure, temperature, and gas detection, in one device. These sensors use materials such as rGO/PU nanofibers and hybrid structures to enhance performance [73, 74]. Innovations in geometry and material engineering have led to highly stretchable and sensitive PDs, which are useful in diverse applications, including optical communications and wearable technology. Despite some challenges with photoresponsiveness, ongoing research continues to improve their efficiency and functionality.

14.5.4.2 Temperature Sensors

Stretchable temperature sensors monitor environmental changes, provide feedback, and protect heat-sensitive electronics. With a range of −10 to +85 °C and sensitivity ≤1.0 °C, innovations in materials and design enhance their performance [75]. Most rely on the thermoresistive effect, where a material's resistivity changes with temperature. For example, buckled thin films, serpentine designs, and coiled structures enhance flexibility. Materials like carbon nanotubes and graphene are also used but need mixing with other materials to improve sensitivity. Recent advancements include sensors with hybrid materials and designs that maintain performance under strain. For example, a stretchable graphene thermistor with a 50% stretchability and a Cu nanowire mesh that can stretch up to 80% without damage [76, 77].

14.5.4.3 Humidity Sensors

Humidity significantly affects precipitation patterns, biospheres, surface hydrology, and the operation of electronics. It impacts human and animal health, causing heat stress in high humidity and various health issues in low humidity. Monitoring humidity levels can provide insights into physiological conditions and aging mechanisms. Humidity sensors measure relative humidity and are categorized by the type of sensing material used (ceramic, semiconductor, polymer) and the sensing mechanism (resistive, capacitive). Recent developments in stretchable humidity sensors have focused on enhancing material selection, design strategies, and performance.

For example, a capacitive-type sensor using CNT micro-yarn and Ecoflex on a PDMS substrate changes capacitance with humidity due to water absorption/desorption [78]. A resistive-type sensor with SWNT/PVA filaments uses PVA's hygroscopicity to alter resistance [79]. Innovations like spiral configurations of spandex-covered yarn coated with humidity-sensitive PANI allow for ultra-stretchability up to 200%. 2D materials like graphene oxide (GO) and reduced graphene oxide (rGO) have gained popularity due to their extensive surface area. A GO-based sensor achieved a 30 ms response and recovery time but limited stretchability [80]. Combining rGO with PU improves flexibility, achieving up to 60% strain without performance loss [81]. Other examples include WS2 and MoS2-based sensors, which offer transparency, flexibility, and improved sensitivity even under mechanical stress.

14.5.4.4 pH Sensors

The pH scale measures the hydrogen ion concentration in water-based solutions, indicating their acidity or alkalinity. Monitoring pH is crucial due to its significant impact on environmental health; for example, ocean pH fluctuations affect marine organisms' resilience. Environmental pH changes, caused by factors like acid rain and pollution, can contaminate water and harm ecosystems. Potentiometric pH sensors, which use ion-sensitive and reference electrodes to measure potential differences, are widely used due to their simplicity [75]. However, traditional glass membranes used in these sensors are fragile. Advances include stretchable sensors using materials like PANI and iridium oxide, and novel approaches such as stretchable hydrogels that provide flexibility and biocompatibility [82, 83]. These sensors, from various designs like serpentine patterns to advanced hydrogels, aim to maintain performance while adapting to environmental and biological conditions.

14.5.4.5 Gas Sensors

Monitoring air quality and toxic gases has become crucial due to the severe health impacts and environmental damage caused by pollutants like PM2.5, which contributes to 3.3 million premature deaths annually, mainly in Asia [84]. Stretchable gas sensors have evolved significantly, featuring three main types: chemiresistors, FET-based sensors, and triboelectric generators. Chemiresistors, like those using ZnO, change resistance based on gas interactions, while FET-based sensors use materials like graphene for gas detection [75]. Triboelectric sensors, such as carbon fiber e-skin, detect gases through triboelectrification. Recent advancements include stretchable sensors with 2D materials (e.g., graphene and rGO) and innovative designs like patterned substrates and nanocomposites. Despite progress, issues like poor response kinetics and humidity interference persist, though advances such as crumpled PbS quantum dots offer improved stability and performance.

14.6 Advantages, Challenges, and Future Perspectives

Nanocomposites offer numerous advantages for wearable monitoring devices due to their high sensitivity, flexibility, and multifunctionality. The high surface area of nanomaterials grants nanocomposites superior sensitivity, making them ideal for detecting minute changes in biometrics. Their flexibility allows seamless integration into wearable devices, ensuring comfort and durability even under strain. The enhanced conductivity provided by nanoparticles like carbon nanotubes or metal nanoparticles is crucial for developing efficient electrodes for biosignal monitoring (ECG, EMG) and bioimpedance measurements. Additionally, nanocomposites exhibit improved mechanical properties, such as strength and elasticity, over traditional polymer matrices. This robustness ensures that wearable devices are not only comfortable but also durable for daily use. Tailoring the sensing properties through different nanofillers enables the detection of specific biomolecules, such as glucose and lactate, enhancing health monitoring capabilities. The lightweight and flexible nature of nanocomposites contributes to the development of unobtrusive devices that integrate seamlessly with the body. Furthermore, the multifunctionality of nanocomposites allows for the combination of features, such as conductivity and antibacterial properties, promoting hygiene and user safety.

Despite significant advancements in nanocomposites for wearable monitoring devices, several challenges persist that hinder their widespread practical application:

Despite their potential, several obstacles prevent nanocomposites from being widely used in wearable technology. Achieving scalable, economical production with reliable quality is a significant challenge, especially for materials like graphene. Another issue is mechanical dependability since it takes a lot of creativity to optimize device architecture while maintaining flexibility and durability under frequent use. Furthermore, because nanoparticles are hydrophobic, surface contamination can impair sensor performance, requiring careful handling and production procedures.

There are additional challenges when integrating wearable sensors with necessary parts like power supplies and data processing devices. Another technical challenge is achieving both high sensitivity and a wide working range, since existing designs frequently break down under extreme pressure or are ineffective at detecting multidirectional strains. Reliable performance requires environmental stability in a variety of variables, such as temperature and humidity, yet this is still difficult to achieve. Furthermore, new solutions like artificial intelligence and IoT integration are required for wireless signal transmission and processing large volumes of data. Figure 14.6 reports the challenges in achieving significant advancements in nanocomposites for wearable monitoring devices for widespread practical applications.

Addressing these challenges requires continued research and innovation in material science, fabrication techniques, and integration strategies to advance the development of reliable, high-performance nanocomposite-based wearable monitoring devices. The future of nanocomposites in wearable monitoring looks promising,

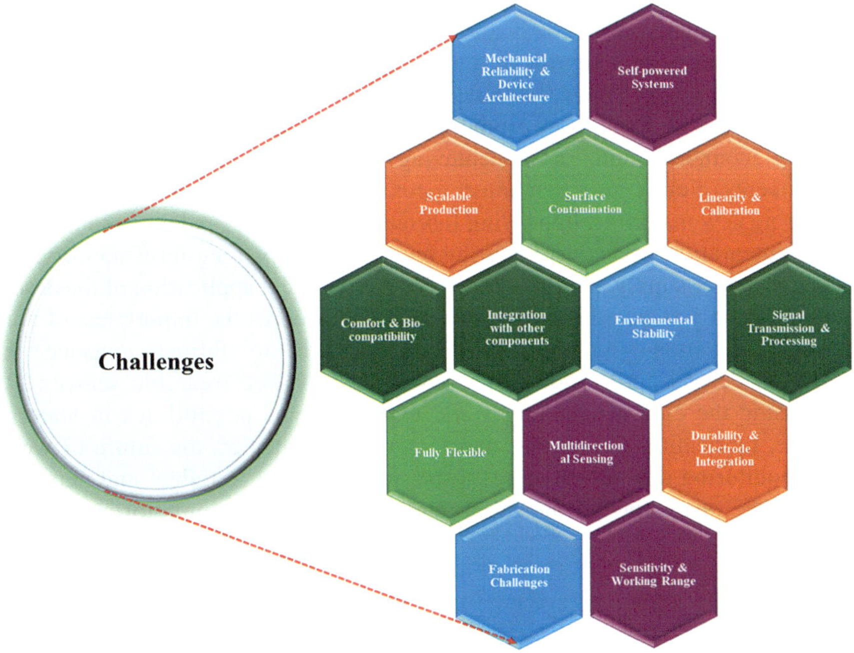

Fig. 14.6 Challenges in achieving significant advancements in nanocomposites for wearable monitoring devices for widespread practical applications

with ongoing research focused on improving material properties, developing new fabrication techniques, and exploring innovative applications. Integration with advanced technologies such as artificial intelligence and the Internet of Things (IoT) will further enhance the capabilities of wearable sensors, making them smarter and more efficient.

14.7 Conclusions

Nanocomposites represent a transformative approach in the development of wearable monitoring devices, offering unmatched performance and new functionalities. Despite the challenges, advancements in nanomaterial synthesis, processing, and device integration continue to drive the field forward, promising a future where wearable technology seamlessly integrates into our daily lives for better health and well-being. The rapid advancements in the development of portable, wearable, and lightweight strain sensors underscore the urgent need for highly efficient and flexible sensing strategies. This chapter has highlighted the potential of polymer nanocomposites due to their unique properties such as high conductivity, large surface area, and versatile morphologies, making them ideal for strain sensing applications. Through various fabrication methodologies and advancements, nanocomposites have shown exceptional capabilities in monitoring subtle and significant physiological signals, thereby enhancing the accuracy and reliability of wearable devices. Despite the progress made, challenges remain in scaling up production, ensuring mechanical reliability, preventing contamination, and achieving seamless integration with other components. Future research must focus on overcoming these obstacles by exploring new materials, improving fabrication processes, and developing innovative integration strategies. Ensuring biocompatibility, long-term stability, and efficient power supply are also critical for the practical application of these sensors, especially in healthcare. This chapter underscores the importance of continued innovation and multidisciplinary efforts to further enhance the performance and applicability of nanocomposite-based wearable sensors. By addressing the current challenges and exploring new possibilities in material science, fabrication techniques, and integration strategies, the future of wearable monitoring devices promises to be more efficient, reliable, and versatile, paving the way for advanced applications in health monitoring, sports, and beyond.

References

1. Liu L, Zhang X. A focused review on the flexible wearable sensors for sports: from kinematics to physiologies. Micromachines. 2022;13 https://doi.org/10.3390/mi13081356.
2. Kanoun O, Bouhamed A, Ramalingame R, Bautista-Quijano JR, Rajendran D, Al-Hamry A. Review on conductive polymer/CNTs nanocomposites based flexible and stretchable strain and pressure sensors. Sensors. 2021;21:341.
3. Costa P, Carvalho MF, Correia V, Viana JC, Lanceros-Mendez S. Polymer nanocomposite-based strain sensors with tailored processability and improved device integration. ACS Appl Nano Mater. 2018;1:3015–25.
4. Gavande V, Mahalingam S, Kim J, Lee W-K. Optimization of UV-curable polyurethane acrylate coatings with hexagonal boron nitride (hBN) for improved mechanical and adhesive properties. Polymers (Basel). 2024;16 https://doi.org/10.3390/polym16172544.
5. Liu H, Gao H, Hu G. Highly sensitive natural rubber/pristine graphene strain sensor prepared by a simple method. Compos Part B Eng. 2019;171:138–45.
6. Gavande V, Lee W-K. Optically transparent PDMS nanocomposites with ultrafine electrospun nanofiber reinforcement. Mol Cryst Liq Cryst. 2023;(1):–9. https://doi.org/10.1080/15421406.2023.2176049.
7. Li Q, Luo S, Wang Y, Wang Q-M. Carbon based polyimide nanocomposites thin film strain sensors fabricated by ink-jet printing method. Sens Actuators A Phys. 2019;300:111664.
8. Wang W, Lu L, Li Z, Lin L, Liang Z, Lu X, Xie Y. Fingerprint-inspired strain sensor with balanced sensitivity and strain range using laser-induced graphene. ACS Appl Mater Interfaces. 2021;14:1315–25.
9. Gong M, Zhang L, Wan P. Polymer nanocomposite meshes for flexible electronic devices. Prog Polym Sci. 2020;107:101279.
10. Alizadeh A, Burns A, Lenigk R, Gettings R, Ashe J, Porter A, McCaul M, Barrett R, Diamond D, White P. A wearable patch for continuous monitoring of sweat electrolytes during exertion. Lab Chip. 2018;18:2632–41.

11. Wang X, Zhang Y, Zhang X, Huo Z, Li X, Que M, Peng Z, Wang H, Pan C. A highly stretchable transparent self-powered triboelectric tactile sensor with metallized nanofibers for wearable electronics. Adv Mater. 2018;30:1706738.
12. Yang Y, Yang X, Tan Y, Yuan Q. Recent progress in flexible and wearable bio-electronics based on nanomaterials. Nano Res. 2017;10:1560–83.
13. Liu C, Han S, Xu H, Wu J, Liu C. Multifunctional highly sensitive multiscale stretchable strain sensor based on a graphene/glycerol–KCl synergistic conductive network. ACS Appl Mater Interfaces. 2018;10:31716–24.
14. Zhu H, Wang X, Liang J, Lv H, Tong H, Ma L, Hu Y, Zhu G, Zhang T, Tie Z. Versatile electronic skins for motion detection of joints enabled by aligned few-walled carbon nanotubes in flexible polymer composites. Adv Funct Mater. 2017;27:1606604.
15. Lim C, Hong YJ, Jung J, Shin Y, Sunwoo S-H, Baik S, Park OK, Choi SH, Hyeon T, Kim JH. Tissue-like skin-device interface for wearable bioelectronics by using ultrasoft, mass-permeable, and low-impedance hydrogels. Sci Adv. 2021;7:eabd3716.
16. Choi C, Lee Y, Cho KW, Koo JH, Kim D-H. Wearable and implantable soft bioelectronics using two-dimensional materials. Acc Chem Res. 2018;52:73–81.
17. Kim J, Jeerapan I, Imani S, Cho TN, Bandodkar A, Cinti S, Mercier PP, Wang J. Noninvasive alcohol monitoring using a wearable tattoo-based iontophoretic-biosensing system. ACS Sens. 2016;1:1011–9.
18. Jia W, Bandodkar AJ, Valdés-Ramírez G, Windmiller JR, Yang Z, Ramírez J, Chan G, Wang J. Electrochemical tattoo biosensors for real-time noninvasive lactate monitoring in human perspiration. Anal Chem. 2013;85:6553–60.
19. Tamayol A, Akbari M, Zilberman Y, Comotto M, Lesha E, Serex L, Bagherifard S, Chen Y, Fu G, Ameri SK. pH-sensing hydrogel fibers: flexible pH-sensing hydrogel fibers for epidermal applications. Adv Healthc Mater. 2016;5:624.
20. Peng B, Zhao F, Ping J, Ying Y. Recent advances in nanomaterial-enabled wearable sensors: material synthesis, sensor design, and personal health monitoring. Small. 2020;16:2002681.
21. Jayathilaka WADM, Qi K, Qin Y, Chinnappan A, Serrano-García W, Baskar C, Wang H, He J, Cui S, Thomas SW. Significance of nanomaterials in wearables: a review on wearable actuators and sensors. Adv Mater. 2019;31:1805921.
22. Dabhade AH, Verma RP, Paramasivan B, Kumawat A, Saha B. Development of silver nanoparticles and aptamer conjugated biosensor for rapid detection of E coli in a water sample. 3 Biotech. 2023;13:244.
23. Mishra S, Saha B. Graphene- polymer nanocomposite-based wearable strain sensors for physiological signal monitoring: recent progress and challenges. Curr Opin Solid State Mater Sci. 2024;31:101174. https://doi.org/10.1016/j.cossms.2024.101174.
24. Peng S, Yu Y, Wu S, Wang C-H. Conductive polymer nanocomposites for stretchable electronics: material selection, design, and applications. ACS Appl Mater Interfaces. 2021;13:43831–54.
25. Raman S, Ravi Sankar A. Intrinsically conducting polymers in flexible and stretchable resistive strain sensors: a review. J Mater Sci. 2022;57:13152–78.
26. Chen Z, Chen Y, Hedenqvist MS, Chen C, Cai C, Li H, Liu H, Fu J. Multifunctional conductive hydrogels and their applications as smart wearable devices. J Mater Chem B. 2021;9:2561–83.
27. Jiang D, Liu Z, Xiao Z, Qian Z, Sun Y, Zeng Z, Wang R. Flexible electronics based on 2D transition metal dichalcogenides. J Mater Chem A Mater. 2022;10:89–121.
28. Singh E, Singh P, Kim KS, Yeom GY, Nalwa HS. Flexible molybdenum disulfide (MoS2) atomic layers for wearable electronics and optoelectronics. ACS Appl Mater Interfaces. 2019;11:11061–105.
29. Hosseini H, Kokabi M, Mousavi SM. Conductive bacterial cellulose/multiwall carbon nanotubes nanocomposite aerogel as a potentially flexible lightweight strain sensor. Carbohydr Polym. 2018;201:228–35.
30. Jeong Y, Gu J, Byun J, Ahn J, Byun J, Kim K, Park J, Ko J, Jeong J, Amjadi M, Park I. Ultra-wide range pressure sensor based on a microstructured conductive nanocomposite for wear-

able workout monitoring. Adv Healthc Mater. 2021;10:2001461. https://doi.org/10.1002/adhm.202001461.
31. Sang M, Kang K, Zhang Y, Zhang H, Kim K, Cho M, Shin J, Hong J-H, Kim T, Lee SK, Yeo W-H, Lee JW, Lee T, Xu B, Yu KJ. Ultrahigh sensitive Au-doped silicon nanomembrane based wearable sensor arrays for continuous skin temperature monitoring with high precision. Adv Mater. 2022;34:2105865. https://doi.org/10.1002/adma.202105865.
32. Tung TT, Tran MT, Pereira ALC, Cordeiro CMB, Nguyen DD, Tai N-H, Tran VV, Hsu C-C, Joshi P, Yoshimura M. Graphene woven fabric-polydimethylsiloxane piezoresistive films for smart multi-stimuli responses. Colloids Surf B Biointerfaces. 2023;221:112940.
33. Peña-Consuegra J, Pagnola MR, Useche J, Madhukar P, Saccone FD, Marrugo AG. Manufacturing and measuring techniques for graphene-silicone-based strain sensors. JOM. 2023;75:631–45.
34. Li L, Meng J, Zhang M, Liu T, Zhang C. Recent advances in conductive polymer hydrogel composites and nanocomposites for flexible electrochemical supercapacitors. Chem Commun. 2022;58:185–207.
35. Yang P, Gao X, Wang L, Wu Q, Chen Z, Lin X. Amperometric sensor for ascorbic acid based on a glassy carbon electrode modified with gold-silver bimetallic nanotubes in a chitosan matrix. Microchim Acta. 2014;181:231–8.
36. Dutta B, Kar E, Bose N, Mukherjee S. NiO@ SiO2/PVDF: a flexible polymer nanocomposite for a high performance human body motion-based energy harvester and tactile e-skin mechanosensor. ACS Sustain Chem Eng. 2018;6:10505–16.
37. Cao J, Lu C, Zhuang J, Liu M, Zhang X, Yu Y, Tao Q. Multiple hydrogen bonding enables the self-healing of sensors for human–machine interactions. Angew Chem. 2017;129:8921–6.
38. Rockwood DN, Preda RC, Yücel T, Wang X, Lovett ML, Kaplan DL. Materials fabrication from Bombyx mori silk fibroin. Nat Protoc. 2011;6:1612–31.
39. Afsarimanesh N, Nag A, Sarkar S, Sabet GS, Han T, Mukhopadhyay SC. A review on fabrication, characterization and implementation of wearable strain sensors. Sensors Actuators A Phys. 2020;315:112355. https://doi.org/10.1016/j.sna.2020.112355.
40. Hou C, Xu Z, Qiu W, Wu R, Wang Y, Xu Q, Liu XY, Guo W. A biodegradable and stretchable protein-based sensor as artificial electronic skin for human motion detection. Small. 2019;15:1805084.
41. Lee J, Lim M, Yoon J, Kim MS, Choi B, Kim DM, Kim DH, Park I, Choi S-J. Transparent, flexible strain sensor based on a solution-processed carbon nanotube network. ACS Appl Mater Interfaces. 2017;9:26279–85. https://doi.org/10.1021/acsami.7b03184.
42. Fortunato M, Bellagamba I, Marra F, Tamburrano A, Sarto MS. Development and characterization of a piezoresistive polyurethane/GNP coating for strain sensing applications. In: 2020 IEEE 20th international conference on nanotechnology (IEEE-NANO). IEEE; 2020. p. 176–9.
43. Gunasekaran HB, Ponnan S, Zheng Y, Laroui A, Wang H, Wu L, Wang J. Facile fabrication of highly sensitive thermoplastic polyurethane sensors with surface-and interface-impregnated 3D conductive networks. ACS Appl Mater Interfaces. 2022;14:22615–25.
44. Gavande V, Nagappan S, Seo B, Cho Y-S, Lee W-K. Transparent nylon 6 nanofibers-reinforced epoxy matrix composites with superior mechanical and thermal properties. Polym Test. 2023;122:108002. https://doi.org/10.1016/j.polymertesting.2023.108002.
45. Gavande V, Nagappan S, Seo B, Lee W-K. A systematic review on green and natural polymeric nanofibers for biomedical applications. Int J Biol Macromol. 2024;262:130135. https://doi.org/10.1016/j.ijbiomac.2024.130135.
46. Wang X, Meng S, Tebyetekerwa M, Li Y, Pionteck J, Sun B, Qin Z, Zhu M. Highly sensitive and stretchable piezoresistive strain sensor based on conductive poly(styrene-butadiene-styrene)/few layer graphene composite fiber. Compos A Appl Sci Manuf. 2018;105:291–9. https://doi.org/10.1016/j.compositesa.2017.11.027.

47. Mohseni Taromsari S, Shi HH, Saadatnia Z, Park CB, Naguib HE. Design and development of ultra-sensitive, dynamically stable, multi-modal GnP@MXene nanohybrid electrospun strain sensors. Chem Eng J. 2022;442:136138. https://doi.org/10.1016/j.cej.2022.136138.
48. Mehmood A, Mubarak NM, Khalid M, Walvekar R, Abdullah EC, Siddiqui MTH, Baloch HA, Nizamuddin S, Mazari S. Graphene based nanomaterials for strain sensor application—a review. J Environ Chem Eng. 2020;8:103743.
49. Ramasamy S, Balan A. Wearable sensors for ECG measurement: a review. Sens Rev. 2018;38:412–9.
50. Park M, Do K, Kim J, Son D, Koo JH, Park J, Song J-K, Kim JH, Lee M, Hyeon T. Oxide nanomembrane hybrids with enhanced mechano-and thermo-sensitivity for semitransparent epidermal electronics. Adv Healthc Mater. 2015;4:992–7.
51. Yao S, Zhu Y. Wearable multifunctional sensors using printed stretchable conductors made of silver nanowires. Nanoscale. 2014;6:2345–52.
52. Zhu X, Ju Y, Chen J, Liu D, Liu H. Nonenzymatic wearable sensor for electrochemical analysis of perspiration glucose. ACS Sens. 2018;3:1135–41.
53. Lee H, Choi TK, Lee YB, Cho HR, Ghaffari R, Wang L, Choi HJ, Chung TD, Lu N, Hyeon T, Choi SH, Kim D-H. A graphene-based electrochemical device with thermoresponsive microneedles for diabetes monitoring and therapy. Nat Nanotechnol. 2016;11:566–72. https://doi.org/10.1038/nnano.2016.38.
54. Roh E, Hwang B-U, Kim D, Kim B-Y, Lee N-E. Stretchable, transparent, ultrasensitive, and patchable strain sensor for human–machine interfaces comprising a nanohybrid of carbon nanotubes and conductive elastomers. ACS Nano. 2015;9:6252–61. https://doi.org/10.1021/acsnano.5b01613.
55. Liu Z, Liu J, Sun T, Zeng D, Yang C, Wang H, Yang C, Guo J, Wu Q, Chen H-J, Xie X. Integrated multiplex sensing bandage for in situ monitoring of early infected wounds. ACS Sens. 2021;6:3112–24. https://doi.org/10.1021/acssensors.1c01279.
56. Li Q, Li J, Tran D, Luo C, Gao Y, Yu C, Xuan F. Engineering of carbon nanotube/polydimethylsiloxane nanocomposites with enhanced sensitivity for wearable motion sensors. J Mater Chem C. 2017;5:11092–9.
57. Sharma S, Chhetry A, Sharifuzzaman M, Yoon H, Park JY. Wearable capacitive pressure sensor based on MXene composite nanofibrous scaffolds for reliable human physiological signal acquisition. ACS Appl Mater Interfaces. 2020;12:22212–24. https://doi.org/10.1021/acsami.0c05819.
58. Ciui B, Martin A, Mishra RK, Nakagawa T, Dawkins TJ, Lyu M, Cristea C, Sandulescu R, Wang J. Chemical sensing at the robot fingertips: toward automated taste discrimination in food samples. ACS Sens. 2018;3:2375–84. https://doi.org/10.1021/acssensors.8b00778.
59. Mannoor MS, Tao H, Clayton JD, Sengupta A, Kaplan DL, Naik RR, Verma N, Omenetto FG, McAlpine MC. Graphene-based wireless bacteria detection on tooth enamel. Nat Commun. 2012;3:763.
60. Kabiri Ameri S, Ho R, Jang H, Tao L, Wang Y, Wang L, Schnyer DM, Akinwande D, Lu N. Graphene electronic tattoo sensors. ACS Nano. 2017;11:7634–41.
61. He J, Xiao P, Lu W, Shi J, Zhang L, Liang Y, Pan C, Kuo S-W, Chen T. A universal high accuracy wearable pulse monitoring system via high sensitivity and large linearity graphene pressure sensor. Nano Energy. 2019;59:422–33. https://doi.org/10.1016/j.nanoen.2019.02.036.
62. Zhao S, Liu R, Fei C, Zia AW, Jing L. Flexible sensor matrix film-based wearable plantar pressure force measurement and analysis system. PLoS One. 2020;15:e0237090.
63. Barratt GK, Bellenger C, Robertson EY, Lane J, Crowther RG. Validation of plantar pressure and reaction force measured by moticon pressure sensor insoles on a Concept2 rowing ergometer. Sensors. 2021;21:2418.
64. Nie B, Huang R, Yao T, Zhang Y, Miao Y, Liu C, Liu J, Chen X. Textile-based wireless pressure sensor array for human-interactive sensing. Adv Funct Mater. 2019;29:1808786.
65. Cho Y, Lee Y, Kim P, Jeong S, Kim K-S. The MSC prosthetic hand: rapid, powerful, and intuitive. IEEE Rob Autom Lett. 2022;7:3170–7.

66. Yang Y, Hou X, Geng W, Mu J, Zhang L, Wang X, He J, Xiong J, Chou X. Human movement monitoring and behavior recognition for intelligent sports using customizable and flexible triboelectric nanogenerator. SCIENCE CHINA Technol Sci. 2022;65:826–36.
67. Tao J, Dong M, Li L, Wang C, Li J, Liu Y, Bao R, Pan C. Real-time pressure mapping smart insole system based on a controllable vertical pore dielectric layer. Microsyst Nanoeng. 2020;6:62. https://doi.org/10.1038/s41378-020-0171-1.
68. Hamidi Rad M, Gremeaux V, Dadashi F, Aminian K. A novel macro-micro approach for swimming analysis in main swimming techniques using IMU sensors. Front Bioeng Biotechnol. 2021;8:597738.
69. Hao J, Zhu Z, Hu C, Liu Z. Photosensitive-stamp-inspired scalable fabrication strategy of wearable sensing arrays for noninvasive real-time sweat analysis. Anal Chem. 2022;94:4547–55.
70. Ho DH, Sun Q, Kim SY, Han JT, Kim DH, Cho JH. Stretchable and multimodal all graphene electronic skin. Adv Mater. 2016;28:2601–8.
71. Lou Z, Chen S, Wang L, Shi R, Li L, Jiang K, Chen D, Shen G. Ultrasensitive and ultraflexible e-skins with dual functionalities for wearable electronics. Nano Energy. 2017;38:28–35.
72. Ai Y, Lou Z, Chen S, Chen D, Wang ZM, Jiang K, Shen G. All rGO-on-PVDF-nanofibers based self-powered electronic skins. Nano Energy. 2017;35:121–7.
73. Yan C, Wang J, Wang X, Kang W, Cui M, Foo CY, Lee PS. An intrinsically stretchable nanowire photodetector with a fully embedded structure. Adv Mater. 2014;26:943–50.
74. Kim M, Kang P, Leem J, Nam S. A stretchable crumpled graphene photodetector with plasmonically enhanced photoresponsivity. Nanoscale. 2017;9:4058–65.
75. Yang Y, Deng ZD. Stretchable sensors for environmental monitoring. Appl Phys Rev. 2019;6:11309. https://doi.org/10.1063/1.5085013.
76. Yan C, Wang J, Lee PS. Stretchable graphene thermistor with tunable thermal index. ACS Nano. 2015;9:2130–7.
77. Han S, Kim MK, Wang B, Wie DS, Wang S, Lee CH. Mechanically reinforced skin-electronics with networked nanocomposite elastomer. Adv Mater. 2016;28:10257–65.
78. Kim SY, Park S, Park HW, Park DH, Jeong Y, Kim DH. Highly sensitive and multimodal all-carbon skin sensors capable of simultaneously detecting tactile and biological stimuli. Adv Mater. 2015;28:4178–85.
79. Zhou G, Byun J-H, Oh Y, Jung B-M, Cha H-J, Seong D-G, Um M-K, Hyun S, Chou T-W. Highly sensitive wearable textile-based humidity sensor made of high-strength, single-walled carbon nanotube/poly (vinyl alcohol) filaments. ACS Appl Mater Interfaces. 2017;9:4788–97.
80. Borini S, White R, Wei D, Astley M, Haque S, Spigone E, Harris N, Kivioja J, Ryhänen T. Ultrafast graphene oxide humidity sensors. ACS Nano. 2013;7:11166–73.
81. Trung TQ, Duy LT, Ramasundaram S, Lee N-E. Transparent, stretchable, and rapid-response humidity sensor for body-attachable wearable electronics. Nano Res. 2017;10:2021–33.
82. Oh SY, Hong SY, Jeong YR, Yun J, Park H, Jin SW, Lee G, Oh JH, Lee H, Lee S-S. Skin-attachable, stretchable electrochemical sweat sensor for glucose and pH detection. ACS Appl Mater Interfaces. 2018;10:13729–40.
83. Chung H, Sulkin MS, Kim J, Goudeseune C, Chao H, Song JW, Yang SY, Hsu Y, Ghaffari R, Efimov IR. Stretchable, multiplexed pH sensors with demonstrations on rabbit and human hearts undergoing ischemia. Adv Healthc Mater. 2014;3:59–68.
84. Lelieveld J, Evans JS, Fnais M, Giannadaki D, Pozzer A. The contribution of outdoor air pollution sources to premature mortality on a global scale. Nature. 2015;525:367–71.

Chapter 15
Clinical Translation of Smart Nanomaterials

Vignesh Mariappan and P. Vinayaga Moorthi

Abstract Smart nanomaterials have emerged as transformative tools in clinical medicine, leading to a paradigm shift from conventional therapy to precision medicine. While nanomaterials in biomedicine have primarily been used for drug delivery, a new nanoscale platform has recently been developed, advancing biomaterials for the prevention, diagnosis, and treatment of diseases. Due to their minute dimension and unique physicochemical nature, these nanomaterials are widely employed in various biological applications, including targeted drug delivery, gene therapy, biosensors, microfluidics, early prognosis, and diagnostics. They play a significant role in extending drug circulation time, enhancing biodistribution, improving solubility, facilitating intracellular transport, and traversing biological membranes. The scientific community is now advancing multifunctional nanomaterials that integrate therapeutic, targeting, and imaging properties. This chapter highlights the classification, characterization, and preclinical development methods of nanomaterials, as well as their significant implication in diagnostics and theranostics. Additionally, it aims to educate and engage the clinical community on the current state and challenges in translating nanomaterials for clinical applications.

Keywords Nanomaterials · Diagnostics · Theranostics · Preclinical · Challenges · Regulations

---

V. Mariappan (✉)
Mahatma Gandhi Medical Advanced Research Institute (MGMARI), Sri Balaji Vidyapeeth (Deemed to be University), Puducherry, India

Disease Modelling & Transmission Section, Laboratory of Virology, Rocky Mountain Laboratories, DIR, NIAID, NIH, Hamilton, Montana, USA
e-mail: vignesh.mariappan@nih.gov

P. Vinayaga Moorthi
Department of Human Genetics and Molecular Biology, Bharathiar University, Coimbatore, Tamil Nadu, India
e-mail: pvmhgmb@buc.edu.in

S. Mondal et al. (eds.), *Smart and Sustainable Nanomaterials in Digital Healthcare and Theranostic*, https://doi.org/10.1007/978-981-95-9386-6_15

15.1 Overview of Nanomaterials

Nanomaterials are defined as materials with at least one of the three dimensions in the nanometric scale, with a size between 1 and 100 nm and a spherical surface area by volume higher than 60 m^2/cm^3 [1]. Compared to their respective particles at a larger scale, they display unique chemical, physical, and biological properties at the nanoscale due to their distinct features and functions [2]. Nanoparticle matter is a unique state at which they exhibit novel electrical, magnetic, and optical characteristics [1, 2]. This makes nanomaterials smart as well as multifunctional as depicted in Fig. 15.1.

Nanotechnology is the study of the synthesis, engineering, and application of nanoparticles (NPs) and materials. Due to the ground-breaking and fascinating applications of nanomaterials, nanotechnology has revolutionized next industrial generations, from agricultural, electronics, energy, and food engineering to cosmetics and biomedicine [3]. In the last four decades, many investigations have been carried out in the field of nanomedicine, from disease detection to treatment and several medical problems such as diagnosis, drug discovery, cancer treatment, and personalized medicine [4]. Therefore, nanomedicine is considered an interdisciplinary field that adopts outcomes or applications of biotechnology, nanotechnology, biomedical robotics, and genetic engineering. This aids in developing numerous nano-based diagnostic kits, including nanosensors, nanoparticle-based imaging, nano-based PCR assays, and lab-on-chip assays that are being commercialized for clinical research and usage. Moreover, medicines encapsulated with liposomal- and polymer-based formulations as well as nanovaccines are recently getting medical

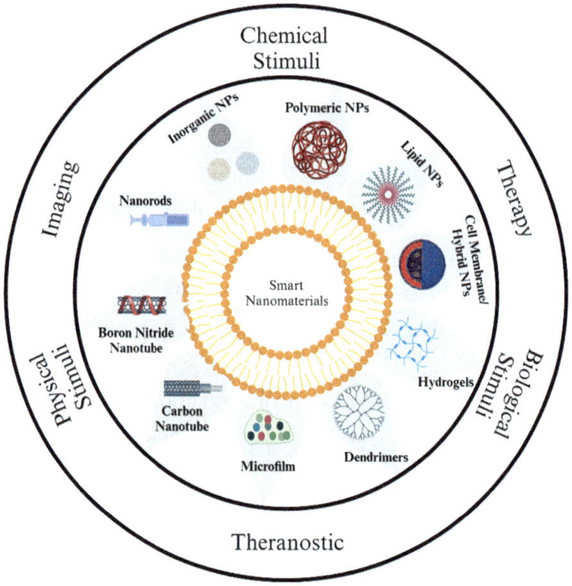

Fig. 15.1 Smart nanomaterials for nanomedicine application: stimuli-responsive, imaging, therapy, and theragnostic

approval for human use [5]. Thus, nano-scaling of medical technologies paves a way to functional effectiveness as well as efficacy, a rapid response rate in most clinical setups [6]. Also, it holds great promise for advancing healthcare, offering new solutions for complex medical challenges, and ushering in an era of more adaptive, tailored, and efficient medical treatments.

15.2 Classification of Nanomaterials and Their Clinical Applications

15.2.1 pH-Responsive Nanomaterials

In normal physiological processes, pH is important, especially for maintaining tissue and cell homeostasis. The pH in the eukaryotic system decreases from 7.4 in the bloodstream to 6.4 in the early endosomal process and reaches below 5 in the lysosomal compartments [7]. In addition, pH is implicated in various pathological conditions such as cancer, inflammation, and infection [8, 9]. In reference to this, it has been reported that the tumor microenvironment may have a slightly acidic pH [9]. This suggests that variation in the pH directly impacts lysosomal catabolism, membrane transport, cell proliferation, receptor cycling, and viral entry into cells [10, 11].

pH-responsive materials can be developed by integrating them into polymer--based nanostructures. This can be designed by altering the surface chemistry, modifying the size or form of particle, or disassembling or releasing cargo. This alteration in nanoparticle function leads to controlled cargo release and optimized cell uptake [12]. As a result, a pH-responsive nanomaterial with pH as a stimulant signal provides a powerful method for engineering disease imaging and therapeutic delivery system. For instance, pH-responsive nanoparticles have been demonstrated to disrupt the endosomal/lysosomal membrane [13], thereby insuring efficient drug delivery to target region of the cell. A list of pH-responsive nanomaterials for drug delivery and therapy is given in Table 15.1.

15.2.2 Temperature-Responsive Nanomaterials

In terms of cellular and physiological processes, the use of thermal energy has been extensively investigated, especially in medical applications for cancer treatment and disease diagnostics [20]. Therefore, heat is regarded as a non-invasive trigger at the site of disease. In cancer treatment, hyperthermia is traditionally referred as a localized or systematic rise in temperature at the tumor by external factors. There are two main categories of local hyperthermia: (i) mild hyperthermia (temperature 41–45 °C) and (ii) thermal ablation (temperature over 50 °C). This application aids in direct destruction of cells as well tissue, matrix component and blood vessels [21]. For

Table 15.1 Advanced pH-based nanomaterial for cancer therapy and drug delivery

Nanomaterials	Encapsulated drug/ strategy	Result	Application	Reference
Functional nanomaterial loaded with pH-responsive prodrug, a GSH--responsive prodrug, folate-receptor targeting polymers, and T1-enhanced magnetic resonance imaging contrast agents	Combrestatin A4 (CA4), doxorubicin (DOX), and Camptothecin (CPT)	Drug release rate increase by 63.4% at pH 6.4 C4 reduced angiogenesis and increased uptake of FTDCAG NPs Increased the intracellular concentration of GSH inside the tumor cells and released CPT and DOX	Chemotherapy	[14]
Magnetic graphene oxide NPs surrounded PLGA polymer (MNP)	5-iodo-2-deoxyuridine (IUdR)	Both in vivo and in vitro data demonstrated prolonged circulation as well as targeted glioma via external magnetic field At pH 5.6, the release rate of IUdR is increased at tumor site than pH 7.4 Under high voltage X-ray, MNP increased apoptosis induced by radiation	Radiotherapy	[15]
Micelle vaccine platform	Poly (2-ethyl-2--oxazoline)-poly (D, L-lactide) (PEOz-PLA)	In an acidic pH, the tertiary amine group in the PEOz backbone become protonated Displayed good laminin target and promoted antigen presentation, complement system activation and dendritic cell maturation	Immunotherapy	[16]

(continued)

Table 15.1 (continued)

Nanomaterials	Encapsulated drug/ strategy	Result	Application	Reference
pH-responsive polymer shielding system	Click reaction between poly(γ-allyl-L--glutamate) and thioglycolic acid or 2-(Boc-amino) ethanethiol	Through fast charge conversion, the NPs released therapeutic drug at the pH below 6.8 In vivo analysis showed higher transfection efficiency and inhibitory effect of tumor growth	Gene therapy	[17]
Block polymer folate PEG-b-poly (asparaginyl--chidamide)	Pyropheophorbide a (Pha)	The NPs showed a steady therapeutic index and minimal cytotoxicity in vitro Further, it reduced implanted tumor growth in melanoma--bearing mice and pulmonary metastasis	Photodynamic therapy	[18]
Hybrid polymer NPs	Hydrophobic PLGA segments, Indocyanine green (ICG) dye, amphiphilic tocopherol PEG succinate, and pH-responsive mPEG-benzoic imine-1-octadecylamine	The NPs killed MCF2 cell and improved anticancer effect when exposed to pH 5.5 and near-infrared (NIR) radiation	Photothermal therapy	[19]

instance, a study demonstrated that DOX in combination with mild localized hyperthermia has enhanced the long- and short-term survival of individual with soft tissue sarcoma when compared to chemotherapy alone [22, 23]. However, one of the major drawbacks of classical hyperthermia is that it can be challenging to heating the local tumor site to optimal temperature without damaging the surrounding healthy tissues. Therefore, novel hyperthermia systems which can distinguish normal and cancer cells are currently under development by employing various applications of nanotechnology [24].

Temperature-responsive or thermo-sensitive nanomaterials are the materials that might potentially target a pre-selected site in response to an alteration in the temperature. A number of factors, including surface characteristics, interfacial structures, and quantum or classical size effects, impact the thermal features of nanomaterials [25]. Despite the fact that many different thermosensitive materials have been described (Table 15.2), thermosensitive polymer-based NPs (micelles and nanogels), liposomes, magnetic NPs (MNPs), gold NPs (GNPs), and suparamagnetic iron oxide (SPIONs) have advanced biomedicine applications in clinical settings [26].

15.2.3 Light-Responsive Nanomaterials

Phototherapy has gained much attraction in recent decades because of its benefits, which include clinical safety, minimal invasiveness, and spatiotemporal addressability [46, 47]. For example, phototherapy has been employed in biomedical engineering to treat seasonal affective disorder [48], non-seasonal depression [49], skin disease [50], and circadian rhythm sleep disturbance [51]. Additionally, it has been a successful tumor-ablating technique with the application of photosensitizers and photothermal conversion agents (PTCAs) [52]. Particularly, light sources such as ultraviolet, visible, and near-infrared light are used in cancer phototherapy. However, biological tissue absorption has limited the depth of tissue penetration for extensive usage of UV and visible light [53]. Because of this, conventional phototherapy is only effective on superficial tumors and may increase the risk of metastasis and recurrence [47, 54]. The low target efficiency caused by the non-specific distribution of the phototherapeutic agent is another important drawback of traditional phototherapy. A list of light-responsive nanomaterials for biomedical applications is represented in Table 15.3.

A number of phototherapeutic nanoagents have been explored and utilized to overcome the aforementioned restriction in cancer phototherapy [16, 55]. For example, studies have demonstrated that specific nanoagent sizes (20–200 nm) are distributed in tumor areas because of their improved permeability and retention features [56, 57]. Thus, nanomaterials could serve as an effective carrier by precisely delivering therapeutic substances like PTCAs, photosensitizers, medications, and genes to the tumor tissue and region, thereby enabling combination and targeted therapy

Table 15.2 Thermo-sensitive or temperature-responsive nanomaterials for diagnostics, imaging, and cancer

Nanomaterial	Encapsulated drug/codelivery	Outcomes	Application	Reference
Photoswitchable multicolor probe with magnetic NPs	Thermochromic dye	Light-dark states and shift in adsorption can be switched by photothermal heating The probes demonstrated high contrast for visualizing cells and deep tissue	Multimodal cellular diagnostics	[27]
Gold nanorod-poly(N--isopropylacrylamide) microgel	–	Increased plasmon resonance shifts	Smart temperature sensor	[28–31]
Gold nanoclusters with thermo-sensitive copolymers	–	Enhanced native fluorescence of gold NPs	Fluorescent live-imaging and nanosenor	[32]
PNIPAM/silver nanoprism	–	Showed 5–10 times thermochromic shift than other PNIPAM composites and exhibited very large ratiometric alteration in scattering in near infrared radiation	Bioimaging as well as NIR labeling and taggants	[33]
Magnetically actuated protease nanosensors	Matrix metalloprotease (MMP)	Remotely triggered at the disease site using an AMF set to 515 kHz and 15 kA/m Detects cleaved substrate (peptides) in urine and protease activity in tumor in vivo	Cancer diagnosis	[34]
Acetylated polyethylenimine--entrapped gold NPs	–	Precisely detected hepatic cancer using negative computed tomography imaging		[35]

(continued)

Table 15.2 (continued)

Nanomaterial	Encapsulated drug/codelivery	Outcomes	Application	Reference
Lyso-thermosensitive liposomal doxorubicin (ThermoDox)	DOX	Increased overall survival rate of hepatocellular cancer patients by 2.1 years	Drug delivery/ nanocarrier	[36]
Heat-activated thermosensitive liposome formulation of CDDP (HTLC)	Cisplatin	Mild hyperthermia along with HTLC triggered effective release of cisplatin in triple negative breast cancer tumor model		[37]
		Effectively delayed the tumor growth of cervical carcinomas in mice model		[38]
Liposome encapsulated with hyaluronic acid	Paciltaxel and Marimastat	Showed an effective release of docetaxel during mild hyperthermia (42 °C) and anti-tumor property in 4Ti tumor-bearing mice model		[39]
Thermosensitive O-maleoyl chitosan micelle conjugated with folate	Erlotinib	At 37 °C, 90% of erlotinib were released with 24 h		[40]
Gold hybrid NPs with chitosan copolymer		Demonstrated higher anti-cancer cytotoxicity effect at 36 °C		[41]
Poly-*N*,*N*′-dimethyl aminoethyl methacrylate smart nanogel	DOX and albumin labeled with radioisotope (^{13}I)	Showed enhanced both chemo and radiotherapy	Chemotherapy and drug delivery	[42]
Water in water thermo--nanoprecipitation nanogel	Etanercept	Demonstrated effective etanercept delivery,temperature--triggered action, and anti-inflammatory effects for psoriasis		[43]
Magneto liposome	Fluorescent dye (Cy5.5) and DOX	Demonstrated higher dual-imaging effect, thermo and chemotherapy	Theranostic	[44]
Theranostic nanosystem	Aptamer probes and gold NPs	Enhanced imaging and photothermal therapy under NIR radiation		[45]

Table 15.3 Light-responsive nanomaterials for immunotherapy and tumor targeting applications

Nanomaterial	Co-delivery	Immunotherapeutic molecule	Significant outcome	Application	Reference
820 nm light-responsive nanoparticle	Docetaxel	CF27, a PD-L1 agonist peptide	Prevented the growth of primary tumor within 24 h by combining photothermal (IR820) therapy Check point (PD-1/PD-L1) blockade inhibitor	Immunotherapy	[62]
NIR light-responsive hydrogel	ICG dye	Resiquimod (R848) and CPG, a TLR agonist	NIR triggered the release of immune component R848 and CPG		[63]
NIR light-responsive nanoparticle	DOX, Verteporfin (VPF), cathepin B-specific cleavable peptide	Anti-PD-L1-antibody	Shown improved retention and permeability DOX and VPF induced immunogenic cell death Prevented tumor growth, recurrence, and metastasis		[64]
Blue-light responsive nanoparticles	–	BMS-1	Showed good PD-1/PD-L1 inhibition and minimal toxicity		[65]

(continued)

Table 15.3 (continued)

Nanomaterial	Co-delivery	Immunotherapeutic molecule	Significant outcome	Application	Reference
Light-inducible nuclear translocation and dimerization (LINTAD) system	–	CAR-T cells	Both in vitro and in vivo, LINTAD CAR T cells demonstrated potent cytotoxicity against cancer cells Serves as an effective non--invasive method for activating inducible CAR T cells and controlling gene expression	Immune modulation	[66]
NIR light-responsive silica--coated upconversion nanoparticle	–	CAR-T cells	Demonstrated phototunable activation of therapeutic T cells to induce tumor cell killing Serve as miniature deep-tissue photo transducer		[67]
Polydopamine nanoparticles coated with macrophage membrane	–	TMP195, TAMs repolarization agent	Enhanced macrophage polarization		[68]
370 nm light-responsive chemically modified α-galactosylceramides	–	–	Controlled production of pro-inflammatory cytokine (IFNγ)		[69]

UV-responsive cationic PAMAM dendrimer	–	Antigen OVA	Induced endosomal escape of OVA and activated a higher production of TNFα from macrophage	Drug delivery	[70]
PLGA-ICG polymeric nanoparticles	ICG dye	Cytomembrane vesicles (CMV, antigen) and outer membrane vesicles (OMV, adjuvant)	OMV-induced immune cytokine and melanoma CMV triggered antitumor immunity Exhibited synergistic antitumor effects		[71]
NIR light-responsive synthetic microorganism	–	PCC 7942, adjuvants	Direct elimination of tumor cells and release of adjuvants to stimulate immune cells		[72]
Manganese-porphyrin metal-organic framework	AS1411 Aptamer (AS1411) with vorinostat and photosensitizer (TCPP)	Manganese ions and tumor--linked antigens	TCPP-mediated photodynamic nuclear DNA damage and cytosolic release under laser irradiation Improved the interferon gene pathways		[73]

[58, 59]. Furthermore, scientists have created NIR-light responsive nanomaterials to address the difficulty of light penetrating deep tissues [60, 61].

15.2.4 Ligand-Functionalized Targeted Nanomaterials

Conventional therapies (such as chemotherapy and radiotherapy) are implicated with increased systematic toxicity, resulting in adverse side effects on normal cells [74]. To address this intrinsic limitation, several nanomedical strategies have been recommended for clinical use and many others are under clinical investigation [75]. One such strategy is ligand-based targeted nanomaterials, which refers to a nanoparticle that has modified surface known as "ligand" that allows it to selectively bind to a target cell or tissue's receptor or target site. This makes it possible to use the specific receptors found on the target cells to deliver medicinal drugs or imaging probes to particular location of the body (such as tumor site) [76]. The specificity of nanomaterial internalization without causing toxicity can be regulated by surface modification and preservation of their distinct characteristics, including shape, morphology, size, surface charge, surface functionalization, hydrophilicity, and hydrophobicity [77–80]. Furthermore, small molecules such as peptides, aptamers, oligosaccharides, proteins, and antibodies can be decorated as a ligand on the nanomaterials [81]. In line with this, researchers have developed nanomaterials with ligands that exhibit differential affinities for cellular proteins and surface molecules [82].

On the other hand, some nanomaterials without functionalized surface could be unstable and exhibit increased surface energy. But such nanomaterials can be stabilized by surface modification with protective coating or capping [83]. In this context, a study that coated albumin onto nanoparticles showed improved active targeting and decreased toxicity [84]. Therefore, surface functionalized nanomaterials result in effective internalization, decreased toxicity, controlled contact with the milieu, and eventually suppress the immune response [85]. Also, to enhance the nanomaterials binding with biological molecules, homo/hetero cross-linkers are adorned with organic functional groups to increase their biocompatibility, decrease cellular damage, and optimal production of reactive oxygen species [86–88]. Table 15.4 represents the recent investigation of surface-modified nanomaterials and their significant outcomes.

15.2.5 Multifunctional Nanomaterials

The next generation of nanomedicine, known as multifunctional nanomaterials (Fig. 15.2), exhibit distinct electric, optical, magnetic, and plasmonic features due to address various applications [101]. Typically, organic nanomaterials (such as carbon nanotubes, dendrimers, and liposomes) are major foundation materials for developing multifunctional nanomaterials [102]. But certain nanomaterials also consist of inorganic materials like metal oxides, semiconductors, mineral and silica. In addition, it is developed using a polymer, linker, protein or medication, imaging agent, and functional group or ligands [101]. A few nanoparticles are naturally multifunctional like gold nanoparticles, which has been studied as possible contrast agents for optical imaging, computed tomography, and photoacoustic imaging [103, 104]. In addition, gold nanoshells and nanocages are frequently utilized in photothermal treatments [102, 105, 106].

Multifunctional nanoparticles are prepared by the flash nanoprecipitation (FNP) process, initially developed by Johnson and Prudhomme to develop

Table 15.4 Surface-modified nanomaterials for biomedical applications

Nanomaterials	Agent/ligand for surface modification	Application	Results	Reference
Gadolinium-doped cerium oxide nanoparticles	Dextran	MRI contrast agent	Exhibited excellent r1 relaxivity, good colloidal stability, and effective internalization into both cancerous and healthy cells	[89]
Iron-oxide nanoparticle	Polyethylene glycol (PEG)		Showed negligible toxicity and higher apoptosis rate in normal L939 cell & HepG2 liver cancer cells, respectively	[90]
Polymer-based upconversion nanoparticle	PEGylated and carboxylic groups	Bioimaging	Showed enhanced cellular uptake and labeling	[91]
Gold-iron oxide nanoparticles	Poly-l-lysine		Increased cellular uptake in breast cancer cells and inhibits NP aggregation. Also, enhanced the MRI image's contrast	[92]

(continued)

Table 15.4 (continued)

Nanomaterials	Agent/ligand for surface modification	Application	Results	Reference
Iron oxide nanoparticles	Polyvinyl alcohol, sorafenib, and aluminum-layered double hydroxide	Drug delivery and nanocarrier	Demonstrated good targeting ability. Also, NPs showed increase antitumor effect and controlled drug release in cancer cell lines	[93]
Gold nanorods	Zeolitic imidazolate framework-8 (ZIF-8) and metal-organic framework		Controlled release of ZIF-8 under NIR stimuli or weakly acidic condition. In addition, it served as potent cancer treatment strategy both in vitro and in vivo	[94]
Ligand switchable nanoparticle (Pep/Gal-PNPs)	Liver-targeting moiety (Gal) and pH-responsive cell-penetrating peptide (Pep)		Caused Pep to extend in an acidic condition, enabling the targeted delivery of nanomaterials to the liver Also, the study used insulin-loaded Pep/Gal-PNPs to show effective intestinal absorption and hepatic deposition of insulin	[95]
Strontium nanoparticles	Transferrin and fibronectin		Showed remarkable increase in gene transfection activity in vitro and in vivo	[96]
Dual-ligand synergistic nanoplatform	Photosensitizer--loaded nanocarrier and a drug-loaded nanocarrier		Demonstrated reduced long-term toxicity	[97]
Iron oxide nanoparticles	pH-responsive poly(aspartic acid) hydrogel	Biocompatibility	Showed no cytotoxicity effect and high colloidal stability in water	[98]
Gold nanoparticles	PEG		Demonstrated a reduced hepatotoxic effect in vivo	[99]
Poly(ethylenimine)-docusate nanoparticles	Fibroin		Decreased the α-mangosteen hematotoxicity	[100]

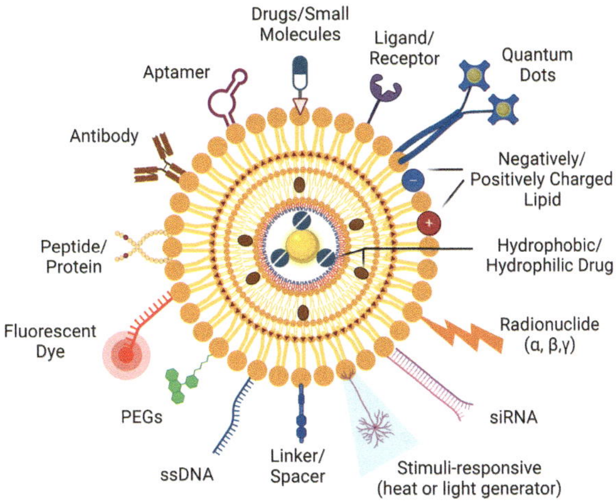

Fig. 15.2 Multifunctional nanoparticle: structural and functional features

hydrophobic drug encapsulation using nanoparticles with a controlled size distribution and high drug payload rate based on a hydrophobic core surrounded by polymers [107]. Another study utilized FNP to create multifunctional particles with surface modification that enable both fluorescent imaging and drug delivery at particular wavelengths simultaneously [108]. Wang and co-workers developed "ChemoRad," a multipurpose nanomaterial that combines chemotherapy and radiation. The ChemoRad nanoparticle is composed of the lecithin lipid monolayer on the surface, hydrophilic PEG shell, hydrophobic and biodegradable polymer, and DMPE-DTPA lipid-chelator layer [109]. In line with this, ChemoRad nanoparticles coated with folate-targeted ligand were used by Wener et al. to treat ovarian cancer [110]. Khdair et al. created a system of multifunctional nanoparticles employing sodium alginate, a natural polymer, to target two medications in one particle: the photodynamic therapy-related methylene blue and the chemotherapy drug doxorubicin to counteract the multidrug resistance effect [111]. Table 15.5 represents the recent updates on multifunctional nanomaterials and their application in drug delivery, therapy, and imaging.

Table 15.5 Advanced multi-functionalized nanomaterials for imaging, drug delivery, and cancer therapeutics

Nanomaterials	Decorated materials/ therapeutic molecules	Significant results	Reference
Oleic acid-capped monodisperse superparamagnetic iron oxide nanocrystals	Gold NP	Enhanced contrast for imaging applications	[112]
Amphiphilic triblock copolymer	Plasmid DNA and paclitaxel	Achieved high efficiency gene transfection and delivery of Paclitaxel both in vivo and in vitro Also, suppressed cancer growth in breast cancer model	[113]
Temperature-sensitive pentablock copolymer with pluronic polymer	Plasmid DNA and paclitaxel	Demonstrated synergistic and sustained delivery of both agents in human ovarian cancer cell lines	[114]
Nanostructured calcium carbonate	Doxorubicin hydrochloride and p53 expression plasmids	Enhanced cell apoptosis in cervical carcinoma HeLa cells	[115]
Triblock copolymers nano-sized micelles	VEGF siRNA and paclitaxel	Exhibited enhanced gene silencing efficacy and improved cellular uptake of paclitaxel	[116, 117]
	Polo-like kinase-1 specific siRNA and paclitaxel	Improved endocytosis and tumor suppression	
Liposome-grafted PEG	Anti-HER2 antibody	Increased cellular uptake and circulation time of NPs in HER2 expressing breast tumor	[118]
Polymeric nanoparticle	Conjugated with BIND-014	Showed 10-times more docetaxel delivery at the tumor site and prolonged circulation as well as retention time	[119, 120]
Magnetic nanoparticle	Fluorescent dye-doped silica ($DySiO_2$)	Detects neuroblastoma via MRI, along with subcellular localization	[121]
	Radionuclides (^{124}I)	Accurately detects lymph node metastasis	
Iron oxide NPs with PEG-grafted chitosan polymer	Tumor targeting moiety and fluorescent dye (Cy5.5)	Highly accumulated in medulloblastoma tumor tissue in vivo model. Further, the signal intensity increased over 50 h and persisted till 70 h	[122]
Iron oxide nanoparticle	^{64}Cu radionuclide and tumor binding RGD peptide	Used as an imaging agent in MRI and PET analyzing neuroblastoma tumors	[123]
Quantum dot-aptamer	DOX and prostate tumor cell-specific aptamer (A10RNA)	Detects the tumor cells' response to the medication	[124]

(continued)

Table 15.5 (continued)

Nanomaterials	Decorated materials/ therapeutic molecules	Significant results	Reference
Gold nanoparticle	Gemcitabine (chemotherapy drug) and EGFR antibody (cetuximab) as a targeting moiety	Showed a significant inhibition of tumor growth in pancreatic cancer model	[125]
Superparamagnetic iron oxide nanoparticles	Mesoporous silica and/or lipid	Improve the biocompatibility of NPs significantly and enhance the suitability of these particles as drug carriers. In addition, the NP showed potential theragnostic application and enhanced contrast agent	[126]
Gadolinium liposomal contrast agent	ICG	Serve as agent for multimodal imaging in diagnosis and therapy of advanced ovarian cancer	[127]
Superparamagnetic iron oxide nanoparticles coated with liposomes	ICG and tumor--targeted agent (RGD)	Noth MRI and NIRF showed clear tumor delineation after administrating NPs	[128]
Gadolinium liposomes	PE-DTPA (chelating Gd + 3)	Exhibited negligible toxicity and side effects in HepG2 cells, liver non-differentiated progenitor HepaRG cells, and HepaRG cells	[129]
Maghemite nanoparticles incorporated in phosphatidylcholine liposomes	–	After internalization, the NPs showed good biological and magnetic properties, thereby enhancing biocompatibility	[130]
MM-DX-929 liposome	Cu-64	PET analysis showed a significant difference colon tumor tissues in animals treated with NPs compared to untreated controls	[131]
Ultra-magnetic liposomes	–	Magnetic targeting efficiency of liposomes was significantly higher in tumor when compared to T_2 contrast agents	[132]

15.3 Preclinical Development

15.3.1 Methods for Developing Smart Nanoparticles

The design, production, characterization, and test of nanomaterials are some of the crucial steps involved in engineering nanomaterials for biomedical applications. There are many different ways to engineer nanomaterials, but they can be broadly categorized into top-down and bottom-up methods.

15.3.1.1 Top-Down Approach

This process is also referred to as destructive since it breaks down bulk materials into smaller ones before turning them into nanomaterials. Top-down processes include lithography, sputtering, electron explosion, arc discharge, laser ablation, thermal decomposition, and mechanical or ball milling [133, 134].

(a) Mechanical or Ball Milling Method

Mechanical or ball milling method was first established by John Benjamin at the International Nickel Company to create strengthened alloys for high-temperature structural applications [135]. The primary goal of milling is to reduce the size of the particles and combine them into new phases. This process involves adding milling medium to a high-energy mill combined with a suitable powder charge (a combination of substances) [136]. Nanomaterials can be produced using a variety of ball milling techniques, where the balls affect the powder charge. Generally, ball milling is a more cost-effective method of producing nanosize grain on a large scale [137]. The energy imparted to the powder by the balls during milling determines the kinetics of mechanical milling [138]. Numerous factors influence the energy transfer, including the type of mill, the powder used to power the milling chamber, the speed at which the mill is operating, the size and distribution of the balls, whether the milling is done dry or wet, the temperature of milling, and the duration of milling [139]. This process is commonly used to develop nano alloys, wear-resistant spray coatings, oxide- and carbide-strengthened aluminum alloys, and other nanocomposite materials [1].

(b) Nanolithography Method

Nanolithography is a field of nanotechnology that involves the art of creating nanostructures on a nanomaterial scale. There are numerous special ways to perform nanolithography. Typically, most nanolithography techniques use light or electrons to create patterns on a substrate. Following this, masks can be added to the photoresist to target this patterning and protect a specific area from incoming light [140]. The preferred method for creating a smaller structure is electron beam lithography. Instead of illuminating the surface with light, this method scans the surface using a highly concentrated electron beam. This approach is referred as photolithography or electron beam lithography [141]. It is frequently used to develop integrated circuits and various parts of semiconductor technology. This aids in creating smaller devices with more compact transistors and circuits, enabling us to improve the power efficiency and performance of the component [142]. Furthermore, this method has been used to construct complex structures, which can be utilized for microelectrochemical or nanoelectrochemical systems [143]. Dip-pen nanolithography (DPN) is another technique in which a solvent meniscus is transferred to ink from the tip of a pen to a substrate. Currently, DNP approach has been advanced from a serial writing tool to massive parallel nanofabrication platform [144, 145].

(c) Laser Ablation Method

Laser ablation is a method for creating nanoparticles that removes materials off the target's surface by applying a very high energy at a precise location to a solid target immersed in a liquid medium [146]. In this process, the target electron absorbs electromagnetic radiation when a laser pulse strikes a bulk material's surface, transferring energy to the material's vibrating lattice. Consequently, material is released from the surface as a plasma plume, which contains nanoparticles [147]. The energy is transferred to the surrounding liquid during the plasma decay, which creates a cavitation bubble and a layer of vapor with a volume roughly equivalent to the plasma [148]. Then, the cavitation bubble periodically expands and contracts until it collapses, at which point nanoparticles are released into the liquid. In general, the ablation rate is affected by various factors such as pulse duration, fluence, wavelength and repetition rate, transmission, liquid chemical composition, and target material light absorption efficiency. Similarly, the characteristics of NPs are also influenced by the liquid medium and laser settings. The criteria for laser ablation are wavelengths ranging from UV-Vis to NIR-IR, a laser fluence roughly consisting of 0.1–100 J/cm^2, pulse lengths ranging from nanoseconds (ns) to picoseconds (ps), and femtoseconds (fs) [149, 150].

(d) Sputtering Method

Sputtering is a physical method of creating nanoparticles that can be collected in a liquid medium. It works by subjecting a target material (made of the desired nanoparticle materials) to an energetic ion bombardment in a vacuum chamber. This causes atoms to be ejected from the target and condense onto a substrate. This process is known as physical vapor deposition. In simple word, it is a technique to deposit thin film of distinct material onto a surface. This method is considered as a clean and unique way to synthesize nanoparticles with high purity since it does not require additional stabilizers or chemical reducing agents [151]. In general, there are two sputtering mechanism theoretical models: (i) Thermal vaporization theory: the target surface is heated to produce vaporization after being bombarded by energetic particles; (ii) Momentum-transfer theory: the atoms' surface emits after the incident particle's kinetic momentum is transferred to the target surface's atoms [152]. Some of the variable that affect the overall yielding of the sputtering process are the quality of the target materials, the crystal structure of the target surface material, the energy of energetic ions or particles, and the reflection angle of the incident particles [153]. Sputtering is frequently employed in vacuum deposition, ion plating, surface science, and the removal of impurities from solid surfaces [154]. Additionally, it is employed in the semiconductor industry and space weathering to etch anisotropy and alter the chemical and physical characteristics of airless bodies, like the moon, respectively [155, 156].

(e) Thermal Decomposition Method

Thermal decomposition is a novel method to develop stable monodispersed nanoparticles. In this process, a chemical precursor compound is heated to a high temperature, causing it to break down and form nanoparticles. This method is frequently used to develop highly uniform and stable nanoparticle in the presence of stabilizing agent within a solvent, allowing for precise regulation over the size and morphology of the resulting nanoparticles [157]. According to Palacious-Hernández et al. and Kino et al., thermal decomposition is a simple and moderate process that doesn't require any raw materials [158, 159]. Likewise, Tran et al. suggested that thermal decomposition is used to manufacture huge quantities of nanoparticles at a single time, in contrast to biological approaches that only produced small numbers [160]. Regarding stabilizer, reports suggested that capping agents, like alkyl amines and carboxylic acids, may impact the production of monodispersed nanoparticles obtained from thermal decomposition [161]. In addition, a number of factors influence the temperature and pressure at which thermal decomposition occurs, including the type of metallic ions present and the force of reactivity with the ligands in coordination compounds [162]. A typical example is the production of iron oxide nanoparticles through thermal degradation of an iron oleate precursor in a solvent with a high boiling point, such as 1-octadecene, with oleic acid serving as the stabilizing surfactant [163].

(f) The Arc Discharge Method

The arc discharge method is a popular technique, where a catalyst is frequently added to the anode to affect the structure of the final nanoparticles. It creates a high-temperature plasma by generating an electric arc between two electrodes, usually made of graphite, which vaporizes the material from the anode (positive electrode). This allows the atoms to condense and form nanoparticles in the surrounding inert gas environment [164, 165]. This method particular known for the production of carbon nanotubes, where a catalyst metal (e.g., iron, nickel, and cobalt) is often mixed with the anode materials to promote the formation of appropriate structure [164]. The most common application of arch discharge method is the production of both single- and multi-walled carbon nanotubes and synthesis of several metal nanoparticles like silver, gold, and copper [166, 167].

15.3.1.2 Bottom-Up Approach

This approach refers to as the constructive method, which create material from atoms to clusters to nanoparticles. Few examples of this approach are sol-gel, spinning, pyrolysis, chemical vapor deposition, and biological synthesis [134, 168, 169].

(a) Sol-Gel Method

This method creates a nanoparticle in a liquid condition and at a low temperature (often below 100 °C). The end product is solid, and this solid product is produced by the polymerization process between the metal in the raw materials. This process involves the following steps [170–172]:

- Mixing: a molecular precursor (metal alkoxide) is dissolved either in water or alcohol.
- Hydrolysis/Alcoholysis: To turn the mixture into gel, it is heated and agitated.

- Drying: A desired application is used to dry the wet gel.
- Powdering and calcining: The dried gel is grounded into a powder and subsequently calcined.

Numerous factors, including the pH, metal alkoxide activity, temperature, the water-to-alkoxide ratio, solvent type, and additive employed, affect the hydrolysis and condensation reaction. Therefore, by altering these factors, materials with unique surface chemistry and microstructure can be created [173]. Certain salts, hydroxides, alkoxides, oxides, acrylates, and amines are utilized in the context of precursors [174]. However, alkoxides are the most often used sol-gel precursors [175]. The sol-gel process has several uses, including: (i) creating complexly shaped optical components; (ii) using the product in unique forms such as aerogel, fibers, and surface coatings; (iii) developing materials with altered physical characteristics like low UV absorption, low thermal expansion coefficient, and high optical transparency; and (iv) developing materials in an amorphous state and applying them to thin layers [173].

(b) Spinning Method

Electrospinning is the widely used "spinning" technique for synthesizing nanoparticles. It is a simple method for creating nanofibrous materials with modifiable architectures and functional characteristics. Typically, a high voltage is applied to a liquid solution containing the required material to create Talyor cone at the needle top from which a charged jet is ejected and solidifies into nanofibers [176, 177]. This is performed in a spinning disc rotator. It is made up of a revolving disc container with a chamber or reactor that allows for the regulation of physical parameters like temperature. This process can be affected by liquid/precursor ratio, disc surface, liquid flow rate, rotation speed, and feed position [1, 134]. Electrospinning can be used to produce nanofiber with several materials like metal, polymers, and ceramics, which can subsequently be treated to isolate the nanoparticles. Moreover, these techniques are employed in various fields, including material science, healthcare, tissue engineering, energy storage, and sensing [178].

(c) Pyrolysis Method

The most widely used pyrolysis technique for creating nanoparticles, known as "spray pyrolysis," involves spraying a precursor solution into a hot environment where the solvent quickly evaporates, causing the dissolved precursor molecules to break down and form nanoparticles through nucleation and growth processes [179]. Flame spray pyrolysis and laser pyrolysis are the two types of pyrolysis techniques. The flame spray pyrolysis method uses a flame as a heating source to achieve a high temperature and a higher production rate [180, 181]. In contrast, laser pyrolysis uses a high-power laser to carefully manage the nucleation processes in order to break down the precursor molecules [182]. Evidence suggests that metals, carbides, nitrides, oxides, and composite nanoparticles are effectively produced by laser pyrolysis [183]. For instance, using laser pyrolysis, silicon carbide, silicon, molybdenum disulfide, and TiO/SiO_2 nanoparticles have been developed for protecting cultural heritage and energy applications [184–186].

(d) Chemical Vapor Deposition (CVD) Method

CVD is a straightforward process that uses chemical processes to deposit a thin layer of vapor species onto surfaces. To synthesize nanoparticles, a controlled gas-phase reaction at high temperatures is usually used. This process entails introducing volatile precursor chemicals into a heated reaction chamber, where they either react or decompose to form nanoparticles that can be deposited onto a substrate or collected as a powder. Numerous intricate elements, including reactor configuration, gas ratios, reactor pressure and gas partial pressures, temperature, and growth line, and reactions that occur inside the CVD reactor [187].

Thermal CVD on metal was initially developed in 1966 to produce a crystalline graphite sheet on a Ni substrate [188]. Afterwards, the Pt surface was used to create a single-layer graphite via hydrocarbon breakdown at 530 °C [189]. The investigation of CVD's potential for creating graphene layer using LPCVD on an Ir substrate progressed after graphene was initially isolated in 2004. Currently, both multi-layer and single-layer graphene films are developed using CVD technique [190]. These days, CVD procedures are divided into seven main categories according to the features of the processing parameters: temperature, precursor type, wall/substrate, depositing time, pressure, gas flow state, and activation source [191, 192]. CVD techniques are recently employed in the fields of electronics (light-emitting diodes, nanoelectrochemical systems, biosensors, and flexible wearable technology) and energy (batteries and supercapacitors) [187]. However, the need for specialized equipment and the extremely poisonous gaseous byproducts are two major drawbacks of CVD [134].

(e) Biosynthesis or Biological Method

The process of biosynthesis is commonly referred to as "green synthesis" because it creates biological and non-toxic nanoparticles. Therefore, green synthesis nanoparticles have special and improved functionalities that make them appropriate for environmental and biological applications. Typically, biological templates (genomic materials), microorganisms (bacteria, fungi, and algae), and other plant components are employed in the green production of nanoparticles [168, 193].

Unique nanostructure materials called biological templates—DNA, RNA, or proteins—are employed in biosensors, bioNEMS, and bioelectronic systems [194, 195]. In particular, proteins are extensively utilized as components in nanocomposite materials [196]. An intracellular protein called ferritin, for example, accumulates iron oxide and releases it under specified conditions. Furthermore, it functions as a buffer in humans, controlling iron overload and shortage [197]. Like biological templates, nanomaterials are made from metal salt aqueous solutions using microorganisms (algae, fungi, and bacteria) [198–200]. For example, *Fusarium oxysporum* is used to manufacture silver nanoparticles [201], the bacteria *Rhodopseuomonas* is utilized to create gold nanoparticles [202], and *magnetotactic* bacteria have been shown to generate magnetic particles in anaerobic environments [203]. However, the fact that certain microorganisms are harmful to humans is a drawback of this technique. Lastly, the development of nanoparticles has made substantial use of plant extracts or plant parts [198]. For example, metal nanoparticles are made from phytochemicals found in plants, such as quinones, organic acids, and flavones [204]. A study has shown that the biomass of the plants *Pelargonium graveolnes* and *Medicago sativa* can be used to create gold nanoparticles [205, 206]. Similarly, bimetallic gold and silver nanoparticles are frequently made from *Azadirachta indica* leaves [207]. Accordingly, *Brassica juncea* and *Helianthus annus* are used to synthesis a number of metallic nanoparticles [208–211].

15.4 Clinical Translation

15.4.1 Overview of Regulatory Pathways of FDA and EMA

The regulatory standards of the FDA mainly focus on the safety, efficacy, and quality of nanomaterials. Particularly, before entering into a clinical trial, the nanomaterials must demonstrate significant preclinical analysis. This comprises both in vitro and in vivo analysis such as biocompatibility, toxicity, and side effects on cells, tissues, and organs. This information aids to determine systemic toxicity, immunotoxicity, targeted toxicity, pharmacokinetics, and biodistribution of nanomaterials [212]. Knowing these parameters allows us to predict the functionality of nanomaterials in the human body. In addition, the FDA underlines the need to consider unique features and behaviors imparted by nanotechnology, since these may affect the safety, effectiveness, and public health impact of the products.

The FDA considers two key points when evaluating a nanotech product: (i) the nanomaterial or end product should have at least one dimension, or surface structure, in the nanoscale range (~1 to 100 nm), and (ii) the nanomaterial or end product should exhibit properties attributable to its dimension(s) [213, 214]. The FDA evaluates the safety, efficacy, and quality of nano-drugs during drug approval. After approval, respective pharmacopeias should develop a product monograph that describes critical quality attributes. These points are further refined by the FDA, which aids in improving the regulatory framework of nanotechnology. Thus, collaboration with regulatory bodies from the initial stages of development is advised to ensure successful translation of nanomedicines [215–217].

On the other hand, EMA has proposed several actions to address the scientific and regulatory challenges posed by complex nanomaterials. Particularly, it includes the pharmacokinetic/pharmacodynamic requirements and long-term profile of nanomedicines. A key focus of EMA is to understand the critical quality attributes of nanomedicine products and their interaction with biological system both in in vitro and in vivo. In addition, the EMA plans to develop and standardize new testing method to assess the quality and safety of nanomedicines that particularly exhibits some unique properties [218, 219]. For the clinical translation, the EMA

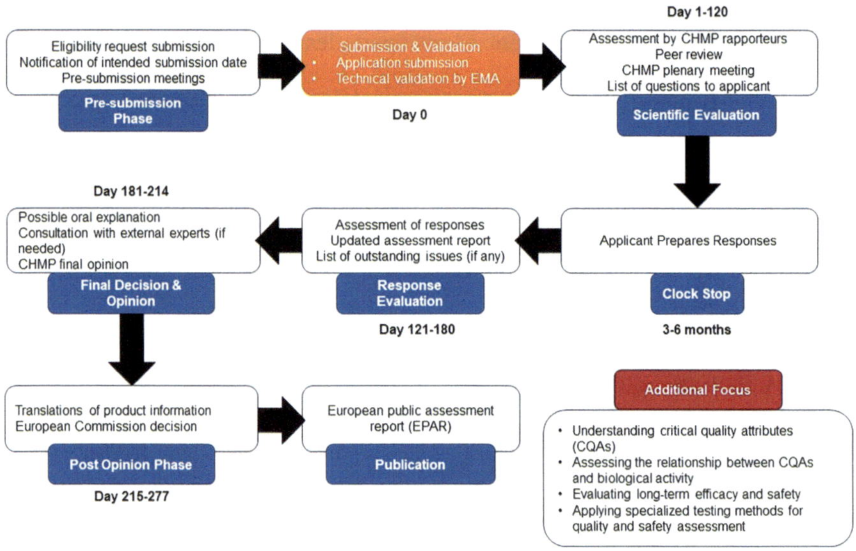

Fig. 15.3 Evaluation process of EMA for the translation of nanomaterials for clinical use

follows a structured evaluation process like pre-submission phases, scientific evaluation, and post-opinion phases (Fig. 15.3). EMA encourages early and frequent dialogue with developers throughout the development process to address these complex issues and facilitate successful clinical translation.

Besides, the International Pharmaceutical Regulators Program (IPRP) is responsible for international pharmaceutical regulation, focusing on issues related to nanotechnological products. The IPRP aims to develop synchronized regulatory frameworks for nanomedicines through cooperation with international regulatory bodies [217]. The lack of specific guidelines for characterization of nanomedicines has led to failures at clinical stages [220, 221]. Thus, defining the parameters (Fig. 15.4) for quality control and safety is crucial for regulatory definition [222].

15.4.2 Challenges in Translation

(a) Financial Challenges

- Securing funding to advance fundamental scientific research into extensive clinical trials is a challenge for many academic researchers and small and medium-sized business (SMEs) members.
- Universities face financial difficulties and pressure to finish the experiment as soon as possible, even if they obtain significant funds by establishing SMEs.

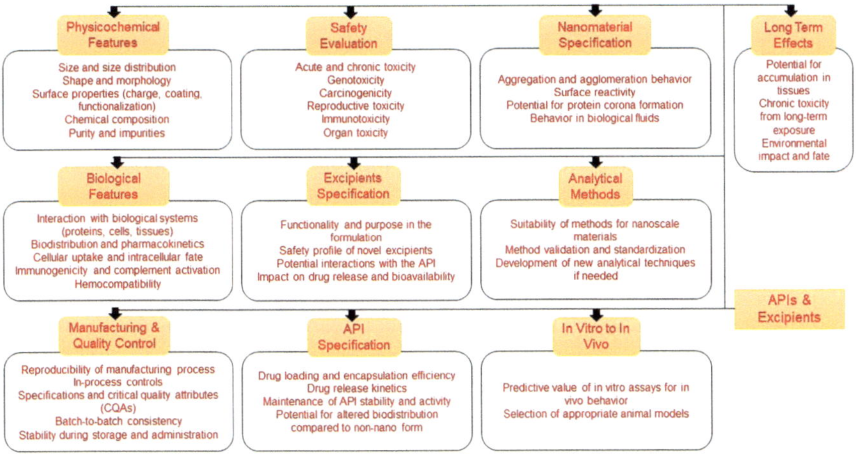

Fig. 15.4 Key parameters and quality control of active pharmaceutical ingredient and excipients

- Lower-than-anticipated patient recruitment makes the trial longer and expensive.
- Most nanomedicines are created for the treatment of cancer. Some nanomedicines may be beneficial for other diseases like diabetes, atherosclerosis, and arthritis. These trials have different primary and secondary goals than clinical trials for cancer, and they frequently require advanced imaging methods, which raises the cost of the trial.
- Numerous national and international funding organizations make significant investments in nanotechnology and nanomedicine by establishing centers of excellence and implementing collaborative funding programs. However, the "rationale of priority setting" at the policy level and the efficiency of distributing available funding among numerous research projects in the field are controversial.
- Some established and traditional pharmaceutical companies have trouble getting funding since they don't support innovative methods for drug delivery and treatment.
- Availability of patent protection for goods under development or investigation influences the researcher's chance of securing the required funds to advance the product into clinical translation and investor's interest.

Therefore, significant financial resources are needed to scale up GMP production of specialized nanomedicine products [223–228].

(b) Ethical Challenges

- Ethical review is based on the assessment of risks and benefits. Risk assessment, benefit/harm, and information gathering are major obstacles in clinical trials of the cutting-edge application of nanotechnology [229].

- Meaningful patient recruitment in the ethical evaluation of trials emphasized the need for a wide stakeholder discussion, and criticized ethics committees for their propensity toward what they saw as excessive caution, particularly when there is lack of treatment option [230].
- Physicians, researchers, and medical professionals may find it difficult to communicate to patients the risk and the improbable likelihood of trial benefit. Particularly, providing scientifically accurate facts without totally destroying patients' hopes is one of their biggest concerns [231].

(c) Regulatory Challenges

- The pre-examination and scientific recommendations of authorities and consultations on new nanodrugs are quite helpful in trial preparation. Nonetheless, regulatory authorities and their specific needs vary on a regional and national level, thereby impact on multicentric trials conducted across nation and worldwide [229].
- Because of lack of experience with nanoparticles and formulation in underdeveloped nations, they provide poor support and advice for clinical trials. This has a big effect on the researcher who uses nanotechnology to treat neglected illnesses [232].
- Another significant obstacle facing European researchers is nanocharacterization and toxicity testing. Therefore, cooperation with the Nanotechnology Characterization Laboratory in the USA may enhance nanocharacterization capabilities in Europe [233].
- Drugs and devices have distinct regulatory pathways. Alteration of these rules over time has a significant impact on product development during the translation process [229].

15.4.3 Case Studies

15.4.3.1 Successful Translation of Smart Nanomaterials to Clinical Application

(a) Case Study I—Lipid Nanoparticles (LNPs) for mRNA Vaccine

In 2018, the FDA approved Onpattro (Patisiran), a first-in-class RNA interference (RNAi) therapeutic drug, to treat polyneuropathy in adults with hereditary transthyretin-mediated (hATTR) amyloidosis. It uses lipid-based nanoparticle technology to deliver siRNA targeting TTR mRNA and reduces the production of TTR protein in the liver as well as decreasing amyloid deposits in peripheral nerves [234–236]. The composition of LNPs is composed of ionizable cationic lipids (Dlin-MC3-DMA), phospholipids, cholesterol, and PEG-modified lipids (PEG2000-C-DMG) [237]. The drug is administered via IV route (0.3 mg/kg for patients <100 kg; 30 mg for patients ≥ 100 kg) every 3 weeks. In a phase III clinical trial, the drug improved muscle strength, sensation, reflexes, and autonomic symptoms compared to placebo in 225 patients [238]. Onpattro is Currently marketed by Alnylam PharmaCeutiCals with an annual cost between $451,430 and $677,145 per patient. Some of the common side effects are infusion-related reactions and reduced serum vitamin A levels [239].

Comirnaty (BNT162b2) is a COVID-19 vaccine developed by BioNTech and Pfizer. The vaccine is formulated with LNPs and nucleoside-modified mRNA, which codes for SARS-CoV-2 spike protein with mutation to stabilize it in the prefusion conformation. The vaccine received emergency use authorization globally in December 2020 [240]. The composition of LNPs includes ionizable cationic lipids (ALC-0315), PEGylated lipids (ALC-0159), phospholipids, and cholesterol. The molecular ratios of the components are 46.3:1.6:9.4:42.7 (cationic:PEG:phospholip id:cholesterol) [241]. In the phase III clinical trial, the vaccine showed 95% efficacy across a diverse population and against severe disease. The vaccine induces robust CD4+ and CD8+ cell expansion, resulting in robust neutralizing antibody and T cell responses. However, the efficacy of the vaccine declines after 6 months [242].

Spikevax (mRNA-1273) is a COVID-19 vaccine developed by Moderna in association with the National Institute of Allergy and Infectious Diseases. It received FDA emergency use approval in December 2020. The vaccine is encapsulated with lipid nanoparticles and encodes the prefusion stabilized spike protein of SARS-CoV-2 [243, 244]. In a phase III clinical trial, the vaccine showed 94.1% efficacy in preventing COVID-19 symptoms, particularly in severe cases. Further, it elicits both neutralizing antibody and T cell responses as well as reducing the viral replication in the respiratory tracts [245]. The LNP protects the mRNA from degradation and increases the cellular uptake. The composition of LNP includes ionizable lipids, phospholipids, cholesterol, and PEG lipids. The ionizable lipid SM102 is used in mRNA-1273. Further, PEG coating aids in preventing aggregation, and increases circulation time and mucus penetration [241].

(b) Case Study II—Iron-Oxide Nanoparticle for MRI Imaging

Ferumoxytol (FE) is an iron replacement product used to treat iron deficiency anemia in individuals with chronic kidney disease. It is sold under the brand name Feraheme and was approved by the FDA in June 2009 [246]. FE consists of a superparamagnetic iron oxide core (Fe_3O_4) nanoparticle surrounded by a semi-synthetic carboxylated coating (size of 30 nm and molecular weight of ~731 KDa), which allows it to be administered at a relatively high dose [247, 248]. Basically, the drug works by restoring iron reserves in the body, thereby producing healthy red blood cells to manage anemia.

Later, it gained significant interest as an off-MRI labeling agent due to its distinct properties and advantages over gadolinium-based contrast agents (GBCAs) [249]. FE is a potent T1 and T2 relaxation agent with a half-life of 14–21 h. This enables a versatile imaging application and steady-state blood volume mapping. Unlike GBCAs, which cause nephrogenic systemic fibrosis, FE can be used in patients with impaired renal function [249, 250]. Currently, FE-enhanced MRI is widely used in magnetic resonance angiography, perfusion-weighted imaging, and the detection and imaging of brain tumors and myocardial inflammation [247, 249–251].

(c) Case Study III—Gold Nanoparticle for Cancer Therapy

AuroLase therapy is a novel nanomedicine-based approach developed by Nanospectra Bioscience for selective thermal ablation of tumors. This therapy utilizes a novel class of nanoparticles known as auroshells to target and destroy cancer cells while minimizing damage to surrounding healthy cells. AuroShells are composed of a silica core coated with a thin gold shell (150 nm) [252]. The NPs are delivered via IV route and accumulate in tumor tissues. When exposed to NIR light (750–800 nm wavelength), they convert the light energy into heat, thereby causing localized thermal ablation of the tumor and its blood supply [253]. Currently, a clinical trial with prostate cancer patients resulted in 87.5% of the lesions in the ablation zone being negative for tumor at 12 months post-treatment [254]. In line with this, initial clinical trials were conducted with patients with recurrent tumors of head and neck carcinomas [252].

(d) Case Study IV—Dendrimers for Drug Delivery in Ocular Disease

Poly(amidoamine) (PAMAM) dendrimers are highly branched, synthetic polymers that have attracted researchers and scientists as a drug delivery system, specifically for ocular disease, including the treatment of uveitis with corticosteroids. PAMAM dendrimers have significantly improved the water solubility of poorly soluble drugs [255]. A study has demonstrated that dendrimers facilitate better corneal penetration of drugs, thereby improving bioavailability [256]. Corticosteroids, such as dexamethasone (DEX), are more commonly used to treat uveitis. In reference to this, DEX-PAMAM-conjugated nanomaterials have shown prolonged release of DEX, potentially reducing dose frequency and improving penetration of corticosteroids through ocular barriers. Particularly, a study showed that PAMAM G3.5 and G4.5 dendrimers conjugated with DEX can increase ocular permeability following subconjunctival injections in rats [257]. In addition, PAMAM dendrimers have been investigated for the delivery of other ocular drugs, such as timolol for glaucoma, with positive results in animal models [258].

(e) Case study V—Polymeric Nanoparticle for Anticancer Drug Delivery

ABRAXANE is an albumin-based nanoparticle drug that delivers hydrophobic drugs to tumor tissue. It was developed by Dr. Neil Desai and Dr. Patrick Soon-Shiong in response to side effects implicated by traditional paclitaxel. Unlike conventional paclitaxel, ABRAXANE eliminated the need of toxic solvent such as Cremophor EL and ethanol. It became the first FDA-approved nano-based drug in cancer treatment [259]. Moreover, it is widely used to treat multiple cancers like metastatic breast cancer [260], non-small cell lung cancer [261], and pancreatic cancer [262].

15.4.3.2 Lessons Learned from Failures or Challenges

- Standardized procedures and regulatory frameworks are required for the biological assessment, production, and characterization of nanomaterials. Translation has been hampered due to distinct regulatory pathways within and between local, regional, and national levels [229].
- Lack of physicochemical and biological characterization of nanoparticles often leads to questions on safety, long-term effects, and scaling up processes. Thus, a detailed investigation, including systemic toxicity, immunotoxicity, pharmacokinetics, biological interaction, and biodistribution of nanomaterials, is required [213, 263].
- Despite the promising results of nanomaterials in vitro, many nanomaterials do not prove effective in clinical trials or animal models. Therefore, a better predictive model needs to be established [264, 265].
- Converting a basic manufacturing process of nanoproduct from a laboratory setup into large-scale industrial production needs potential funding resources as well as investors' interest [266, 267].
- Batch-to-batch variation impacts the safety and efficiency of specialized nanoproducts during the scale-up process. Thus, rigorous and robust quality control measures are required [268, 269].

15.5 Future Directions

15.5.1 Research and Development Needs

Although nanoparticles have shown encouraging outcomes in lab settings, their long-term impacts and interactions with biological systems are still unclear, which fuels discussion over their biocompatibility and biodegradability. Therefore, researchers are encouraged to develop nanoparticles that can be efficiently broken down and eliminated from the body without any adverse effects [270–272]. Similarly, it is necessary to increase the target efficiency of smart nanoparticles. Particularly, the nanomaterials must be enhanced or decorated with potential tumor-specific ligands and explore their targeting mechanism to overcome obstacles like the blood-brain barriers [273, 274]. In addition, the safety and effectiveness of nano-based therapies are affected by batch-to-batch variation. Thus, designing a stable nanomaterial with a cost-effective approach is crucial [268, 269]. Furthermore, a uniform regulatory framework is necessary to guarantee the effectiveness and safety of these cutting-edge nanomaterials in all countries [229].

15.5.2 Emerging Technologies

The development of multifunctional nanomaterials that respond to various stimuli, such as pH, temperature, enzymes, and redox processes, is considered one of the major advancements in emerging nanotechnologies [275–277]. Using this approach, scientists have engineered specialized nanomaterials that can perform both therapeutic and diagnostic functions simultaneously [278, 279]. In a similar vein, researchers are integrating machine learning models with artificial intelligence, a strategy known as nanoparticle informatics, to enhance the behavior and design of nanomaterials [280, 281].

On the other hand, the development of biomimetic and bioinspired nanoparticles is another advancement of cutting-edge technology in the field of nanomedicine [282, 283]. For instance, studies have created cell-membrane-coated nanoparticles that resemble the surface characteristics of normal cells, thereby modulating the immune response in the biological system [284, 285]. Additionally, DNA-based nanoparticles are currently being developed with tunable size, shape, and functionality that are extensively employed in biosensors and drug delivery systems [286–288].

15.6 Conclusion

Nanomedicine has significantly enhanced diagnosis, target delivery, imaging, and theranostic applications. Despite the promising results and advancements that have been achieved, there remain persistent challenges associated with the regulatory framework governing these technologies, as well as concerns regarding the stability, design, long-term safety, and overall efficacy of the nanomaterials. To tackle these multifaceted challenges, it is imperative to leverage the capabilities of artificial intelligence and machine learning algorithms. Additionally, the successful transition of sophisticated smart nanomaterials from basic scientific research into practical clinical applications necessitates a robust and synergistic cooperation of diverse range of stakeholders, including academic institutions, researchers, financial investors, government officials, regulatory bodies, and policymakers. Ultimately, the concerted efforts of these various entities will be crucial in overcoming existing barriers and in paving the way for the future integration of nanotechnology into everyday medical practice, thereby enhancing patient care and therapeutic outcomes on a global scale.

Acknowledgments We thank Sri Balaji Vidyapeeth (Deemed to be University) and Bharathiar University for providing infrastructure facilities for the preparation of this chapter. Vignesh Mariappan completed majority of this work at Sri Balaji Vidyapeeth (Deemed to be University). The author's (Vignesh Mariappan) current affiliation with the National Institute of Health is provided for identification purpose only. The NIH had no role in conception, execution, or funding for this book chapter.

References

1. Mekuye B, Abera B. Nanomaterials: an overview of synthesis, classification, characterization, and applications. Nano Select. 2023;4:486–501.
2. Joudeh N, Linke D. Nanoparticle classification, physicochemical properties, characterization, and applications: a comprehensive review for biologists. J Nanobiotechnol. 2022;20:262.
3. Malik S, Muhammad K, Waheed Y. Nanotechnology: a revolution in modern industry. Molecules. 2023;28:661.
4. Haleem A, Javaid M, Singh RP, et al. Applications of nanotechnology in medical field: a brief review. Glob Health J. 2023;7:70–7.
5. Dessale M, Mengistu G, Mengist HM. Nanotechnology: a promising approach for cancer diagnosis, therapeutics and theragnosis. Int J Nanomed. 2022;17:3735–49.
6. Fox KE, Tran NL, Nguyen TA, et al. Surface modification of medical devices at nanoscale—recent development and translational perspectives. In: Biomaterials in translational medicine. Elsevier. p. 163–89.
7. Such GK, Yan Y, Johnston APR, et al. Interfacing materials science and biology for drug carrier design. Adv Mater. 2015;27:2278–97.
8. Hajjar S, Zhou X. pH sensing at the intersection of tissue homeostasis and inflammation. Trends Immunol. 2023;44:807–25.
9. Hosonuma M, Yoshimura K. Association between pH regulation of the tumor microenvironment and immunological state. Front Oncol. 2023;13:1175563.
10. Izumi H, Torigoe T, Ishiguchi H, et al. Cellular pH regulators: potentially promising molecular targets for cancer chemotherapy. Cancer Treat Rev. 2003;29:541–9.
11. Maxfield FR, McGraw TE. Endocytic recycling. Nat Rev Mol Cell Biol. 2004;5:121–32.
12. Deirram N, Zhang C, Kermaniyan SS, et al. pH-responsive polymer nanoparticles for drug delivery. Macromol Rapid Commun. 2019;40:1800917.
13. Ade C, Brodszkij E, Thingholm B, et al. Small organic catalase mimic encapsulated in micellar artificial organelles as reactive oxygen species scavengers. ACS Appl Polym Mater. 2019;1:1532–9.
14. Wang N, Liu C, Yao W, et al. A traceable, GSH/pH dual-responsive nanoparticles with spatiotemporally controlled multiple drugs release ability to enhance antitumor efficacy. Colloids Surf B Biointerfaces. 2021;205:111866.
15. Shirvalilou S, Khoei S, Khoee S, et al. Enhancement radiation-induced apoptosis in C6 glioma tumor-bearing rats via pH-responsive magnetic graphene oxide nanocarrier. J Photochem Photobiol B Biol. 2020;205:111827.
16. Li C, Lu Y, Chen Q, et al. Tailored polymers with complement activation ability to improve antitumor immunity. Mol Pharm. 2019;16:2648–60.
17. Chen J, Guo Z, Jiao Z, et al. Poly(L -glutamic acid)-based Zwitterionic polymer in a charge conversional shielding system for gene therapy of malignant tumors. ACS Appl Mater Interfaces. 2020;12:19295–306.
18. Ma Z, Hu P, Guo C, et al. Folate-mediated and pH-responsive chidamide-bound micelles encapsulating photosensitizers for tumor-targeting photodynamic therapy. Int J Nanomed. 2019;14:5527–40.
19. Ting C-W, Chou Y-H, Huang S-Y, et al. Indocyanine green-carrying polymeric nanoparticles with acid-triggered detachable PEG coating and drug release for boosting cancer photothermal therapy. Colloids Surf B Biointerfaces. 2021;208:112048.

20. Tannock IF, Rotin D. Acid pH in tumors and its potential for therapeutic exploitation. Cancer Res. 1989;49:4373–84.
21. Roti Roti JL. Cellular responses to hyperthermia (40–46 °C): cell killing and molecular events. Int J Hyperth. 2008;24:3–15.
22. Issels RD, Lindner LH, Verweij J, et al. Neo-adjuvant chemotherapy alone or with regional hyperthermia for localised high-risk soft-tissue sarcoma: a randomised phase 3 multicentre study. Lancet Oncol. 2010;11:561–70.
23. Issels RD, Lindner LH, Verweij J, et al. Effect of neoadjuvant chemotherapy plus regional hyperthermia on long-term outcomes among patients with localized high-risk soft tissue sarcoma: the EORTC 62961-ESHO 95 randomized clinical trial. JAMA Oncol. 2018;4:483.
24. Beik J, Abed Z, Ghoreishi FS, et al. Nanotechnology in hyperthermia cancer therapy: from fundamental principles to advanced applications. J Control Release. 2016;235:205–21.
25. Sánchez-Moreno P, De Vicente J, Nardecchia S, et al. Thermo-sensitive nanomaterials: recent advance in synthesis and biomedical applications. Nanomaterials. 2018;8:935.
26. Amin M, Huang W, Seynhaeve ALB, et al. Hyperthermia and temperature-sensitive nanomaterials for spatiotemporal drug delivery to solid tumors. Pharmaceutics. 2020;12:1007.
27. Harrington WN, Haji MR, Galanzha EI, et al. Photoswitchable non-fluorescent thermochromic dye-nanoparticle hybrid probes. Sci Rep. 2016;6:36417.
28. Ding T, Rudrum AW, Herrmann LO, et al. Polymer-assisted self-assembly of gold nanoparticle monolayers and their dynamical switching. Nanoscale. 2016;8:15864–9.
29. Fernández-López C, Polavarapu L, Solís DM, et al. Gold Nanorod–pNIPAM hybrids with reversible Plasmon coupling: synthesis, modeling, and SERS properties. ACS Appl Mater Interfaces. 2015;7:12530–8.
30. Manikas AC, Romeo G, Papa A, et al. Highly efficient surface-enhanced Raman scattering substrate formulation by self-assembled gold nanoparticles physisorbed on poly(*N* -isopropylacrylamide) thermoresponsive hydrogels. Langmuir. 2014;30:3869–75.
31. Zhang C-L, Cao F-H, Wang J-L, et al. Highly stimuli-responsive au nanorods/poly(*N* -isopropylacrylamide) (PNIPAM) composite hydrogel for smart switch. ACS Appl Mater Interfaces. 2017;9:24857–63.
32. Hembury M, Beztsinna N, Asadi H, et al. Luminescent gold nanocluster-decorated polymeric hybrid particles with assembly-induced emission. Biomacromolecules. 2018;19:2841–8.
33. Samai S, Qian Z, Ling J, et al. Optical properties of reconfigurable polymer/silver Nanoprism hybrids: tunable color and infrared scattering contrast. ACS Appl Mater Interfaces. 2018;10:8976–84.
34. Schuerle S, Dudani JS, Christiansen MG, et al. Magnetically actuated protease sensors for in vivo tumor profiling. Nano Lett. 2016;16:6303–10.
35. Zhou B, Xiong Z, Wang P, et al. Acetylated polyethylenimine-entrapped gold nanoparticles enable negative computed tomography imaging of orthotopic hepatic carcinoma. Langmuir. 2018;34:8701–7.
36. Tak WY, Lin S-M, Wang Y, et al. Phase III HEAT study adding lyso-thermosensitive liposomal doxorubicin to radiofrequency ablation in patients with unresectable hepatocellular carcinoma lesions. Clin Cancer Res. 2018;24:73–83.
37. Dunne M, Dou YN, Drake DM, et al. Hyperthermia-mediated drug delivery induces biological effects at the tumor and molecular levels that improve cisplatin efficacy in triple negative breast cancer. J Control Release. 2018;282:35–45.
38. Dou YN, Zheng J, Foltz WD, et al. Heat-activated thermosensitive liposomal cisplatin (HTLC) results in effective growth delay of cervical carcinoma in mice. J Control Release. 2014;178:69–78.
39. Lv Y, Xu C, Zhao X, et al. Nanoplatform assembled from a CD44-targeted prodrug and smart liposomes for dual targeting of tumor microenvironment and cancer cells. ACS Nano. 2018;12:1519–36.

40. Fathi M, Zangabad PS, Aghanejad A, et al. Folate-conjugated thermosensitive O-maleoyl modified chitosan micellar nanoparticles for targeted delivery of erlotinib. Carbohydr Polym. 2017;172:130–41.
41. Fathi M, Sahandi Zangabad P, Barar J, et al. Thermo-sensitive chitosan copolymer-gold hybrid nanoparticles as a nanocarrier for delivery of erlotinib. Int J Biol Macromol. 2018;106:266–76.
42. Maiti D, Chao Y, Dong Z, et al. Development of a thermosensitive protein conjugated nanogel for enhanced radio-chemotherapy of cancer. Nanoscale. 2018;10:13976–85.
43. Giulbudagian M, Yealland G, Hönzke S, et al. Breaking the barrier – potent anti-inflammatory activity following efficient topical delivery of Etanercept using thermoresponsive nanogels. Theranostics. 2018;8:450–63.
44. Guo Y, Zhang Y, Ma J, et al. Light/magnetic hyperthermia triggered drug released from multi-functional thermo-sensitive magnetoliposomes for precise cancer synergetic theranostics. J Control Release. 2018;272:145–58.
45. Shi H, Ye X, He X, et al. Au@Ag/Au nanoparticles assembled with activatable aptamer probes as smart "nano-doctors" for image-guided cancer thermotherapy. Nanoscale. 2014;6:8754.
46. Shanmugam V, Selvakumar S, Yeh C-S. Near-infrared light-responsive nanomaterials in cancer therapeutics. Chem Soc Rev. 2014;43:6254–87.
47. Xie Z, Fan T, An J, et al. Emerging combination strategies with phototherapy in cancer nanomedicine. Chem Soc Rev. 2020;49:8065–87.
48. Campbell PD, Miller AM, Woesner ME. Bright light therapy: seasonal affective disorder and beyond. Einstein J Biol Med. 2017;32:E13–25.
49. Perera S, Eisen R, Bhatt M, et al. Light therapy for non-seasonal depression: systematic review and meta-analysis. BJPsych Open. 2016;2:116–26.
50. Jagdeo J, Austin E, Mamalis A, et al. Light-emitting diodes in dermatology: a systematic review of randomized controlled trials. Lasers Surg Med. 2018;50:613–28.
51. Dodson ER, Zee PC. Therapeutics for circadian rhythm sleep disorders. Sleep Med Clin. 2010;5:701–15.
52. Qiu M, Ren WX, Jeong T, et al. Omnipotent phosphorene: a next-generation, two-dimensional nanoplatform for multidisciplinary biomedical applications. Chem Soc Rev. 2018;47:5588–601.
53. Lee G-H, Moon H, Kim H, et al. Multifunctional materials for implantable and wearable photonic healthcare devices. Nat Rev Mater. 2020;5:149–65.
54. Zhou Z, Song J, Nie L, et al. Reactive oxygen species generating systems meeting challenges of photodynamic cancer therapy. Chem Soc Rev. 2016;45:6597–626.
55. Chen J, Fan T, Xie Z, et al. Advances in nanomaterials for photodynamic therapy applications: status and challenges. Biomaterials. 2020;237:119827.
56. Dai Y, Xu C, Sun X, et al. Nanoparticle design strategies for enhanced anticancer therapy by exploiting the tumour microenvironment. Chem Soc Rev. 2017;46:3830–52.
57. Torchilin V. Tumor delivery of macromolecular drugs based on the EPR effect. Adv Drug Deliv Rev. 2011;63:131–5.
58. Deng S, Li X, Liu S, et al. Codelivery of CRISPR-Cas9 and chlorin e6 for spatially controlled tumor-specific gene editing with synergistic drug effects. Sci Adv. 2020;6:eabb4005.
59. Nakielski P, Pawłowska S, Rinoldi C, et al. Multifunctional platform based on electrospun nanofibers and plasmonic hydrogel: a smart nanostructured pillow for near-infrared light-driven biomedical applications. ACS Appl Mater Interfaces. 2020;12:54328–42.
60. Zheng B, Bai Y, Chen H, et al. Near-infrared light-excited upconverting persistent nanophosphors in vivo for imaging-guided cell therapy. ACS Appl Mater Interfaces. 2018;10:19514–22.
61. Chen S, Weitemier AZ, Zeng X, et al. Near-infrared deep brain stimulation via upconversion nanoparticle–mediated optogenetics. Science. 2018;359:679–84.
62. Peng J, Yang Q, Xiao Y, et al. Tumor microenvironment responsive drug-dye-peptide nanoassembly for enhanced tumor-targeting, penetration, and photo-chemo-immunotherapy. Adv Funct Mater. 2019;29:1900004.

63. Jia YP, Shi K, Yang F, et al. Multifunctional nanoparticle loaded injectable thermoresponsive hydrogel as NIR controlled release platform for local Photothermal immunotherapy to prevent breast cancer postoperative recurrence and metastases. Adv Funct Mater. 2020;30:2001059.
64. Choi J, Shim MK, Yang S, et al. Visible-light-triggered prodrug nanoparticles combine chemotherapy and photodynamic therapy to potentiate checkpoint blockade cancer immunotherapy. ACS Nano. 2021;15:12086–98.
65. Liu Y, Long K, Kang W, et al. Optochemical control of immune checkpoint blockade via light-triggered PD-L1 dimerization. Adv NanoBiomed Res. 2022;2:2200017.
66. Huang Z, Wu Y, Allen ME, et al. Engineering light-controllable CAR T cells for cancer immunotherapy. Sci Adv. 2020;6:eaay9209.
67. Nguyen NT, Huang K, Zeng H, et al. Nano-optogenetic engineering of CAR T cells for precision immunotherapy with enhanced safety. Nat Nanotechnol. 2021;16:1424–34.
68. Yue Y, Li F, Li Y, et al. Biomimetic nanoparticles carrying a repolarization agent of tumor-associated macrophages for remodeling of the inflammatory microenvironment following Photothermal therapy. ACS Nano. 2021;15:15166–79.
69. Hartrampf N, Seki T, Baumann A, et al. Optical control of cytokine production using photoswitchable galactosylceramides. Chem A Eur J. 2020;26:4476–9.
70. Song Y, Chen Y, Li P, et al. Photoresponsive polypeptide-glycosylated Dendron Amphiphiles: UV-triggered Polymersomes, OVA release, and in vitro enhanced uptake and immune response. Biomacromolecules. 2020;21:5345–57.
71. Chen Q, Huang G, Wu W, et al. A hybrid eukaryotic–prokaryotic nanoplatform with photothermal modality for enhanced antitumor vaccination. Adv Mater. 2020;32:1908185.
72. Wang H, Guo Y, Gan S, et al. Photosynthetic microorganisms-based biophotothermal therapy with enhanced immune response. Small. 2021;17:2007734.
73. Zhao X, Zhang K, Wang Y, et al. Intracellular self-assembly driven nucleus-targeted photo-immune stimulator with chromatin Decompaction function for robust innate and adaptive antitumor immunity. Adv Funct Mater. 2022;32:2108883.
74. Zhao Z, Ukidve A, Kim J, et al. Targeting strategies for tissue-specific drug delivery. Cell. 2020;181:151–67.
75. Ahmad E, Ali A, Fatima MT, et al. Ligand decorated biodegradable nanomedicine in the treatment of cancer. Pharmacol Res. 2021;167:105544.
76. Friedman A, Claypool S, Liu R. The smart targeting of nanoparticles. CPD. 2013;19:6315–29.
77. Emami F, Banstola A, Vatanara A, et al. Doxorubicin and anti-PD-L1 antibody conjugated gold nanoparticles for colorectal cancer photochemotherapy. Mol Pharm. 2019;16:1184–99.
78. Santos-Rasera JR, Sant'Anna Neto A, Rosim Monteiro RT, et al. Toxicity, bioaccumulation and biotransformation of Cu oxide nanoparticles in *Daphnia magna*. Environ Sci Nano. 2019;6:2897–906.
79. Rees P, Wills JW, Brown MR, et al. The origin of heterogeneous nanoparticle uptake by cells. Nat Commun. 2019;10:2341.
80. Liu T, Bai R, Zhou H, et al. The effect of size and surface ligands of iron oxide nanoparticles on blood compatibility. RSC Adv. 2020;10:7559–69.
81. Borowik A, Butowska K, Konkel K, et al. The impact of surface functionalization on the biophysical properties of silver nanoparticles. Nano. 2019;9:973.
82. Mout R, Moyano DF, Rana S, et al. Surface functionalization of nanoparticles for nanomedicine. Chem Soc Rev. 2012;41:2539.
83. Wieszczycka K, Staszak K, Woźniak-Budych MJ, et al. Surface functionalization – the way for advanced applications of smart materials. Coord Chem Rev. 2021;436:213846.
84. Sanità G, Armanetti P, Silvestri B, et al. Albumin-modified melanin-silica hybrid nanoparticles target breast cancer cells via a SPARC-dependent mechanism. Front Bioeng Biotechnol. 2020;8:765.
85. Khan SS, Ullah I, Ullah S, et al. Recent advances in the surface functionalization of nanomaterials for antimicrobial applications. Materials. 2021;14:6932.

86. Ahmad F, Salem-Bekhit MM, Khan F, et al. Unique properties of surface-functionalized nanoparticles for bio-application: functionalization mechanisms and importance in application. Nano. 2022;12:1333.
87. Jiang Y, Li Y, Richard C, et al. Hemocompatibility investigation and improvement of near-infrared persistent luminescent nanoparticle $ZnGa_2\ O_4:Cr^{3+}$ by surface PEGylation. J Mater Chem B. 2019;7:3796–803.
88. Passos Gibson V, Nunes JBB, Falcao DQ, et al. Lipid coating of chitosan Nanogels for improved colloidal stability and in vitro biocompatibility. AAPS PharmSciTech. 2021;22:159.
89. Popov AL, Abakumov MA, Savintseva IV, et al. Biocompatible dextran-coated gadolinium-doped cerium oxide nanoparticles as MRI contrast agents with high T_1 relaxivity and selective cytotoxicity to cancer cells. J Mater Chem B. 2021;9:6586–99.
90. Karahaliloglu Z, Kilicay E, Hazer B. PLinaS-g-PEG coated magnetic nanoparticles as a contrast agent for hepatocellular carcinoma diagnosis. J Biomater Sci Polym Ed. 2020;31:1580–603.
91. Klimkevicius V, Voronovic E, Jarockyte G, et al. Polymer brush coated upconverting nanoparticles with improved colloidal stability and cellular labeling. J Mater Chem B. 2022;10:625–36.
92. Abedin MR, Umapathi S, Mahendrakar H, et al. Polymer coated gold-ferric oxide superparamagnetic nanoparticles for theranostic applications. J Nanobiotechnol. 2018;16:80.
93. Ebadi M, Buskaran K, Bullo S, et al. Drug delivery system based on magnetic iron oxide nanoparticles coated with (polyvinyl alcohol-zinc/aluminium-layered double hydroxide-sorafenib). Alex Eng J. 2021;60:733–47.
94. Huang J, Xu Z, Jiang Y, et al. Metal organic framework-coated gold nanorod as an on-demand drug delivery platform for chemo-photothermal cancer therapy. J Nanobiotechnol. 2021;19:219.
95. Yang T, Wang A, Nie D, et al. Ligand-switchable nanoparticles resembling viral surface for sequential drug delivery and improved oral insulin therapy. Nat Commun. 2022;13:6649.
96. Bakhtiar A, Liew QX, Ng KY, et al. Active targeting via ligand-anchored pH-responsive strontium nanoparticles for efficient nucleic acid delivery into breast cancer cells. J Pharm Investig. 2022;52:243–57.
97. Luo F, Zhong T, Chen Y, et al. Dual-ligand synergistic targeting anti-tumor Nanoplatforms with Cascade-responsive drug release. Pharmaceutics. 2023;15:2014.
98. Vega-Chacón J, Arbeláez MIA, Jorge JH, et al. pH-responsive poly(aspartic acid) hydrogel-coated magnetite nanoparticles for biomedical applications. Mater Sci Eng C. 2017;77:366–73.
99. Patlolla AK, Shinde AK, Tchounwou PB. A comparison of poly-ethylene-glycol-coated and uncoated gold nanoparticle-mediated hepatotoxicity and oxidative stress in Sprague Dawley rats. Int J Nanomed. 2019;14:639–47.
100. Pham DT, Tiyaboonchai W. Fibroin-coated poly(ethylenimine)-docusate nanoparticles as a novel drug delivery system. Curr Sci. 2021;121:775.
101. Alivisatos P. The use of nanocrystals in biological detection. Nat Biotechnol. 2004;22:47–52.
102. De Dios AS, Díaz-García ME. Multifunctional nanoparticles: analytical prospects. Anal Chim Acta. 2010;666:1–22.
103. Gobin AM, Lee MH, Halas NJ, et al. Near-infrared resonant nanoshells for combined optical imaging and photothermal cancer therapy. Nano Lett. 2007;7:1929–34.
104. Popovtzer R, Agrawal A, Kotov NA, et al. Targeted gold nanoparticles enable molecular CT imaging of cancer. Nano Lett. 2008;8:4593–6.
105. Huang X, El-Sayed IH, Qian W, et al. Cancer cell imaging and photothermal therapy in the near-infrared region by using gold nanorods. J Am Chem Soc. 2006;128:2115–20.
106. Hirsch LR, Stafford RJ, Bankson JA, et al. Nanoshell-mediated near-infrared thermal therapy of tumors under magnetic resonance guidance. Proc Natl Acad Sci USA. 2003;100:13549–54.
107. Johnson BK, Prud'homme RK. Flash NanoPrecipitation of organic actives and block copolymers using a confined impinging jets mixer. Aust J Chem. 2003;56:1021.

108. Akbulut M, Ginart P, Gindy ME, et al. Generic method of preparing multifunctional fluorescent nanoparticles using flash NanoPrecipitation. Adv Funct Mater. 2009;19:718–25.
109. Wang AZ, Yuet K, Zhang L, et al. Chemorad nanoparticles: a novel multifunctional nanoparticle platform for targeted delivery of concurrent chemoradiation. Nanomedicine. 2010;5:361–8.
110. Werner ME, Karve S, Sukumar R, et al. Folate-targeted nanoparticle delivery of chemo- and radiotherapeutics for the treatment of ovarian cancer peritoneal metastasis. Biomaterials. 2011;32:8548–54.
111. Khdair A, Di Chen, Patil Y, et al. Nanoparticle-mediated combination chemotherapy and photodynamic therapy overcomes tumor drug resistance. J Control Release. 2010;141:137–44.
112. Jin Y, Jia C, Huang S-W, et al. Multifunctional nanoparticles as coupled contrast agents. Nat Commun. 2010;1:41.
113. Wang Y, Gao S, Ye W-H, et al. Co-delivery of drugs and DNA from cationic core–shell nanoparticles self-assembled from a biodegradable copolymer. Nature Mater. 2006;5:791–6.
114. Zhang B, Jia F, Fleming MQ, et al. Injectable self-assembled block copolymers for sustained gene and drug co-delivery: an in vitro study. Int J Pharm. 2012;427:88–96.
115. Chen S, Zhao D, Li F, et al. Co-delivery of genes and drugs with nanostructured calcium carbonate for cancer therapy. RSC Adv. 2012;2:1820.
116. Zhu C, Jung S, Luo S, et al. Co-delivery of siRNA and paclitaxel into cancer cells by biodegradable cationic micelles based on PDMAEMA–PCL–PDMAEMA triblock copolymers. Biomaterials. 2010;31:2408–16.
117. Sun T-M, Du J-Z, Yao Y-D, et al. Simultaneous delivery of siRNA and paclitaxel *via* a "two-in-one" Micelleplex promotes synergistic tumor suppression. ACS Nano. 2011;5:1483–94.
118. Kirpotin DB, Drummond DC, Shao Y, et al. Antibody targeting of long-circulating lipidic nanoparticles does not increase tumor localization but does increase internalization in animal models. Cancer Res. 2006;66:6732–40.
119. Hrkach J, Von Hoff D, Ali MM, et al. Preclinical development and clinical translation of a PSMA-targeted docetaxel nanoparticle with a differentiated pharmacological profile. Sci Transl Med. 4. Epub ahead of print 4 April 2012. https://doi.org/10.1126/scitranslmed.3003651.
120. Sanna V, Siddiqui IA, Sechi M, et al. Nanoformulation of natural products for prevention and therapy of prostate cancer. Cancer Lett. 2013;334:142–51.
121. Cheon J, Lee J-H. Synergistically integrated nanoparticles as multimodal probes for nanobiotechnology. Acc Chem Res. 2008;41:1630–40.
122. Veiseh O, Sun C, Fang C, et al. Specific targeting of brain tumors with an optical/magnetic resonance imaging nanoprobe across the blood-brain barrier. Cancer Res. 2009;69:6200–7.
123. Lee H-Y, Li Z, Chen K, et al. PET/MRI dual-modality tumor imaging using arginine-glycine-aspartic (RGD)–conjugated radiolabeled iron oxide nanoparticles. J Nucl Med. 2008;49:1371–9.
124. Bagalkot V, Zhang L, Levy-Nissenbaum E, et al. Quantum dot−Aptamer conjugates for synchronous cancer imaging, therapy, and sensing of drug delivery based on bi-fluorescence resonance energy transfer. Nano Lett. 2007;7:3065–70.
125. Patra CR, Bhattacharya R, Wang E, et al. Targeted delivery of gemcitabine to pancreatic adenocarcinoma using Cetuximab as a targeting agent. Cancer Res. 2008;68:1970–8.
126. Patil-Sen Y, Torino E, De Sarno F, et al. Biocompatible superparamagnetic core-shell nanoparticles for potential use in hyperthermia-enabled drug release and as an enhanced contrast agent. Nanotechnology. 2020;31:375102.
127. Ravoori MK, Singh S, Bhavane R, et al. Multimodal magnetic resonance and near-infrared-fluorescent imaging of intraperitoneal ovarian cancer using a dual-mode-dual-gadolinium liposomal contrast agent. Sci Rep. 2016;6:38991.
128. Chen Q, Shang W, Zeng C, et al. Theranostic imaging of liver cancer using targeted optical/MRI dual-modal probes. Oncotarget. 2017;8:32741–51.

129. Šimečková P, Hubatka F, Kotouček J, et al. Gadolinium labelled nanoliposomes as the platform for MRI theranostics: in vitro safety study in liver cells and macrophages. Sci Rep. 2020;10:4780.
130. Lorente C, Cabeza L, Clares B, et al. Formulation and in vitro evaluation of magnetoliposomes as a potential nanotool in colorectal cancer therapy. Colloids Surf B: Biointerfaces. 2018;171:553–65.
131. Blocker SJ, Douglas KA, Polin LA, et al. Liposomal[64] Cu-PET imaging of anti-VEGF drug effects on Liposomal delivery to colon cancer xenografts. Theranostics. 2017;7:4229–39.
132. Thébault CJ, Ramniceanu G, Michel A, et al. In vivo evaluation of magnetic targeting in mice colon tumors with ultra-magnetic liposomes monitored by MRI. Mol Imaging Biol. 2019;21:269–78.
133. Baig N, Kammakakam I, Falath W. Nanomaterials: a review of synthesis methods, properties, recent progress, and challenges. Mater Adv. 2021;2:1821–71.
134. Ijaz I, Gilani E, Nazir A, et al. Detail review on chemical, physical and green synthesis, classification, characterizations and applications of nanoparticles. Green Chem Lett Rev. 2020;13:223–45.
135. Benjamin JS. Dispersion strengthened superalloys by mechanical alloying. Metall Trans. 1970;1:2943–51.
136. Koch CC, Whittenberger JD. Mechanical milling/alloying of intermetallics. Intermetallics. 1996;4:339–55.
137. Janot R, Guerard D. Ball-milling in liquid media applications to the preparation of anodic materials for lithium-ion batteries. Prog Mater Sci. 2005;50:1–92.
138. Tjong SC, Chen H. Nanocrystalline materials and coatings. Mater Sci Eng R Rep. 2004;45:1–88.
139. Benjamin JS. Mechanical alloying—a perspective. Metal Powder Rep. 1990;45:122–7.
140. Pimpin A, Srituravanich W. Review on micro- and nanolithography techniques and their applications. Eng J. 2012;16:37–56.
141. Chen Y. Nanofabrication by electron beam lithography and its applications: a review. Microelectron Eng. 2015;135:57–72.
142. Murr LE. Photolithography applied to integrated circuit (IC) microfabrication. In: Handbook of materials structures, properties, processing and performance. Cham: Springer International Publishing. p. 607–12.
143. Rassaei L, Singh PS, Lemay SG. Lithography-based nanoelectrochemistry. Anal Chem. 2011;83:3974–80.
144. Liu G, Petrosko SH, Zheng Z, et al. Evolution of dip-pen nanolithography (DPN): from molecular patterning to materials discovery. Chem Rev. 2020;120:6009–47.
145. Bhagoria P, Mathew Sebastian E, Kumar Jain S, et al. Nanolithography and its alternate techniques. Mater Today Proc. 2020;26:3048–53.
146. Balachandran A, Sreenilayam SP, Madanan K, et al. Nanoparticle production via laser ablation synthesis in solution method and printed electronic application – a brief review. Results Eng. 2022;16:100646.
147. Shih C-Y, Streubel R, Heberle J, et al. Two mechanisms of nanoparticle generation in picosecond laser ablation in liquids: the origin of the bimodal size distribution. Nanoscale. 2018;10:6900–10.
148. Zhang D, Gökce B, Barcikowski S. Laser synthesis and processing of colloids: fundamentals and applications. Chem Rev. 2017;117:3990–4103.
149. Walter JG, Petersen S, Stahl F, et al. Laser ablation-based one-step generation and biofunctionalization of gold nanoparticles conjugated with aptamers. J Nanobiotechnol. 2010;8:21.
150. Zhang J, Chaker M, Ma D. Pulsed laser ablation based synthesis of colloidal metal nanoparticles for catalytic applications. J Colloid Interface Sci. 2017;489:138–49.
151. Meischein M, Ludwig A. Upscaling nanoparticle synthesis by sputter deposition in ionic liquids. J Nanopart Res. 2021;23:129.

152. Mattox DM. Physical sputtering and sputter deposition (Sputtering). In: Handbook of physical vapor deposition (PVD) processing. Elsevier. p. 237–86.
153. Hamadi O. Fundamentals of plasma sputtering. Epub ahead of print 2015. https://doi.org/10.13140/RG.2.1.3855.5605.
154. Sergievskaya A, Chauvin A, Konstantinidis S. Sputtering onto liquids: a critical review. Beilstein J Nanotechnol. 2022;13:10–53.
155. Kelly JJ, Philipsen HGG. Anisotropy in the wet-etching of semiconductors. Curr Opinion Solid State Mater Sci. 2005;9:84–90.
156. Szabo PS, Biber H, Jäggi N, et al. Experimental insights into space weathering of Phobos: laboratory investigation of sputtering by atomic and molecular planetary ions. JGR Planets. 2020;125:e2020JE006583.
157. Salavati-Niasari M, Davar F, Mazaheri M. Synthesis of Mn3O4 nanoparticles by thermal decomposition of a [bis(salicylidiminato)manganese(II)] complex. Polyhedron. 2008;27:3467–71.
158. Palacios-Hernández T, Hirata-Flores GA, Contreras-López OE, et al. Synthesis of Cu and Co metal oxide nanoparticles from thermal decomposition of tartrate complexes. Inorg Chim Acta. 2012;392:277–82.
159. Kino T, Kuzuya T, Itoh K, et al. Synthesis of chalcopyrite nanoparticles via thermal decomposition of metal-thiolate. Mater Trans. 2008;49:435–8.
160. Tran QH, Nguyen VQ, Le A-T. Silver nanoparticles: synthesis, properties, toxicology, applications and perspectives. Adv Nat Sci Nanosci Nanotechnol. 2013;4:033001.
161. Askerzade I. Anisotropic Eliashberg equations and influence of multiband effects. In: Unconventional superconductors. Berlin/Heidelberg: Springer Berlin Heidelberg. p. 95–140.
162. Kelly CHW, Lein M. Choosing the right precursor for thermal decomposition solution-phase synthesis of iron nanoparticles: tunable dissociation energies of ferrocene derivatives. Phys Chem Chem Phys. 2016;18:32448–57.
163. Lassenberger A, Grünewald TA, Van Oostrum PDJ, et al. Monodisperse iron oxide nanoparticles by thermal decomposition: elucidating particle formation by second-resolved in situ small-angle X-ray scattering. Chem Mater. 2017;29:4511–22.
164. Sharma R, Sharma AK, Sharma V. Synthesis of carbon nanotubes by arc-discharge and chemical vapor deposition method with analysis of its morphology, dispersion and functionalization characteristics. Cogent Eng. 2015;2:1094017.
165. Das R, Shahnavaz Z, Ali ME, et al. Can we optimize arc discharge and laser ablation for well-controlled carbon nanotube synthesis? Nanoscale Res Lett. 2016;11:510.
166. Jabłońska J, Jankowski K, Tomasik M, et al. Preparation of silver nanoparticles in a high voltage AC arc in water. SN Appl Sci. 2021;3:244.
167. Elwakil BH, Toderas M, El-Khatib M. Arc discharge rapid synthesis of engineered copper oxides nano shapes with potent antibacterial activity against multi-drug resistant bacteria. Sci Rep. 2022;12:20209.
168. Kolahalam LA, Kasi Viswanath IV, Diwakar BS, et al. Review on nanomaterials: synthesis and applications. Mater Today Proc. 2019;18:2182–90.
169. Oner GA, Nadaroglu H, Acar V, et al. Flexural and thermal characterization of epoxy composites reinforced with nanoparticles synthesized from waste walnut husk with green synthesis method. Biomass Conv Bioref. 2024;14:20201–12.
170. Chen R, Cheng Y, Wang P, et al. Facile synthesis of a sandwiched Ti3C2Tx MXene/nZVI/fungal hypha nanofiber hybrid membrane for enhanced removal of Be(II) from Be(NH) complexing solutions. Chem Eng J. 2021;421:129682.
171. Wang M, Jiang C, Zhang S, et al. Reversible calcium alloying enables a practical room-temperature rechargeable calcium-ion battery with a high discharge voltage. Nat Chem. 2018;10:667–72.
172. Zhang X, Tang Y, Zhang F, et al. A novel Aluminum–Graphite Dual-Ion battery. Adv Energy Mater. 2016;6:1502588.

173. Bokov D, Turki Jalil A, Chupradit S, et al. Nanomaterial by sol-gel method: synthesis and application. Adv Mater Sci Eng. 2021;2021:5102014.
174. Li B, Wang X, Yan M, et al. Preparation and characterization of nano-TiO2 powder. Mater Chem Phys. 2003;78:184–8.
175. Jaroenworaluck A, Sunsaneeyametha W, Kosachan N, et al. Characteristics of silica-coated TiO_2 and its UV absorption for sunscreen cosmetic applications. Surf Interface Anal. 2006;38:473–7.
176. Li H, Xu M, Shi R, et al. Advances in electrostatic spinning of polymer fibers functionalized with metal-based nanocrystals and biomedical applications. Molecules. 2022;27:5548.
177. Masoumi S, O'Shaughnessy S, Pakdel A. Organic-based flexible thermoelectric generators: from materials to devices. Nano Energy. 2022;92:106774.
178. Zhang S, Jia Z, Liu T, et al. Electrospinning nanoparticles-based materials interfaces for sensor applications. Sensors. 2019;19:3977.
179. Workie AB, Ningsih HS, Shih S-J. An comprehensive review on the spray pyrolysis technique: historical context, operational factors, classifications, and product applications. J Anal Appl Pyrolysis. 2023;170:105915.
180. Meierhofer F, Mädler L, Fritsching U. Nanoparticle evolution in flame spray pyrolysis—process design via experimental and computational analysis. AICHE J. 2020;66:e16885.
181. Gröhn AJ, Pratsinis SE, Sánchez-Ferrer A, et al. Scale-up of nanoparticle synthesis by flame spray pyrolysis: the high-temperature particle residence time. Ind Eng Chem Res. 2014;53:10734–42.
182. Kumari S, Raturi S, Kulshrestha S, et al. A comprehensive review on various techniques used for synthesizing nanoparticles. J Mater Res Technol. 2023;27:1739–63.
183. Reau A, Guizard B, Mengeot C, et al. Large scale production of nanoparticles by laser pyrolysis. Mater Sci Forum 2007; 534–536: 85–88.
184. Maskrot H, Herlin-Boime N, Leconte Y, et al. Blue TiO_{2-x} /SiO_2 nanoparticles by laser pyrolysis. J Nanopart Res. 2006;8:351–60.
185. Swihart MT. Vapor-phase synthesis of nanoparticles. Curr Opin Colloid Interface Sci. 2003;8:127–33.
186. D'Amato R, Falconieri M, Gagliardi S, et al. Synthesis of ceramic nanoparticles by laser pyrolysis: from research to applications. J Anal Appl Pyrolysis. 2013;104:461–9.
187. Saeed M, Alshammari Y, Majeed SA, et al. Chemical vapour deposition of graphene—synthesis, characterisation, and applications: a review. Molecules. 2020;25:3856.
188. Karu AE, Beer M. Pyrolytic formation of highly crystalline graphite films. J Appl Phys. 1966;37:2179–81.
189. Land TA, Michely T, Behm RJ, et al. STM investigation of single layer graphite structures produced on Pt(111) by hydrocarbon decomposition. Surf Sci. 1992;264:261–70.
190. Coraux J, N'Diaye AT, Busse C, et al. Structural coherency of graphene on Ir(111). Nano Lett. 2008;8:565–70.
191. Xu Y, Yan X-T. Chemical vapour deposition. London: Springer London. Epub ahead of print 2010. https://doi.org/10.1007/978-1-84882-894-0.
192. Ferrari AC, Bonaccorso F, Fal'ko V, et al. Science and technology roadmap for graphene, related two-dimensional crystals, and hybrid systems. Nanoscale. 2015;7:4598–810.
193. Karunakaran G, Sudha KG, Ali S, et al. Biosynthesis of nanoparticles from various biological sources and its biomedical applications. Molecules. 2023;28:4527.
194. Mozneb M, Mirtaheri E, Sanabria AO, et al. Bioelectronic properties of DNA, protein, cells and their applications for diagnostic medical devices. Biosens Bioelectron. 2020;167:112441.
195. Santhanam M, Algov I, Alfonta L. DNA/RNA electrochemical biosensing devices a future replacement of PCR methods for a fast epidemic containment. Sensors. 2020;20:4648.
196. Wang Z, Kang S, Cao S, et al. Protein-based functional nanocomposites. MRS Bull. 2020;45:1017–26.
197. Sudarev VV, Dolotova SM, Bukhalovich SM, et al. Ferritin self-assembly, structure, function, and biotechnological applications. Int J Biol Macromol. 2023;224:319–43.

198. Mariappan V, Moorthi PV. An overview of naturally synthesized metallic nanoparticles. J App Pharm Sci. Epub ahead of print 2017. https://doi.org/10.7324/JAPS.2017.70634.
199. Ying S, Guan Z, Ofoegbu PC, et al. Green synthesis of nanoparticles: current developments and limitations. Environ Technol Innovation. 2022;26:102336.
200. Singh NA, Narang J, Garg D, et al. Nanoparticles synthesis via microorganisms and their prospective applications in agriculture. Plant Nano Biol. 2023;5:100047.
201. Basavaraja S, Balaji SD, Lagashetty A, et al. Extracellular biosynthesis of silver nanoparticles using the fungus Fusarium semitectum. Mater Res Bull. 2008;43:1164–70.
202. He S, Guo Z, Zhang Y, et al. Biosynthesis of gold nanoparticles using the bacteria Rhodopseudomonas capsulata. Mater Lett. 2007;61:3984–7.
203. Araujo A, Abreu F, Silva K, et al. Magnetotactic bacteria as potential sources of bioproducts. Mar Drugs. 2015;13:389–430.
204. Habeeb Rahuman HB, Dhandapani R, Narayanan S, et al. Medicinal plants mediated the green synthesis of silver nanoparticles and their biomedical applications. IET Nanobiotechnol. 2022;16:115–44.
205. Zeiri Y, Elia P, Zach R, et al. Green synthesis of gold nanoparticles using plant extracts as reducing agents. IntJ Nanomed. 2014;9:4007.
206. Kokina I, Plaksenkova I, Jankovskis L, et al. New insights on biosynthesis of nanoparticles using plants emphasizing the use of Alfalfa (Medicago sativa L.). J Nanotechnol. 2024;2024:1–24.
207. Shankar SS, Rai A, Ahmad A, et al. Rapid synthesis of Au, Ag, and bimetallic Au core–Ag shell nanoparticles using Neem (Azadirachta indica) leaf broth. J Colloid Interface Sci. 2004;275:496–502.
208. Siddiqi KS, Husen A. Engineered gold nanoparticles and plant adaptation potential. Nanoscale Res Lett. 2016;11:400.
209. Arora S, Sharma P, Kumar S, et al. Gold-nanoparticle induced enhancement in growth and seed yield of Brassica juncea. Plant Growth Regul. 2012;66:303–10.
210. Mohammadi H, Amani-Ghadim AR, Matin AA, et al. Fe0 nanoparticles improve physiological and antioxidative attributes of sunflower (Helianthus annuus) plants grown in soil spiked with hexavalent chromium. 3 Biotech. 2020;10:19.
211. Kariyanna G, Siddegowda SB, Shivram AK, et al. Helianthus-annuus assisted synthesis of ZrO_2 nanoparticles: enhanced electrochemical, photoluminescent, and optical properties. Chem Phys Mater. 2023;2:148–54.
212. Sun L, Liu H, Ye Y, et al. Smart nanoparticles for cancer therapy. Sig Transduct Target Ther. 2023;8:418.
213. Đorđević S, Gonzalez MM, Conejos-Sánchez I, et al. Current hurdles to the translation of nanomedicines from bench to the clinic. Drug Deliv and Transl Res. 2022;12:500–25.
214. Liao J, Yuan M, Xu Z, et al. Editorial: smart nanomaterials for biosensing and therapy applications, volume II. Front Bioeng Biotechnol. 2024;12:1387969.
215. Center for Drug Evaluation and Research. Drug products, including biological products, that contain nanomaterials – guidance for industry. 2022. https://www.fda.gov/regulatory--information/search-fda-guidance-documents/drug-products-including-biological-products-contain-nanomaterials-guidance-industry. Accessed 25 Nov 2024.
216. Center for Drug Evaluation and Research. Liposome drug products: chemistry, manufacturing, and controls; human pharmacokinetics and bioavailability; and labeling documentation. 2021. https://www.fda.gov/regulatory-information/search-fda-guidance-documents/liposome-drug-products-chemistry-manufacturing-and-controls-human-pharmacokinetics-and. Accessed 9 July 2024.
217. European Commission. Joint Research Centre. Global summit on regulatory science 2019 nanotechnology and nanoplastics: perspectives on nanotechnology and nanoplastics. LU: Publications Office; 2020. https://data.europa.eu/doi/10.2760/517689. Accessed 9 July 2024.
218. Regulatory science strategy | European Medicines Agency (EMA). 2020. https://www.ema.europa.eu/en/about-us/how-we-work/regulatory-science-strategy. Accessed 25 Nov 2024.

219. Hines PA, Gonzalez-Quevedo R, Lambert AIOM, et al. Regulatory science to 2025: an analysis of stakeholder responses to the European medicines agency's strategy. Front Med (Lausanne). 2020;7:508.
220. Sainz V, Conniot J, Matos AI, et al. Regulatory aspects on nanomedicines. Biochem Biophys Res Commun. 2015;468:504–10.
221. Gaspar RS, Florindo HF, Silva LC, et al. Regulatory aspects of oncologicals: nanosystems main challenges. In: Alonso MJ, Garcia-Fuentes M, editors. Nano-oncologicals. Cham: Springer International Publishing. p. 425–52.
222. Center for Drug Evaluation and Research. Q7 good manufacturing practice guidance for active pharmaceutical ingredients guidance for industry. 2020. https://www.fda.gov/regulatory-information/search-fda-guidance-documents/q7-good-manufacturing-practice-guidance-active-pharmaceutical-ingredients-guidance-industry. Accessed 25 Nov 2024.
223. Satalkar P, Elger BS, Shaw DM. Defining nano, nanotechnology and nanomedicine: why should it matter? Sci Eng Ethics. 2016;22:1255–76.
224. Patton MQ. Qualitative research & evaluation methods: integrating theory and practice. 4th ed. Thousand Oaks: SAGE Publications, Inc.; 2015.
225. de Melo-Martín I, Hellmers N, Henchcliffe C. First-in-human cell transplant trials in Parkinson's disease: the need for an improved informed consent process. Parkinsonism Relat Disord. 2015;21:829–32.
226. Chapman AR, Scala CC. Evaluating the first-in-human clinical trial of a human embryonic stem cell-based therapy. Kennedy Inst Ethics J. 2012;22:243–61.
227. Delivering nanomedicines to patients: a practical guide – PubMed. https://pubmed.ncbi.nlm.nih.gov/25724929/. Accessed 25 Nov 2024.
228. Desai N. Challenges in development of nanoparticle-based therapeutics. AAPS J. 2012;14:282–95.
229. Tinkle S, McNeil SE, Mühlebach S, et al. Nanomedicines: addressing the scientific and regulatory gap. Ann NY Acad Sci. 2014;1313:35–56.
230. Genske A, Engel-Glatter S. Rethinking risk assessment for emerging technology first-in-human trials. Med Health Care Philos. 2016;19:125–39.
231. Zamboni WC, Torchilin V, Patri AK, et al. Best practices in cancer nanotechnology: perspective from NCI nanotechnology alliance. Clin Cancer Res. 2012;18:3229–41.
232. Farjadian F, Ghasemi A, Gohari O, et al. Nanopharmaceuticals and nanomedicines currently on the market: challenges and opportunities. Nanomedicine (Lond). 2019;14:93–126.
233. Satalkar P, Elger BS, Hunziker P, et al. Challenges of clinical translation in nanomedicine: a qualitative study. Nanomedicine. 2016;12:893–900.
234. Commissioner O of the. FDA approves first-of-its kind targeted RNA-based therapy to treat a rare disease. FDA; 2020. https://www.fda.gov/news-events/press-announcements/fda-approves-first-its-kind-targeted-rna-based-therapy-treat-rare-disease. Accessed 28 Nov 2024.
235. Onpattro | European Medicines Agency (EMA). 2018. https://www.ema.europa.eu/en/medicines/human/EPAR/onpattro. Accessed 28 Nov 2024.
236. Urits I, Swanson D, Swett MC, et al. A review of Patisiran (ONPATTRO®) for the treatment of polyneuropathy in people with hereditary transthyretin amyloidosis. Neurol Ther. 2020;9:301–15.
237. Akinc A, Maier MA, Manoharan M, et al. The Onpattro story and the clinical translation of nanomedicines containing nucleic acid-based drugs. Nat Nanotechnol. 2019;14:1084–7.
238. Adams D, Gonzalez-Duarte A, O'Riordan WD, et al. Patisiran, an RNAi therapeutic, for hereditary transthyretin amyloidosis. N Engl J Med. 2018;379:11–21.
239. Onpattro (patisiran) FDA Approval History. Drugs.com. https://www.drugs.com/history/onpattro.html. Accessed 28 Nov 2024.
240. Commissioner O of the. FDA approves first COVID-19 vaccine. FDA; 2024. https://www.fda.gov/news-events/press-announcements/fda-approves-first-covid-19-vaccine. Accessed 28 Nov 2024.

241. Khurana A, Allawadhi P, Khurana I, et al. Role of nanotechnology behind the success of mRNA vaccines for COVID-19. Nano Today. 2021;38:101142.
242. Polack FP, Thomas SJ, Kitchin N, et al. Safety and efficacy of the BNT162b2 mRNA Covid-19 vaccine. N Engl J Med. 2020;383:2603–15.
243. Moderna Announces FDA Authorization of Moderna COVID-19 Vaccine in U.S., https://investors.modernatx.com/news/news-details/2020/Moderna-Announces-FDA-Authorization-of-Moderna-COVID-19-Vaccine-in-U.S/default.aspx. Accessed 28 Nov 2024.
244. Albert-Ludwigs-Universität Freiburg, Germany, Fortner A, Schumacher D, et al. First COVID-19 vaccines receiving the US FDA and EMA emergency use authorization. Discoveries (Craiova). 2021;9:e122.
245. Baden LR, El Sahly HM, Essink B, et al. Efficacy and safety of the mRNA-1273 SARS-CoV-2 vaccine. N Engl J Med. 2021;384:403–16.
246. Lu M, Cohen MH, Rieves D, et al. FDA report: Ferumoxytol for intravenous iron therapy in adult patients with chronic kidney disease. Am J Hematol. 2010;85:315–9.
247. Si G, Du Y, Tang P, et al. Unveiling the next generation of MRI contrast agents: current insights and perspectives on ferumoxytol-enhanced MRI. Natl Sci Rev. 2024;11:nwae057.
248. Petronek MS, Teferi N, Lee C-Y, et al. MRI detection and therapeutic enhancement of Ferumoxytol internalization in glioblastoma cells. Nano. 2024;14:189.
249. Toth GB, Varallyay CG, Horvath A, et al. Current and potential imaging applications of ferumoxytol for magnetic resonance imaging. Kidney Int. 2017;92:47–66.
250. Finn JP, Nguyen K, Hu P. Ferumoxytol vs. Gadolinium agents for contrast-enhanced MRI: thoughts on evolving indications, risks, and benefits. Magn Reson Imaging. 2017;46:919–23.
251. Bashir MR, Bhatti L, Marin D, et al. Emerging applications for ferumoxytol as a contrast agent in MRI. Magn Reson Imaging. 2015;41:884–98.
252. Nanospectra biosciences, Inc. A pilot study of AuroLase(tm) therapy in patients with refractory and/or Recurrent Tumors of the Head and Neck. Clinical Trial Registration NCT00848042. 2016. clinicaltrials.gov, https://clinicaltrials.gov/study/NCT00848042. Accessed 29 Nov 2024.
253. Lin AY, Yang E, Rink JS, et al. Photoablation with the Aurolase system reduces T cell exhaustion and synergizes with immunotherapies in lymphoma. Blood. 2023;142:2825.
254. Sung D, Sanchez A, Tward JD. Successful salvage brachytherapy after infusion of gold AuroShell nanoshells for localized prostate cancer in a human patient. Adv Radiat Oncol. 2023;8:101202.
255. Wang J, Li B, Qiu L, et al. Dendrimer-based drug delivery systems: history, challenges, and latest developments. J Biol Eng. 2022;16:18.
256. Dhull A, Yu C, Wilmoth AH, et al. Dendrimers in corneal drug delivery: recent developments and translational opportunities. Pharmaceutics. 2023;15:1591.
257. Yavuz B, Bozdağ Pehlivan S, Sümer Bolu B, et al. Dexamethasone – PAMAM dendrimer conjugates for retinal delivery: preparation, characterization and *in vivo* evaluation. J Pharm Pharmacol. 2016;68:1010–20.
258. Lancina MG, Wang J, Williamson GS, et al. DenTimol as a Dendrimeric Timolol analogue for glaucoma therapy: synthesis and preliminary efficacy and safety assessment. Mol Pharm. 2018;15:2883–9.
259. Abraxane approved for metastatic pancreatic cancer. Cancer Discov. 2013;3:OF3.
260. De Luca R, Profita G, Cicero G. Nab-paclitaxel in pretreated metastatic breast cancer: evaluation of activity, safety, and quality of life. OTT. 2019;12:1621–7.
261. Blair HA, Deeks ED. Albumin-bound paclitaxel: a review in non-small cell lung cancer. Drugs. 2015;75:2017–24.
262. Von Hoff DD, Ervin T, Arena FP, et al. Increased survival in pancreatic cancer with nab-paclitaxel plus gemcitabine. N Engl J Med. 2013;369:1691–703.
263. Xuan L, Ju Z, Skonieczna M, et al. Nanoparticles-induced potential toxicity on human health: applications, toxicity mechanisms, and evaluation models. MedComm (2020). 2023;4:e327.

264. Yang L, Wang H, Leng D, et al. Machine learning applications in nanomaterials: recent advances and future perspectives. Chem Eng J. 2024;500:156687.
265. Jeon S, Jun E, Chang H, et al. Prediction the clinical EPR effect of nanoparticles in patient-derived xenograft models. J Control Release. 2022;351:37–49.
266. Charitidis CA, Georgiou P, Koklioti MA, et al. Manufacturing nanomaterials: from research to industry. Manuf Rev. 2014;1:11.
267. Rambaran T, Schirhagl R. Nanotechnology from lab to industry – a look at current trends. Nanoscale Adv. 4:3664–75.
268. Souto EB, Silva GF, Dias-Ferreira J, et al. Nanopharmaceutics: part II—production scales and clinically compliant production methods. Nanomaterials (Basel). 2020;10:455.
269. Liu X, Meng H. Consideration for the scale-up manufacture of nanotherapeutics—a critical step for technology transfer. VIEW. 2021;2:20200190.
270. Martínez-Ballesta M, Gil-Izquierdo Á, García-Viguera C, et al. Nanoparticles and controlled delivery for bioactive compounds: outlining challenges for new "smart-foods" for health. Foods. 2018;7:72.
271. Li Y, Jacques S, Gaikwad H, et al. Inhibition of acute complement responses towards bolus-injected nanoparticles using targeted short-circulating regulatory proteins. Nat Nanotechnol. 2024;19:246–54.
272. Rasmussen JW, Martinez E, Louka P, et al. Zinc oxide nanoparticles for selective destruction of tumor cells and potential for drug delivery applications. Expert Opin Drug Deliv. 2010;7:1063–77.
273. Liu H-J, Xu P. Strategies to overcome/penetrate the BBB for systemic nanoparticle delivery to the brain/brain tumor. Adv Drug Deliv Rev. 2022;191:114619.
274. Pinheiro RGR, Coutinho AJ, Pinheiro M, et al. Nanoparticles for targeted brain drug delivery: what do we know? Int J Mol Sci. 2021;22:11654.
275. Lee J, Lee H, Kim HJ, et al. Quantification of doping state of redox sensitive nanoparticles for probing the invasiveness of cancer cells using surface enhanced Raman scattering. Mater Today Bio. 2022;14:100241.
276. Shrestha B, Wang L, Brey EM, et al. Smart nanoparticles for chemo-based combinational therapy. Pharmaceutics. 2021;13:853.
277. Majumder J, Minko T. Multifunctional and stimuli-responsive nanocarriers for targeted therapeutic delivery. Expert Opin Drug Deliv. 2021;18:205–27.
278. Hosseini SM, Mohammadnejad J, Salamat S, et al. Theranostic polymeric nanoparticles as a new approach in cancer therapy and diagnosis: a review. Mater Today Chem. 2023;29:101400.
279. Shabani L, Abbasi M, Azarnew Z, et al. Neuro-nanotechnology: diagnostic and therapeutic nano-based strategies in applied neuroscience. Biomed Eng Online. 2023;22:1.
280. Adir O, Poley M, Chen G, et al. Integrating artificial intelligence and nanotechnology for precision cancer medicine. Adv Mater. 2019;32:e1901989.
281. Tripathy A, Patne AY, Mohapatra S, et al. Convergence of nanotechnology and machine learning: the state of the art, challenges, and perspectives. IJMS. 2024;25:12368.
282. Wu G, Hui X, Hu L, et al. Recent advancement of bioinspired nanomaterials and their applications: a review. Front Bioeng Biotechnol. 2022;10:952523.
283. Bigham A, Zarepour A, Safarkhani M, et al. Inspired by nature: bioinspired and biomimetic photocatalysts for biomedical applications. Nano Mater Sci. 2024:S2589965124000175.
284. Kroll AV, Fang RH, Zhang L. Biointerfacing and applications of cell membrane-coated nanoparticles. Bioconjug Chem. 2017;28:23–32.
285. Desai N, Tambe V, Pofali P, et al. Cell membrane-coated nanoparticles: a new frontier in immunomodulation. Adv NanoBiomed Res. 2024;4:2400012.
286. Yuwen L, Zhang S, Chao J. Recent advances in DNA nanotechnology-enabled biosensors for virus detection. Biosensors (Basel). 2023;13:822.

287. Abu-Salah KM, Zourob MM, Mouffouk F, et al. DNA-based nanobiosensors as an emerging platform for detection of disease. Sensors (Basel). 2015;15:14539–68.
288. Zhang Y, Tian X, Wang Z, et al. Advanced applications of DNA nanostructures dominated by DNA origami in antitumor drug delivery. Front Mol Biosci. 2023;10:1239952.

Chapter 16
Smart and Sustainable Nanomaterials: Challenges, Safety, and Ethical Considerations

Dipanwita Bhattacharya, Annada Das, and Souti Prasad Sarkhel

Abstract Nanotechnology has revolutionized diverse fields through groundbreaking advancements in the design, modeling, fabrication, and characterization of nanomaterials and nanocrystals. Its applications are widespread and include electronics, nanomedicine, food processing, and environmental engineering. The unique properties of nanomaterials, arising from their "nano"-scale dimensions and enhanced stability, have enabled breakthroughs in drug delivery systems, biosensing technologies, and food safety protocols. These advancements hold immense promise for addressing global health disparities, particularly in resource-limited settings, by facilitating early disease diagnosis, efficient drug delivery, and improved patient outcomes. However, these innovations also present significant challenges, including safety concerns, ethical dilemmas, the potential toxicity of nanomaterials, and growing concerns regarding their environmental impact and sustainability. Currently, a considerable gap exists in the formulation of universally accepted standardized protocols and a coherent classification system for developing and understanding various nanomaterials and their mechanisms of action. This inconsistency hinders progress within the field. To fully realize the potential of nanotechnology while mitigating associated risks, it is crucial to implement standardized assessment methodologies, conduct rigorous *in vitro* and *in vivo* clinical trials, and foster enhanced collaboration with national and international regulatory agencies. A comprehensive approach is vital, encompassing stringent global safety standards, transparent communication, and thorough ethical review processes. The regulatory

D. Bhattacharya (✉)
Department of Livestock Products Technology, Faculty of Veterinary & Animal Sciences, Banaras Hindu University, Rajiv Gandhi South Campus, Mirzapur, U.P., India

A. Das
Department of Livestock Products Technology, Institute of Veterinary Science and Animal Husbandry, Siksha 'O' Anusandhan University, Bhubaneswar, Odisha, India

S. P. Sarkhel
Department of Veterinary Parasitology, Faculty of Veterinary & Animal Sciences, Rajiv Gandhi South Campus, Banaras Hindu University, Mirzapur, U.P., India

S. Mondal et al. (eds.), *Smart and Sustainable Nanomaterials in Digital Healthcare and Theranostic*, https://doi.org/10.1007/978-981-95-9386-6_16

landscape surrounding nanomaterials is complex, with varying standards across jurisdictions. Therefore, establishing universal and effective regulatory frameworks is essential to ensure the safety and efficacy of nanomaterials in healthcare, environmental, and food applications. Against this backdrop, this chapter explores the complexities of nanomaterials, focusing on their biomedical applications, the challenges they present, safety issues, and ethical considerations.

Keywords Nanomaterial · Safety · Health · Ethics · Environment · Regulatory · Risks

16.1 Introduction

Nanotechnology has profoundly transformed human life, integrating seamlessly into daily routines and enhancing convenience, efficiency, and comfort. The application of nanotechnology is ubiquitous, ranging from nanomemory chips powering our smartphones to ultrafine particles of zinc oxide and titanium dioxide in sunscreen lotions. Its applications span diverse sectors, including textiles, automotive, sports equipment, and healthcare, where it has enabled advancements such as strain-resistant fabrics, scratch-resistant coatings, improved sports equipment, and targeted drug delivery. The emergence of nanomaterials as versatile tools has driven innovation across various scientific disciplines. The journey from bulky first-generation computers to slim laptops, the transition from bulk matter to "nano" carbon dots in chemistry, the exploration of nanoscale structures through advanced microscopy in physics, and the investigation of complex biomolecules at the atomic level in biology collectively underscore the evolution of nanotechnology. This evolution has revolutionized fields such as materials science, physics, chemistry, computer science, engineering, biomedical sciences, and environmental science. By enabling precise manipulation of matter at the nanoscale, nanotechnology has significantly increased the quality of human life by translating scientific breakthroughs from the laboratory "bench" to "bedside" and has opened new frontiers for research and development, leading to groundbreaking discoveries and applications.

The Greek word "nano"" means "dwarf", referring to a very small size, depicting one thousand millionths of a meter (10^{-9} m) [1, 2]. Owing to their unique properties derived from their nanoscale dimensions (1–100 nm), nanomaterials have revolutionized fields ranging from medicine, electronics, food, and energy to environmental monitoring in recent decades [3, 4]. Many ancient studies have utilized nanocomposites and nanoparticles, thus confirming the long history of nanomaterial usage. The "Lycurgus cup" at the British Museum is the oldest example of dichroic glass made up of Au-Ag nanocomposites [5–7]. Some other interesting examples include the "stained-glass windows" of the late medieval church that altered color due to light reflections [8–10], glowing and glittering "lustre ceramic" used in the Islamic world that contained Ag or Cu nanoparticles [11, 12], Italian "Renaissance pottery" during the sixteenth century [2, 13], "Damascus sabre blades" where cementite nanowires and carbon nanotubes were used to provide durability, suppleness and extraordinarily sharp edges [2, 11, 12, 14], Michel Faraday's study demonstrating unique optical properties of gold nanoparticles in "Ruby" gold in 1857 [15, 16], etc. However, the American Physicist, Nobel laureate, and father of modern nanotechnology Richard Feynman's lecture titled "There is plenty of room at the bottom" led to the hypothesis "Why can't we write the entire 24 volumes of the Encyclopedia Britannica on the head of a pin?" that introduced the concept of nanotechnology in 1959 [2, 17]. The term "nanotechnology" was coined by Norio Taniguchi in 1974 [18]. The inventions of scanning tunneling microscopy (STM) [19], atomic force microscopy (AFM), and scanning probe microscopy (SPM) [20] have also shed light on the development of modern nanotechnology. The discovery of fullerenes or buckyballs in 1985 [19], carbon nanotubes in 1991 [20], carbon dots (c-dots) and graphene in 2004 [21, 22], the creation of the historic International Business Machines (IBM) logo utilizing 35 xenon atoms by Don Eigler in 1990 [11, 23], Paul Rothemund's "scaffolded DNA origami" in 2006 [24], nanopharmaceuticals, nanobiochips, nanoelectrodes, nanobiosensors, etc., opened new possibilities for applying nanomaterials in various fields.

Innovative nanomaterials, including nanoparticles, nanotubes, and nanocomposites, have been engineered to possess large surface area-to-volume ratios; tunable optical, electrical, and magnetic properties; and biocompatibility [25, 26]. These characteristics make them ideal candidates for developing biosensors with a wide range of applications. Smart and sustainable nanomaterial-based biosensors, devices, and compounds are being utilized in healthcare for point-of-care testing and disease diagnosis [27], drug delivery under nanomedicine [28], nano-oncology [29], biomolecular imaging [30], etc. Biosensors based on plasmonic nanoparticles have been developed for rapid cancer diagnosis [31]. Nanomaterials with antimicrobial activities are being explored as alternative antimicrobials for combating antimicrobial resistance (AMR) in multidrug-resistant (MDR) bacteria [32, 33]. Nanomaterials are also used as cardiovascular biomarkers [34] and for the treatment of neurogenerative disorders [35]. Additionally, nanomaterials have potential uses in the fields of molecular biotechnology, nanoinformatics, environmental surveillance, food safety, and quality control [36, 37]. Nanoinformatics improves the nanomodeling of tumor cells and aids in the detection of drug-resistant tumor cells, thereby facilitating chemotherapy [38]. In environmental science, carbon nanotubes and graphene-based smart nanomaterials are used as powerful tools for real-time monitoring by quantifying pollutants, toxins, residues, and pathogens in air, water, and soil [39]. Similarly, smart and sustainable nanomaterials play crucial roles in ensuring the quality and safety of food products from "farm to fork", thereby safeguarding public health and building consumer trust. Nanomaterial-based smart biosensors aid in the rapid detection of foodborne pathogens such as *E. coli, Salmonella* spp., *Listeria* spp., toxins, allergens, residues, adulterants, and contaminants [40]. Nanoparticles such as TiO_2, ZnO, and nanomaterial composites containing green nanoparticles with antimicrobial and antioxidant activities are also being utilized in food packaging [41–43]. In the field of nanomedicine, diverse research has been conducted for advanced target-specific drug delivery systems with better accuracy, absorbability, controlled release, long-term stability, etc. Modern nanomedicine offers significant potential for anticancer therapies and has demonstrated notable efficacy in improving the bioavailability and dissolution properties crucial for chemotherapy. Moreover, nanoscience is pivotal in the extensive application of early disease diagnosis.

While offering substantial advantages, nanotechnology also presents significant challenges. The diverse adoption of nanomaterials also highlights the associated hurdles, safety concerns, and ethical considerations, which must be carefully addressed. One of the significant challenges is the development of robust and reliable nanomaterial-based sensors that exhibit high sensitivity, specificity, and reproducibility across different matrices and environmental conditions [44, 45]. Safety considerations include the adverse physicochemical properties of engineered nanomaterials that might be toxic or could pose a health risk or hazard to humans and the environment [46, 47]. Ethical considerations surrounding smart nanomaterials include equity and access, privacy, consent, data ownership, long-term application, the potential for misuse or unintended consequences [48, 49], etc. Furthermore, understanding the challenges, safety concerns, and ethical considerations associated with smart and sustainable nanomaterials may provide new opportunities to address these pitfalls. Through collective, integrated, and proactive measures, we can effectively harness nanoscience's transformative potential while safeguarding human and environmental health and upholding ethical principles.

Therefore, to develop safe and effective nanomaterials, several critical concerns, including toxicity, immune responses, potential health effects, and ethical implications, must be addressed. These challenges significantly influence regulatory standards, which require thorough evaluation and transparent communication. By addressing these issues directly, we can foster public trust and encourage broader acceptance of nanomaterials. In light of this context, this chapter examines the intricacies, safety issues, and ethical implications related to the growing application of nanomaterials, with the goal of developing smart and sustainable strategies for a range of human and environmental challenges. Furthermore, we investigate the application of nanotechnology in drug delivery, biosensing, food safety, and nanomedicine, providing valuable insights into the intricate challenges and opportunities present across diverse scientific and interdisciplinary fields.

16.2 Nanoparticles in Nanomedicine: A Success Story

Nanotechnology has been effectively utilized in developed nations to enhance medical care, facilitating the early detection of life-threatening diseases and controlling their spread, which in turn improves patient outcomes. In stark contrast, when mortality rates are compared between developed and developing countries, the latter suffer from significantly higher casualties across various age groups. This disparity can be attributed to a lack of essential resources in developing nations, such as safe drinking water, adequate nutrition, accessible healthcare, equitable social services, and a clean environment. These critical deficiencies present substantial challenges to public health in these regions. To address this crisis, harnessing the potential of advanced nanoscience, particularly in nanomedicine and biomedical diagnostics, is essential. By prioritizing enhancements in safety, intelligent design, and sustainable nanotechnologies over traditional methods while also improving affordability, we can help bridge the healthcare gap, regardless of economic constraints [57–59].

A diverse array of nanodrug delivery carriers encapsulate therapeutic agents, bioactive peptides, antimicrobials, phytomedicines, and nutraceuticals for efficient transport to specific cells within the body (Table 16.1). These nanocarriers increase the bioavailability, insolubility, controlled release, and stability of mixed drug formulations and increase drug absorption and bioefficacy [59]. Nanomedicines have demonstrated remarkable potential in treating early-stage cancer, improving chemotherapy precision, and enabling noninvasive imaging through MRI (Fig. 16.1) [57]. In addition, nanocarriers deliver drugs to their payloads and can interact and integrate with the surrounding microenvironment and respond accordingly. This interaction could lead to advancements in diagnostic and theranostic concepts [60]. Improving imaging modalities and therapeutic approaches has strengthened the development of nanotheranostics for better preclinical and clinical outcomes [60]. Moreover, they show promise in addressing infertility, contraceptive management, wound healing, and chronic conditions such as diabetes, asthma, myocardial ischemia, rheumatoid arthritis, irritable bowel syndrome, and neurodegenerative diseases [57, 61]. By replacing traditional carriers with responsive polymeric nanocarriers, quantum dots, liposomes, nanocrystals, micelles, carbon dots, nanoemulsions, hydrogels, dendrimers, and magnetic nanoparticles, drug and nutraceutical delivery is significantly enhanced with prolonged stability and targeted organ distribution (Table 16.1). Advanced nanotechnology-based laboratory screening has revolutionized the early diagnosis of tuberculosis, HIV, endometriosis, uterine fibroids, autoimmune disorders, and numerous other diseases [55, 57]. To further propel this field, bionanotechnology will be instrumental in genetic engineering, tissue engineering, gene repair, and the development of polymeric therapeutics for gene vaccines to address genetic disorders and viral infections, including cystic fibrosis, cancer, and immune disorders [51].

16.3 Nanotechnology: Ethical Concerns

Nanotechnology has become a major driver of innovation across diverse scientific disciplines, demonstrating its immense potential. Its impact spans various sectors, ranging from nanodrug delivery systems in nanomedicine to advancements in disease diagnostics and enhancements in agricultural productivity. Additionally, it has transformed the packaging industry through the advancement of intelligent and smart packaging materials, contributed to the development of designer foods, and enabled innovative waste management solutions, all while supporting ecological balance [57]. However, as the fusion of science and innovation propels

Table 16.1 Examples of important approved and experimental nanocarriers along with their potential applications

Nanoparticles	Characteristics	Applications	References
Liposomes (Approved by FDA & EMA)	Spherical vesicle with phospholipid and cholesterol bilayer membrane; in the core hydrophilic drugs can bind, and in lipid bilayer membrane, hydrophobic components can bind; 90–150 nm in size	Vehicle for cancer vaccine Antigen-specific immune responses Delivery of genetic materials (DNA, mRNA) Onpattro containing Patisiran sodium—FDA-approved MARQIBO (vincristine sulphate liposome injection)—FDA-approved	[50–52]
Micelles (FDA approved)	Amphiphilic polymers are used; Hydrophobic internal core that may encapsulate drugs with lesser aqueous solubility; outer surface allows dissolution in aqueous solutions	Easily penetrate the endothelial cell junction Chemotherapy in cancer treatments (Estrasorb, Oxaliplatin, Cisplatin, etc.)	[50, 53]
Protein nanoparticles	Protein carriers conjugate to active protein therapeutics; reduced toxicity; improved solubility	Improved drug delivery system without much need of toxic solvent (Abraxane approved by FDA, albumen-bound paclitaxel shows improved drug delivery and tumor inhibition, better pharmacokinetics).	[54]
Inorganic nanoparticles	Metal and metal oxide are used for therapeutic and imaging.; due to slow dissolution, better drug administration property; paracellular & transcytosis in vivo transportation system; no clear information on toxicity	Venofer and Ferrlecit are iron oxide-based nanodrugs used to treat anemia and chronic kidney disease (FDA-approved); Cornell dots are silica nanoparticles designed for fluorescence imaging; No approval by the FDA for gold nanoparticles in therapeutics.	[54, 55]
Quantum dots	Semiconductor nanocrystals (2–10 nm); emissions in the near-infrared region (< 650 nm); lower absorption by tissues	Conjugated QDs with immunoglobulin aptamer, proteins for detection and diagnosis of early-stage cancer (biomarker-specific) Biomedical imaging Drug delivery	[50, 55]

(continued)

Table 16.1 (continued)

Nanoparticles	Characteristics	Applications	References
Carbon nanotubes	Folded graphene sheet into tube; single-walled or multiple-walled needle-like structures; nanoscale size; biocompatible & good electrical conductivity	Deliver target-specific drugs, biomolecules Transporting gene, proteins, anticancer therapeutics—surface functionalization, better absorption (e.g. silibinin drug loaded in chitosan-coated multiple-walled CNTs; Droxidopa-loaded CNTs)	[50, 51]
Dendrimers	Dendritic effect on medicine delivery; made up of sugar, nucleotides, amino acids; poly (acyl thiourea, poly thiourea-isothiocyanate-amine coupling & thiol-methacrylate Michael addition reaction; three-dimensional structure; globular tree-like structure; mono-dispersibility	Effective in chemotherapeutic drug delivery and diagnosis; effective transdermal transportation of drugs Increased absorption of anticancer drugs, better stability, increased half-life Useful in MRI Limited clinical uses because of amine groups that show toxicity; modification is needed for clinical purposes, e.g., L-lysine dendrimer containing SN-38	[50, 51, 55]
Hydrogels	Make crosslinks of hydrophilic polymer chains that may trap multiple drugs, three-dimensional structures; biocompatible	Lesser toxic effect Controlled drug release property, longer stability, high absorption Effective for cancer treatment pH responsiveness, heat sensitive Wound healing	[50, 51, 56]
Fullerenes	Allotropes of carbon act as a scaffold for drug formulation	Effective for treatment of cancer, HIV Sustained release properties of drugs at the targeted site Maintain the drug concentrations at the targeted site Lack of pharmacokinetics information Cost issue	[51, 56]

(continued)

Table 16.1 (continued)

Nanoparticles	Characteristics	Applications	References
Polymeric nanoparticles	Colloidal, biodegradable polymeric structure in the form of nanocapsule or nanoemulsion	Effective drug delivery system Antimicrobial components carrier For example, chitosan-based nanoparticle containing curcumin-antimicrobial; ofloxacin loaded polycaprolactone-effective drug release; cyclosporin nanoemulsion-chronic dry eye treatment Plegridy-multiple sclerosis; Somavert-acromegaly (FDA-approved)	[51–53]

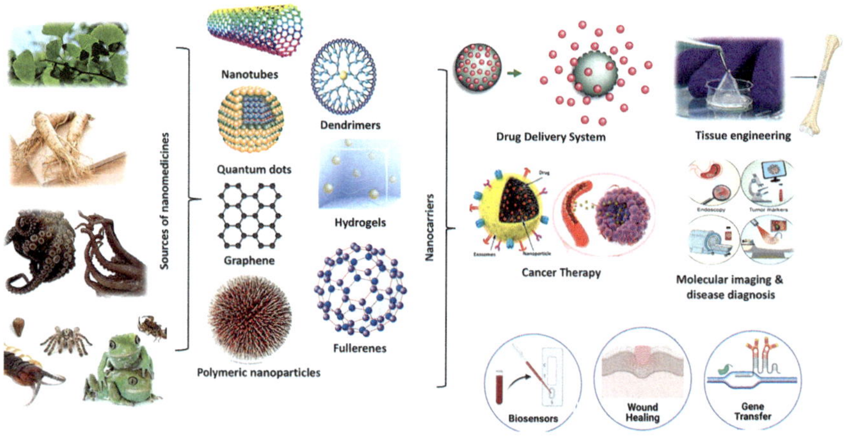

Fig. 16.1 Applications of nanomaterials in biomedicines

technological advances, it is essential to balance this progress with robust ethical considerations, stringent safety standards, and effective regulatory structures [58]. This balanced strategy encourages sustainable development and builds public trust in emerging technologies through an interdisciplinary approach that impacts society [59]. Thus, cultivating and sustaining public confidence requires increasing collaboration among scientists, researchers, policymakers, regulatory bodies, industry leaders, and stakeholders. By maximizing benefits while minimizing risks to human health, the environment, and animal welfare, we can responsibly tap into the full potential of nanotechnology [62]. Moreover, ethical assessments are crucial to ensure that nanotechnology products undergo thorough safety and efficacy evaluations prior to market release. A strong regulatory and safety framework is necessary for mitigating potential risks linked to laboratory-derived technologies. Addressing ethical issues and establishing solid regulatory structures are essential for

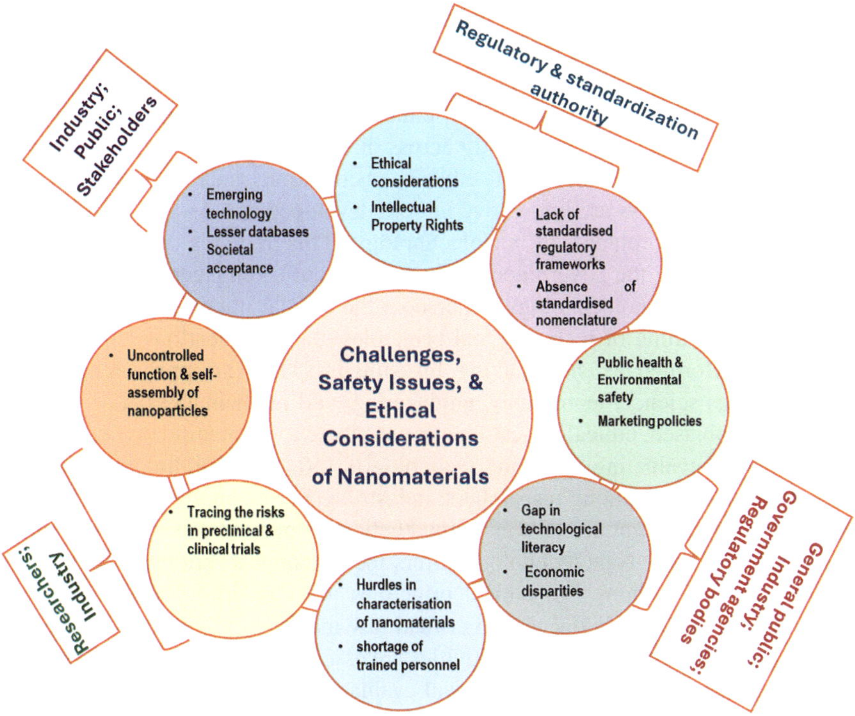

Fig. 16.2 Challenges, safety, and ethical considerations of emerging nanomaterials

responsible technology transfer and advancement [62]. Nevertheless, laboratory-based research inherently involves identified and unidentified risks that need careful management to avert unforeseen challenges (Fig. 16.2). Thus, effective technology transfer calls for open dialogue among researchers, industry leaders, policymakers, consumers, and government agencies to address ethical concerns and foster public confidence. Clear communication regarding the possible risks and advantages of using nanotechnology in daily life is crucial for gaining broader public acceptance of advanced science-based technologies [57, 63].

16.3.1 Identifying Ethical Considerations

As nanotechnology promises significant advancements across diverse scientific disciplines and seeks greater integration into society, it is essential to consider the potential psychosocial, demographic, and cultural implications. Understanding public perceptions of such technological innovations is crucial for their successful adoption. The lack of a clear definition for nanotechnology-derived products and uncertainty about their mechanisms contribute to public apprehension regarding safety and risks [63]. The rapid and ongoing convergence of nanoscience with fields such as molecular biotechnology, bioinformatics, and materials science, among others, has generated a complex ethical landscape. While this interdisciplinary fusion offers immense potential, it also raises ethical concerns [57]. Importantly, ethical considerations may vary significantly across different disciplines within the broad field of nanotechnology. Addressing ethical considerations and implementing robust regulatory frameworks are imperative in both developed and developing nations to foster societal acceptance of nanotechnology. This requires a comprehensive approach involving the government, industry, and public engagement [57]. Recent advancements in nanotechnology underscore the critical importance of enhancing public understanding of technological principles, their applications, and potential impacts for informed decision-making. Investing in STEM (an approach to learning that integrates science, technology, engineering, and mathematics) education and promoting unbiased, ethical education can contribute to a scientifically literate public capable of evaluating emerging technologies [50, 63]. Building trust requires collaborative efforts among researchers, industry, government, media, and the public. Transparent communication and empathetic engagement can overcome public skepticism [57, 58]. Nanotechnology offers the potential to bridge economic disparities between nations, but ethical principles must guide its development and application [57]. Ensuring access to critical raw materials, environmental sustainability, and respect for cultural sensitivities are essential components of responsible nanotechnology [64]. Continuous ethical evaluation is essential to ensure that the benefits of nanotechnology are maximized while minimizing its potential risks.

16.3.2 Ethical Implications of Nanotechnology Applications: Specific Issues

Nanotechnology has infiltrated nearly every sphere of scientific research and development. The rapid pace of technological advancement in laboratories has precipitated a host of ethical concerns related to developmental progress, cytological evaluation of toxicity, and product introduction. While superficial successes in specific areas might initially appear promising, a deeper ethical evaluation is imperative, considering sociological, demographic, and dormant risk and trust factors [63, 65, 66].

16.3.2.1 Health

Although nanoparticles have long been integral to technological advancement, their continually evolving structural characteristics, ambiguous definitions, and absence of comprehensive regulatory frameworks at both the national and international levels have prompted public apprehension. The remarkable progress in nanomedicine can be attributed to its unique properties, including variable crystalline structures, atomic stability, sterility, high purity, enhanced solubility, increased surface area, improved bioavailability, reduced viscosity, sustained drug delivery, and precision release capabilities [67]. As a result, nanomedicine plays a crucial role in the early diagnosis and treatment of diseases. Despite these significant strides, pressing ethical concerns surrounding nanomedicine persist, particularly concerning the safety assessments of these technologies, their interactions with human health systems and the environment, the potential toxicity of engineered nanoparticles, and the biosafety challenges that arise with stem cell research [59]. Traditionally, research has focused on the toxicological evaluation of nanoparticles, paying considerable attention to their chemical compositions, surfactants, cosurfactants, and stabilizers. Nevertheless, existing evaluation methods often overlook the atomic components present on nanoparticle surfaces. Additionally, the small size, composition, and high surface-to-volume ratio of nanomaterials enable them to cross biological barriers such as the blood–brain barrier, placenta, and skin through inhalation, ingestion, and skin contact, which poses critical concerns about the potential for long-term systemic toxicity and adverse health effects [68]. The migratory properties of nanoparticles, alongside altered pharmacokinetics and the potential risks of cytotoxicity, immunotoxicity, and genotoxicity, highlight the need for rigorous scrutiny and thorough investigations and the establishment of revised regulatory standards aimed at safeguarding public health and environmental integrity [69]. Moreover, the unpredictable interactions of nanomaterials with biological systems can engender cellular damage, compromise the body's defense mechanisms, provoke inflammation, induce oxidative stress, and contribute to bioaccumulation. Despite these inherent risks, nanomedicine and nanotechnology products have garnered FDA approval, and numerous innovations are at the cusp of commercialization. Consequently, to facilitate informed decision-making, it is crucial to ensure clear communication regarding the composition, biomechanisms, reactive and barrier properties, safety precautions, potential side effects, and manufacturing processes associated with nanomedicine to consumers [57–59].

16.3.2.2 Environmental

Ethical considerations extend to the sustainable utilization of natural resources. Many developing nations rich in inorganic and organic materials face the dilemma of exporting these valuable assets or harnessing them for domestic industrialization, economic growth, and environmental protection [58]. Consequently, nanotechnology has emerged as a potential avenue for developing alternative materials. For example, polysaccharide-based hydrogels and nanocrystals derived from natural resources are being explored as drug, vaccine, and immunity booster carriers. A critical environmental concern is the potential for nanomaterial release during manufacturing, use, and disposal. Improper disposal from consumer goods, agriculture, industry, medicine, and wastewater treatment can lead to nanomaterial accumulation in soil and water bodies, disrupting ecosystems and biodiversity [70]. The persistence of nanoparticles in soil, water, and air raises concerns about long-term environmental impacts. Furthermore, water contamination by nanowastes can negatively impact aquatic organisms, disrupting population dynamics and the ecological balance. The potential for bioaccumulation and biomagnification through the food chain due to nanoparticle ingestion from contaminated soil and water is a significant concern [71]. The persistence of nanoparticles in these environments or their transformation in the environment poses long-term risks, including altered properties that can harm flora and fauna. The indiscriminate use of silver nanoparticles in food, medicine, and consumer products has increased concerns about antimicrobial resistance (AMR) and ecological toxicity [72].

16.3.2.3 Occupational

The occupational health and safety of workers involved in the production, handling, and disposal of nanomaterials are paramount concerns. Continuous exposure to airborne nanoparticles within manufacturing units can result in respiratory allergies, skin irritation, pigmentation, and other systemic health issues [63]. Implementing effective prevention and control measures, utilizing personal protective equipment, and conducting regular health checkups are essential to safeguarding worker health and mitigating occupational hazards in nanoparticle manufacturing facilities [57].

16.3.2.4 Biomedical

The ever-expanding field of biomedical engineering has witnessed robust integration of electromagnetic screening fields, highly conductive nanometals, and nanomagnetic particles. However, this technological advancement has introduced novel occupational hazards for laboratory technicians and other personnel. The landscape of materials employed in this domain is continually evolving. While conventional materials such as metals are being increasingly replaced by carbon nanotubes and fullerenes owing to their superior mechanical properties and electron affinity [73] and semiconductor nanocrystals (quantum dots) are supplanting organic dyes owing to their enhanced emission properties and reduced tissue absorption [68], the ethical implications of utilizing these materials must be carefully considered. The unique physicochemical properties of these "smart" and "sustainable" nanomaterials, which are distinct from their bulk counterparts, raise significant concerns about human health and environmental safety [64]. For example, carbon nanotubes and graphene, which are commonly employed in biomedical applications, share structural similarities with asbestos and have been linked to respiratory risks. These emerging threats underscore the urgent need for stringent ethical guidelines governing the development and application of nanomaterials in biomedical engineering. Given these challenges, a substantial increase in ethical standards is imperative for the responsible utilization of these materials in nanotechnology.

16.3.2.5 Patents

Patents are of paramount importance in nanomedicine, granting developers a government-sanctioned monopoly that incentivizes research and development investment. This exclusive right enables the recoupment of research and development investments, protection from generic competition, and enhanced investor credibility, facilitating funding acquisition. In addition to product exclusivity, patents on fundamental technology components can confer control over specific nanomedicine industry sectors and generate revenue through licensing [65]. While patents undeniably stimulate innovation and shape the nanomedicine industry [50, 57], concerns about patent misuse, such as excessive fees or overly broad claims, can hinder innovation. Challenges arise when multiple entities, including researchers, institutions, and industry partners, contest ownership of a particular invention, particularly in gene therapy and genetic vaccine development. The partial determination of ownership is crucial, and legal complexities, inaccessibility, and high costs associated with intellectual property rights can hinder innovation [50]. These challenges can limit the availability of new innovations in resource-constrained countries, impacting public health. To address these challenges, a comprehensive overview of the regulatory framework is necessary. This process should involve bioethicists, researchers, industry representatives, and other relevant stakeholders to establish a balanced intellectual property rights system within the nanosystem domain [65].

16.3.2.6 Electronics

The rapid advancement of electronic and computerized technology has led to the development of increasingly streamlined and efficient devices with sophisticated data analysis capabilities. Among these innovations are radio frequency identifiers (RFIDs), small microchip-based devices capable of autonomous information collection and processing for biosensing applications. While these technological advancements have replaced human activities in numerous domains through computerized tools, robotic systems, and software, they have also raised significant privacy concerns. The increasing miniaturization and ubiquity of electronic devices have endowed them with potent monitoring capabilities, leading to questions about their potential control over individuals [58]. Consequently, a critical examination of ethical implications and a subsequent update of regulatory frameworks have become necessary to address public safety concerns stemming from the potential displacement of human decision-making by device-based data analysis, storage, control, and monitoring.

16.3.2.7 Military

A significant ethical challenge arises from the potential misuse of nanotechnology for the development of more potent biological, chemical, and missile-based weaponry. Additionally, the dual-use nature of nanotechnological innovations presents a complex ethical dilemma. While military advancements can enhance public and soldier safety, the associated societal concerns necessitate careful consideration in future research and development programs [63, 74].

16.4 Regulatory Aspects and Safety Concerns

Nanotechnology advancements have promising applications in healthcare, electronics, environmental monitoring, and food safety. Integrating smart and sustainable nanomaterials in biosensors can revolutionize medicine, disease diagnosis, environmental surveillance, and food quality control. However, there are significant regulatory and safety concerns surrounding their use and disposal, representing a critical intersection of technological innovation, environmental protection, and public health [75]. The regulatory landscape and safety considerations pertinent to smart and sustainable nanomaterials are discussed below.

16.4.1 Global Regulatory Landscape

The regulatory landscape governing nanomaterials is complex and varies across different jurisdictions, regions, and sectors. While some developed countries have established comprehensive regulations, others are still developing approaches. However, all regulatory bodies require the labelling of products containing nanomaterials to aid in making informed decisions for consumers and ensuring the safety of public health and the environment [76]. The countries leading from the front in nanomaterial regulation include the United States of America (USA), the European Union (EU), Canada, Australia, and Japan [77]. Internationally, the regulations on nanomaterial use and disposal, as given by organizations, agencies and bodies such as the Codex Alimentarius Commission (CAC), the United States Food and Drug Administration (US-FDA), the European Medicines Agency (EMA), the European Food Safety Authority (EFSA), the European Chemicals Agency (ECHA), and the United States-Environmental Protection Agency (EPA), are widely followed [76, 78]. All types of nanoparticles, whether used as diagnostic or therapeutic agents, must be thoroughly screened and evaluated for their various mechanisms of action to ensure human health security, especially before the introduction of novel materials [60]. These materials adhere to various regulatory guidelines and legislative principles, depending on their different modes of action, which can be physical, mechanical, chemical, or pharmacological. Their mechanisms distinguish whether they are classified as medical devices or therapeutics, leading to variations in their regulatory requirements [60]. Complexity arises in regulatory principles when these products fall as "borderline products" intermixed with different angles of mechanisms of action. The International Organization for Standardization (ISO) has developed standards such as ISO/TS 80004–1, which provides terminology and definitions for nanomaterials used in nanotechnology-based products [79]. In the USA, the regulations concerning nanomaterials fall under existing laws such as the Toxic Substance Control Act (TSCA), Federal Food, Drug, and Cosmetic Act (FFDCA), Federal Insecticide, Fungicide, and Rodenticide Act (FIFRA), and Nanotechnology Research and Development Act (NRDA) [80, 81]. The EU employs precautionary approaches through regulations such as Registration, Evaluation, Authorization, and Restriction of Chemicals (REACH) [82]. The EU's REACH regulation now explicitly covers nanoforms, requiring companies to report information related to nanomaterials [83]. Additionally, the EU has specific provisions for regulations related to nanomaterials under the Cosmetics Regulation and Biocidal Products Regulation (BPR) [84]. In the United Kingdom (UK), the Food Standards Agency (FSA), Department for Environment, Food and Rural Affairs (DEFRA), and Health and Safety Executive (HSE) provide guidelines and regulations on the safe use of nanomaterials in various settings [85]. In India, the Indian Pharmacopoeia Commission (IPC) guidelines for nanoparticle characterization (2019) provide a regulatory framework for the characterization and use of nanoparticles [76]. Similarly, several countries, such as China, Canada, Australia, Brazil, Mexico, and other Latin American countries, are developing new guidelines or refining their existing regulations tailored to nanomaterials. Above all, maintaining stringent regulations on different medicinal products or medical devices is very challenging, as these systems with novel compounds may show wide variations in reactivity and spatial dynamics in living systems. Hence, it is important to fabricate different classifications or nomenclatures of nanomaterials in different fields on the basis of their actions and integrity mechanisms with their hosts. Centralized regulatory frameworks based on FDA or EMA principles for various nanomaterials should be periodically restructured. Preclinical trials, monitoring task forces, and regular centralized discussions are recommended during the investigational phase of any new device or drug application before market release [60].

16.4.2 Regulatory Aspects of Smart and Sustainable Nanomaterials in Different Sectors

In the healthcare sector, regulatory agencies such as the US FDA and EMA play crucial roles in reassessing the safety and efficacy of nanomaterial-based medicines and biomedical devices [86]. Several nanomedicines are available on the market that the FDA regulates, and few are in progress with clinical trials. These agencies require extensive preclinical and clinical surveys to assess the risks and benefits associated with nanomedicines, dosages, drug delivery systems, biosensors used for disease diagnosis, etc. [87]. The major challenge faced by producers is the lack of uniform standardized characterization protocols to evaluate the mutable morphological, diverse functional, and toxicological properties of particular nanodrugs. Regulatory authorities are expected to collaborate in the early screening of the potential toxicity and compatibility of nanodrugs and their design materials. Owing to their uncertain transformation, aggregation, individual design, and developmental phases, no strict regulatory guidelines could have been implemented to classify them and mitigate these challenges. It is important to revise traditional regulatory frameworks and implement strict FDA regulatory guidelines in nanomedicine to prioritize human health and safety. Presently, reformed regulatory frameworks are crucial for overseeing the development of gene vaccines and genetic engineering models, which present challenges regarding patient safety, privacy, autonomy, and potential adverse outcomes on the global platform [62].

Environmental regulatory frameworks exist to ensure the safe use and disposal of nanomaterials in environmental monitoring applications. Agencies such as the EPA in the USA and the ECHA in the EU regulate the manufacture, import, and use of nanomaterials to mitigate potential risks to human health and the environment [88, 89]. These agencies set rules for producers of smart and sustainable nanomaterial-based products, requiring comprehensive ethical risk assessments and information on properties, exposure pathways, potential environmental hazards, and waste utilization possibilities.

In the food sector, regulatory agencies, viz., the US FDA and the EFSA, oversee the underlying regulations and safety aspects of the nanomaterials used in food packaging, food additives, and quality control biosensors in the USA and EU, respectively [90]. These agencies evaluate the potential risks posed by nanomaterials to human health and the environment and establish guidelines for safe use in food products [91]. Nanomaterials such as TiO_2 as a whitening agent in candies, chewing gums, and powdered sugar, ZnO as a food colorant and dietary supplement, iron oxide as a food colorant, and nanosized silica as an anticaking agent in coffee creamers have been approved by the US FDA [76]. In India, the FSSAI regulations on food additive (2011) species concern food additives, including those derived from nanotechnology in food products [92]. Additionally, international organizations such as the CAC, a joint FAO-WHO body, provide guidelines on the risk assessment and regulatory oversight of nanomaterials in food products [93].

16.5 Risk Assessment and Management of Safety Concerns

Despite efforts to establish regulatory frameworks for nanomaterials, challenges such as a lack of standardization methods for safety assessment, a limited understanding of long-term environmental impacts, gaps in regulatory oversights, etc., persist for their effective implementation [85, 94]. Furthermore, nanomaterials possess novel properties that could pose risks not addressed by traditional risk assessment methods [95]. Addressing the risks associated with nanomaterials is essential for realizing their potential benefits while minimizing the risks to human health and the environment. A multifaceted approach encompassing robust regulations, rigorous risk assessment, and stakeholder engagement is paramount to the safe, sustainable, healthier, and more resilient future of nanotechnology [96]. The entire risk assessment process, especially when used to address the safety concerns associated with smart and sustainable nanomaterials, involves the following steps.

16.5.1 Characterization and Standardization

Nanomaterials are engineered substances with at least one dimension within the nanoscale range, typically up to 100 nanometers, and are often designed to exploit size-dependent properties. While this is the general scientific definition, the regulatory stances of the FDA and EMA are less specific. Nanomaterials may encompass particles up to 1000 nanometers in size for drug products if their size is intentionally manipulated to achieve particular functionalities. Accurate characterization of nanomaterials is paramount for assessing their safety and efficacy [97]. Structural parameters, including size distribution, surface area, surface charge, and chemical composition, significantly influence the toxicological profile of nanomaterials [26]. Standardized characterization methodologies are essential for consistent risk assessment, and guidelines for good manufacturing practices (GMPs) and good laboratory practices (GLPs) should be followed [60, 98, 99]. Recognizing the nascent nature of nanotechnology in medicine, the FDA issued guidelines for drug products containing nanomaterials in 2022. This guidance emphasizes nanomaterial component characterization, control, and testing, differentiating between intentionally engineered and naturally occurring nanoscale structures. Premarket submissions for drug products incorporating nanomaterials must comprehensively describe their composition, size, shape, stability, and additional attributes, such as drug substance assays, release profiles, and material compatibility, as relevant to the specific product and its intended use.

16.5.2 Life Cycle Analysis (LCA)

Life cycle assessment (LCA) is a critical tool for evaluating the environmental and health impacts of nanomaterials throughout their lifecycle [76], from raw material extraction to production, use, and disposal. This analysis aids in identifying potential risks and opportunities for risk mitigation, informing decision-making regarding the development of safe and sustainable nanomaterials [100]. Ensuring the quality and efficacy of pharmaceutical products demands rigorous evaluation throughout their lifecycle. Dissolution/in vitro release testing is essential for ensuring consistent product quality and clinical performance. Additionally, assessing the immunogenicity risk on a case-by-case basis is crucial during product development and throughout its lifecycle, considering the potential severity and likelihood of immune responses.

16.5.3 Safe-by-Design Approach

A "safe-by-design" approach, which integrates safety considerations into nanomaterial product design and manufacturing, is crucial for developing safer alternatives to conventional nanomaterials [101]. By carefully selecting low-toxicity materials, optimizing particle size and surface properties, and minimizing release potential, manufacturers can significantly mitigate the risks associated with nanomaterial production and use [102, 103]. Early identification of critical quality attributes (CQAs) is pivotal for efficient in-process control implementation during manufacturing. A robust design control strategy provides invaluable process knowledge, especially in areas with a limited understanding of variability, scale effects, and safety parameters. This approach ensures product safety and efficacy. Clinical studies for nanomaterial-based drug products must demonstrate noninferiority to the reference drug for regulatory approval. If superiority is claimed, additional studies are necessary. A sequential noninferiority and superiority design can be employed when the applicant believes that their nanomaterial-based drug offers increased efficacy. A scientifically justified noninferiority margin is essential for detecting meaningful differences in efficacy and safety between new and existing drugs.

16.5.4 Risk Assessment

Risk assessment is a scientific approach involving data collection, analysis, and regulatory recommendations to evaluate the potential adverse effects of nanomaterials on human health and the environment [104, 105]. Understanding the characteristics of a nanomaterial, including its properties, strength, stability, and quality, is crucial for assessing its impact on product performance. Identifying critical quality attributes (CQAs) and their influence on the functions of nanomaterials is essential. Moreover, potential risks associated with changes in nanomaterial properties must be defined. Risk assessments should elucidate the relationships among a nanomaterial's structure, function, and critical attributes, guiding control strategies during development and manufacturing. Moreover, risk assessments must consider the potential enhancement of immune responses to nanomaterials for vaccines or biological products incorporating nonbiological nanomaterials. These products may elicit immune reactions distinct from those elicited by the biological component alone, necessitating specific evaluation.

16.5.5 Risk Management

The risk management of nanomaterials is a policy-driven approach that necessitates legislative frameworks encompassing guideline formulation, regulatory measures, risk reduction targets, and preventative/control strategies for identified nanomaterial-associated risks [106, 107]. Following a comprehensive assessment of nanomaterial lifecycle risk, appropriate mitigation measures must be implemented to ensure safe production, handling, and disposal. Traditional chemical risk management principles, adapted for the medical sector, emphasize a "safe-by-design" philosophy and a hierarchical control approach (substitution, technical, organizational, and personal protective measures), as outlined by NIOSH (2013). To address nanomaterial hazards proactively, private industries should prioritize the elimination or substitution of harmful components through the "safe-by-material design" (SbMD) concept. This approach, which draws inspiration from drug development safety practices, aims to control nanobio interactions from early research and development (R&D) stages [108]. Like risk reduction strategies in drug discovery and advanced therapy medicinal products (ATMPs), the SbMD approach seeks to replace hazardous materials with safer alternatives [109]. This approach integrates safety into manufacturing by incorporating safety criteria into quality assurance and good manufacturing practices (GMPs). The "Safe-by-Design (SbD) Implementation Concept" from the EU FP7 ProSafe project provides a framework for early-stage R&D decision-making, utilizing predictive toxicology tools to optimize safety assessments and reduce costs. Effective SbD implementation hinges on robust risk assessment tools and formal safety reviews throughout product development. In alignment with the FDA and EMA guidelines for ATMPs, SbD for nanomaterials incorporates process analytical control (PAC) strategies, in silico tools (e.g., nano-QSARs), and additional characterization/toxicity testing in the pilot phase to ensure product quality and safety. Regulatory frameworks for nanomaterial risk management are evolving. The ATMP guideline [110] mandates a risk management plan (RMP) for market authorization, encompassing safety specifications, pharmacovigilance, and risk minimization. Medical devices (MDs) require postmarket risk management files, incorporating risk–benefit analyses and risk minimization strategies. To enhance benefit-risk assessment, the EMA introduced multicriteria decision analysis (MCDA) frameworks such as PrOACT-URL and PhRMA BRAT [111, 112]. The UMBRA framework aims to unify various methodologies into a structured decision-making process [113]. Despite advancements, standardization challenges persist for endpoints such as drug release and nanomedicine–immune system interactions [114]. EU-funded projects such as BIORIMA and REFINE address these gaps by developing robust test methods for nanomedicines. ISO 14971:2007, endorsed by international agencies, provides a risk management framework for medical devices, aligning with EU directives. Anticipated revisions will accommodate the latest EU Medical Device Regulation [109].

16.5.6 Risk Communication

Effective communication of nanomaterial-associated risks is crucial for informed decision-making among researchers, stakeholders, policymakers, regulatory authorities, industry personnel, and the public [115]. A risk management framework can serve as a valuable tool for conducting benefit-risk assessments, analyzing risks, evaluating supply chain processes for bionanomaterial-based products, and gathering data on nanomedicine and other nanoderived product applications [111]. This framework necessitates assessing toxicological parameters, environmental risks, and occupational hazards and conducting intrinsic and extrinsic risk analyses. Comprehensive documentation of this information is essential for producers and patients to understand these products. Establishing new regulatory standards and guidelines for risk communication and management is paramount to improve the public perception and acceptance of nanomaterials. The transparent dissemination of scientific findings and regulatory updates concerning nanomaterial-related risks is essential for fostering public trust and awareness [116, 117]. Effective communication of the risks associated with nanomaterials is essential for informed decision-making by stakeholders, policymakers, industry personnel, and the public. The transparent dissemination of scientific findings and regulatory updates on risks related to nanomaterials fosters trust and creates awareness among the general public.

16.6 Challenges and Future Prospects

Nanotechnology-related risks, particularly in nanomedicine, encompass a wide range of concerns. These include pharmacological efficacy, toxicological effects, long-term immunological issues, biological system barrier properties, stability and sterility challenges, privacy concerns, and psychological impacts on consumers [118]. Rigorous evaluation at every stage of manufacturing and clinical trials is essential, including advanced preclinical studies employing *in vitro*, *in vivo*, and *ex vivo* models. Comprehensive investigations into biophysical, biomechanical, biodistribution, and pharmacokinetic properties, in addition to assessments of specific and nonspecific binding affinities and intracellular trafficking mechanisms, are needed to elucidate potential nanotechnology-related risks. Harmonized standards and refined regulations are necessary to dispel unfounded concerns. Transparent, detailed analyses and research will clarify the complex interplay of risks and regulatory challenges, paving the way to successfully translate nanomaterials into practical applications. Contemporary nanotechnology holds immense promise for revolutionizing healthcare through advancements in early cancer diagnosis enabled by nanoprobe biomarkers, cancer immunotherapy via gene therapy-based vaccines, targeted drug delivery systems employing nanorobots, and enhanced assisted reproductive technologies utilizing nanoimaging. Additionally, nanotechnology offers potential solutions to infertility through gene editing and repair techniques. Integrating artificial intelligence for data management and analysis further augments these capabilities. Collectively, these innovations may pave the way for a future characterized by improved human health, reduced dependency, and a more integrated and secure society [73, 119]. Novel nanotechnological approaches involving the encapsulation of live, gut-protective probiotic microorganisms within composite polysaccharide microbeads to establish a probiotic drug delivery system hold promise for enhancing public gut health and digestive well-being. Furthermore, the development of intelligent drug delivery systems responsive to pH, specific enzymes, temperature, and electrical stimuli predicts the potential of nanomedicine to deliver personalized or "curated" treatments for individual patients [53]. The inherent adaptability and transformability of nanomaterials offer potential advantages in identifying and mitigating risks that may arise during and after treatment. A robust regulatory framework is imperative to ensure that ethical considerations are comprehensively addressed throughout the nanomaterial lifecycle, from the inception of laboratory research to the culmination of commercial production [52]. This underscores the need for extensive research to address the ethical and regulatory complexities of nanotechnology.

16.7 Conclusion

Nanotechnology has the potential to revolutionize society, with applications ranging from healthcare and electronics to environmental sustainability. The integration of nanotechnology into human life, exemplified by advancements in artificial intelligence, nanorobotics, and nanochip-based smart devices and the reutilization of nanowaste in environmental systems, promises a symbiotic relationship characterized by efficiency and sustainability. The pursuit of nanotechnology research and development on a global scale is driven by its capacity to address previously insurmountable challenges. However, the rapid evolution of nanotechnology has also led to concerns regarding safety and efficacy. The growing concerns regarding safety and potential risks associated with nanotechnology necessitate comprehensive dialogue among a diverse array of stakeholders, including researchers, developers, academics, policymakers, biotechnologists, bioethicists, pharmaceutical representatives, national and international regulatory bodies, end-users, government officials, and legislators. A comprehensive understanding of the interactions between specific nanoparticles and human organs, tissues, and cells is crucial. This includes investigating alterations in the physicochemical properties of nanomaterials, their ability to penetrate biological barriers, the retention of residual impurities, metabolic pathways, and potential environmental impacts. Nanotheranostics and nanomedicine, which are prime examples of the impact of nanotechnology, have demonstrated remarkable potential in improving human health. However, its widespread adoption necessitates a collaborative effort among researchers, policymakers, and healthcare professionals to address emerging ethical dilemmas and establish clear safety and efficacy standards. By fostering a global commitment toward innovative and sustainable "nano" innovation, the field of nanotechnology can be harnessed to create a future characterized by improved human well-being and environmental sustainability. The ethical implications of nanotechnology necessitate rigorous evaluation to prevent potential catastrophic consequences for human health, psychosocial well-being, and ecological balance. A robust regulatory framework incorporating strengthened legislation, guidelines, and safety protocols is therefore essential to address ethical concerns and ensure the responsible conduct of nanoscience research, ultimately paving the way for a better nanoworld.

References

1. Ahire SA, Bachhav AA, Pawar TB, et al. The augmentation of nanotechnology era: a concise review on fundamental concepts of nanotechnology and applications in material science and technology. Results Chem. 2022;4 https://doi.org/10.1016/j.rechem.2022.100633.
2. Bayda S, Adeel M, Tuccinardi T, et al. The history of nanoscience and nanotechnology: From chemical–physical applications to nanomedicine. Molecules. 2019;25:112. https://doi.org/10.3390/molecules25010112.
3. Asha AB, Narain R. Nanomaterials properties. In: Polymer science and nanotechnology. Elsevier; 2020. p. 343–59.
4. Joudeh N, Linke D. Nanoparticle classification, physicochemical properties, characterization, and applications: a comprehensive review for biologists. J Nanobiotechnol. 2022;20 https://doi.org/10.1186/s12951-022-01477-8.
5. Mehmood U, Yasmeen S, Nazar R, Tiwari SK. Metallic nanoparticles: status and Prospect. In: Nanoparticles reinforced metal nanocomposites: mechanical performance and durability; 2023. p. 127–59. https://doi.org/10.1007/978-981-19-9729-7_5.
6. Montanarella F, Kovalenko MV. Three millennia of nanocrystals. ACS Nano. 2022;16:5085–102. https://doi.org/10.1021/acsnano.1c11159.
7. Mehmood U, Yasmeen S, Nazar R, Tiwari SK. Effects of nano reinforcing/matrix interaction on chemical, thermal and mechanical properties of epoxy nanocomposites. J Compos Mater. 2023;55:127–59. https://doi.org/10.1007/978-981-19-9729-7_5.
8. Kumar T, Pandey RK, Kumar R, et al. Historical perspective of nanotechnology and functionalized nanomaterials. In: Materials horizons: From nature to nanomaterials part F1329; 2024. p. 3–24. https://doi.org/10.1007/978-981-99-3021-0_1.
9. Patin M, Nys K, Thienpont H, Meulebroeck W. Prestige markers in art: subtle stratagems in material selection for fifteenth-century stained-glass windows. Herit Sci. 2022;10 https://doi.org/10.1186/s40494-022-00698-2.
10. Parker JM, Martlew D. Stained glass windows. In: Encyclopedia of glass science, technology, history, and culture. Wiley; 2021. p. 1341–59.
11. Gupta PK. Introduction and historical background. In: Nanotoxicology in nanobiomedicine. Cham: Springer International Publishing; 2023. p. 1–22.
12. Litter MI, Ahmad A. Industrial applications of nanoparticles: a prospective overview. Boca Raton: CRC Press; 2023.
13. Fatima A, Islam MU, Ahmad MW. Traditional and recently advanced synthetic routes of the metal oxide materials. In: Renewable polymers and polymer-metal oxide composites: synthesis, properties, and applications; 2022. p. 79–99. https://doi.org/10.1016/B978-0-323-85155-8.00004-2.
14. Jetha KL, Vyas A, Teli D, et al. History of nanoparticles. In: Nanocarrier vaccines. Wiley; 2024. p. 1–23.

15. Dvorsky R, Svoboda L, Bednář J. Nanoparticles' preparation, properties, interactions and self-organization. In: Springer briefs in applied sciences and technology; 2022. p. 1–41. https://doi.org/10.1007/978-3-030-89144-2_1.
16. Dhumale VA, Gangwar RK, Pande N. Importance of gold nanoparticles for detection of toxic heavy metal ions and vital role in biomedical applications. Mater Res Innov. 2021;25:354–62. https://doi.org/10.1080/14328917.2020.1825770.
17. Feynman RP. There's plenty of room at the bottom. In: Micromechanics and MEMS: Classic and seminal papers to 1990; 1997. p. 2–9. https://doi.org/10.1109/9780470545263.sect1.
18. Srivastava S, Bhargava A. Green nanotechnology: an overview. In: Green nanoparticles: the future of nanobiotechnology; 2022. p. 1–13. https://doi.org/10.1007/978-981-16-7106-7_1.
19. Ghosh D, Dutta G, Sugumaran A, et al (2023) Fullerenes: Bucky balls in the therapeutic application. 1–25. https://doi.org/10.1007/978-3-031-28263-8_1
20. Alosime EM. A review on surface functionalization of carbon nanotubes: methods and applications. Discover Nano. 2023;18 https://doi.org/10.1186/s11671-023-03789-6.
21. Dugam S, Nangare S, Patil P, Jadhav N. Carbon dots: a novel trend in pharmaceutical applications. Ann Pharm Fr. 2021;79:335–45. https://doi.org/10.1016/j.pharma.2020.12.002.
22. Fang Z, Xing Q, Fernandez D, et al. A mini review on two-dimensional nanomaterial assembly. Nano Res. 2020;13:1179–90. https://doi.org/10.1007/s12274-019-2559-5.
23. Mishra S, Sharma V, Gupta R. Toxicity, legal and health aspects of nanomaterials. In: Handbook of green and sustainable nanotechnology; 2022. p. 1–39. https://doi.org/10.1007/978-3-030-69023-6_104-1.
24. Han SP, Maune H, Bockrath MW. DNA-guided self-assembly of carbon nanotube electronics. In: Springer Series in Materials Science 284. 2021. pp. 481–501. https://doi.org/10.1007/978-3-030-18778-1_21
25. Khan S, Hossain MK. Classification and properties of nanoparticles. In: Nanoparticle-based polymer composites; 2022. p. 15–54. https://doi.org/10.1016/B978-0-12-824272-8.00009-9.
26. Abbasi R, Shineh G, Mobaraki M, et al. Structural parameters of nanoparticles affecting their toxicity for biomedical applications: a review. J Nanopart Res. 2023;25 https://doi.org/10.1007/s11051-023-05690-w.
27. Deyasi A, Basak A, Sarkar A. Application of nanomaterial-based biosensors for healthcare diagnostics. Smart Innov Syst Technol. 2023;322:103–22. https://doi.org/10.1007/978-981-19-7107-5_6.
28. Shinde MU, Patwekar M, Patwekar F, et al. Nanomaterials: a potential hope for life sciences from bench to bedside. J Nanomater. 2022;2022 https://doi.org/10.1155/2022/5968131.
29. Li Y, Zheng X, Chu Q. Bio-based nanomaterials for cancer therapy. Nano Today. 2021;38 https://doi.org/10.1016/j.nantod.2021.101134.
30. Singhal J, Verma S, Kumar S, Mehrotra D. Recent advances in nano-bio-sensing fabrication technology for the detection of oral cancer. Mol Biotechnol. 2021;63:339–62. https://doi.org/10.1007/s12033-021-00306-x.
31. Agrawal N, Saxena R, Singh L, et al. Recent advancements in plasmonic optical biosensors: a review. ISSS J Micro Smart Syst. 2022;11:31–42. https://doi.org/10.1007/s41683-021-00079-0.
32. Sharma P, Goyal D, Chudasama B. Nanostrategies against rising antimicrobial resistance (AMR)-metallic nanoparticles as Nanoweapon. In: Emerging modalities in mitigation of antimicrobial resistance; 2022. p. 541–62. https://doi.org/10.1007/978-3-030-84126-3_25.
33. Mubeen B, Ansar AN, Rasool R, et al. Nanotechnology as a novel approach in combating microbes providing an alternative to antibiotics. Antibiotics. 2021;10 https://doi.org/10.3390/antibiotics10121473.
34. Azzouz A, Hejji L, Sonne C, et al. Nanomaterial-based aptasensors as an efficient substitute for cardiovascular disease diagnosis: future of smart biosensors. Biosens Bioelectron. 2021;193 https://doi.org/10.1016/j.bios.2021.113617.

35. Kumar A, Chaudhary RK, Singh R, et al. Nanotheranostic applications for detection and targeting neurodegenerative diseases. Front Neurosci. 2020;14 https://doi.org/10.3389/fnins.2020.00305.
36. Balasamy S, Sekaran S, Eswaramoorthy R. Supporting nanotechnology safety through nanoinformatics. In: Green nanoremediation: sustainable management of environmental pollution; 2023. p. 313–32. https://doi.org/10.1007/978-3-031-30558-0_14.
37. Mukherjee K, Bhadaria H, Pillai S, et al. Nano-informatics: studies on Nano information platforms and their application in various sectors. In: Biological applications of nanoparticles; 2023. p. 163–76. https://doi.org/10.1007/978-981-99-3629-8_10.
38. Maurya SK, Budhalakoti B, Bhatrola K, et al. Nano-engineered material and remediation strategy. In: Environmental footprints and eco-design of products and processes; 2023. p. 179–99. https://doi.org/10.1007/978-981-19-7978-1_9.
39. Zahra Q ul A, Fang X, Luo Z, et al. Graphene based nanohybrid aptasensors in environmental monitoring: concepts, design and future outlook. Crit Rev Anal Chem. 2023;53:1433–54. https://doi.org/10.1080/10408347.2022.2025758.
40. Nanda PK, Bhattacharya D, Das JK, et al. Emerging role of biosensors and chemical indicators to monitor the quality and safety of meat and meat products. Chemosensors. 2022;10 https://doi.org/10.3390/chemosensors10080322.
41. Islamipour Z, Zare EN, Salimi F, et al. Biodegradable antibacterial and antioxidant nanocomposite films based on dextrin for bioactive food packaging. J Nanostructure Chem. 2022;12:991–1006. https://doi.org/10.1007/s40097-022-00491-4.
42. Vieira IRS, de Carvalho APA, Conte-Junior CA. Recent advances in biobased and biodegradable polymer nanocomposites, nanoparticles, and natural antioxidants for antibacterial and antioxidant food packaging applications. Compr Rev Food Sci Food Saf. 2022;21:3673–716. https://doi.org/10.1111/1541-4337.12990.
43. Wu M, Zhou Z, Yang J, et al. ZnO nanoparticles stabilized oregano essential oil Pickering emulsion for functional cellulose nanofibrils packaging films with antimicrobial and antioxidant activity. Int J Biol Macromol. 2021;190:433–40. https://doi.org/10.1016/j.ijbiomac.2021.08.210.
44. Sui X, Downing JR, Hersam MC, Chen J. Additive manufacturing and applications of nanomaterial-based sensors. Mater Today. 2021;48:135–54. https://doi.org/10.1016/j.mattod.2021.02.001.
45. Lee YY, Sriram B, Wang SF, et al. Advanced nanomaterial-based biosensors for N-terminal pro-brain natriuretic peptide biomarker detection: Progress and future challenges in cardiovascular disease diagnostics. Nanomaterials. 2024;14 https://doi.org/10.3390/nano14020153.
46. Gottardo S, Mech A, Drbohlavová J, et al. Towards safe and sustainable innovation in nanotechnology: state-of-play for smart nanomaterials. NanoImpact. 2021;21:100297. https://doi.org/10.1016/j.impact.2021.100297.
47. Kaur J, Singh H, Khatri M. Regulatory considerations for safety of nanomaterials. In: Nanomedicine for Bioactives: Healthcare applications; 2020. p. 431–50. https://doi.org/10.1007/978-981-15-1664-1_17.
48. Srivastava S. Ethical issues regarding the use of nanobiotechnology-based products. In: Nanobiotechnology for the livestock industry. Elsevier; 2023. p. 435–73.
49. Saheb T, Saheb T, Carpenter DO. Mapping research strands of ethics of artificial intelligence in healthcare: a bibliometric and content analysis. Comput Biol Med. 2021;135 https://doi.org/10.1016/j.compbiomed.2021.104660.
50. Souto EB, Blanco-Llamero C, Krambeck K, Kiran NS, Yashaswini C, Postwala H, et al. Regulatory insights into nanomedicine and gene vaccine innovation: safety assessment, challenges, and regulatory perspectives. Acta Biomater. 2024;180:1.
51. Sultana N, Waheed A, Ali A, Jahan S, Aqil M, Sultana Y, Mujeeb M. Exploring new frontiers in drug delivery with minimally invasive microneedles: fabrication techniques, biomedical applications, and regulatory aspects. Expert Opin Drug Deliv. 2023;20(6):739–55.

52. Thapa RK, Kim JO. Nanomedicine-based commercial formulations: current developments and future prospects. J Pharm Investig. 2023;53(1):19–33.
53. Ventola CL. Progress in nanomedicine: approved and investigational nanodrugs. Pharm Ther. 2017;42(12):742.
54. Bobo D, Robinson KJ, Islam J, Thurecht KJ, Corrie SR. Nanoparticle-based medicines: a review of FDA-approved materials and clinical trials to date. Pharm Res. 2016;33:2373–87.
55. Patra JK, Das G, Fraceto LF, Campos EVR, Rodriguez-Torres MDP, Acosta-Torres LS, et al. Nano based drug delivery systems: recent developments and future prospects. J Nanobiotechnol. 2018;16:1–33.
56. Singh AP, Biswas A, Shukla A, Maiti P. Targeted therapy in chronic diseases using nanomaterial-based drug delivery vehicles. Signal Transduct Target Ther. 2019;4(1):33.
57. Atalla K, Chaudhary A, Mehrnoosh Eshaghian-Wilner M, et al. Wireless computing in medicine: from Nano to cloud with ethical and legal implications. 2016.
58. Schummer J. The global institutionalization of nanotechnology research: a bibliometric approach to the assessment of science policy. Scientometrics. 2007;70:669–92.
59. Mohi-ud-din R, Mir RH, Pottoo FH, et al. Nanophytomedicine ethical issues, regulatory aspects, and challenges. In: Nanophytomedicine. Singapore: Springer Singapore; 2020. p. 173–92.
60. Gawne PJ, Ferreira M, Papaluca M, et al. New opportunities and old challenges in the clinical translation of nanotheranostics. Nat Rev Mater. 2023;8:783–98. https://doi.org/10.1038/s41578-023-00581-x.
61. Luo X, Jia K, Xing J, Yi J. The utilization of nanotechnology in the female reproductive system and related disorders. Heliyon. 2024;10:e25477.
62. Gordijn B, De Vries R, O'Mathúna DP. Ethical issues in nanotechnology. In: The Sage handbook of health care ethics. London: Sage; 2011. p. 402–12.
63. Kamarulzaman NA, Lee KE, Siow KS, Mokhtar M. Public benefit and risk perceptions of nanotechnology development: psychological and sociological aspects. Technol Soc. 2020;62 https://doi.org/10.1016/j.techsoc.2020.101329.
64. Bleeker EAJ, Swart E, Braakhuis H, et al. Towards harmonisation of testing of nanomaterials for EU regulatory requirements on chemical safety—a proposal for further actions. Regul Toxicol Pharmacol. 2023;139 https://doi.org/10.1016/j.yrtph.2023.105360.
65. Ten Have H. Nanotechnologies, ethics and politics. UNESCO Pub; 2007.
66. Atalla K, Chaudhary A, Mehrnoosh Eshaghian-Wilner M, et al. Wireless computing in medicine: from Nano to cloud with ethical and legal implications. 2021.
67. Capon A, Gillespie J, Rolfe M, Smith W. Perceptions of risk from nanotechnologies and trust in stakeholders: a cross sectional study of public, academic, government and business attitudes. BMC Public Health. 2015;15:1–13.
68. Dave V, Sur S, Gupta N. 9 Current framework, ethical consideration and future challenges of regulatory approach for nano-based products. 2021.
69. Alberto Ferreira MM, António Filipe J. Ethical considerations on nanotechnology.
70. Babatunde DE, Denwigwe IH, Babatunde OM, et al. Environmental and societal impact of nanotechnology. IEEE Access. 2020;8:4640–67.
71. Kiran V, Harini K, Thirumalai A, et al. Nanotechnology's role in ensuring food safety and security. Biocatal Agric Biotechnol. 2024;58:103220.
72. Verma SK, Nandi A, Simnani FZ, et al. In silico nanotoxicology: the computational biology state of art for nanomaterial safety assessments. Mater Des. 2023;235:112452.
73. Bhattacharya B, Roy P, Bhattacharya S, et al. Nanotechnology and sustainable development. In: Engineered nanomaterials for sustainable agricultural production, soil improvement and stress management. Elsevier; 2022. p. 431–45.
74. Wang R, Bush-Evans R, Arden-Close E, et al. Transparency in persuasive technology, immersive technology, and online marketing: facilitating users' informed decision making and practical implications. Comput Human Behav. 2023;139:107545. https://doi.org/10.1016/j.chb.2022.107545.

75. Jain A, Ranjan S, Dasgupta N, Ramalingam C. Nanomaterials in food and agriculture: an overview on their safety concerns and regulatory issues. Crit Rev Food Sci Nutr. 2018;58:297–317. https://doi.org/10.1080/10408398.2016.1160363.
76. Kumari R, Suman K, Karmakar S, et al. Regulation and safety measures for nanotechnology-based agri-products. Front Genome Ed. 2023;5 https://doi.org/10.3389/fgeed.2023.1200987.
77. Mishra AK, Das R, Sahoo S, Biswal B. Global regulations and legislations on nanoparticles usage and application in diverse horizons. Compr Anal Chem. 2022;99:261–90. https://doi.org/10.1016/bs.coac.2021.12.004.
78. Konstantopoulos G, Koumoulos EP, Charitidis CA. Digital innovation enabled nanomaterial manufacturing; machine learning strategies and green perspectives. Nanomaterials. 2022;12 https://doi.org/10.3390/nano12152646.
79. Dubey N, Dubey N. Current regulatory framework in nanotechnology and medicine. In: Nanotechnology in medicine: toxicity and safety; 2021. p. 373–406. https://doi.org/10.1002/9781119769897.ch17.
80. Sorensen RM, Kanwar RS, Jovanovi B. Past, present, and possible future policies on plastic use in the United States, particularly microplastics and nanoplastics: a review. Integr Environ Assess Manag. 2023;19:474–88. https://doi.org/10.1002/ieam.4678.
81. Stretz HA, Ambuken P V., Kumar G, et al. Regulatory and environmental issues of nanotechnology safety. In: Nanotechnology safety. pp. 43–56. 2013. https://doi.org/10.1016/B978-0-444-59438-9.00004-7
82. García-Fernández AJ. Ecotoxicological risk assessment in the context of different EU regulations. In: Methods in pharmacology and toxicology; 2020. p. 3–25. https://doi.org/10.1007/978-1-0716-0150-1_1.
83. Saldívar-Tanaka L, Hansen SF. Should the precautionary principle be implemented in Europe with regard to nanomaterials? Expert interviews. J Nanopart Res. 2021;23 https://doi.org/10.1007/s11051-021-05173-w.
84. Brinch A, Hansen SF, Hartmann NB, Baun A. EU regulation of nanobiocides: challenges in implementing the biocidal product regulation (BPR). Nano. 2016;6 https://doi.org/10.3390/nano6020033.
85. Chávez-Hernández JA, Velarde-Salcedo AJ, Navarro-Tovar G, Gonzalez C. Safe nanomaterials: from their use, application, and disposal to regulations. Nanoscale Adv. 2024;6:1583–610. https://doi.org/10.1039/d3na01097j.
86. Maji I, Mahajan S, Sriram A, et al. Nanotoxicology: toxicity and safety issues of nanoparticles. In: Multifunctional nanocarriers; 2022. p. 461–74. https://doi.org/10.1016/B978-0-323-85041-4.00017-2.
87. Kannan B, Nandagawale A, Karnati P, et al. Regulatory barriers to the marketing authorization of nanodrug delivery system. In: Nanotechnology and drug delivery; 2023. p. 61–100. https://doi.org/10.1201/9781003430407-2.
88. Karim ME. Functional nanomaterials: selected legal and regulatory issues. In: Handbook of Functionalized Nanomaterials for Industrial Applications; 2020. p. 983–94. https://doi.org/10.1016/B978-0-12-816787-8.00030-2.
89. Creutzenberg O. Nanoparticles and their regulation. In: Regulatory toxicology. 2021. pp. 1–17. https://doi.org/10.1007/978-3-642-36206-4_122-1
90. Allan J, Belz S, Hoeveler A, et al. Regulatory landscape of nanotechnology and nanoplastics from a global perspective. Regul Toxicol Pharmacol. 2021;122 https://doi.org/10.1016/j.yrtph.2021.104885.
91. Kaur G, Singh K. Nanotechnology in the food sector. In: Emerging technologies in food science. Singapore: Springer Singapore; 2020. p. 15–36.
92. Saikanth DRK, Gawande V, Chaithanya G, et al. Development and current state of nanotechnology in the agricultural and food sectors: a review. Int J Environ Climate Chang. 2023;13:1602–12. https://doi.org/10.9734/ijecc/2023/v13i92392.

93. Tarhan Ö, Yardımcı AI. Regulatory principles on food nano-particles legislated by international organizations. In: Safety and regulatory issues of nanoencapsulated food ingredients; 2021. p. 251–90. https://doi.org/10.1016/B978-0-12-815725-1.00008-2.
94. Ramachandran G, Wolf SM, Paradise J, et al. Recommendations for oversight of nanobiotechnology: dynamic oversight for complex and convergent technology. J Nanopart Res. 2011;13:1345–71. https://doi.org/10.1007/s11051-011-0233-2.
95. Bragard C, Halldorsson TI, Hernandez-Jerez A, et al. Guidance on risk assessment of nanomaterials to be applied in the food and feed chain: human and animal health. EFSA J. 2019;13:1–11.
96. Gana M, Isibor PO, Damisa JI, et al. Nanoparticle-based remediation and environmental cleanup. In: Environmental nanotoxicology; 2024. p. 161–81. https://doi.org/10.1007/978-3-031-54154-4_9.
97. Johnston LJ, Gonzalez-Rojano N, Wilkinson KJ, Xing B. Key challenges for evaluation of the safety of engineered nanomaterials. NanoImpact. 2020;18 https://doi.org/10.1016/j.impact.2020.100219.
98. Adegbeye MJ, Elghandour MMMY, Reddy PRK, et al. Potential of silver nanoparticles for veterinary applications in livestock performance and health. Silver nanomaterials for agri-food applications. 2021:657–83. https://doi.org/10.1016/B978-0-12-823528-7.00022-6.
99. Forest V. Experimental and computational nanotoxicology— complementary approaches for nanomaterial hazard assessment. Nano. 2022;12 https://doi.org/10.3390/nano12081346.
100. Nizam NUM, Hanafiah MM, Woon KS. A content review of life cycle assessment of nanomaterials: current practices, challenges, and future prospects. Nano. 2021;11 https://doi.org/10.3390/nano11123324.
101. Trump BD, Antunes D, Palma-Oliveira J, et al. Safety-by-design and engineered nanomaterials: the need to move from theory to practice. Environ Syst Decis. 2024;44:177–88. https://doi.org/10.1007/s10669-023-09927-w.
102. Salieri B, Barruetabeña L, Rodríguez-Llopis I, et al. Integrative approach in a safe by design context combining risk, life cycle and socio-economic assessment for safer and sustainable nanomaterials. NanoImpact. 2021;23 https://doi.org/10.1016/j.impact.2021.100335.
103. Ruijter N, Soeteman-Hernández LG, Carrière M, et al. The state of the art and challenges of in vitro methods for human hazard assessment of nanomaterials in the context of safe-by-design. Nano. 2023;13 https://doi.org/10.3390/nano13030472.
104. Kaur A, Singh H. Nanomaterials in environment: sources, risk assessment, and safety aspect. 2023. pp. 75–93
105. Karahalil B. Risk assessment and risk management of functionalized nanomaterials. In: Handbook of functionalized nanomaterials: environmental health and safety: a volume in micro and nano technologies; 2021. p. 309–20. https://doi.org/10.1016/B978-0-12-822415-1.00007-X.
106. Hwang M, Lee EJ, Kweon SY, et al. Risk assessment principle for engineered nanotechnology: in food and drug. Toxicol Res. 2012;28:73–9. https://doi.org/10.5487/TR.2012.28.2.073.
107. Rodríguez H. Nanotechnology and risk governance in the European Union: the constitution of safety in highly promoted and contested innovation areas. NanoEthics. 2018;12:5–26. https://doi.org/10.1007/s11569-017-0296-3.
108. Hjorth R, van Hove L, Wickson F. What can Nanosafety learn from drug development? The feasibility of "safety by design". Nanotoxicology. 2017;11:305–12. https://doi.org/10.1080/17435390.2017.1299891.
109. Giubilato E, Cazzagon V, Amorim MJ, Blosi M, Bouillard J, Bouwmeester H, Costa AL, Fadeel B, Fernandes TF, Fito C, Hauser M. Risk management framework for nano-biomaterials used in medical devices and advanced therapy medicinal products. Materials. 2020;13(20):4532.
110. European Medicines Agency (EMA). Guideline on safety and efficacy follow-up—risk management of advanced therapy medicinal products. London: European Medicines Agency; 2008.

111. Coplan PM, Noel RA, Levitan BS, Ferguson J, Mussen F. Development of a framework for enhancing the transparency, reproducibility and communication of the benefit-risk balance of medicines. Clin Pharmacol Ther. 2011;89:312–5. https://doi.org/10.1038/clpt.2010.291.
112. European medicines agency (EMA). European medicines agency benefit-risk methodology project- description of the current practice of benefit-risk assessment for cetralised procedure products in the EU regulatory network—summary of original report. Reproduction. 2010;44:2–4.
113. McAuslane N, Leong J, Liberti L, Walker S. The benefit-risk assessment of medicines. Ther Innov Regul Sci. 2017;51:635–44. https://doi.org/10.1177/2168479017696260.
114. Halamoda-Kenzaoui B, Holzwarth U, Roebben G, Bogni A, Bremer-Hoffmann S. Mapping of the available standards against the regulatory needs for nanomedicines. Wiley Interdiscip Rev Nanomed Nanobiotechnol. 2019;11(1):e1531.
115. Isigonis P, Hristozov D, Benighaus C, et al. Risk governance of nanomaterials: review of criteria and tools for risk communication, evaluation, and mitigation. Nano. 2019;9 https://doi.org/10.3390/nano9050696.
116. Bostrom A, Löfstedt RE. Nanotechnology risk communication past and prologue. Risk Anal. 2010;30:1645–62. https://doi.org/10.1111/j.1539-6924.2010.01521.x.
117. Porcari A, Borsella E, Benighaus C, et al. From risk perception to risk governance in nanotechnology: a multi-stakeholder study. J Nanopart Res. 2019;21 https://doi.org/10.1007/s11051-019-4689-9.
118. Costa S, Vilas-Boas V, Lebre F, et al. Microfluidic-based skin-on-chip systems for safety assessment of nanomaterials. Trends Biotechnol. 2023;41:1282–98.
119. Afzal O, Altamimi AS, Nadeem MS, Alzarea SI, Almalki WH, Tariq A, et al. Nanoparticles in drug delivery: from history to therapeutic applications. Nano. 2022;12(24):4494.

Chapter 17
Nanomaterials in Healthcare: Regulatory Aspects and Safety Perspectives

Bimal Rajchal, Yub Narayan Thapa, Deepshikha Karki, Vimal Katiyar, and Rameshwar Adhikari

Abstract The integration of nanotechnology into the healthcare system has led to the emergence of nanomedicine that offers transformative potential in advanced diagnostics, targeted drug delivery, and tissue engineering. However, the unique properties of nanoparticles, which enable their widespread application, also allow them to infiltrate living systems and ecosystems through various pathways. This has raised significant concerns about their safety, toxicity, and environmental impact.

B. Rajchal
Central Department of Chemistry, Tribhuvan University, Kirtipur, Kathmandu, Nepal

Research Centre for Applied Science and Technology (RECAST), Tribhuvan University, Kirtipur, Kathmandu, Nepal

Nepal Polymer Institute (NPI), Kirtipur, Kathmandu, Nepal

Department of Chemistry, Bhaktapur Multiple Campus, Tribhuvan University, Bhaktapur, Bagmati Province, Nepal

Y. N. Thapa
Central Department of Chemistry, Tribhuvan University, Kirtipur, Kathmandu, Nepal

Research Centre for Applied Science and Technology (RECAST), Tribhuvan University, Kirtipur, Kathmandu, Nepal

Nepal Polymer Institute (NPI), Kirtipur, Kathmandu, Nepal

Department of Chemistry, Tribhuvan Multiple Campus, Tribhuvan University, Tansen, Palpa, Lumbini Province, Nepal

D. Karki
Central Department of Chemistry, Tribhuvan University, Kirtipur, Kathmandu, Nepal

Research Centre for Applied Science and Technology (RECAST), Tribhuvan University, Kirtipur, Kathmandu, Nepal

Nepal Polymer Institute (NPI), Kirtipur, Kathmandu, Nepal

V. Katiyar
Department of Chemical Engineering, Indian Institute of Technology Guwahati, Guwahati, Assam, India

S. Mondal et al. (eds.), *Smart and Sustainable Nanomaterials in Digital Healthcare and Theranostic*, https://doi.org/10.1007/978-981-95-9386-6_17

These risks underscore the urgent need for robust regulatory frameworks and comprehensive guidelines to guarantee nanomedicine's safe development and use. International agencies such as the United States Food and Drug Administration (FDA), European Medicines Agency (EMA), World Health Organization (WHO), Organization for Economic Cooperation and Development (OECD), National Institute for Food and Drug Control (NIFDC) in China, and the Therapeutic Goods Association (TGA) in Australia are actively working on establishing effective risk assessment frameworks and regulatory landscapes for nanomaterials. These initiatives aim to evaluate potential hazards, exposure risks, and long-term impacts associated with nanoparticles. This chapter highlights the need for collaborative international efforts to develop standardized regulations, enabling the safe and sustainable integration of nanomaterials into healthcare while minimizing risks to human health and the environment.

Keywords Nanomedicine · Regulatory frameworks · Risk Assessment · Nanoparticle safety · Nanotoxicity · Regulatory agencies

17.1 Introduction and Overview

The entire scientific community was left astonished when Richard Feynman, in 1959, gave a talk, "*There's Plenty of Room at the Bottom*," envisioning the "dwarf" world that felt like science fiction [1]. In 1974, Norio Taniguchi coined the term "nanotechnology" in his article "On the Basic Concept of Nanotechnology," emphasizing the control of matter on a nanoscale [2]. Gerd Binnig and Heinrich Rohrer invented the scanning tunnelling microscope in 1981 which made manipulation of individual atoms possible [3]. Following this, in 1986, Eric Drexler highlighted the potential of creating novel materials with unique features in a famous book, "Engines of Creation: The Coming Era of Nanotechnology" [4]. Since then, the world of "Nanoscience" and "Nanotechnologies" gained popularity and brought revolution in the fields of inventions, discoveries, and developments. Nanoscience involves the study of nanomaterials, while nanotechnologies refer to the practical application of nanoscience [5].

R. Adhikari (✉)
Central Department of Chemistry, Tribhuvan University, Kirtipur, Kathmandu, Nepal

Research Centre for Applied Science and Technology (RECAST), Tribhuvan University, Kirtipur, Kathmandu, Nepal

Nepal Polymer Institute (NPI), Kirtipur, Kathmandu, Nepal

Department of Chemical Engineering, Indian Institute of Technology Guwahati, Guwahati, Assam, India
e-mail: rameshwar.adhikari@cdc.tu.edu.np

Nanomaterials (NMs), with at least one of their dimensions less than 100 nm, exhibit unique physical, chemical, optical, electrical, and magnetic properties than their bulk counterparts. The reduced size, greater surface area, and quantum effects are the three main reasons for their enhanced mechanical strength, increased chemical reactivity, and improved electrical, magnetic, and optical properties [5]. These properties, on one hand, make nanomaterials applicable in a variety of sectors such as medicine, energy, environment, industries, communication, agriculture, transport, household products, and consumer products to bring out revolution in an unprecedented manner [6]. At the same time the same properties of nanomaterials, particularly engineered one, have also raised serious concerns about their potential risks, safety, and toxicity [7]. It has thus necessitated regulatory frameworks and risk management strategies to ensure their safe and sustainable production as well as applications [8].

The principles of nanotechnology have been merged with medicine to form a completely new avenue in healthcare called nanomedicine [9]. It opens up new possibilities for detection of diseases, treatment plans, drug delivery methods, tissue engineering, and the regeneration of injured tissues by interacting with biological systems at the cellular and molecular levels with nanoscale instruments, devices, and structures [10]. Quantum dots, metal oxide nanoparticles, and fluorescent nanoparticles are examples of nanoparticles that function as contrast agents to improve fluorescence imaging, magnetic resonance imaging (MRI), and computed tomography (CT) imaging. The exceptional brightness, stability, and adjustable features of these nanoparticles allow for accurate and real-time imaging of cells, tissues, and even molecular events [11]. Similarly, surface-functionalized nanoparticles act as carriers of therapeutic drugs for their targeted and controlled delivery to the desired site while minimizing side effects and enhancing treatment efficiency [12, 13]. Additionally, the three-dimensional scaffolds, hydrogels, and nanofibers made of nanomaterials create an extracellular matrix-like environment that aids in the regeneration and repair of injured bodily tissues and organs [14]. Thus, the fusion of nanotechnology with medicine has caused a dramatic transformation that has given rise to the nano revolution in medicine [15].

However, a number of issues and concerns, such as the toxicity and safety of nanomaterials, must be carefully examined and resolved in order to guarantee their biocompatibility, long-term benefits, and broad use [7]. Because of their minute size, nanoparticles enter living systems very easily through the respiratory tract, oral, or dermal routes (Fig. 17.1). Inside living systems, these particles may accumulate at cellular junctions or enter the cell and get localized in the nucleus. It causes chronic health issues, including cytotoxicity, genotoxicity, and oxidative stress [16, 17].

Similarly, nanoparticles can enter various ecosystems through several routes such as consumer products, industrial discharges, and wastewater (Fig. 17.2). Once these particles enter the ecosystem, they may accumulate in the food chain or contaminate environmental components, posing risks to organisms [17–19]. It is thus

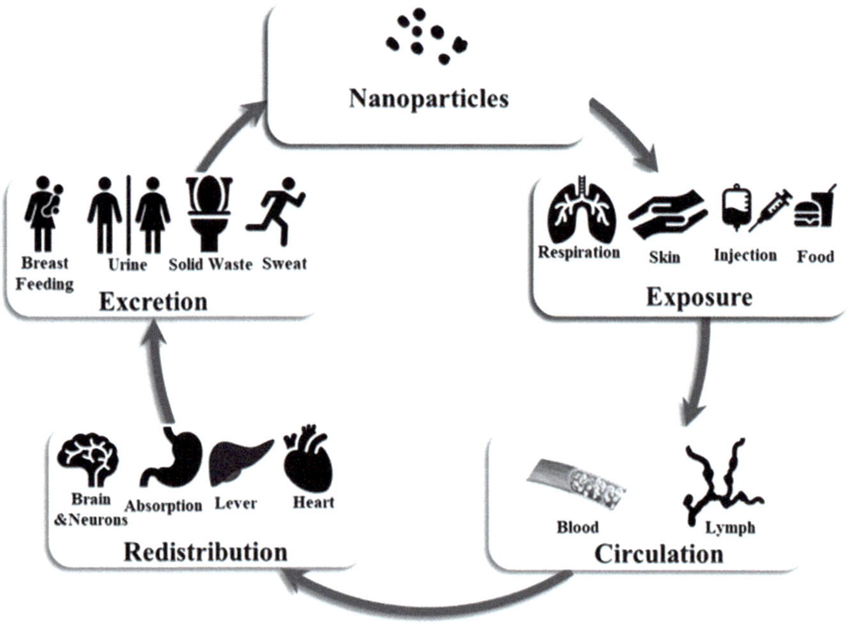

Fig. 17.1 Nanomaterial's cycle through human body. (Reproduced with permission from [17])

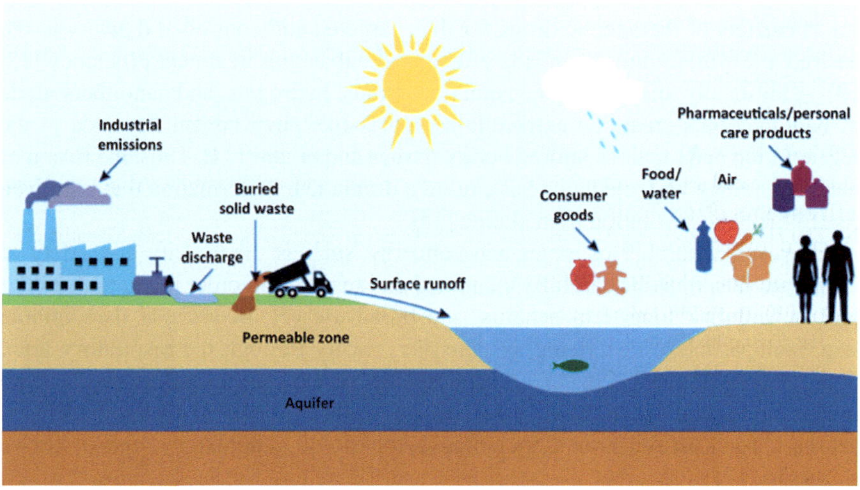

Fig. 17.2 Nanomaterial's pathways through the environment. (Reproduced with permission from [18])

essential to evaluate the potential health and environmental risks of nanomaterials in terms of risk assessment and then provide appropriate frameworks for their effective regulation [8].

Risk assessment of nanomaterials involves identification of potential hazards (e.g., toxicity and reactivity) of nanomaterials, determination of their dose-response relationship, evaluation of human and environmental exposure to nanomaterials, and estimation of the overall risks of nanomaterials [20]. To accomplish those assessments, several programs and regulatory efforts have been carried out by many international organizations like ISO (International Organization for Standardization), OECD (Organization for Economic Co-operation and Development), and SAICM (Strategic Approach to International Chemicals Management) [21, 22]. Further, varieties of regulatory approaches have also been developed and implemented in different regions of the globe based on their original ground. For instance, the European Union has integrated regulatory frameworks for nanomaterials with REACH (Registration, Evaluation, Authorization, and Restriction of Chemicals) and CLP (Classification, Labelling, and Packaging of Substances and Mixtures) regulations [23]. Similarly, in the United States, agencies like EPA (Environmental Protection Agency), FDA (Food and Drug Administration), and OSHA (Occupational Safety and Health Administration) are working on the regulation of nanomaterials [24]. Likewise, Japan's Ministry of Economy, Trade and Industry (METI), China's Ministry of Ecology and Environment (MEE), and Australia's National Industrial Chemicals Notification and Assessment Scheme (NICNAS) in the Asia-Pacific countries are also working seriously in regulating engineered nanomaterials [25].

The advancement of nanomaterials, nanoscience, and nanotechnology has thus offered enumerable benefits to humankind and various aspects related to human life including society and the environment. But, at the same time, it has also posed potential dangers to human health and the environment. Therefore, there is a need for effective regulations to manage the safety issues and risks associated with nanomaterials and ensure their safe development and applications. For this purpose, effective regulatory frameworks for nanomaterials should be developed and implemented by collaborative research initiatives, collective efforts, and international cooperation among different national and international governments as well as non-government organizations.

17.2 Safety Concerns and Risk Assessments

Nanomaterials hold immense potential in revolutionizing healthcare with improved theragnosis. The euphoria with the advent of these NMs has also awakened the scientific fraternity towards the deleterious effects of these particles. They exhibit unique properties compared to their larger counterpart. These materials are small enough with a large surface area to interact with the biological system differently and unpredictably compared to traditional drugs. So, they are prone to causing chronic health risks [26]. This raises concerns regarding their safe use and potential toxicity, inflammation, and immune response. The development and the use of these particles as nanomedicine is in the toddling stage, and their detailed behaviour in human health and the environment is still not fully understood. The traditional toxicity testing protocols are not sufficient enough to capture the complex behaviour of these materials.

Risk assessment is a systematic process of identifying, analysing, and evaluating the possible risks associated with a product. It is an understanding of how the newly developed NMs might interact with the body and what potential risks they might pose. The foremost step of this process is to identify the hazards associated with NMs. This step involves identifying all the possible hazards associated with considering their physical and chemical properties, their potential routes of exposure, and their intended use. This step is followed by estimating the likelihood of occurrence of hazard and severity, considering factors such as dose, duration of exposure, and the susceptibility of an individual. Finally, based on the characterization of risks, strategies to minimize or eliminate the potential risks are developed.

17.2.1 Potential Risks Associated with NMs

The fusion of nanotechnology and material science with pharmaceuticals and biomedical science has led to the discovery of nanomedicines. These are used in diagnosis (such as imaging and medical biosensors), regenerative medicine (such as bone and cartilage regeneration, dentistry, etc.), and in therapy (drug delivery, phototherapy, immunotherapy) [27]. However, there are potential risks associated with them, as no particles are entirely inert and even at low concentrations can exhibit harmful health effects [28]. They can penetrate the cellular structures in various organs due to their smaller size compared to cells and cell organelles via circulatory, nervous, and lymphatic systems [29]. They interfere with the physiological functions and induce tissue inflammation, abnormal cell behaviour, and even cell death [30].

They pose genotoxicity and mutagenicity by either directly interfering with our DNA or disrupting cell division [31, 32]. The harmful effects of NMs can be caused not only by their direct interaction with cells but also indirectly through the activation of immune cells like macrophages and neutrophils, which release reactive oxygen species (ROS) that can damage the surrounding tissues [33, 34]. Various types of NMs, such as quantum dots (QDs), metallic, magnetic, silica, and carbon-based NMs, have been extensively used as biosensors, imaging, and drug carriers [35]. However, they are prone to imposing toxicity. QDs disrupt mitochondrial function and damage DNA [36]. Similarly, carbon-based NMs interfere the cell signalling [37]. Nevertheless, all the nanoparticles do not show adverse health effects. Their toxicity depends on various factors like size, surface charge, crystallinity, and

Table 17.1 Potential risks of different kinds of nanomaterials

Category	Nanomaterials	Specific risks	References
Human health risks	Carbon nanotubes	Cytotoxicity and genotoxicity such as DNA damage, granulomas, and cancer	[38]
	TiO_2 and silica nanoparticles	Respiratory issues such as pulmonary inflammation and fibrosis	[39, 40]
	ZnO NPs	Skin penetration and irritation including dermatitis	[41]
	Gold NPs	Neurotoxicity and neuronal damage	[42]
	Silver NPs	Allergic reactions like immune hypersensitivity	[43]
	Quantum dots	Bioaccumulation in liver, kidney, and spleen	[44]
Environmental risks	Silver NPs	Accumulation in aquatic food chains	[45]
	TiO_2 and ZnO NPs	Ecotoxicity causing disruption of aquatic life	[46]
	Carbon nanomaterials	Harms soil microbes causing soil fertility impairment	[47]
	Quantum dots	Long-term contamination in water and soil ecosystems	[48, 49]
	Metal NPs	Assimilate through different levels of the food chain	[50]
	Nanoparticles from combustion	Impacts air quality by accumulating particulate matter	[51]

composition. Moreover, the toxicity of any NMs is also determined by the genetic complement of an individual [28].

As mentioned in Table 17.1, the risks associated with nanomaterials can be categorized under two classes: human health risks and environmental risks. Human health risks involve risks related to cytotoxicity and genotoxicity, respiratory issues, skin penetration and irritation, neurotoxicity, allergic reactions, and bioaccumulation in delicate organs of the human body that are caused by various carbon nanomaterials, quantum dots, and metallic and metal oxide nanomaterials. Similarly, the environmental risks of nanomaterials include ecotoxicity, contaminations of water, soil, and air, and accumulation and assimilation of various nanoparticles in the food chain.

17.2.2 Mechanism of Nanotoxicity

Understanding the underlying mechanism of nanotoxicity is very crucial for risk assessment and the development of safe and efficient nanomedicines. NMs interact with the cells and develop various adverse effects due to the generation of reactive oxygen species like hydrogen peroxide, superoxide, and hydroxyl radicals, leading to oxidative stress [52]. This oxidative stress may cause cellular and mitochondrial

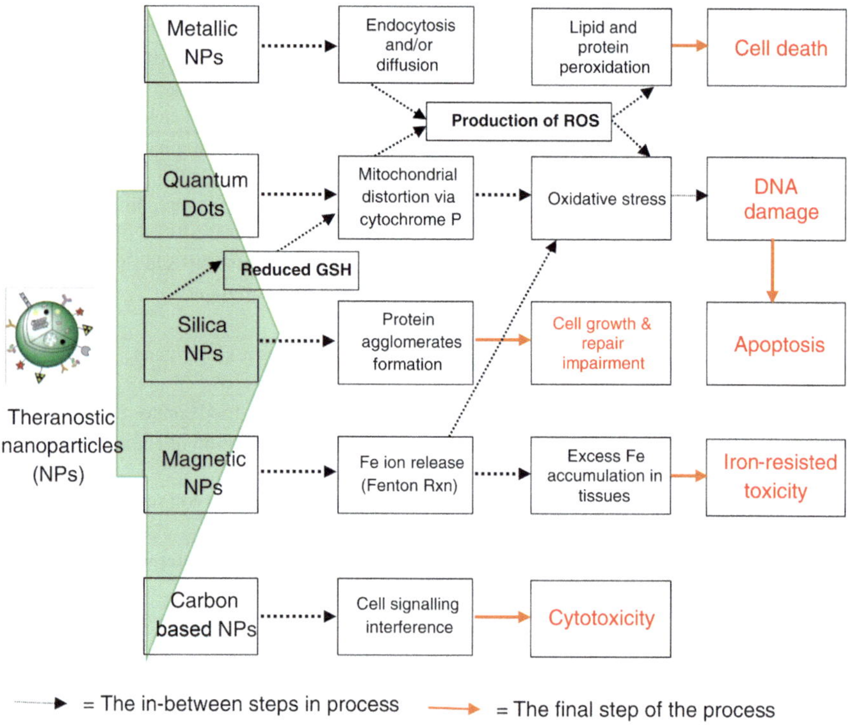

Fig. 17.3 Schematic illustration of the mechanism of nanotoxicity. (Reproduced with permission from [54])

dysfunction, autophagy, apoptosis, genotoxicity, and organelle dysfunction and trigger inflammatory responses in cells and tissues [53]. The possible mechanism of nanotoxicity of various types of NMs is depicted in Fig. 17.3.

17.2.3 Pharmacokinetics of NMs

Mapping the path and changes occurring in the body, right from their absorption to excretion, is crucial in understanding the risks related to the use of NMs. However, the fate of these particles in the body is quite unclear. They interact with bionanointerfaces inside the body, which is a very complicated process and makes safety assessments quite challenging [55].

Pharmacokinetics examines how the body absorbs, distributes, metabolizes, and finally eliminates drugs from the body. It is crucial to assess the therapeutic efficacy and the toxicity of NMs administered into the body. The pharmacokinetics of NMs are dependent on various factors like shape and size, surface properties, composition, and administration route [54].

Toxicokinetics deals with how the body absorbs, metabolizes, distributes, accumulates, and eliminates NMs and the potential toxic effects associated with them [56, 57]. Understanding these processes is crucial for the health risk assessment of these NMs.

17.2.3.1 Absorption

The first step of toxicokinetics is the absorption of NMs into the human body, which depends on the amount ingested and the physical and chemical characteristics. The absorption of these particles depends on the administration route into the body, size, and the surface charges [58]. The cellular uptake of such NMs is greatly influenced by their size. Smaller particles are absorbed more than larger ones. The positively charged NMs are absorbed through the gastrointestinal (GI) tract in comparison to negative and neutral ones [59].

17.2.3.2 Distribution

The NMs are distributed to different parts of the body from the site of absorption. Once in the systemic circulation, these particles interact with coagulation factors, plasma proteins, and the blood cells [60]. The distribution of these particles depends on the size, charge, and functional coating. Smaller particles are prone to being distributed in various organs like the kidneys, liver, spleen, lungs, and even the brain. On the contrary, larger remains solely on the GI tract [61].

17.2.3.3 Metabolism

Functionalized NMs are considered to be metabolized compared to inert NMs such as silver and gold NPs [60]. The enzymes in the body bind these NMs and metabolize them. The protein cap of functionalized quantum dots can be broken down by the protein proteases, for instance [62]. However, the distinctive mechanism of such metabolism demands further in vivo studies. NMs that are hard to degrade by the intracellular processes, such as inert gold NMs, remain in the liver for pretty much longer time [63].

17.2.3.4 Accumulation

The NMs administered into the body accumulate at several parts of the body, such as the lungs, liver, intestine, brain, and heart. Toxicity is usually negligible at low concentrations or a single dose. At higher concentrations or with chronic exposure, however, large amounts of NMs accumulate at several sites of the body, comprising additional risks.

17.2.3.5 Elimination

It is a crucial process, as the NMs retained in the body can increase the severity of toxicity. The primary route of excretion of these NMs is urine, followed by bile and faeces as other elimination routes. Smaller NMs are preferentially eliminated by the renal route, whereas the larger ones are eliminated through hepatic as it involves little cellular metabolism. The chemical composition and the size influence the excretion of NMs.

A schematic representation of the pharmacokinetics of NMs is depicted in Fig. 17.4.

17.2.4 Risk Assessment Methodologies

One of the foremost challenges for the researchers, industry, and regulators is the dilemma in classifying and testing protocols for the developed new NMs before the products are commercially available in the market [65]. Most importantly, there are challenges in the safety assessment of smart and sustainable nanomaterials due to

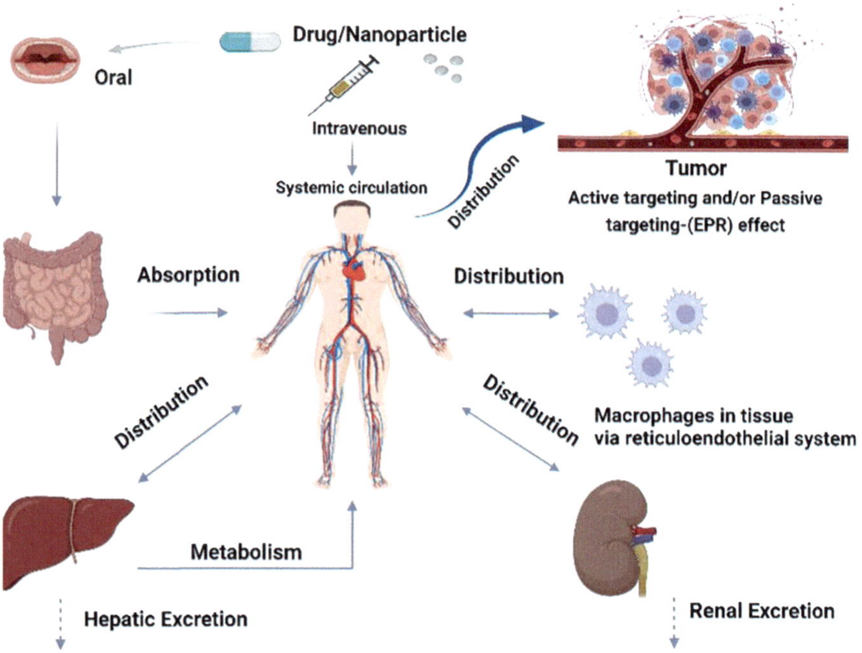

Fig. 17.4 Schematic diagram illustrating the pharmacokinetics of nanomaterials. (Reproduced with permission from [64])

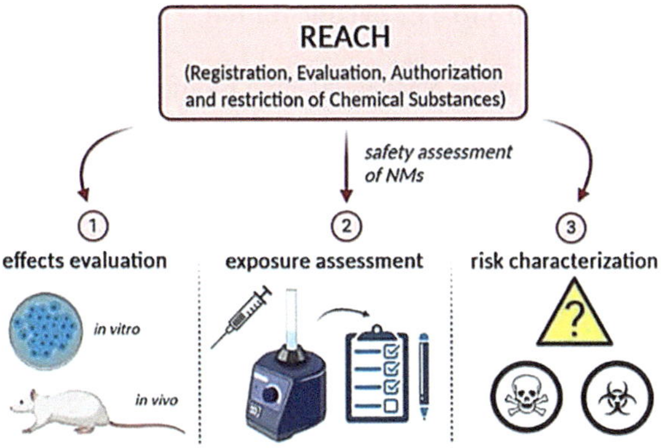

Fig. 17.5 Risk assessment based on REACH requirements. (Reproduced with permission from [66])

factors like complex behaviour and limited data. Similarly, it is crucial to determine whether the existing toxicology knowledge is sufficient enough to assess the safety of NMs. Risk assessment methodologies based on REACH requirements involve evaluation of effects, exposure assessment, and risk characterization (Fig. 17.5). Evaluation of effects includes experimental studies in vitro and in vivo conditions. Exposure assessment involves the identification of all possible sources of exposure, while risk characterization includes proper selection of testing strategies for risk prevention [66].

Nevertheless, nanomedicines are currently subjected to different tests, including physical, in vitro, in vivo, and computer-simulated assessments.

17.2.4.1 Physicochemical Characterization

Assessment of various physicochemical properties of the NMs is crucial before their use in nanomedicine. Particle size, shape, surface charge, composition, stability in solution, agglomeration tendency, etc., affect medical efficacy as well as the toxicity level as they affect the responses within the biological systems [67]. The cellular toxicity level of these particles is size-dependent. A study confirmed that smaller particles pose greater toxicity. Kim and his co-workers observed that silver nanoparticles measuring 10 nm induced greater apoptosis compared to 50 and 100 nm particles. Such small-sized particles induce ROS production and lactate dehydrogenase (LDH) release and apoptosis [68].

The concentration of NMs also affects the toxicity, as observed in the titanium dioxide nanocrystals, which are prone to damaging DNA, lipid peroxidation, and micronuclei formation even at very low concentrations (1 μL/mL) [69]. The chemical composition of the NMs affects their biodegradability. Organic-based NMs with hydrolysable bonds like esters, ortho-esters, and anhydrides are biodegradable compared to their inorganic counterparts. This biodegradability helps to eliminate NMs from the body, thereby reducing long-term toxicity [70].

17.2.4.2 In Vitro Experimentation

The behaviour of NMs is affected by the biological environment. Their behaviour must be assessed mimicking in vivo conditions as closely as possible [71]. Thus, in vitro models are frequently used by the NMs manufacturers and government bodies for the assessment of toxicity and the evaluation of risk associated with their use. This provides the first information about the toxicity of nanomaterials. The foremost evaluation of toxicity involves the change in cell membrane integrity, disruption of the cytoskeleton, and the impairment of the structure and functions of organelles. Trypan blue, tetrazolium reduction assay, neutral red uptake assay, lactate dehydrogenase (LDH) assay, adenosine triphosphate (ATP) assay, dichloro-dihydro-fluorescein diacetate (DCFH-DA) assay, etc., are used for the in vitro toxicity analysis of NMs [53]. In the trypan blue assay, a cell suspension is exposed to the dye with NMs. The cytoplasm of dead cells turns blue, whereas the viable cells possess clear cytoplasm. Then light microscopy is used to determine the ratio of stained and unstained cells that assess the toxicity. Similarly, the tetrazolium reduction assay involves the measurement of the activity of mitochondrial dehydrogenase enzymes in living cells. These enzymes convert tetrazolium salts like 3-(4,5-dimethylthiazol-2-yl)-2,5-diphenyltetrazolium bromide (MTT) into a purple-coloured formazan product through succinate dehydrogenase, and upon its measurement, it gives the cell viability. On the other hand, the LDH assay measures the release of LDH from the damaged cells, which catalyses a reaction to develop a coloured product. The intensity of the colour is proportional to the concentration of LDH released, indicating cell damage, and is determined colorimetrically.

In vitro, cytotoxicity provides invaluable information about the safety of NMs. However, oversimplification of the biological system, lack of physiological relevance, ignoring of immune response, etc., are some limitations that such an assay inherits. Thus, such tests are complemented with in vivo studies for a better understanding of nanomedicine safety and efficacy.

17.2.4.3 In Vivo Model

The cytotoxicity of the NMs is tested on animal models before exploiting them on humans due to physiological, ethical, economic, and logistical reasons [66]. Commonly, rodents, rabbits, and dogs are used for short-duration to long-duration tests of acute toxicity to chronic toxicity. Illness, morbidity, or mortality of these animal models are observed along with skin, eyes, respiration, nervous system, and feeding behaviour abnormalities after administration of NMs. In recent times, tiny water creatures like Daphnia, a type of plankton, have been used for nanotoxicity assays.

Despite their significant biological dissimilarities with humans, these tests primarily act as pre-screening checks [72]. Major biological models currently used for the evaluation of the toxicity of NMs are given in Table 17.2.

Table 17.2 Biological models for the evaluation of nanotoxicity

Type of model		Advantages	Limits	Applications
***In Vitro* Models**	Cell culture (line cells/primary cells)	Easy to use protocols	Far from *in vivo* conditions	Cell proliferation
		Cost and time effectiveness		Cell viability
		High throughput		Cell apoptosis
				Oxidative stress
				Genotoxicity
				Immunotoxicity
	Co-culture	In vivo-like-cell-cell interactions so more relevant than traditional cell culture	Far from *in vivo* conditions	Cell proliferation
			Heterogeneity	Cell viability
				Cell apoptosis
				Oxidative stress
				Genotoxicity
				Immunotoxicity
	Spheroid tissues	3D microarchitecture	Lower reproducibility	Cell proliferation
		More *in vivo* complexity	Simplified 3D architecture	Cell viability
		Nutrient and oxygen gradient		Cell apoptosis
				Oxidative stress
				Genotoxicity
				Immunotoxicity
	Precision-cut tissue slices Liver	Compatible with various tissues samples and animal species	Tissue damage due to slicing process	Histological analysis
		Close to/respect tissue native architecture		
		High reproducibility	Intrinsic inflammatory responses	
			Limited number of slices per organ	
***In Vivo* Models**	Small animal models (rodents, rabbits)	Similar routes of Human exposure	Far from Human (species variability)	Toxicokinetic parameters analysis
		More ethical than large animal models		

(continued)

Table 17.2 (continued)

Type of model		Advantages	Limits	Applications
		Dosages from biological fluid (blood, plasma, urine ...)	High cost	Systemic toxicity assessment
		Tissue biopsies	Time intensive	
	Aquatic models (Planktonic crustaceans, Zebrafish ...)	High throughput	Limited routes of exposure	Embryotoxicity evaluation
		Pre-screening tests	Far from Human (species variability)	
		Rapid developmental process		

Reproduced with permission from [71]

However, the response of humans differs from that of animals used for in vivo studies. Moreover, the subjective effects like headache, nausea, and dizziness as well as mental health, can't be revealed from animal studies. Thus, the real-life patient scenario is more complicated and demands more understanding and tests.

17.2.4.4 Computational Simulation for Toxicity Assessment (In Silico Assay)

In vitro and in vivo cytotoxicity testing of NMs is cumbersome and is highly costly and time-consuming. Another approach to testing includes the use of in silico models and computer algorithms to predict the toxic effects of NMs. It simulates the interactions between the NMs and the biological systems and assesses safety. Quantitative structure-activity relationships (QSARs) modelling, predictive toxicology modelling, physiologically based pharmacokinetic (PBPK) modelling, etc., are used in standalone or in combination that provides a comprehensive assessment of nanotoxicity. QSAR is the most successful computational model that aims to define mathematical dependencies between the biological activity of nanomaterials toxicity and molecular descriptors of nanomaterials (Fig. 17.6) [73].

Thus, the nanosafety of these NMs is investigated through a series of processes that includes physicochemical characterization, in vitro screening, nano QSAR modelling, and finally in vivo validation.

Although significant strides have been made in developing smart NMs, the clinical translation of NMs is a great challenge due to limited safety assessment by the available traditional preclinical tests. The current assessment technologies and the guidelines are not sufficient to assure the safe use of these smart NMs in healthcare and theragnostic. Thus, there is a need for standardized testing protocols for safety

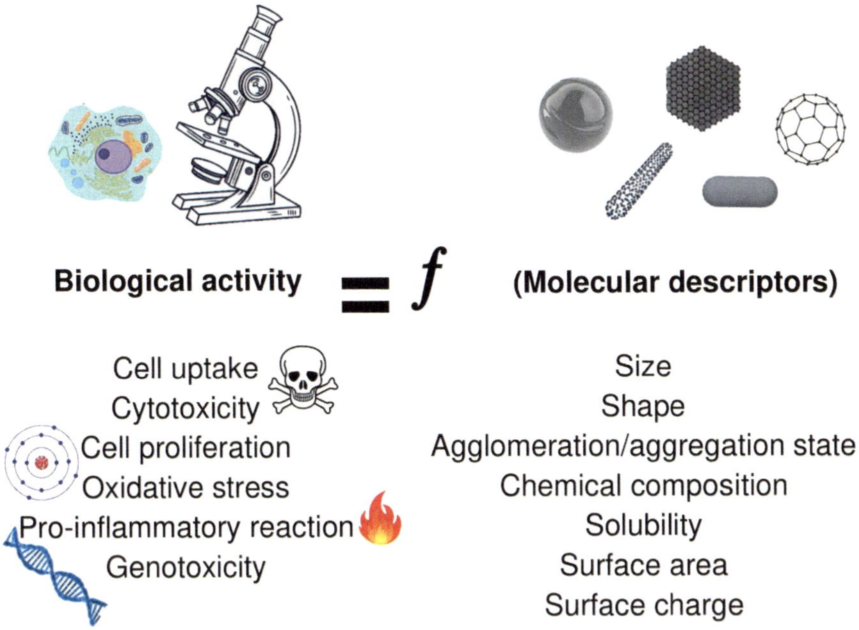

Fig. 17.6 QSAR model showing mathematical dependencies between biological activity and molecular descriptors of nanomaterials. (Reproduced with permission from [73])

evaluation. Comprehensive knowledge of toxicities of each NMs is warranted before their clinical applications. Scientists, government officials, policymakers, and industrialists must work collaboratively for the safe and beneficial development of smart and sustainable NMs in health care and theragnostic.

17.3 Regulatory Landscape

17.3.1 Overview

The regulatory landscape encompasses the comprehensive framework that includes the creation, implementation, and enforcement of regulations for the development, production, approval, commercialization, and monitoring of products. This involves the enactment of laws by legislative bodies, the issuance of policies and guidelines, the development of standards and protocols by regulatory agencies, and the monitoring of compliance and enforcement by stakeholders. The regulatory landscape ensures the safety, effectiveness, and quality of products for consumers, serving as a crucial element of responsibility and ethical practice beyond just a legal framework [74].

In the context of nanomedicine, the regulatory landscape includes a complex array of laws, policies, guidelines, agencies, and practices that regulate the development, approval, and monitoring of nanomedicine products to address the unique challenges and risks associated with their nanoscale properties [75]. Nanomaterials are being used in nanomedicine for diagnostic (nanodiagnosis) applications, controlled drug delivery (nanotherapy), and regenerative medicine. Recently, theranostics—a combination of diagnosis and therapy—has emerged in the medical field, with nanomedicine driving significant changes in clinical settings by presenting innovative drugs for both diagnosis and treatment of diseases [76].

The design and discovery of these novel medicines have successfully addressed complex medical challenges, but their distinctive nanoscale properties raise important questions about safety, efficacy, and quality. This necessitates a specific regulatory framework for nanomedicine. Traditional regulatory frameworks for conventional pharmaceuticals and medical devices are not sufficient to address the risks associated with nanomedicine, requiring revisions and amendments [77]. Important aspects to consider in developing the regulatory framework for nanomedicine are briefly discussed below.

17.3.1.1 Physicochemical Characterization

The characterization of nanomaterials, from their design to the evaluation of their in vitro and in vivo performance, helps to understand their behaviour and interactions in biological systems. It includes determination of characteristics like particle size, shape, size distribution, structure, composition, porosity, surface area, surface chemistry, zeta potential, solubility, photocatalytic ability, and more [76, 77].

17.3.1.2 Manufacturing Practices and Quality Control

To ensure consistent quality standards of nanomedicine, good manufacturing practice is crucial. The quality should actually be built on inside nanomedicine. For this purpose, manufacturers are required to implement rigorous control over the entire production process. It involves the identification and stringent regulation of critical quality attributes of nanomedicine, such as the selection of raw materials, processing parameters, manufacturing process, quality testing, and packaging [76, 77].

17.3.1.3 Efficacy and Clinical Trials

The efficacy of nanomedicine relies on its preclinical and clinical trials as well as understanding of pharmacokinetics (the way nanomedicine interacts with body systems) and pharmacodynamics (effects of nanomedicine on body systems). Preclinical and clinical trials involve thorough biocompatibility testing and mechanism of action of nanomedicine by both in vivo and selected in vitro studies [76, 77].

17.3.1.4 Post-market Surveillance

After the nanomedicine product is approved and dispatched for use, regular surveillance on their adverse effects and risks on consumers should be done by the manufacturers. Further, strategies to mitigate the risks also need to be outlined and implemented to ensure the safety of the product [76, 77].

17.3.1.5 International Harmonization

It refers to the collaboration between various regulatory agencies and research institutions across the world for effective and standard regulation of nanomedicine. It also ensures funding for further research and development on the safety and efficacy of nanomedicine [76, 77].

17.3.2 Regulatory Agencies Involved in Regulation of Nanomedicine

To address the risks posed by nanomedicine, several agencies are playing a vital role across the world in regulating the development, approval, and monitoring of nanomedicine products by formulating specific policies and guidelines. Some forefront agencies and their major works are highlighted below [76, 78].

17.3.2.1 United States Food and Drug Administration (FDA)

The United States Food and Drug Administration is an accountable federal agency for safeguarding public health by ensuring that pharmaceuticals, medical devices, tobacco products, foods, cosmetics, biological products, and radiation-emitting products are safe, effective, and secure. The office of regulatory affairs under the FDA is an authorized body that examines, approves, and monitors all drugs and devices, including nanomedicine products for public use in the United States, by enforcing federal acts and laws. It issues guidance documents on the characterization of nanomaterials, emphasizing the importance of a case-by-case assessment. It also collaborates with other government agencies, academic institutions, and international regulatory bodies to advance the science of nanomedicine and develop better regulatory approaches [78, 79].

17.3.2.2 European Medicines Agency (EMA)

It is a responsible decentralized agency of the European Union that monitors the safety, scientific assessment, and use of medicines. It safeguards public and animal health in EU member states by guaranteeing the safety, efficacy, and quality of medications sold in the EU market. It has several scientific committees, working parties, and regulatory networks for conducting scientific research, developing guidelines and setting standards of medicines, and evaluating and monitoring pharmaceuticals [78, 80].

17.3.2.3 World Health Organization (WHO)

WHO is an organization of the United Nations that does not directly regulate nanomedicines but plays a vital role in setting global standards, guidelines, and frameworks for the safe use of nanomaterials in medicine. It facilitates collaboration between member states, regulatory bodies, and international organizations to harmonize the regulation of nanomedicines globally. WHO's International Program on Chemical Safety (IPCS) is an example of such collaboration. It also provides technical assistance to its member countries to help them develop regulatory frameworks for nanomedicine and conduct research in nanomedicine, particularly in the area of global health challenges [81].

17.3.2.4 Organization for Economic Cooperation and Development (OECD)

OECD, an international organization basically working on social, economic, and environmental issues, helps shape the global regulatory landscape for nanomedicine by promoting international cooperation, developing standardized testing guidelines, and supporting the harmonization of regulatory approaches to nanomedicine. It places emphasis on the environmental health and safety aspects of nanomaterials. It also provides technical assistance to member and non-member countries to help them build capacity in regulating nanomedicine [82].

17.3.2.5 National Institutes for Food and Drug Control (NIFDC)

The NIFDC, an organization under the National Medical Products Administration (NMPA) in China, is responsible for ensuring the safety, efficacy, and quality of pharmaceuticals, including nanomedicines. It is involved in the formulation and implementation of national policies and guidelines that govern the production, testing, and approval of nanomedicines and their ethical and social implications in China. It conducts research on nanotechnology and its applications in medicine, contributing to the scientific understanding of nanomedicine. It also offers technical support and collaborative research in the field of nanomedicine among stakeholders in China [83].

17.3.2.6 The Therapeutic Goods Administration (TGA)

TGA is a government organization of Australia responsible for the evaluation, assessment, and monitoring of therapeutic goods. It ensures the healthy and safe lives of Australian citizens by regulating commercial medications, medical devices, and biologicals. It develops, implements, and monitors guidelines for manufacturing, labelling, packaging, and distributing therapeutic goods inside Australia [78, 84].

17.3.3 Legal Regulations of Nanomedicine

Various acts, regulations, and guidelines have been developed worldwide to regulate nanomedicine and nanomedicine products. Some significant legal regulations of nanomedicine are presented below.

17.3.3.1 U.S. Food and Drug Administration (FDA) Regulations

The FDA regulates nanomedicine under its existing frameworks for drugs, biologics, medical devices, and combination products. The main aspects of FDA regulation related to nanomedicine are listed below [85]:

(a) Nanomedicine products aimed to diagnose, cure, alleviate, treat, or prevent disease are considered drugs or biologics and must fulfil all the norms set by the Food, Drug, and Cosmetic Act (FDCA) and the Public Health Service Act (PHSA).
(b) The development and evaluation of drugs and biologics containing nanomaterials must follow the "Drug Products, Including Biological Products, that Contain Nanomaterials" document 2022.
(c) Preclinical and clinical testing standards for nanomedicine products are the same as those for conventional medical products; however, additional studies may be required to assess nanotechnology-specific problems such as biodistribution, toxicity, and long-term consequences.
(d) Depending on the kind of product, nanomedicine products may be reviewed under the New Drug Application (NDA), Biologics License Application (BLA), or Premarket Approval (PMA) pathways.

(e) It is mandatory for manufacturers to report adverse events, and the FDA reserves the right to monitor these reports for any safety signals about the unique features of nanomaterials.
(f) The FDA can collaborate with international regulatory organizations to harmonize standards and exchange information on the regulation of nanomedicines.

17.3.3.2 Toxic Substances Control Act (TSCA) Regulations

Although there are no specific regulations assigned for nanomedicine, TSCA regulates the production and use of chemicals, including nanomaterials, in the United States. The key points of regulation are listed below [86]:

(a) Pre-manufacturing notices (PMN), which include information on chemical identification, production, volume, by-products, use, and disposal, are required for the manufacture and import of nanomaterials.
(b) The EPA evaluates the potential hazards to human health and the environment from the usage of nanomaterials and has the authority to issue a significant new user rule (SNUR).
(c) The EPA may impose restrictions on the production, use, or disposal of nanomaterials if it is deemed to pose unreasonable hazards to human health and the environment.
(d) Some TSCA regulations may not apply to nanomaterials that are solely utilized exclusively for research and development.
(e) Companies that violate the nanomaterials-related provisions of the TSCA may be subject to fines and prohibitions on further operations.
(f) The EPA may collaborate with the FDA to ensure that nanomedicine products are properly regulated under the Federal Food, Drug, and Cosmetic Act (FDCA) as well as the TSCA.

17.3.3.3 REACH (Registration, Evaluation, Authorization, and Restriction of Chemicals) Regulations

The production and use of chemical substances, including nanomaterials, are controlled by REACH regulations in the European Union. However, there is no specific regulation for nanomedicine products. The main points of REACH regulations are listed below [23, 87]:

(a) REACH defines nanomaterials as materials with peculiar qualities that require detailed information on their attributes, like particle size distribution, shape, and surface chemistry.
(b) The manufacturer or importer of nanomaterials must register with the European Chemicals Agency (ECHA) and provide information about their properties, applications, and dangers.

(c) ECHA evaluates the registered nanomaterials by performing Chemical Safety Assessment (CSA) to verify compliance and assess potential risks. ECHA reserves the right to ask for additional information or tests to address any uncertainties regarding the nanomaterial.
(d) Nanomaterials having carcinogenicity, mutagenicity, or reproductive toxicity are categorized as substances of very high concern (SVHCs) and may require authorization for specific applications.
(e) ECHA monitors the safety of registered nanomaterials and reserves the right to ban their production, usage, or sale if they are found to pose intolerable risks to human health and the environment.
(f) Safety Data Sheets (SDS) for nanomaterials, which include instructions on safe handling, storage, disposal, and emergency measures, must be provided by manufacturers and suppliers.
(g) By the Classification, Labelling, and Packaging (CLP) regulation, hazardous nanomaterials must be categorized and labelled to inform users of their potential risks.
(h) Nanomaterials used in medical products might also be regulated under other EU laws, such as the Medical Devices Regulation (MDR).

17.3.3.4 OECD (Organization for Economic Co-operation and Development) Guidelines

OECD provides guidelines and frameworks that are often used as references for the safe handling and regulation of nanomaterials, including those used in nanomedicine. An overview of OECD guidelines applicable to nanomedicine is presented below [82]:

(a) Because of their unique properties, including surface area, particle size, and shape, nanomaterials require different testing methodologies. It includes testing for physicochemical properties, ecotoxicity, and implications on human health.
(b) Precise safety assessment requires proper sample preparation, particularly in medical applications where complex interaction with biological systems may occur.
(c) Nanomaterials must be classified based on their physical and chemical properties as well as possible effects on the environment and human health.
(d) In vitro assays and in silico models can be applied as alternative testing techniques for the safety assessment of nanomaterials.
(e) Public engagement is encouraged in the development of nanotechnology regulations.

17.3.3.5 NMPA (National Medical Products Administration) Regulations

In China, the NMPA is the regulatory body responsible for regulating the safety, efficacy, and quality of medical products, including nanomedicine. The following regulations and guidelines established by the NMPA are relevant to the development, approval, and management of nanomedicines [88]:

(a) The Drug Administration Law governs the approval, manufacturing, distribution, and supervision of drugs, including nanomedicines. It provides the legal framework for ensuring that all drugs, including nanomedicine, are safe, effective, and of high quality.
(b) Nanomedicines are considered new drugs and must undergo rigorous evaluation, including preclinical and clinical testing, before receiving market approval.
(c) Nanomedicine manufacturers must comply with China's Good Manufacturing Practices (GMP) standards, which ensure that pharmaceuticals are reliably produced and controlled according to quality standards.
(d) Before being commercialized in China, nanomedicines must be registered with the NMPA and provide information on their composition, manufacturing process, clinical trial results, and safety data.
(e) Packaging of nanomedicines must comply with NMPA standards to guarantee the stability and integrity of the product throughout its shelf life.
(f) Nanomedicine manufacturers are required to evaluate and reduce the environmental impact of their products, particularly with regard to the release of nanomaterials during production and disposal.
(g) An ethical assessment is required for research involving nanomedicines in order to ensure the protection of the rights and safety of participants.
(h) NMPA may collaborate with international regulatory bodies and participate in global initiatives to harmonize the regulation of nanomedicines.

17.4 Conclusion

Nanomedicine offers unprecedented opportunities for diagnosis, treatment, and drug delivery, yet the unique properties of nanomaterials also pose distinct safety challenges that require careful consideration. Unlike traditional pharmaceuticals, nanomedicines exhibit behaviours at the nanoscale that can lead to unexpected biological interactions, toxicity, and long-term effects. Addressing these concerns necessitates a comprehensive regulatory framework that is both flexible and robust, capable of evolving alongside technological innovations.

One of the major concerns in nanomedicine is the potential for unforeseen toxicological impacts. Nanomaterials may interact with biological systems in ways that are not yet fully understood, leading to concerns about bioaccumulation, oxidative stress, and immune responses. These risks underscore the importance of developing and implementing advanced safety assessment methods that go beyond conventional protocols. Regulatory bodies must prioritize the establishment of standardized testing procedures specifically designed to evaluate the unique features of nanomedicines, such as their size, shape, surface charge, and chemical composition.

The regulatory landscape for nanomedicine is still in its formative stages, with different regions adopting varying approaches to oversight. This lack of harmonization can create significant obstacles to the global development and commercialization of nanomedicine products. Therefore, international collaboration is essential to create unified regulatory standards that facilitate the safe and efficient introduction of nanomedicines into the market. Such collaboration should also focus on fostering innovation while ensuring rigorous safety evaluations are in place to protect public health.

To effectively manage the safety concerns and regulatory challenges of nanomedicine, a proactive and adaptive approach is required. Continuous post-market surveillance, coupled with ongoing research into the long-term effects of nanomedicine, will be critical in ensuring that these products are both safe and effective. By striking the right balance between innovation and regulation, the potential of nanomedicine can be fully realized, leading to transformative improvements in healthcare outcomes while maintaining the highest standards of patient safety.

References

1. Eberhard WG, Wcislo WT. Plenty of room at the bottom? Am Sci. 2012;100:226–33. https://doi.org/10.1511/2012.96.226.
2. Taniguchi N. On the basic concept of "Nano-technology." Proc Intl Conf Prod Eng Tokyo, Part II. 1974.
3. Binnig G, Rohrer H, Gerber C, Weibel E. Tunneling through a controllable vacuum gap. Appl Phys Lett. 1982;40:178–80. https://doi.org/10.1063/1.92999.
4. Unbounding the future: The nanotechnology revolution. Precis Eng. 1991;13:309. https://doi.org/10.1016/0141-6359(91)90088-z.
5. Dowling A, Clift R, Grobert N, Hutton D, Oliver R, O'neill O, et al. Nanoscience and nanotechnologies: opportunities and uncertainties. Lond R Soc R Acad Eng Rep. 2004;46:617.
6. Elzein B. Nano revolution: "Tiny tech, big impact: how nanotechnology is driving SDGs progress". Heliyon. 2024;10 https://doi.org/10.1016/j.heliyon.2024.e31393.
7. Linkov I, Satterstrom FK, Corey LM. Nanotoxicology and nanomedicine: making hard decisions. Nanomed Nanotechnol Biol Med. 2008;4:167–71. https://doi.org/10.1016/j.nano.2008.01.001.
8. Oomen AG, Steinhäuser KG, Bleeker EAJ, van Broekhuizen F, Sips A, Dekkers S, et al. Risk assessment frameworks for nanomaterials: scope, link to regulations, applicability, and outline for future directions in view of needed increase in efficiency. NanoImpact. 2018;9:1–13. https://doi.org/10.1016/j.impact.2017.09.001.
9. Mago A, Junaid Tahir M, Arslan Khan M, Abbasher Hussien Mohamed Ahmed K, Usman Munir M. Nanomedicine: advancement in healthcare. Ann Med Surg. 2022;79:104078. https://doi.org/10.1016/j.amsu.2022.104078.
10. Shehata M, Shaker MA, Rahman SA, Abdul MI, Shaker MA. Nanomedicines: challenges and perspectives for future nanotechnology in the healthcare system. Sci Res Essays. 2019;14:32–8. https://doi.org/10.5897/sre2019.6604.

11. Rao Y, Kumar A. Devices of nanomedicine for anti-cancerous drug delivery system. Asian J Pharm Inven. 2013;1.
12. Ahmad N, Gopinath P. Intelligent nanomaterials for drug delivery applications. 2020.
13. Solaiman SM, Yamauchi Y, Kim JH, Horvat J, Dou SX, Alici G, et al. Nanotechnology and its medical applications: revisiting public policies from a regulatory perspective in Australia. Nanotechnol Rev. 2017;6:255–69. https://doi.org/10.1515/ntrev-2016-0095.
14. Shrivastava S, Dash D. Applying nanotechnology to human health: revolution in biomedical sciences. J Nanotechnol. 2009;2009:1–14. https://doi.org/10.1155/2009/184702.
15. Ferrari M, Philibert MA, Sanhai WR. Nanomedicine and society. Clin Pharmacol Ther. 2009;85:466–7. https://doi.org/10.1038/clpt.2008.276.
16. El-Kalliny AS, Abdel-Wahed MS, El-Zahhar AA, Hamza IA, Gad-Allah TA. Nanomaterials: a review of emerging contaminants with potential health or environmental impact. Discov Nano. 2023;181:1–21. https://doi.org/10.1186/S11671-023-03787-8.
17. Malakar A, Kanel SR, Ray C, Snow DD, Nadagouda MN. Nanomaterials in the environment, human exposure pathway, and health effects: a review. Sci Total Environ. Elsevier. 2021;759:143470. https://doi.org/10.1016/J.SCITOTENV.2020.143470.
18. Kurwadkar S, Pugh K, Gupta A, Ingole S. Nanoparticles in the environment: occurrence, distribution, and risks. J Hazard Toxic Radioact Waste. 2015;19:1–9. https://doi.org/10.1061/(asce)hz.2153-5515.0000258.
19. Shao C, Zhao H, Wang P. Recent development in functional nanomaterials for sustainable and smart agricultural chemical technologies. Nano Converg. 2022;9:1–17. https://doi.org/10.1186/S40580-022-00302-0/FIGURES/6.
20. Hristozov D, Gottardo S, Semenzin E, Oomen A, Bos P, Peijnenburg W, et al. Frameworks and tools for risk assessment of manufactured nanomaterials. Environ Int. 2016;95:36–53. https://doi.org/10.1016/j.envint.2016.07.016.
21. Frameworks R, Nanotechnology FOR, Foods IN. Regulatory Frameworks for Nanotechnology in Foods and medical products. 2013.
22. Laux P, Tentschert J, Riebeling C, Braeuning A, Creutzenberg O, Epp A, et al. Nanomaterials: certain aspects of application, risk assessment and risk communication. Arch Toxicol. 2018;92:121–41. https://doi.org/10.1007/s00204-017-2144-1.
23. Rauscher H, Rasmussen K, Sokull-Klüttgen B. Regulatory aspects of nanomaterials in the EU. Chemie-Ingenieur. 2017;89:224–31. https://doi.org/10.1002/cite.201600076.
24. Chávez-Hernández JA, Velarde-Salcedo AJ, Navarro-Tovar G, Gonzalez C. Safe nanomaterials: from their use, application, and disposal to regulations. Nanoscale Adv. 2024;6:1583–610. https://doi.org/10.1039/D3NA01097J.
25. Karim E. Nanotechnology safety in Asian perspective: a legal. Analysis. 2014:1–6.
26. Peters K, Unger RE, Gatti AM, Monari E, Kirkpatrick CJ. Effects of nano-scaled particles on endothelial cell functions in vitro. Trans - 7th World Biomater Congr. 2004;5:1881.
27. Smolkova B, Dusinska M, Gabelova A. Nanomedicine and epigenome. Possible health risks. Elsevier Ltd. 2017;109 https://doi.org/10.1016/j.fct.2017.07.020.
28. Buzea C, Pacheco II, Robbie K. Nanomaterials and nanoparticles: sources and toxicity. Biointerphases. 2007;2:MR17–71. https://doi.org/10.1116/1.2815690.
29. Medina C, Santos-Martinez MJ, Radomski A, Corrigan OI, Radomski MW. Nanoparticles: pharmacological and toxicological significance. Br J Pharmacol. 2007;150:552–8. https://doi.org/10.1038/sj.bjp.0707130.
30. Wei A, Mehtala JG, Patri AK. Challenges and opportunities in the advancement of nanomedicines. J Control Release. 2012;164:236–46. https://doi.org/10.1016/j.jconrel.2012.10.007.
31. Kumar A, Dhawan A. Genotoxic and carcinogenic potential of engineered nanoparticles: an update. Arch Toxicol. 2013;87:1883–900. https://doi.org/10.1007/s00204-013-1128-z.
32. Magdolenova Z, Collins A, Kumar A, Dhawan A, Stone V, Dusinska M. Mechanisms of genotoxicity. A review of in vitro and in vivo studies with engineered nanoparticles. Nanotoxicology. 2014;8:233–78. https://doi.org/10.3109/17435390.2013.773464.

33. Dusinska M, Boland S, Saunders M, Juillerat-Jeanneret L, Tran L, Pojana G, et al. Towards an alternative testing strategy for nanomaterials used in nanomedicine: lessons from NanoTEST. Nanotoxicology. 2015;9:118–32. https://doi.org/10.3109/17435390.2014.991431
.
34. Stone V, Johnston H, Schins RPF. Development of in vitro systems for nanotoxicology: methodological considerations in vitro methods for nanotoxicology Vicki Stone et al. Crit Rev Toxicol. 2009;39:613–26. https://doi.org/10.1080/10408440903120975.
35. Chen X. Nanoplatform-based molecular imaging. John Wiley & Sons, Inc.; 2011.
36. Nguyen KC, Rippstein P, Tayabali AF, Willmore WG. Mitochondrial toxicity of cadmium telluride quantum dot nanoparticles in mammalian hepatocytes. Toxicol Sci. 2015;146:31–42. https://doi.org/10.1093/toxsci/kfv068.
37. Yildirimer L, Thanh NTK, Loizidou M, Seifalian AM. Toxicological considerations of clinically applicable nanoparticles. Nano Today. 2011;6:585–607. https://doi.org/10.1016/j.nantod.2011.10.001.
38. Lam CW, James JT, McCluskey R, Hunter RL. Pulmonary toxicity of single-wall carbon nanotubes in mice 7 and 90 days after intractracheal instillation. Toxicol Sci. 2004;77:126–34. https://doi.org/10.1093/toxsci/kfg243.
39. Oberdörster G, Sharp Z, Atudorei V, Elder A, Gelein R, Lunts A, et al. Extrapulmonary translocation of ultrafine carbon particles following whole-body inhalation exposure of rats. J Toxicol Environ Health. 2002;65:1531–43. https://doi.org/10.1080/00984100290071658.
40. Warheit DB, Webb TR, Colvin VL, Reed KL, Sayes CM. Pulmonary bioassay studies with nanoscale and fine-quartz particles in rats: toxicity is not dependent upon particle size but on surface characteristics. Toxicol Sci. 2007;95:270–80. https://doi.org/10.1093/toxsci/kfl128.
41. Baroli B, Ennas MG, Loffredo F, Isola M, Pinna R, López-Quintela MA. Penetration of metallic nanoparticles in human full-thickness skin. J Invest Dermatol. 2007;127:1701–12. https://doi.org/10.1038/sj.jid.5700733.
42. Oberdörster G, Sharp Z, Atudorei V, Elder A, Gelein R, Kreyling W, et al. Translocation of inhaled ultrafine particles to the brain. Inhal Toxicol. 2004;16:437–45. https://doi.org/10.1080/08958370490439597.
43. Chuang HC, Hsiao TC, Wu CK, Chang HH, Lee CH, Chang CC, et al. Allergenicity and toxicology of inhaled silver nanoparticles in allergen-provocation mice models. Int J Nanomedicine. 2013;8:4495. https://doi.org/10.2147/IJN.S52239.
44. Das K, Meena R, Gaharwar US, Priyadarshini E, Rawat K, Paulraj R, et al. Bioaccumulation of CdSe quantum dots show biochemical and oxidative damage in Wistar rats. Oxidative Med Cell Longev. 2023;2023:7707452. https://doi.org/10.1155/2023/7707452.
45. Babaei M, Tayemeh MB, Jo MS, Yu IJ, Johari SA. Trophic transfer and toxicity of silver nanoparticles along a phytoplankton-zooplankton-fish food chain. Sci Total Environ. 2022;842 https://doi.org/10.1016/J.SCITOTENV.2022.156807.
46. Wang F, Zhou L, Mu D, Zhang H, Zhang G, Huang X, et al. Current research on ecotoxicity of metal-based nanoparticles: from exposure pathways, ecotoxicological effects to toxicity mechanisms. Front Public Health. 2024;12:1390099. https://doi.org/10.3389/FPUBH.2024.1390099/BIBTEX.
47. Yang X, Zhang X, Shu X, Zhang W, Kai J, Tang M, et al. Effects of multi-walled carbon nanotubes in soil on earthworm growth and reproduction, enzymatic activities, and metabolomics. Ecotoxicol Environ Saf. 2022;246:114158. https://doi.org/10.1016/J.ECOENV.2022.114158.
48. Giroux MS, Zahra Z, Salawu OA, Burgess RM, Ho KT, Adeleye AS. Assessing the environmental effects related to quantum dot structure, function, Synthesis and Exposure. Environ Sci Nano. 2022;9:867. https://doi.org/10.1039/D1EN00712B.
49. Wang X, Wu T. An update on the biological effects of quantum dots: from environmental fate to risk assessment based on multiple biological models. Sci Total Environ. 2023;879:163166. https://doi.org/10.1016/J.SCITOTENV.2023.163166.

50. Isibor PO, Oyegbade SA, Oni JG, Ahmed WW, Abiodun EO, Oyewole OA. Nanoparticles in food chains: bioaccumulation and trophic transfer. Environ Nanotoxicol. 2024:203–33. https://doi.org/10.1007/978-3-031-54154-4_11.
51. Ilyasu US, Aworunse OS, Olusanya CS, Isibor PO, Gana M, Oyewole OA. Nanoparticles in air and their impact on air quality. Environ Nanotoxicol. 2024:183–202. https://doi.org/10.1007/978-3-031-54154-4_10.
52. Starkov AA. The role of mitochondria in reactive oxygen species metabolism and signaling. Ann N Y Acad Sci. 2008;1147:37–52. https://doi.org/10.1196/annals.1427.015.
53. Patel G, Patra C, Srinivas SP, Kumawat M, Navya PN, Daima HK. Methods to evaluate the toxicity of engineered nanomaterials for biomedical applications: a review. Environ Chem Lett. 2021;19:4253–74. https://doi.org/10.1007/s10311-021-01280-1.
54. Kang H, Mintri S, Menon AV, Lee HY, Choi HS, Kim J. Pharmacokinetics, pharmacodynamics and toxicology of theranostic nanoparticles Homan. Nanoscale. 2015:7. https://doi.org/10.1039/x0xx00000x.
55. Dickinson AM, Godden JM, Lanovyk K, Ahmed SS. Assessing the safety of nanomedicines: a mini review. Appl Vitr Toxicol. 2019;5:114–22. https://doi.org/10.1089/aivt.2019.0009.
56. Zhao J, Castranova V. Toxicology of nanomaterials used in nanomedicine. J Toxicol Environ Health. 2011;14:593–632. https://doi.org/10.1080/10937404.2011.615113.
57. Ozbek O, Genc DE, Ulgen K O. Advances in physiologically based pharmacokinetic (PBPK) modeling of nanomaterials. ACS Pharmacol Transl Sci. 2024; https://doi.org/10.1021/acsptsci.4c00250.
58. Hamidi M, Azadi A, Rafiei P, Ashrafi H. A pharmacokinetic overview of Nanotechnology-based drug delivery systems: an ADME-oriented approach. Crit Rev Ther Drug Carrier Syst. 2013;30:435–67. https://doi.org/10.1615/CritRevTherDrugCarrierSyst.2013007419.
59. Florence AT. Nanoparticle uptake by the oral route: fulfilling its potential? Drug Discov Today Technol. 2005;2:75–81. https://doi.org/10.1016/j.ddtec.2005.05.019.
60. Hagens WI, Oomen AG, de Jong WH, Cassee FR, Sips AJAM. What do we (need to) know about the kinetic properties of nanoparticles in the body? Regul Toxicol Pharmacol. 2007;49:217–29. https://doi.org/10.1016/j.yrtph.2007.07.006.
61. Hillyer JF, Albrecht RM. Gastrointestinal persorption and tissue distribution of differently sized colloidal gold nanoparticles. J Pharm Sci. 2001;90:1927–36. https://doi.org/10.1002/jps.1143.
62. Hardman R. A toxicologic review of quantum dots: toxicity depends on physicochemical and environmental factors. Environ Health Perspect. 2006;114:165–72. https://doi.org/10.1289/ehp.8284.
63. Wang B, He X, Zhang Z, Zhao Y, Feng W. Metabolism of nanomaterials in vivo: blood circulation and organ clearance. Acc Chem Res. 2013;46:761–9. https://doi.org/10.1021/ar2003336.
64. Alghamdi MA, Fallica AN, Virzì N, Kesharwani P, Pittalà V, Greish K. The promise of nanotechnology in personalized medicine. J Pers Med. 2022;12 https://doi.org/10.3390/jpm12050673.
65. Bobo D, Robinson KJ, Islam J, Thurecht KJ, Corrie SR. Nanoparticle-based medicines: a review of FDA-approved materials and clinical trials to date. Pharm Res. 2016;33:2373–87. https://doi.org/10.1007/s11095-016-1958-5.
66. Zielińska A, Costa B, Ferreira MV, Miguéis D, Louros JMS, Durazzo A, et al. Nanotoxicology and nanosafety: safety-by-design and testing at a glance. Int J Environ Res Public Health. 2020;17:1–22. https://doi.org/10.3390/ijerph17134657.
67. Gulati K, Scimeca JC, Ivanovski S, Verron E. Double-edged sword: therapeutic efficacy versus toxicity evaluations of doped titanium implants. Drug Discov Today. 2021;26:2734–42. https://doi.org/10.1016/j.drudis.2021.07.004.
68. Kim TH, Kim M, Park HS, Shin US, Gong MS, Kim HW. Size-dependent cellular toxicity of silver nanoparticles. J Biomed Mater Res. 2012;100(A):1033–43. https://doi.org/10.1002/jbm.a.34053.

69. Shukla RK, Kumar A, Gurbani D, Pandey AK, Singh S, Dhawan A. TiO2 nanoparticles induce oxidative DNA damage and apoptosis in human liver cells. Nanotoxicology. 2013;7:48–60. https://doi.org/10.3109/17435390.2011.629747.
70. Wang S, Kim G, Lee YEK, Hah HJ, Ethirajan M, Pandey RK, et al. Multifunctional biodegradable polyacrylamide nanocarriers for cancer theranostics-A "see and treat" strategy. ACS Nano. 2012;6:6843–51. https://doi.org/10.1021/nn301633m.
71. Scimeca JC, Verron E. Nano-engineered biomaterials: safety matters and toxicity evaluation. Mater Today Adv. 2022;15:100260. https://doi.org/10.1016/j.mtadv.2022.100260.
72. Baun A, Hartmann NB, Grieger K, Kusk KO. Ecotoxicity of engineered nanoparticles to aquatic invertebrates: a brief review and recommendations for future toxicity testing. Ecotoxicology. 2008;17:387–95. https://doi.org/10.1007/s10646-008-0208-y.
73. Forest V. Experimental and computational nanotoxicology— complementary approaches for nanomaterial hazard assessment. Nano. 2022;12 https://doi.org/10.3390/nano12081346.
74. Beetler DJ, Di Florio DN, Law EW, Groen CM, Windebank AJ, Peterson QP, et al. The evolving regulatory landscape in regenerative medicine. Mol Asp Med. 2023;91 https://doi.org/10.1016/j.mam.2022.101138.
75. Sainz V, Conniot J, Matos AI, Peres C, Zupančič E, Moura L, et al. Regulatory aspects on nanomedicines. Biochem Biophys Res Commun. 2015;468:504–10. https://doi.org/10.1016/j.bbrc.2015.08.023.
76. Foulkes R, Man E, Thind J, Yeung S, Joy A, Hoskins C. The regulation of nanomaterials and nanomedicines for clinical application: current and future perspectives. Biomater Sci. 2020;8:4653–64. https://doi.org/10.1039/d0bm00558d.
77. Soares S, Sousa J, Pais A, Vitorino C. Nanomedicine: principles, properties, and regulatory issues. Front Chem. 2018;6:1–15. https://doi.org/10.3389/fchem.2018.00360.
78. Tambe V, Maheshwari R, Chourasiya Y, Choudhury H, Gorain B, Tekade RK. Clinical aspects and regulatory requirements for nanomedicines. Elsevier Inc.; 2018. https://doi.org/10.1016/B978-0-12-817909-3.00018-2.
79. FDA. n.d. **https://www.fda.gov/about-fda**. Accessed 22 Aug 2024.
80. European Medicines Agency (EMA). n.d. **https://www.ema.europa.eu/en/about-us**. Accessed 22 Aug 2024.
81. Who we are. n.d. **https://www.who.int/about/who-we-are**. Accessed 22 Aug 2024.
82. The OECD Guidelines - OECD Watch. n.d. **https://www.oecdwatch.org/oecd-ncps/the--oecd-guidelines-for-mnes/**. Accessed 22 Aug 2024.
83. National Institutes for Food and Drug Control (Center for Medical Device Standards Management of NMPA, National Institute for Drug Control). n.d. **https://english.nmpa.gov.cn/2019-07/19/c_389166.htm**. Accessed 22 Aug 2024.
84. About us | Therapeutic Goods Administration (TGA). n.d. **https://www.tga.gov.au/about-tga**. Accessed 22 Aug 2024.
85. Paradise J. Regulating nanomedicine at the Food and Drug Administration. AMA J Ethics. 2019;21:E347–55.
86. Chemicals E and Manual I. EPA/OECA/OC/MAMPD effective date: May 1, 2022 TSCA New and Existing Chemicals Inspection Manual OECA-MANL-2021-001-R0 2022.
87. The REACH Regulation : A regulation that concerns ALL of us. Stands for … n.d.
88. Yang Y. China NMPA reform and new regulations/guidelines/requirements. PharmaSUG. 2019:1–11.

Chapter 18
Smart Sustainable Nanomaterials-Based Biosensing Technology: Future Trends and Innovations in the Field

Vinith Kumar, Shashank, Jayant Haridas Pisal, Angelene Hannah Jebarani D, Mayank Roy Chowdhury, and Sudarshana Deepa Vijaykumar

Abstract In the era of ever-growing human population, the emergence of neoteric ailments and sundry pandemics is not uncommon. Contemporary healthcare practices are focused on finding effective solutions to combat such diseases with ease. The unique properties of nanomaterials make them versatile candidates for use in diagnostic and therapeutic procedures. Of late, the development and application of biosensors has substantiated to be a pivotal frontier in healthcare and theragnosis. Biosensing technologies aid in the diagnosis, monitoring, and prevention of disease states. In this chapter, we discuss on the spectrum of smart and sustainable nanomaterials availed for use in the design of biosensors. The future trends and innovations in the application of biosensing devices for healthcare, such as miniaturization, point-of-care testing, smartphone integration, and others have been discussed. Further, it provides insights on the challenges related to use of nano-based biosensors for healthcare and theragnosis.

Keywords Nanotechnology · Sensors · Biosensing · Sustainable nanomaterials · Healthcare

V. Kumar · Shashank · J. H. Pisal · M. R. Chowdhury · S. D. Vijaykumar (✉)
Department of Biotechnology, National Institute of Technology Andhra Pradesh, Tadepalligudem, India
e-mail: sudarshanadeepa@nitandhra.ac.in

A. H. Jebarani D
Department of Biotechnology, National Institute of Technology Andhra Pradesh, Tadepalligudem, India

Department of Biotechnology, Vel Tech High Tech Dr. Rangarajan Dr. Sakunthala Engineering College, Chennai, Tamil Nadu, India

S. Mondal et al. (eds.), *Smart and Sustainable Nanomaterials in Digital Healthcare and Theranostic*, https://doi.org/10.1007/978-981-95-9386-6_18

18.1 Introduction

Biosensors, which convert biological responses into electrical signals, are crucial in modern medicine. They are widely used to detect and monitor various biological markers, from glucose levels in diabetics to variations in specific target protein markers of diseases such as cancer and infectious diseases. The introduction of nanomaterials—materials engineered at the nanoscale—has significantly improved the capabilities of these biosensors. Nanomaterials' unique properties, such as high surface area, tunable physical characteristics, and enhanced chemical reactivity, enable exceptional sensitivity and specificity in biosensing applications [59].

Smart sustainable nanomaterials are the next frontier in this domain. These materials are designed to perform specific functions competently and sustainably, leveraging renewable resources, reducing waste, and minimizing energy consumption, in alignment with global sustainability goals. In healthcare, these materials promise to develop diagnostic tools that are not only highly effective but also environmentally friendly [70]. The intersection of biosensors and smart sustainable nanomaterials is transforming healthcare diagnostics and monitoring. The fusion of nanotechnology with biological sensing mechanisms has led to the development of innovative solutions that enhance the precision, efficiency, and sustainability of medical diagnostics. The various types of sustainable nanomaterials used in biosensing including carbon nanostructures, known for their exceptional electrical properties [48]; inorganic nanomaterials, valued for their stability and diverse functionalities [40]; organic nanomaterials, which are versatile and biocompatible [8]; and bio-derived smart nanostructures, which integrate biological molecules for enhanced performance [25] have been detailed.

Further, imminent trends and innovations in the field of smart biosensors with distinctive features for targeted applications are set to revolutionize healthcare. For instance, multifunctionality in biosensors will allow the simultaneous detection of multiple biomarkers, enhancing diagnostic accuracy [64]; miniaturization and wearability will enable continuous monitoring through compact and comfortable devices [32]; point-of-care and remote sensing technologies will bring diagnostic capabilities directly to patients, facilitating timely interventions [47]; high-throughput screening will accelerate drug discovery and personalized medicine [55]; and integration with smartphones will make biosensing more accessible and user-friendly [65]. Additionally, the incorporation of artificial intelligence and data analytics will improve the interpretation of complex biological data, leading to more informed clinical decisions [15]. These adaptations are expected to play a major role in elevating the potential application of biosensors.

Nevertheless, as with any incipient technology, several challenges need to be addressed to achieve widespread adoption of these smart biosensing systems. The general concerns include scalability, cost-effectiveness, and regulatory approval of smart sustainable nanomaterials [20]. However, it can be appreciated that significant opportunities exist to enhance the design, functionality, and integration of these biosensors within the current healthcare infrastructure (Table 18.1).

Table 18.1 Opportunities in adopting smart sustainable nanomaterials

Challenge	Description	Potential solutions
Scalability	Difficulty in mass production	Advanced manufacturing techniques
Cost-effectiveness	High cost of materials and production	Economies of scale, cost-efficient synthesis methods
Regulatory approval	Regulatory hurdles and compliance issues	Clear guidelines, thorough testing

This chapter aims to provide a comprehensive overview of the current state-of-the-art in smart sustainable nanomaterial-based biosensing technology, explore future trends and innovations, and discuss the challenges along with the opportunities that lie ahead. By focusing on these aspects, we seek to highlight the potential impact of these advanced smart biosensing systems on creating a more efficient, accessible, and sustainable healthcare system.

18.2 Sustainable Nanomaterials in Biosensing

The advancement of biosensing technologies has been significantly propelled by the integration of nanotechnology, particularly through the use of sustainable nanomaterials. These materials, engineered at the nanoscale, offer unique properties, which collectively improve the sensitivity, specificity, and overall performance of biosensors. This section explores the various types of sustainable nanomaterials utilized in biosensing, alongside the latest scientific advancements in each domain.

18.2.1 Carbon Nanostructures

Carbon nanostructures, such as graphene, carbon nanotubes (CNTs), and carbon dots, have drawn significant interest for use in biosensors due to remarkable properties, including the sizeable surface area, extensive electrical conductivity, and inherent compatibility with biological specimens. The common carbon materials, their key properties, and potential applications are discussed.

Graphene is a single layer of carbon atoms arranged in a hexagonal lattice, renowned for its extraordinary electronic properties, such as high electron mobility and significant surface-to-volume ratio. These attributes make graphene an excellent material for biosensors aimed at detecting various biomolecules at low concentrations. Recent studies have highlighted the efficacy of graphene-based biosensors in detecting glucose, DNA, and proteins, underscoring their potential in medical diagnostics [71].

Carbon nanotubes (CNTs) are typically built from rolled-up graphene sheet structures and therefore demonstrate remarkable mechanical strength and electrical properties. Functionalization of CNTs with biomolecules has resulted in the fabrication of sensors that detect biomarkers with high specificity for use in the diagnosis of diseases such as cancer and diabetes. The integration of CNTs into flexible, wearable biosensors represents a burgeoning area of research, aiming to facilitate real-time health monitoring and personalized medicine [36].

18.2.2 Inorganic Nanomaterials

Inorganic nanomaterials, including metal and metal oxide nanoparticles, quantum dots, and silica nanoparticles, are favored in biosensing due to their diverse functionalities and robust stability. Some conventional nano inorganic materials, their key properties, and potential applications are discussed.

Metal nanoparticles, such as gold and silver nanoparticles, owing to their optical and electronic material properties are extensively utilized in biosensing applications. These nanoparticles can significantly enhance the signal in detection methods such as surface plasmon resonance (SPR) and electrochemical sensing. Gold nanoparticles, in particular, have been effectively employed for the detection of pathogens, nucleic acids, and proteins [62].

Quantum dots (QDs), semiconductor nanocrystals, exhibit size-dependent optical properties, including bright and stable fluorescence. QDs are instrumental in fluorescence-based biosensors for detecting biomolecules with high sensitivity. Their tuneable emission wavelengths facilitate multiplexed detection, crucial for comprehensive diagnostic assays [7].

18.2.3 Organic Nanomaterials

Organic nanomaterials, such as polymers, dendrimers, and liposomes, are highly versatile and biocompatible, making them a material of choice for a variety of biosensing applications. Examples of nanoscale organic materials, their key properties, and potential applications are discussed.

Polymers, including polyaniline and polypyrrole, are essentially used in electrochemical biosensors due to the materials' superior conductance and their ease of functionalization. These polymers can be modified with enzymes, antibodies, or DNA to create highly specific sensors for detecting glucose, cholesterol, and various biomarkers [46].

Dendrimers, highly branched, tree-like macromolecules, possess multiple functional groups that allow for the attachment of various biomolecules, enhancing the sensitivity and specificity of biosensors. Dendrimer-based biosensors have shown promise in detecting cancer biomarkers and pathogens [54].

18.2.4 Bio-derived Smart Nanostructures

Bio-derived smart nanostructures, which integrate biological molecules with nanomaterials, represent an innovative approach to biosensing. These materials leverage the natural recognition capabilities of biological molecules, such as proteins, DNA, and enzymes, to achieve highly specific and sensitive detection. Some of the generic biological materials used in biosensing, their key properties, and potential applications are discussed.

Enzyme-based nanostructures combine enzymes with nanoparticles or nanofibers to create biosensors with enhanced catalytic activity. These sensors have largely been reported for use in the detection of glucose, cholesterol, and lactate in clinical diagnostics [24].

DNA-based nanostructures, such as DNA origami, utilize the self-assembling properties of DNA to create highly ordered nanostructures. These structures can be functionalized with fluorescent probes or electrochemical tags for detecting nucleic acids and proteins. DNA-based biosensors offer high specificity and can be employed for detecting genetic disorders and infectious diseases [63].

The integration of smart sustainable nanomaterials with sensing systems has proven to be without a doubt a fortunate thing for applications in healthcare, considering both for diagnosis and theragnosis. Furthermore, continued research and development in this area are expected to yield even more innovative solutions, contributing to more efficient, accurate, and sustainable healthcare systems.

18.3 Smart Biosensors: Trends and Innovations

18.3.1 Multifunctionality

Unquestionably, the unique qualities of smart nanomaterials, in particular, the potential to accomplish multiple functions with a single material, make them applicable in the healthcare industry. For instance, surface plasmons are light-interacting oscillations that are restricted to conducting materials' surfaces, and when the real part of the dielectric function drops to zero, a resonance in the absorption takes place at the plasmon frequency in the material [23]. This phenomenon known as surface plasmon resonance (SPR) has been largely used in biosensors for the analysis of many analytes, including harmful microorganisms. Further, a number of innovative biosensors based on the manipulation of various nanoparticle parameters (particle size, shape, composition, and surrounding medium) have been designed for label-free detection, in addition to the variety of working principles used, especially in single-nanoparticle-based detections and live-cell imaging applications [42]. The sensitivity of localized surface plasmon resonance (LSPR)-based nanobiosensors may be enhanced by regulating and adjusting the optical characteristics outlined in the physical theories related to the material characteristics, including composition, size, shape, and material of noble metal nanoparticles. Importantly, in clinical and biomedical applications, LSPR-based nano-biosensors exhibit promise as potent instruments for addressing complex issues related to biosensing [22].

The advent of nano-biosensing has also demonstrated efficacy in the detection of viruses and has drawn great interest from researchers in viral biosensing, especially since the SARS-CoV-2 global pandemic. The method essentially applies the use of cost-effective technologies such as affinity nano-biosensing, nanowire-based biosensors, fiberoptic nano-biosensors, etc. [52]. Further, the detection of various viruses, including HIV, Ebola, Zika, Influenza, Hepatitis B, etc., has been extensively studied through the help of nano-biosensors [51].

Of late, the use of electrochemical nano-biosensors for biomolecule detection has been largely described in the literature. Despite their excellent selectivity, enzymatic sensors have drawbacks like instability, strenuous modification procedures, and significant microenvironmental influences. In contrast, non-enzymatic electrochemical sensors offer good stability, have straightforward modification processes, and lesser external influences. For example, hydrogen peroxide, glucose, and dopamine levels have been effectively detected using enzyme-free electrochemical sensors [74]. Several techniques, including electrochemical and optical methods, have been used to detect glucose. Advanced glucose sensors with greater sensitivity and simplicity have been made possible by the invention of novel transducers using nanomaterials that incorporate fluorescence methods [5].

18.3.2 Point of Care and Remote Sensing

Point-of-care testing (POCT) is a laboratory-medicine discipline that has seen rapid evolution in terms of analytical scope and clinical application. The limitations of conventional laboratory-based testing could be overcome by using point-of-care (PoC) diagnostic platforms, which include remote sensing, a method used for acquisition of data without being in contact. PoC essentially integrates elements of biotechnology, nanotechnology and sensor technology, providing a way for faster, cost-effective, and more accessible diagnostics (Fig. 18.1).

Nanomaterials-based biosensors have been reported to be useful in rapid breast cancer detection. Typically, easily portable and simple nano-biosensors were designed with CA15–33 antibody loaded onto screen-printed Au electrodes for immunoassay-based detection of breast cancer [53]. The instant and accurate measurement of blood glucose level can be achieved by convergence of nanomaterial-based biosensor with electrochemical principles. The changes in the charge or pH near the electrode surface or as measured through a field-effect transistor (FET) can be correlated with the variation in glucose concentration [29]. Likewise, optical nano-biosensors have proven to be a promising platform for PoC detection of cardiovascular disease biomarkers with a low detection limit [60]. These nano-biosensors have evolved as a self-diagnostic platform that ensures real-time in-situ analysis and plays a vital role in the public health control system as they enable the

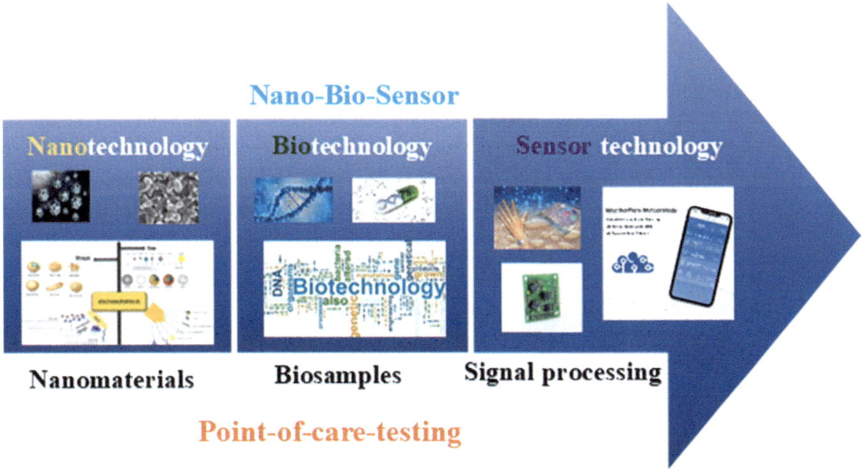

Fig. 18.1 Nano-biosensor and PoC

early detection of deadly diseases through continuous health monitoring technologies and prevent the spread of infectious diseases including COVID-19, HIV, avian influenza, cholera, malaria, severe respiratory syndrome, dengue and viral hepatitis. The integration of nano-materials and advance biosensing technologies further can provide easily accessible, more accurate, and faster IVD-based POCT solutions [18, 31]. The properties of nano-biosensors such as the ability to detect and measure the content of specific proteins or molecules that act as biomarkers make them advantageous in PoC diagnosis of neurodegenerative disorders including Parkinson's disease and Alzheimer's disease. Additionally, the nano-biosensors bind selectively to the biomarkers such as tau protein and amyloid beta peptides providing non-invasive and rapid method for early detection of diseases [13].

More importantly, the use of nanozymes (nanomaterial-based artificial enzymes) in PoC diagnostics is revolutionizing the biosensing technology. These natural enzyme mimetic synthetic materials have various advantages such as low cost, greater robustness, and enhanced stability making them perfect components for developing user-friendly and portable diagnostic devices. Nanozymes can be linked to various materials including metals, metal oxides, and metal-organic frameworks, enabling the design of biosensors that are highly versatile and capable of meeting the criteria assured by the World Health Organization (WHO) such as user friendliness, ease of deliverance to end users, robustness, rapidness, equipment-free, affordability, specificity, and sensitivity. Though nanozymes have potential applications in PoC diagnostics for achieving reliable and consistent performance, there are challenges in optimizing the properties of nanozymes with relevance to environmental conditions (pH and temperature), surface charge, size, and shape. Continued research is required to fill these gaps, such that nanozyme-based biosensors can have high-impact PoC solutions that improve outcomes and accessibility, specifically in the era of limited resources [10].

The biosensors based on nanomaterials that exhibit SPR effect are known as plasmonic biosensors, which can be fitted within small and portable devices for POCT due to their extraordinary sensitivities and versatile designs [28]. An alternative signal transduction pattern containing lateral flow immunoassay (LFIA)-based POC nano-sensors has the potential to break the barriers toward commercialization in terms of practicality, sensitivity, and specificity [41]. As such, the development of nanomaterial-based biosensors for PoC diagnostics has led to a high standard of healthcare management. Yet, there is a need to develop novel nano biosensors for PoC diagnosis of various diseases in order to achieve more accurate, sustainable, remote sensing, and continuous monitoring in patients and also to scale up their applicability from lab scale to the hospital scale.

18.3.3 High-Throughput Screening

High-throughput screening (HTS) is a characterization technique used in the field of biopolymer detection, and is a notable feature of the present as well as future bio-detecting technologies, which can accurately and easily detect the targets. It also serves as the best alternative for traditional methods of detection as it saves lots of time, cost, and provides efficient results. For instance, gold nanoparticles (Au NPs), which are usually a part of the HTS technology, are known for their specific feature of combining biomolecules while not changing their own characteristics, by which they could be decorated in various ways and create different detection methods to achieve high accuracy and efficiency, also serving as an important visual detection method to classify the existence of targets. In the same way, for the detection of proteins, gold nanoparticles are indispensable indicators. Although it is usually only used for preliminary visual detection, it has considerable high-throughput detection characteristics, which can detect markers in a wide range of people simultaneously, while ensuring substantial accuracy of detection. Similarly, for proteins, labelling with gold nanoparticles is only a modification of the protein surface and will not change its properties, which also makes gold nanoparticles a common way of use as an intermediate for binding or interacting with proteins such as fluorescent groups. At the same time, the resonance characteristics of Au NPs have been applied in protein detection very commonly, that is, gold nanoparticles produce different colors in different volumes due to the resonance effect with incident light, which is of great significance in qualitative and semi-quantitative detection. Further, the gold nanoparticles mainly play the role of assisting connection, and can also perform visual pre-inspection, which is an excellent collaborator of high-throughput technology [49].

In today's biomedical applications, fluorescence, whether radio-fluorescence, fluorescence carried by cellular and subcellular proteins, or fluorescence emitted by fluorophores is the primary phenomenon used to detect proteins of interest in order to construct high-throughput characterizations. Measuring fluorescence with a fluorometer can help identify the existence and specific concentration of the target protein, resulting in an efficient, orderly, and high-throughput assay. The fluorescence method based on gold nanoparticles will not interfere with normal visual detection, and the measurement of fluorescence can be automatically done using special instruments, which can accurately determine the concentration of protein solution and also determine whether it is damaged or mutated while being efficient. Usually, in order to achieve high-throughput detection, the method of dual fluorescent modification groups is adopted, using a fluorescent quenching group and a fluorescent emitting group, respectively [44].

In addition to fluorescence-related methods, Au NP-based high-throughput screening still has other methods. Another method for establishing high-throughput characterization is the radiation method, which requires the use of radiolabeled amino acids. Typically, the Au NPs labelled with amino acids for the detection of specific cells is the latest state-of-the-art detection method. For example, antibodies conjugated to gold coupled with silver valorization were used in histochemistry and later in dot and blot assay. In addition, the property of gold nanoparticles in temperature conduction can also be used in high-throughput technologies, and has been applied as emerging technology in some fields, such as LAMP technology. Gold nanoparticle-based high-throughput characterization technology, which is still an innovation, is widely used in pharmaceutical industry, clinical and biomonitoring, and has promising future use to help develop these fields. In addition, this kind of technology has helped a lot during the COVID-19 pandemic, and is ready for usage in similar epidemic prevention [72].

An array of functionalized single-walled carbon nanotubes (SWCNTs) used in a combinatorial HTS and precipitation-based strategies provides different optical responses by which the target analyte can be characterized. This optical response provided by the nano-biosensor typically is a spectral fingerprint of the analyte. For example, HTS-based near-infrared (NIR) spectroscopy has been employed to measure the optical responses (variations in wavelength and intensity of emission) of about 132 complexes formed by SWCNTs and ssDNA in the presence of analytes including endometrial and ovarian cancer protein biomarkers and 10% fetal bovine serum [26]. Further, the nano-biosensors are not employed only in health sector, but also has its own importance in the field of agriculture and environment. For example, biotic and abiotic stresses are the major causes of crop yield and growth, and typically are increased in intensity and frequency with change in climatic conditions. Efficient delivery of pesticides and nutrients along with precise management of scarce water resources helps overcome this challenge and improve agricultural output. Real-time management of plant health plays a crucial role in achieving this, where the role of nanomaterial-based biosensors is to build communication between electronic devices and plant in order to optimize crop yield and growth in response to resource scarcity and environmental stresses. The nano-biosensors along with phenotyping and agricultural devices translate plant chemical signals into digital form to monitor plant health in real time. This technique enables high-throughput screening of chemical phenotypes to screen the stress-tolerant plant varieties [17].

Further, gold nanoparticles continue to drive technological and scientific innovations paving the way for HTS. Also, fluorescent carbon nanotubes are powerful building blocks for sensors and their huge chemical design space makes them an ideal platform for high-throughput approaches. The innovative methodology involving SWCNT offers high-throughput screening of mutated sequences and is marked as a significant advancement in biosensor development. The applications of nanomaterial-based biosensing approach are not narrowed down to health sector alone, and find place in a wide range including real-time plant health monitoring. Therefore, it is evident that they might have potential benefits in other real-world problems as well.

18.3.4 Smartphone Integration

The use of smartphone has become ubiquitous. Handheld detectors, test strips, and sensor chips are few nano-biosensors which are integrated with smartphone due to their properties like availability and portability. A wide variety of smartphone-integrated nano-biosensors have been used for disease and disaster prevention. Smartphones play a key role in optical and electrochemical detection, for example, smartphone aids the integration of electrochemical sensor, Internet of Things (IoT), and remote sensing. Smartphones act as the core of detection system to control, real-time display, and calculate the responses due to their numerous features including convenient operation, excellent computing capacities, high resolution imaging, high popularity, and open-source operation systems. To facilitate in situ detection, smartphone-integrated electrochemical devices are converged with interdigital electrodes and screen-printed electrode. Varieties of smartphone-integrated impedance systems were developed by using different nanomaterials as electrodes like gold nanoparticles, 3-aminophenylboronic acid nanocomposites, carbon nanotubes, graphene, and zinc oxide nanoparticles. Various bio-detection and biosensors with different electrodes are used to detect human serum albumin, bovine serum albumin, trinitrotoluene, and acetone. Uric acid, glucose, dopamine, levodopa, and ascorbic acid content in human system can be monitored using an amperometry-integrated smartphone system. These smartphone-integrated electrochemical biosensors find their application in POCT due to their miniature size and portability [27].

Smartphone-integrated devices (SIDs) are also used for monitoring cardiovascular diseases (CVDs) in PoC. Using smartphone as the source of power, microfluidic devices have also been shown to perform ELISA. Smartphones and their camera have been used for flow cytometric and digital microscopic applications at the PoC for the detection of biological samples including pathogens and healthy cells. Smartphones act as a public awareness platform ensuring public health security. The signs and symptoms of CVDs can be obtained by apps including My Life, My Heart, and MobilePAL. This helps to prevent and cure the initial-stage diseases. SIDs have changed the common health practices and provided an appropriate detection and cure options at the doorstep of public [68].

Smartphones can also be integrated with paper-based platforms, for example, in lateral flow assays (LFA) for the qualitative and quantitative measurement of analytes in complex mixtures. Usually, smartphone integration with LFAs facilitates the analysis and visualization of data. Few examples of LFA platforms include merging of nanobodies specific to ligand-coated quantum beads for early detection of CVDs and malaria and an antibody-conjugated gold nanoparticles-based LFA membrane to detect cortisol (stress hormone) in human serum using the principle of chemiluminescence. Specialized software is required to be operated in order to integrate LFAs into smartphones using cameras and scanners. Moreover, the reliability of results while translating data into digital form may be affected because of the paper platform, flash limitations, and smartphone camera [1]. To summarize, the technological developments in smartphone have allowed a greater multiplicity for communication of devices with each other avoiding human interference. Smartphone integration with nano-biosensors has opened doors for real-world data interpretation, making them significantly important in the health, food, and environmental sciences.

18.3.5 Artificial Intelligence and Data Analytics

Artificial Intelligence (AI) is a technological domain wherein computer systems emulate human cognitive capabilities to execute tasks previously reliant on human intellect. Referred to as smart machines, these entities exhibit the intelligence to autonomously perform cognitive functions. The intersection of AI and nanotechnology has notably influenced the evolution of medical diagnosis, enhancing the quality of diagnostic devices through advanced material construction and heightened functional sophistication. This collaboration has positively impacted medical diagnostics, enabling devices to detect and diagnose conditions with greater precision and depth. The incorporation of nanoscale materials has contributed to heightened device sensitivity, while AI-driven functionalities have elevated diagnostic capabilities, marking a significant stride in advancing healthcare technologies.

The integration of nano-biosensors and machine learning (ML) algorithms helps to overcome the drawbacks of traditional biosensors. Specifically, the evolution of electrochemical nano-biosensors from conventional to wearable and portable forms provides applications in food, health, and environmental sectors. Nanomaterial-based biosensors conjugated with AI are called AI-biosensors. These AI-biosensors have potential role in pathogen (bacteria, virus) detection, hazardous chemical analyte quantification, and early disease diagnosis. Optimization of parameters such as selection of analyte and design of electrode in order to enhance the performance of nano-biosensor is said to be achieved by the fusion of these biosensors with AI tools like ML. The diagnostic precision is significantly improved with the conjugation of biosensors with AI as it fills the gap between data acquisition and interpretation. Integration of non-invasive nano-biosensors and ML has led to healthcare and medical revolution [56].

Unfortunately, the unclear decision-making and ambiguous processes affect the reliability of ML systems, hence often they are referred to as "black boxes" in nature. Therefore, to improve comprehension, the focus has shifted toward explainable ML in recent days. Explainable ML enhances the interpretability of the model by allowing the algorithms to track and rationalize the decision-making processes.

For example, model frameworks such as Model Understanding through Subspace Explanations (MUSE) provides platform for scientists to include extra constraints to output explanations that include specific features of interest. Additionally, SHapley Additive exPlanations (SHAP) is a method that helps to characterize the relative significance of input characteristics for a designed model, which can be easily analyzed along with domain knowledge in order to screen the selected input features of scientific relevance. A small subset of a sample or a single sample can be interpreted using these tools which generate selective analysis of various input feature subspaces. With the help of these explainable ML algorithms, models with superior confidence in scientific soundness and robustness can be built enabling their real-time fusion into food, health, and environmental sectors and normalizing their use [38]. Ultimately, the applications of AI in the field of biosensing are immense and rapidly increasing which includes Internet of Things (IoT), ML, DL, big data, and analytics. The fusion of machine learning algorithms and cutting-edge PoC enables early diagnosis of deadly disorders with greater affordability and accuracy. Nano-biosensors with the assistance of drones, AI, and cloud computing are rapidly replacing the traditional methods of disease diagnosis.

18.3.6 Microarray Integration

A precise monitoring of cytokines during the onset of a disease is an essential aspect to be looked into for understanding the underlying mechanisms of the disease; therefore, a quick and efficient monitoring becomes essential for the same. A promising method to close this technical gap is LSPR-based microfluidic optical biosensing, which may enable sensor miniaturization and real-time refractometric detection of biomolecular binding on a metallic nanoparticle surface, both of which could result in quick and sample-saving analyte analysis. A high sensitivity detection of cytokines as low as 5 pg/mL from a 1 μL serum sample has been made possible, with an acceptable range of percent recovery of cytokines [6].

Similarly, the initial bacterial concentrations in the sample, which were as low as 2.8 ± 19.6 colony-forming units per milliliter, could be quickly and quantitatively assessed using signal analysis of SPR responses. The findings collectively demonstrated how straightforward, user-friendly, fluidic-less, and low-tech microarrays may be applied to raw materials and provide, in a single assay, both qualitative and quantitative data about bacterial contamination [3].

18.3.7 Miniaturization and Wearability

Miniaturization of tools in analytical biology requires a micro/nanofabricated design. The device must have satisfactory selectivity, stability, and sensitivity. Therefore, a combinatory action of nano-biosensing with microfluidic systems will be useful [75]. The nano-biosensing tools have always proved to be beneficial. Some of the reasons have been listed below:

- The nano-level design of the biosensor facilitates improved and unusual, optical, mechanical, catalytic, and electronic properties as compared to a bulk design. They have been a focus of researchers because of possessing approximately the same size as the biomolecules they interact with. They can be used to attain a tunable nanostructure using the constituent metal to obtain suitable selective and sensitive target molecule detection [57].
- Biomolecules can become concentrated on a nanostructure leading to a better response time as compared to a bulk design [58].
- The local refractive index may change if target molecules are present close to the nanoparticle surface [69].
- The ratio of a sensor's output signal to a change in one of its characteristics—likely brought on by a quantity of analyte material attached to the sensor—is known as the sensor's internal sensitivity. The advantage of a miniature design is the increase in sensitivity [2].
- The miniature design helps to obtain exceptional properties, like quantum mechanics effect, enhanced stability and reactivity, and a large surface-to-volume area.

In the optical devices, the use of biosensors is being explored for applications in biological processes. To bind the streptavidin molecules at the nanoscale, the sensor surface was earlier functionalized via biotinylation [21]. Miniaturizing the biosensor dimensions into the nanoscale has been identified as a strategy for addressing the functional requirements of point-of-care and wearable biosensors. Further, when used in immobilization form, the receptor's stability and activity must be maintained during the immobilization process, which must also be steady and repeatable. The method provides a helpful way of detecting biomolecules such as DNA without the need for labelling. Also, the induced surface tension created when molecules attach to a surface is the basis for the operation of nanomechanical biosensors. Detection of single-base mismatches in oligonucleotide hybridization is an application of the concept [35].

In addition, the wearability of nano-biosensors is an efficient non-invasive strategy being explored. The technology is valuable for measuring the biochemical parameters of an individual [73]. One of the most advanced devices include wearable electrocardiogram (ECG) sensing shirt, which has an effective activity even during the vigorous activity of an individual [37]. Not only the assessment of physical parameters, but the measurement of chemical and biological parameters (transcutaneous oxygen monitoring, multiplexed in situ perspiration analysis) are also made possible [16, 45].

18.3.7.1 Epidermal-Based Sensors

The assessment of healing biomarkers in skin wound exudates and histologically examination of full-thickness skin wounds grafted with either unidirectional or multidirectional artificial dermis were made possible by nano-biosensors [4].

General mechanism of epidermal-based sensors is the utilization of sweat to analyze the concentration of various analytes. The electrochemical signals obtained from the analytes are used for data extrapolation [12]. Epidermal electronic system (EES) is a setup which can be used to match the mass density and mechanical stiffness of the epidermis. The adhesion method can be manually improved or simply by van der Waals forces for specialized systems like graphene-based epidermal sensor system (GESS), where the sensor is adhered like a temporary skin-tattoo [43].

Recently, epithelial growth factor receptor (EGFR) markers were created using customized synthetic nanobodies [9] which involved two platforms for label-free electrochemical detection of the) biomarker. In order to link the anti-EGFR nanobody (Nb) and create nano-biocomposites for the electrochemical impedance spectroscopy (EIS) detection of the EGFR biomarker, screen-printed carbon electrodes (SPCE) were decorated with either poly (thiophene acetic acid) (PTAA) or NiO nanoparticles (NPs). The human epidermal growth factor receptor (HER-II) biomarker in breast cancer serum (BCS) can be investigated for cancer diagnosis through a glass-based nano-biosensor [30].

18.3.7.2 Wrist Patches

The skin has the external layer of epidermis, which is utilized in case of epidermal-based nano-biosensors for detection of various components for various components. However, the lack of methods for mounting the tiny electronic component on a thin substrate that can gather sweat-related data and analyze it appropriately makes it more challenging to obtain information about sweat metabolite concentrations from skin. To overcome this limitation, a patch-type biosensor was devised for tangling with the non-uniform skin topography suitably. The wearable patches are low weight and provide easy integration. They do not need the calibration stage because their quantitative recognition method and sensing principle rely on the coupled electrodes. Few non-invasive sensors are non-enzymatic, but the majority are enzymatic [11]. A patch-based wearable nano-biosensor can also be prepared as a hydrogel film. The ideal area of attachment is considered to be the one that perspires the most during the day (e.g., palm, back of palm, fingertips, etc.) The hydrogel is responsible for collecting the released sweat over the skin, through which the analytes are stored in the patches. Diffusion of metabolites from sweat to hydrogels, which efficiently catch and gather analytes in the patches, is facilitated by a watery interface. [39]. A new kind of small-molecule hydrogel plasmonic nano sensors for histamine detection: Asp-capped AuNPs (Asp-AuNPs) serve as both the colorants for histamine molecules and the detecting components in this nano sensor [61]. There is a growing emphasis on flexible sensing, as evidenced by the several skin-interfaced wearable-patch or sensor systems that are now in development.

18.3.7.3 Iontophoresis-Based Biosensors

There are multiple applications for the utility of iontophoresis-based biosensors. A wearable aptamer nano-biosensor that interfaces with the skin and uses target-induced strand displacement to automatically and non-invasively measures estradiol through in situ sweat analysis is a popular one [67]. Capillary bursting valves, autonomous sweat induction at rest through iontophoresis, real-time estradiol analysis and calibration with concurrently collected multivariate data (temperature, pH, and ionic strength), signal processing, and wireless communication with a user interface are the mechanisms that govern the precise microfluidic sweat sampling. By delivering a low-level current between two dermal electrodes, the noninvasive technique known as reverse iontophoresis can enable the controlled transport of biomolecules up to 20KDa in size over the skin barrier. Following sample collection at the electrode location, they can either be monitored on-site or sent to a sensor via a microfluidic channel [19].

18.3.7.4 Saliva-Sensing Wearable Biosensors

The physicochemical characteristics of carbon nanomaterials, such as their large surface area, which enables functionalization and immobilization of biological molecules, high electron mobility, and exceptional conductivity, make them great tools for substance detection. They are utilized for salivary-based detection, which is used for detection of saliva for antigens, cancer biomarkers, dopamine, glucose, sialic acid, etc. The materials employed for the purpose include carbon nanotubes, graphene, graphene oxide, carbon dots, and others [14]. For the label-free monitoring of the stress hormone cortisol levels in saliva samples throughout the day, a portable multiplexed platform based on an array of nanowire sensors is helpful. Particular DNA aptamer sequences can be employed as receptors to bring the complex "target-receptor" closer to the nanowire surface in order to effectively quantify cortisol using field effect transistors (FETs) [33].

18.4 Challenges and Opportunities

The most important difficulties to be resolved before these devices become commercially viable are the growing public and regulatory concerns over the lack of worldwide criteria for assessing the safety of nano-biosensors (Fig. 18.2). The field has been showing a slow rise in popularity due to multiple factors like imprecise particle size due to inconsistent synthesis protocols, viability of the business, and various others [34]. With respect to the uncommon application of nano-biosensors as efficient tools implemented in food industry, the challenges faced have been classified into: (a) economic issues; (b) legal issues; (c) technical issues; (d) ethical

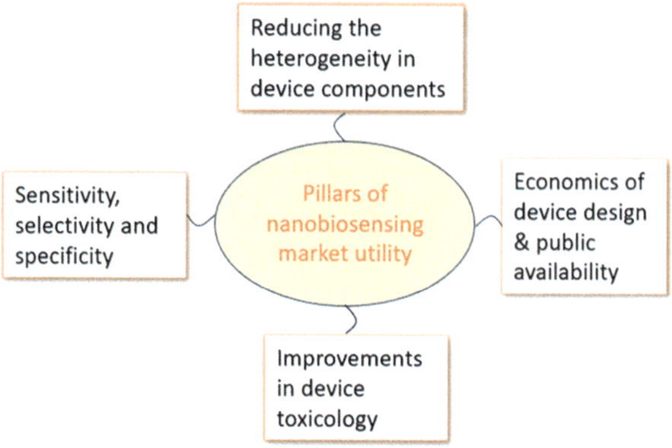

Fig. 18.2 Pillars of nano-biosensing market utility: Description of factors that affect the commercialization of the nano-biosensors

issues; (e) regulatory issues; (f) political issues, and (g) environmental health and safety issues [66].

In fact, when the nano-biosensing concept was applied to the detection of COVID-19, the tools lacked satisfactory selectivity. Making sure the monolayer of probes that target the selected biomarkers on the analyte is adequately adsorbed on the sensor surface usually results in acceptable selectivity. Due to the presence of mutations in the main CoV mRNA and proteins, nano-biosensors led to a raise of the diagnostic error in clinical samples. Also, the nano-biosensors show a lesser precision due to the selection of sample source taken for analysis. These limitations pose a requirement for a design, which shows the performance and accuracy as achieved by the blood sugar sensors [53]. Likewise, the detection of long non-coding RNAs (lncRNAs) has a limitation of instable design and significant bioactivity. Hence, a reproducible design with a biodegradable nature could be looked into for an in-situ detection of lncRNAs [50].

Because of their special characteristics (high surface-to-volume ratio, changeable composition, etc.), nanomaterials may raise issues with application, including their toxicity. Therefore, it is necessary to more precisely evaluate their effects on the environment in terms of their size, dose patterns, accumulation characteristics, immunological response, and retention duration. The concentration of antibodies with the homologous proteins will be an ever-lasting challenge with the current nano-biosensors. Although the presence of proteins that have a least non-specific binding may seem as a solution, this may not always be the case. Therefore, a requirement of high sensitivity cannot be compromised for the acceptable design of nano-biosensors. Further, with the growing population, there is a growing need for the development of a new-generation of devices, which could cope with the uprising demands of the public. Hence, we have a need for the development of a portable, affordable point-of-care testing (POCT) equipment that generates an accurate result at high efficiency. Also, it is essential to ensure that the use of nanoparticles does not cause any human cytotoxicity or hamper the remaining metabolic activities of the biological system.

18.5 Conclusion

Of late, there has been a growing increase in the need of finding effective solutions for both existing and emerging diseases. Essentially, the recent impact of the COVID-19 pandemic has triggered the search for developing smart solutions based on technology for enhancing the convenience of diagnostics. In context, the application of biosensing techniques has received significant attention and the integration of nanomaterials has further advanced its use in medical and related-healthcare applications. In summary, the chapter presents an overview of the various nanomaterials that have been applied in the development of sustainable nano-biosensors. Further, the current trends and possible future modernizations have been discussed in brief to gain a comprehensive understanding of the status of nano-biosensing research and application in real-world applications. Finally, the challenges and opportunities associated with the use of the nanomaterial-based sensing technology for biological applications have also been detailed.

References

1. Beduk T, et al. Smartphone-based multiplexed biosensing tools for health monitoring. Biosensors. 2022;12(8):583. https://doi.org/10.3390/bios12080583.
2. Bellan LM, Wu D, Langer RS. Current trends in nanobiosensor technology. WIREs Nanomed Nanobiotechnol. 2011;3(3):229–46. https://doi.org/10.1002/wnan.136.
3. Bouguelia S, et al. On-chip microbial culture for the specific detection of very low levels of bacteria. Lab Chip. 2013;13(20):4024. https://doi.org/10.1039/c3lc50473e.
4. Casadiegos S, Bustos RH, Fontanilla MR. Comparative evaluation of healing biomarkers in skin wound exudates using a nanobiosensor and histological analysis of full-thickness skin wounds grafted with multidirectional or unidirectional artificial dermis. J Tissue Eng Regen Med. 2018;12(12):2299–308. https://doi.org/10.1002/term.2762.
5. Chen L, Hwang E, Zhang J. Fluorescent nanobiosensors for sensing glucose. Sensors. 2018;18(5):1440. https://doi.org/10.3390/s18051440.
6. Chen P, et al. Multiplex serum cytokine immunoassay using nanoplasmonic biosensor microarrays. ACS Nano. 2015;9(4):4173–81. https://doi.org/10.1021/acsnano.5b00396.
7. Chen Y, et al. Quantum dots in fluorescent biosensing: current trends and future perspectives. Nano Today. 2024;46:233–49.
8. Chen Y, et al. Advances in organic nanomaterials for biosensing applications. Chem Soc Rev. 2022;51(3):1117–42.
9. Cruz-Pacheco AF, et al. Engineered synthetic nanobody-based biosensors for electrochemical detection of epidermal growth factor receptor. Chem Eng J. 2023;465:142941. https://doi.org/10.1016/j.cej.2023.142941.
10. Das B, et al. Nanozymes in point-of-care diagnosis: an emerging futuristic approach for biosensing. Nano-Micro Lett. 2021;13(1):193. https://doi.org/10.1007/s40820-021-00717-0.
11. Das R, Nag S, Banerjee P. Electrochemical nanosensors for sensitization of sweat metabolites: from concept mapping to personalized health monitoring. Molecules. 2023;28(3):1259. https://doi.org/10.3390/molecules28031259.
12. Dervisevic M, et al. Skin in the diagnostics game: wearable biosensor nano- and microsystems for medical diagnostics. Nano Today. 2020;30:100828. https://doi.org/10.1016/j.nantod.2019.100828.

13. Dhahi TS, et al. Application of Nanobiosensor engineering in the diagnosis of neurodegenerative disorders. Results Eng. 2024;24:102790. https://doi.org/10.1016/j.rineng.2024.102790.
14. Ehtesabi H. Carbon nanomaterials for salivary-based biosensors: a review. Mater Today Chem. 2020;17:100342. https://doi.org/10.1016/j.mtchem.2020.100342.
15. Esteva A, et al. Artificial intelligence in healthcare: past, present, and future. Annu Rev Biomed Eng. 2022;24(1):25–48.
16. Gao W, et al. Fully integrated wearable sensor arrays for multiplexed in situ perspiration analysis. Nature. 2016;529(7587):509–14. https://doi.org/10.1038/nature16521.
17. Giraldo JP, Kruss S. Nanosensors for monitoring plant health. Nat Nanotechnol. 2023;18(2):107–8. https://doi.org/10.1038/s41565-022-01307-w.
18. Gowri A, Ashwin Kumar N, Suresh Anand BS. Recent advances in nanomaterials based biosensors for point of care (PoC) diagnosis of Covid-19 - a minireview. Trends Anal Chem. 2021;137:116205. https://doi.org/10.1016/j.trac.2021.116205.
19. Gupta NK, Hwang Y, Cameron BD. The use of reverse iontophoresis based surface plasmon resonance for the development of a noninvasive real time transdermal biomarker sensor. In: Coté GL, editor. Proceedings of SPIE - The International Society for Optical Engineering; 2016. p. 971503. https://doi.org/10.1117/12.2208918.
20. Hibbitts A, et al. Regulatory considerations for nanomaterials in healthcare applications. Nano Today. 2022;37:101064.
21. Hong J, et al. A Mach-Zehnder interferometer based on silicon oxides for biosensor applications. Anal Chim Acta. 2006;573–574:97–103. https://doi.org/10.1016/j.aca.2006.04.045.
22. Hong Y, et al. Nanobiosensors based on localized surface plasmon resonance for biomarker detection. J Nanomat. Edited by M.A. Correa-Duarte. 2012;2012(1) https://doi.org/10.1155/2012/759830.
23. Hou W, Cronin SB. A review of surface plasmon resonance-enhanced photocatalysis. Adv Funct Mater. 2013;23(13):1612–9. https://doi.org/10.1002/adfm.201202148.
24. Huang J, et al. Enzyme-based nanostructures for biosensing applications: advances and challenges. J Mater Chem B. 2024;12(9):113956.
25. Huang J, et al. Bio-derived smart nanostructures for advanced biosensing applications. ACS Nano. 2021;15(4):7546–61.
26. Jeong S, et al. High throughput evolution of DNA-assembled carbon nanotubes for neurochemical optical nanosensors. ECS Meet Abstr. 2022;MA2022-01(8):704. https://doi.org/10.1149/MA2022-018704mtgabs.
27. Ji D, et al. Smartphone-based electrochemical system for biosensors and biodetection. Methods Mol Biol. 2022;2393:493–514. https://doi.org/10.1007/978-1-0716-1803-5_26.
28. Jin C, et al. Plasmonic nanosensors for point-of-care biomarker detection. Mater Today Bio. 2022;14:100263. https://doi.org/10.1016/j.mtbio.2022.100263.
29. Khosravi Ardakani H, et al. Recent progress in nanobiosensors for precise detection of blood glucose level. Biochem Res Int. Edited by Z. Huyut. 2022;2022:1–12. https://doi.org/10.1155/2022/2964705.
30. Khosroshahi ME, Chabok R, Chung N. Glass-based nanobiosensor immobilized with oriented antibody-conjugated gold nanourchin for targeted detection of breast cancer biomarker in serum using FT-NIR and SERS. Plasmonics. 2023;18(6):2155–76. https://doi.org/10.1007/s11468-023-01929-3.
31. Kim C, et al. Advancements in nanobiosensor technologies for in-vitro diagnostics to point of care testing. Heliyon. 2024;10(22):e40306. https://doi.org/10.1016/j.heliyon.2024.e40306.
32. Kim J, et al. Wearable biosensors for personalized health monitoring: current status and future challenges. Adv Funct Mater. 2022;32(9):2108565.
33. Klinghammer S, et al. Nanosensor-based real-time monitoring of stress biomarkers in human saliva using a portable measurement system. ACS Sens. 2020;5(12):4081–91. https://doi.org/10.1021/acssensors.0c02267.

34. Kulkarni MB, Ayachit NH, Aminabhavi TM. Recent advancements in nanobiosensors: current trends, challenges, applications, and future scope. Biosensors. 2022;12(10):892. https://doi.org/10.3390/bios12100892.
35. Lechuga LM, et al. Nanobiosensors based on optoelectronic and nanomechanical transducers for genomic and proteomic applications. Rev Mex Fís. 2006;52(2):94–8.
36. Lee J, et al. Carbon nanotubes in wearable biosensors: applications and future perspectives. Adv Healthc Mater. 2023;12(5):2108565.
37. Lee Y-D, Chung W-Y. Wireless sensor network based wearable smart shirt for ubiquitous health and activity monitoring. Sensors Actuators B Chem. 2009;140(2):390–5. https://doi.org/10.1016/j.snb.2009.04.040.
38. Leong SX, et al. Emerging nanosensor platforms and machine learning strategies toward rapid, point-of-need small-molecule metabolite detection and monitoring. Chem Sci. 2022;13(37):11009–29. https://doi.org/10.1039/D2SC02981B.
39. Lin P-H, et al. Wearable hydrogel patch with noninvasive, electrochemical glucose sensor for natural sweat detection. Talanta. 2022;241:123187. https://doi.org/10.1016/j.talanta.2021.123187.
40. Liu J, et al. Inorganic nanomaterials for biosensing: current progress and future perspectives. Mater Today. 2021;46:233–49.
41. Liu S, et al. Evaluation of the multidimensional enhanced lateral flow immunoassay in point-of-care nanosensors. ACS Nano. 2024;18(40):27167–205. https://doi.org/10.1021/acsnano.4c06564.
42. Long Y-T, Jing C. Localized surface plasmon resonance based nanobiosensors. Berlin, Heidelberg: Springer Berlin Heidelberg (SpringerBriefs in Molecular Science); 2014. https://doi.org/10.1007/978-3-642-54795-9.
43. Lu N, et al. Epidermal electronic systems for sensing and therapy. In: Varadan VK, editor. Proceedings of SPIE - The International Society for Optical Engineering; 2017. p. 101670J. https://doi.org/10.1117/12.2261755.
44. Metternich JT, et al. High-throughput approaches to engineer fluorescent nanosensors. Adv Mater [Preprint]. 2024; https://doi.org/10.1002/adma.202411067.
45. Mitsubayashi K, et al. Wearable and flexible oxygen sensor for transcutaneous oxygen monitoring. Sensors Actuators B Chem. 2003;95(1–3):373–7. https://doi.org/10.1016/S0925-4005(03)00441-6.
46. Nguyen T, et al. Conductive polymers in electrochemical biosensors: recent advances and future directions. Chem Soc Rev. 2024;53(3):1117–42.
47. Nguyen T, et al. Point-of-care diagnostics: recent advances and future trends. Biosens Bioelectron. 2023;198:113850.
48. Novoselov KS, et al. Graphene-based materials for biosensing applications. Nat Rev Mater. 2021;6(5):382–401.
49. Rodriguez-Saona L, et al. Miniaturization of optical sensors and their potential for high-throughput screening of foods. Curr Opin Food Sci. 2020;31:136–50. https://doi.org/10.1016/j.cofs.2020.04.008.
50. Sargazi S, et al. Opportunities and challenges of using high-sensitivity nanobiosensors to detect long noncoding RNAs: a preliminary review. Int J Biol Macromol. 2022;205:304–15. https://doi.org/10.1016/j.ijbiomac.2022.02.082.
51. Saylan Y, Denizli A. Virus detection using nanosensors. In: Nanosensors for smart cities. Elsevier; 2020. p. 501–11. https://doi.org/10.1016/B978-0-12-819870-4.00038-4.
52. Shand H, et al. New age detection of viruses: the nano-biosensors. Front Nanotechnol. 2022;3 https://doi.org/10.3389/fnano.2021.814550.
53. Sharifi M, et al. Rapid diagnostics of coronavirus disease 2019 in early stages using nanobiosensors: challenges and opportunities. Talanta. 2021;223:121704. https://doi.org/10.1016/j.talanta.2020.121704.
54. Shin DM, et al. Dendrimer-based biosensors for the detection of disease biomarkers: current status and future prospects. ACS Nano. 2024;18(4):7546–61.

55. Shin DM, et al. High-throughput screening for nanomedicine development. Nano Today. 2023;42:101176.
56. Shirgir B, Dimililer K, Asir S. Applications of artificial intelligence in biosensors. In: Intelligent informatics; 2025. p. 299–315. https://doi.org/10.1007/978-981-97-2147-4_21.
57. Stuart DA, et al. Biological applications of localised surface plasmonic phenomenae. IEE Proc Nanobiotechnol. 2005;152(1):13. https://doi.org/10.1049/ip-nbt:20045012.
58. Svedendahl M, et al. Refractometric sensing using propagating versus localized surface plasmons: a direct comparison. Nano Lett. 2009;9(12):4428–33. https://doi.org/10.1021/nl902721z.
59. Tiwari JN, et al. Smart nanomaterials for advanced biosensing applications. Nat Rev Mat. 2020;5(1):5–20.
60. Vairaperumal T, Huang C-C, Liu P-Y. Optical nanobiosensor-based point-of-care testing for cardiovascular disease biomarkers. ACS Appl Bio Mater. 2023;6(7):2591–613. https://doi.org/10.1021/acsabm.3c00223.
61. Wang F, et al. A stable and specific hydrogel-based plasmonic nanosensor for histamine detection. Microchem J. 2024a;207:112047. https://doi.org/10.1016/j.microc.2024.112047.
62. Wang J, et al. Gold nanoparticles for biosensing applications: advances and challenges. Biosens Bioelectron. 2024b;98(3):113850.
63. Wang Q, et al. DNA-based nanostructures in biosensing: current trends and future perspectives. Nat Rev Mater. 2024c;7(5):382–401.
64. Wang Q, et al. Multifunctional biosensors for simultaneous detection of multiple biomarkers: recent advances and future challenges. Biosens Bioelectron. 2023;202:113956.
65. Xu L, et al. Smartphone-integrated biosensors for health monitoring: state-of-the-art and future perspectives. Biosens Bioelectron. 2022;187:113321.
66. Yang T, Duncan TV. Challenges and potential solutions for nanosensors intended for use with foods. Nat Nanotechnol. 2021;16(3):251–65. https://doi.org/10.1038/s41565-021-00867-7.
67. Ye C, et al. A wearable aptamer nanobiosensor for non-invasive female hormone monitoring. Nat Nanotechnol. 2024;19(3):330–7. https://doi.org/10.1038/s41565-023-01513-0.
68. Younis MR, et al. Smartphone-based biosensors. In: Nanobiosensors. Wiley; 2020. p. 357–87. https://doi.org/10.1002/9783527345137.ch15.
69. Zalyubovskiy SJ, et al. Theoretical limit of localized surface plasmon resonance sensitivity to local refractive index change and its comparison to conventional surface plasmon resonance sensor. J Opt Soc Am A. 2012;29(6):994. https://doi.org/10.1364/JOSAA.29.000994.
70. Zhang H, et al. Sustainable nanomaterials for biosensing applications: design, synthesis, and implementation. Adv Sci. 2022;9(5):2103452.
71. Zhang H, et al. Advances in graphene-based biosensors for medical diagnostics. J Nanomater. 2024;45(2):345–62.
72. Zhang Y, et al. Sensitive and rapid on-site detection of SARS-CoV-2 using a gold nanoparticle-based high-throughput platform coupled with CRISPR/Cas12-assisted RT-LAMP. Sensors Actuators B Chem. 2021;345:130411. https://doi.org/10.1016/j.snb.2021.130411.
73. Zhao C, et al. A thread-based wearable sweat nanobiosensor. Biosens Bioelectron. 2021;188:113270. https://doi.org/10.1016/j.bios.2021.113270.
74. Zhu C, et al. Electrochemical sensors and biosensors based on nanomaterials and nanostructures. Anal Chem. 2015;87(1):230–49. https://doi.org/10.1021/ac5039863.
75. Ziegler C, Göpel W. Biosensor development. Curr Opin Chem Biol. 1998;2(5):585–91. https://doi.org/10.1016/S1367-5931(98)80087-2.

GPSR Compliance

The European Union's (EU) General Product Safety Regulation (GPSR) is a set of rules that requires consumer products to be safe and our obligations to ensure this.

If you have any concerns about our products, you can contact us on ProductSafety@springernature.com

In case Publisher is established outside the EU, the EU authorized representative is:

Springer Nature Customer Service Center GmbH
Europaplatz 3
69115 Heidelberg, Germany

Batch number: 10732076

Printed by Printforce, the Netherlands